AF844426

A TEXTBOOK OF HISTOLOGY

Donike Demelezi

ALLIED
HEALTH
PRESS

A Textbook of Histology

Author: **Donike Demelezi**

Allied Health Press
4164 Lakeshore Road
Burlington ON L7L 1A4
Canada
www.alliedhealthpress.com
Email: orders@arclereducation.com

© 2025 Allied Health Press
ISBN: 978-1-77956-240-1

This book contains information obtained from highly regarded resources. Reprinted material sources are indicated and copyright remains with the original owners. Copyright for images and other graphics remains with the original owners as indicated. A Wide variety of references are listed. Reasonable efforts have been made to publish reliable data. Authors or Editors or Publishers are not responsible for the accuracy of the information in the published chapters or consequences of their use. The publisher assumes no responsibility for any damage or grievance to the persons or property arising out of the use of any materials, instructions, methods or thoughts in the book. The authors or editors and the publisher have attempted to trace the copyright holders of all material reproduced in this publication and apologize to copyright holders if permission has not been obtained. If any copyright holder has not been acknowledged, please write to us so we may rectify.

General Disclaimer:

This book is a summation of information from different sources and encompasses a wide range of medical conditions, the latest therapy methods, principals and techniques that are used in current practice, at the time of publication. This book offers general information with educational purposes, it is not to be applied or relied on for any diagnostic or treatment purposes. Please do not use the data/matter as a substitute for professional diagnosis and treatment. Please consult your healthcare provider or a licensed physician before making any healthcare queries or treatment choices. The medical information and research findings presented in this book are for educational purposes only and should not be used for the treatment of specific individual patients, as individual cases may vary. The author(s), editors(s) and publisher cannot be held accountable and make no guarantees that the information provided in this book will apply to each and individual patient. This book is meant to serve as a basic guideline and other relevant literature sources should be used for more specific information. This text can be a vital resource for students, trainees, and practitioners, covering essential topics. This book encompasses a wide range of medical conditions and the latest therapy options used in current practice. Through the utilization of many different medical studies this book provides the basics of different medical conditions, which can be used as a basic guide from where medical students, trainees and practitioners can extract necessary information. Further, some of the books have graphic images to explain anatomy for medical/educational purposes only. Hence, the book is intended for students or teachers/staff or individuals with a mature outlook looking to learn or enhance their knowledge.

Notice: Registered trademark of products or corporate names are used only for explanation and identification without intent of infringement.

Allied Health Press publishes wide variety of books and eBooks. For more information about Allied Health Press and its products, visit our website at www.alliedhealthpress.com

ABOUT THE AUTHOR

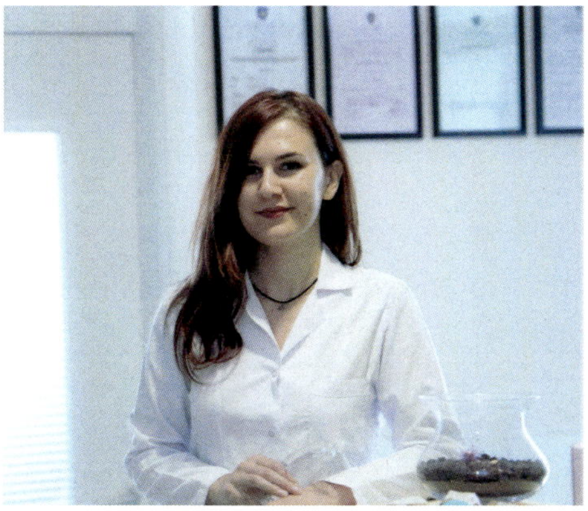

Donikë Demelezi is a dedicated medical doctor with a diverse background in pathology, general practice, and research. Currently serving as a Resident of Pathology and Cytodiagnostics at the University Clinical Center of Kosovo in Pristina, she meticulously analyzes bodily fluids and tissue specimens, compiles pathology reports, and engages in research. Previously, Donikë honed her clinical skills as a General Practitioner, where she assessed and treated patients during COVID-19 pandemic. Donikë's academic journey includes earning her MD degree from the University "Hasan Prishtina", Faculty of Medicine in Pristina. She furthered her knowledge through research summer school at the University of Angers in France. Committed to continuous learning, Donikë actively participates in extracurricular activities. Alongside her professional endeavors, she dedicates her time to volunteering with organizations like the Red Cross of Kosovo. Donikë's passion for medicine, coupled with her diverse experiences, shapes her into a compassionate and skilled healthcare professional.

Word Roots, Prefixes, and Suffixes by Chapter

Chapter 1 Organization and Structure of Cells

Uni-: Meaning "one," often used in terms like "unicellular" (one cell).

Multi-: Meaning "many," as in "multicellular" (many cells).

Pro-: Meaning "before" or "primary," as in "prokaryotic" (before the nucleus).

Euk-: From the Greek "eu," meaning "true," as in "eukaryotic" (true nucleus).

-cyte: Meaning "cell," used in terms like "erythrocyte" (red blood cell).

-some: Meaning "body" or "structure," as in "chromosome" (colored body).

-logy: Meaning "study of," as in "cytology" (the study of cells).

-genesis: Meaning "creation" or "formation," as in "cytogenesis" (formation of cells).

Chapter 2 Epithelium and General Connective Tissues

"theli": Derived from the Greek "thele," meaning "nipple" or "tissue."

"epi-": A Greek prefix meaning "upon," "over," or "above."

"-um": A Latin suffix typically used to denote a singular noun, often indicating a tissue or structure.

Chapter 3 Special Connective Tissue

Tissue (a group of cells that perform a similar function)

Cartilage (flexible connective tissue found in various parts of the body)

Bone (hard connective tissue that forms the skeleton)

Adipose (fat tissue)

Fibro (fibrous connective tissue)

Elastic (ability to stretch and return to original shape)

Adipo- (related to fat)

Chondro- (related to cartilage)

Osteo- (related to bone)

Fibro- (related to fibers)

Hemo- (related to blood)

Chapter 4 Nerve and Muscle

Nerv-: This is the root word related to nerves or the nervous system.

Neuro-: A prefix meaning "nerve" or "nervous system." Commonly used in terms like "neuroscience" or "neurobiology."

-itis: A suffix meaning inflammation, as in "neuritis" (inflammation of a nerve).

-pathy: A suffix meaning disease or disorder, as in "neuropathy" (nerve disease).

-algia: A suffix meaning pain, as in "neuralgia" (nerve pain).

-gram: A suffix meaning a record or image, as in "neurogram" (a record of nerve activity).

-ectomy: A suffix meaning surgical removal, as in "neurectomy" (removal of a nerve).

Chapter 5 Cardiovascular and Lymph Vascular Systems

Inter-: between (e.g., "interventricular" meaning between the ventricles)

Peri-: around (e.g., "pericardium" meaning around the heart)

Tachy-: fast (e.g., "tachycardia" meaning fast heart rate)

Brady-: slow (e.g., "bradycardia" meaning slow heart rate)

-opathy: disease or condition (e.g., "cardiomyopathy" meaning disease of the heart muscle)

-gram: a record or image (e.g., "angiogram" meaning an image of blood vessels)

-graphy: the process of recording (e.g., "angiography" meaning the process of imaging blood vessels)

-scope: an instrument for viewing (e.g., "endoscope" used in procedures involving the heart)

-emia: blood condition (e.g., "anemia" meaning a deficiency of red cells in the blood)

Chapter 6 Sensory System

Vestibul - balance or equilibrium (e.g., vestibular)

Hyper- - over, excessive (e.g., hypersensitivity)

Hypo- - under, below normal (e.g., hyposensitivity)

Multi- - many (e.g., multisensory)

Inter- - between (e.g., intersensory)

-tion - the action or result of (e.g., sensation, perception)

-ive - having the nature of (e.g., sensitive, receptive)

-al - relating to (e.g., sensory, visual)

-logy - study of (e.g., neurology, psychology)

-pathy - disease or disorder (e.g., neuropathy)

Chapter 7 Respiratory and Digestive System

Pulmon/o: lungs

Pneum/o: air, lung

Bronch/o: bronchi (airways)

Laryng/o: larynx (voice box)

Trache/o: trachea (windpipe)

Alveol/o: alveoli (air sacs)

Ox/o: oxygen

Capn/o: carbon dioxide

-itis: inflammation

-ectomy: surgical removal

-gram: record or image

-scopy: viewing or examination

-pnea: breathing

-capnia: carbon dioxide level

Chapter 8 Urinary and Reproductive System

Urin/o - urine

Ren/o - kidney

Nephr/o - kidney

Cyst/o - bladder

Urethr/o - urethra

Lith/o - stone

Olig/o - few or little

-itis - inflammation

-ectomy - surgical removal

-oma - tumor

-osis - condition or disease

-pathy - disease

-plasia - formation or development

Table of Contents

LIST OF FIGURES

LIST OF TABLES

PREFACE

Histology refers to the study of the morphology of cells within their natural tissue environment. As a biomedical discipline, it dates back to the development of first microscopes which allowed to override the physical visual limitation of the human eye. Since the first observations, it was understood that cell shape predicts function and, therefore, shape alterations can identify and explain dysfunction and diseases. The advancements in morphological investigation techniques have allowed to extend our understanding of the shape-function relationships close to the molecular level of organization of tissues, as well as to derive reliable data not only from fixed, and hence static, biological samples but also living cells and tissues and even for extended time periods. These modern approaches, which encompass quantitative microscopy, precision microscopy, and dynamic microscopy, represent the new frontier of morphology.

In medicine, histology plays a vital role in diagnosing diseases, monitoring treatments, and predicting therapy outcomes. Medical professionals use various techniques, including staining, microscopy, and immunohistochemistry, to analyze tissues and organs at a microscopic level. Similarly, biologists use histology to study plant and animal cells, tissues, and organs and understand their structure and function. They employ staining, microscopy, and immunohistochemistry to analyze how these components work together.

In veterinary science, histology helps diagnose and treat diseases in animals, with professionals using staining, microscopy, and immunohistochemistry to analyze tissues and organs. Dentists also rely on histology to understand the oral cavity's tissues and organs, aiding in diagnosing and treating oral diseases. They use staining, microscopy, and immunohistochemistry to analyze tissues and organs in the mouth. Histology involves preparing tissue specimens for microscopic examination. This includes fixing tissues with solutions like formalin, embedding them in wax or resin, cutting thin sections with a microtome, staining them with techniques like Hematoxylin and Eosin (H&E), and mounting them on glass slides for examination under a microscope.

This book summarizes how microscopy techniques have evolved to properly face the challenges of biomedical sciences, thus transforming Histology from a merely qualitative discipline, that played an ancillary role to traditional 'major' sciences such as Anatomy, to a modern experimental science capable of driving knowledge progress in Biology and Medicine.

It aims to provide a comprehensive and accessible overview of histology, catering to students, professionals, and enthusiasts interested in understanding the intricate structures and functions of tissues and organs at a microscopic level.

This book serves as a valuable resource for students embarking on their histology journey, offering a solid foundation in the subject's fundamentals. It also serves as a refresher for seasoned professionals, providing updated insights into histological techniques and applications.

Through clear explanations, detailed illustrations, and real-world examples, this book strives to make histology relatable and relevant. It examines the significance of histology in various fields, such as medicine, biology, veterinary science, and dentistry, highlighting its crucial role in disease diagnosis, treatment monitoring, and therapy prediction.

By the end of this book, readers will have gained a profound appreciation for the complexities of tissues and organs, understanding how their structures are intricately linked to their functions. They will be equipped with the knowledge and skills to interpret histological specimens effectively, paving the way for further exploration and discovery in the fascinating world of histology.

Chapter 1

ORGANIZATION AND STRUCTURE OF CELLS

Contents

Introduction

Multicellular organisms consist of two distinct structural elements: cells and the intercellular (extracellular) substances. Cells are the basic building blocks of living organisms and exhibit various specialized functions that are crucial for the individual's survival. Every cell is a discrete entity, possessing all the necessary apparatus for autonomous existence, and is isolated from its environment by its own cell membrane. The human body is estimated to be composed of approximately 80 to 100 trillion cells (Akamatsu et al., 2013).

Orientation and Directional Terms

Term	Definition	Illustration
Cytoplasmic Organelles	Specialized structures within a cell that perform distinct functions, such as energy production and protein synthesis.	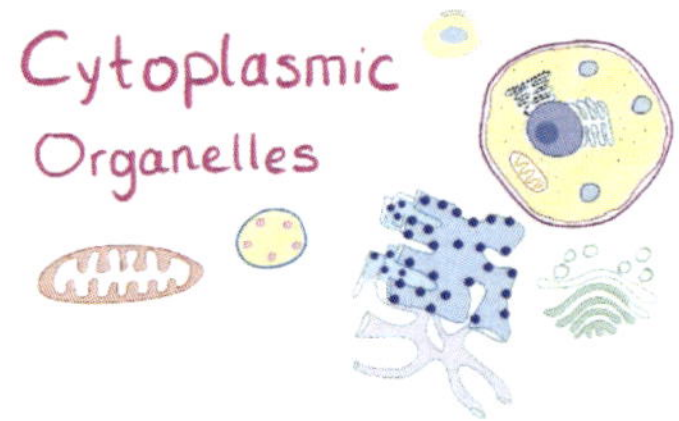
Cytoskeleton	A network of protein filaments and tubules that provide structural support, shape, and movement to the cell.	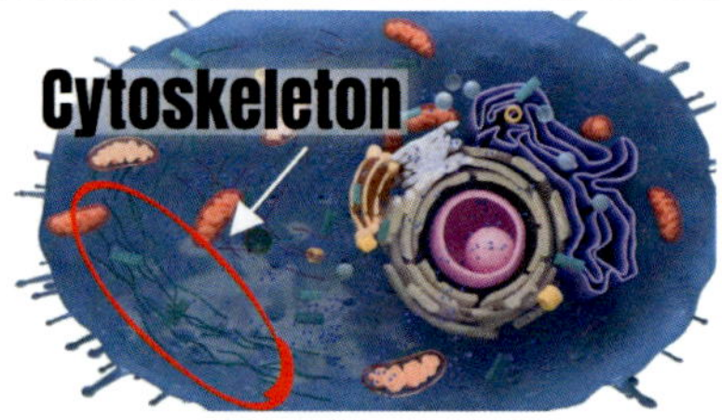
Ribosome	A ribosome is the cellular machinery responsible for making proteins.	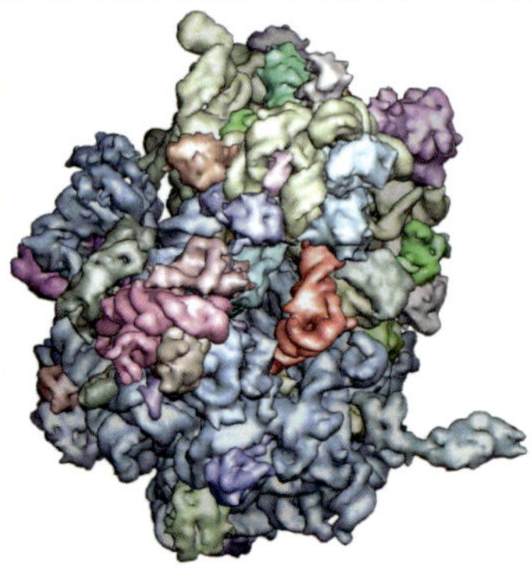
Mitochondria	Mitochondria are membrane-bound cell organelles (mitochondrion, singular) that generate most of the chemical energy needed to power the cell's biochemical reactions.	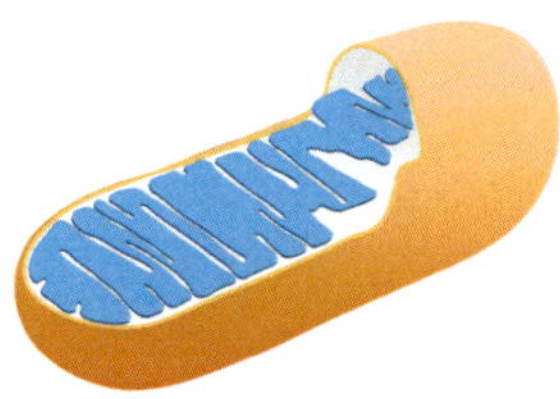
Nuclear Envelope	A double membrane that surrounds the nucleus, separating it from the cytoplasm and regulating the movement of materials in and out of the nucleus.	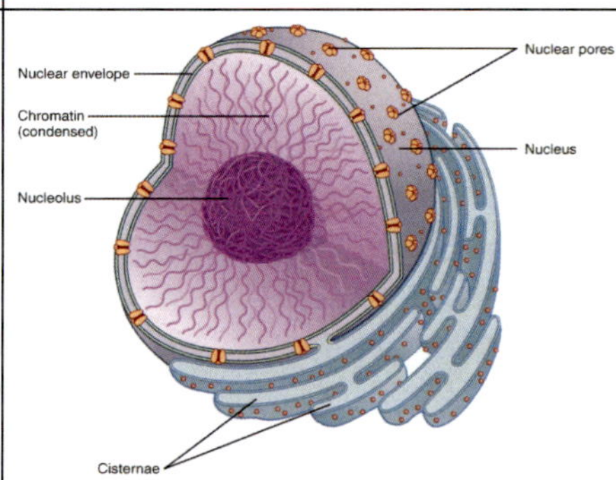

1.1. Protoplasm

Protoplasm, the vital substance found within a cell, is composed of protein, carbohydrate, lipid, nucleic acids, and inorganic materials that are distributed in water, resulting in the formation of an intricate, partially fluid gel. The viscosity of protoplasm varies among different cells and can transition from a viscous to a more fluid state. Protein, either on its own or in conjunction with lipids or carbohydrates, constitutes the primary structural element of the cell and the substances that exist between cells. Enzymes and numerous hormones are classified as proteins (Al-Alawi et al., 2014). Glucose is the primary **source** of energy in human cells, while glycogen serves as the stored form of glucose. The primary components of intercellular substances that bind cells together are complexes of carbohydrates and proteins. Hormones and antibodies are formed by other carbohydrate-protein complexes. Lipids function as a **source** of energy and play crucial roles in providing structure. They are also key constituents of cellular membrane systems.

Nucleic acids are classified into two distinct categories. Deoxyribonucleic acid (DNA) is the genetic material primarily located in the nucleus, although it can also be found in other parts of the cell. Ribonucleic acid (RNA) is found in both the cytoplasm and nucleus and serves as a carrier of information from the nucleus to the cytoplasm. Additionally, it functions as a blueprint for the production of proteins within the cell. Inorganic materials are essential constituents of protoplasm, alongside proteins, carbohydrates, and lipids. Physiological processes cannot occur without these inorganic materials. The inorganic constituents found in protoplasm include calcium, potassium, sodium, and magnesium in the form of carbonates, chlorides, phosphates, and sulfates. Additionally, there are small amounts of iron, copper, and iodine, as well as trace elements like cobalt, manganese, zinc, and other metals. Inorganic materials serve various functions, such as regulating intracellular and extracellular osmotic pressures, transmitting nerve impulses, facilitating muscle contraction, promoting cell adhesion, activating enzymes, facilitating oxygen transport, and maintaining tissue rigidity, particularly in bones. Approximately 75% of protoplasm consists of water. Some of the water is unbound and can be used as a solvent for different metabolic processes, while the rest is attached to protein (Altman et al., 1981).

1.1.1. Properties of Protoplasm

Protoplasm possesses various physiological properties that differentiate it from inanimate matter. All living cells exhibit these characteristics, although in certain cells, a specific characteristic may be emphasized. Irritability is an inherent characteristic of all living cells and pertains to their capacity to react to a stimulus. Conductivity is the capacity of a cell to transmit a stimulus from its point of origin to another point on its surface or to other cells. Conductivity is a characteristic that all cells possess, but it is most prominently developed in nerve tissue, similar to irritability. Contractility refers to the capacity of a cell to alter its shape in response to a stimulus, typically resulting in a reduction in the length of the cell in a particular direction. This characteristic is most conspicuous in muscle tissue. Absorption refers to the process by which substances are transported across the cell membrane and into the cell's interior, where they can be utilized in various ways. All cells possess the capacity to uptake substances, with certain cells exhibiting a high degree of selectivity in this process. Metabolism is the cellular capacity to decompose absorbed substances to generate energy (Ammit et al., 2000). Secretion is the cellular process of producing and releasing substances that are intended for use in other parts of the body. Excretion is the process of removing metabolic waste products from cells. An organism can grow either by augmenting the cytoplasmic volume within existing cells or by proliferating the number of cells. Cell size is constrained by the need to maintain efficient nutrient and oxygen delivery to the cells' interior. Once a certain size threshold is reached, the growth of protoplasm is achieved by the reproduction (division) of cells.

1.1.2. Organization of Protoplasm

While cells may vary in terms of their size, shape, and function, the protoplasm of every cell is composed of two primary components: the nucleus and the cytoplasm. The nucleus houses the hereditary or genetic material and is fully encased by cytoplasm, with a nuclear envelope acting as a barrier between the two. The cytoplasm is enclosed by a plasmalemma, also known as the cell membrane, which acts as a barrier between the cell and its surroundings. The cytoplasm contains various organelles and inclusions. Organelles are intricately structured, living components of the cytoplasm that carry out precise functions within the cell. Inclusions typically refer to non-reactive cellular products or metabolites that are frequently transient components. The majority, although not all, of the organelles, are structures enclosed by a membrane. Their size and concentration differ depending on the specific type and level of activity of the cell. Organelles are typically found in specific regions of the cytoplasm to maintain their separation from other cellular components and their associated metabolic activities. The maintenance of cell shape is facilitated by a three-dimensional cytoskeleton, which offers structural support to the cell and plays a role in cell motility and intracellular transport. The cytoskeleton is composed of diverse microfilaments and microtubules. The organelles and inclusions are held in suspension within a shapeless substance known as the cytoplasmic matrix, also referred to as cytosol. The karyolymph is a structureless ground substance that contains suspended nuclear material. Aside from their distinct locations, karyolymph and cytosol seem to be functionally identical (An et al., 2007).

1.2. Cytoplasmic Organelles

Organelles are specialized structures within a cell that carry out specific functions and are essential components of the cell's living matter. Organelles consist of various structures, including the plasmalemma, granular and smooth forms of endoplasmic reticulum, ribosomes, Golgi complexes, mitochondria, lysosomes, peroxisomes, and centrioles. Several organelles are enclosed by membranes that bear a resemblance to the cell's own boundary, known as the plasmalemma. These membranes, such as the cell membrane, are biologically active layers that are crucial for the cell's survival. The electron micrographs reveal that the membranes possess a trilaminar structure, which comprises inner and outer dense lines that are separated by a light zone. The trilaminar structure, which is present in all biological cell membranes, is commonly referred to as a unit membrane (Aszodi et al., 2006). The thickness of the unit membrane differs among organelles and is typically highest where it constitutes the plasmalemma. Although the physical appearance of the membranes of various organelles may show only slight differences in structure, they exhibit significant variations in terms of their chemical composition, enzymatic properties, and functions. The membranous organelles function to segregate the interior of the cell into distinct functional units, ensuring that the biochemical processes taking place in one organelle do not disrupt those happening in neighboring organelles (Azazi et al., 2014).

1.2.1. Plasmalemma (Cell Membrane)

The plasmalemma surrounding each cell has a trilaminar structure and is 8 to 10 nm thick. The visual representation consists of two compact lines, each with a width of 3 nm, with a distinct gap of 2 to 4 nm between them. The plasmalemma consists of proteins, lipids, glycolipids, and carbohydrates. The plasmalemma is composed of lipids, which make up approximately 50% of its mass. These lipids can be categorized into three main classes: phospholipids, glycolipids, and cholesterol. Phospholipids are the most prevalent among these. Researchers have identified four primary categories of phospholipids in the plasmalemma. The compounds mentioned are sphingomyelin, phosphatidylserine, phosphatidylcholine, and phosphatidylethanolamine. Every phospholipid molecule possesses a polar head region that carries an electric charge, as well as an uncharged, nonpolar tail region composed of two fatty acid chains (Bakakos et al., 2019). The polar heads are hydrophilic and, therefore, reside on both the inner and outer surfaces of the plasmalemma.

The hydrophobic nonpolar tail regions align themselves in the central part of the plasmalemma. The outcome is the formation of a phospholipid bilayer consisting of two parallel layers of phospholipid molecules arranged in a tail-to-tail configuration. In this bilayer, the hydrocarbon (fatty acid) chains are oriented towards the interior, while the polar groups are oriented towards the exterior. Phosphatidylcholine and sphingomyelin are typically present in the outer layer of the cell membrane, known as the plasmalemma. On the other hand, phosphatidylethanolamine and phosphatidylserine are situated in the inner layer, which is adjacent to the cytosol. The plasmalemma exhibits fluidity as a result of the lateral mobility of neighboring phospholipid molecules. Thus, breaks and tears in the phospholipids seal naturally because of their polar nature. Cholesterol molecules in the plasmalemma restrict the sideways movement of phospholipids and enhance the mechanical stability of the plasmalemma (Baum and Duffy, 2011). Due to the polar lipid composition of the plasmalemma, it is highly permeable to substances like oxygen, nitrogen, and small, uncharged molecules. It exhibits impermeability to charged ions such as potassium, sodium, chloride, calcium, larger uncharged molecules, and all charged large molecules. The entry of these substances into the cell is contingent upon integral proteins located on the plasmalemma. Glycolipids, which are lipids that have sugar residues attached to them, make up approximately 10% of the lipids that form the plasmalemma. The sugar residues of this lipid class typically protrude from the outer surface of the cell membrane and play a role in giving the cell surface a negative charge. Glycolipids play a crucial role in facilitating communication between cells and the surrounding interstitial matrix.

Additionally, they may contribute to immune responses. Glycosphingolipids, also known as glycolipids, are primarily derived from ceramide. Gangliosides and galactocerebrosides are significant glycolipids found in the plasmalemma. They serve as major constituents of nerve cell membranes and myelin, respectively. While membrane lipids provide the basic structure of the bilayered plasmalemma, it is primarily membrane proteins that carry out its specialized functions. Proteins make up approximately 50% of the plasmalemma by weight (Bortolozzo et al., 2018). Membrane proteins can undergo lateral movement within the lipid bilayer of the cell's surface, as long as they are not bound to filamentous proteins in the underlying cytoplasm. Membrane proteins have various functions such as transporting molecules in and out of cells (membrane pump proteins, ion-channel proteins, carrier proteins), serving as receptors for chemical signals between cells (hormone receptors), producing messenger molecules that spread into the cytoplasm, connecting elements of the cytoskeleton to the cell membrane, attaching cells to the extracellular matrix (cell adhesion molecules), and potentially exhibiting specific enzymatic activity when stimulated (Bousquet et al., 1990). Membrane proteins can be classified into two fundamental categories: integral proteins and peripheral proteins. There are different types of integral and peripheral membrane proteins (**Figure 1.1**).

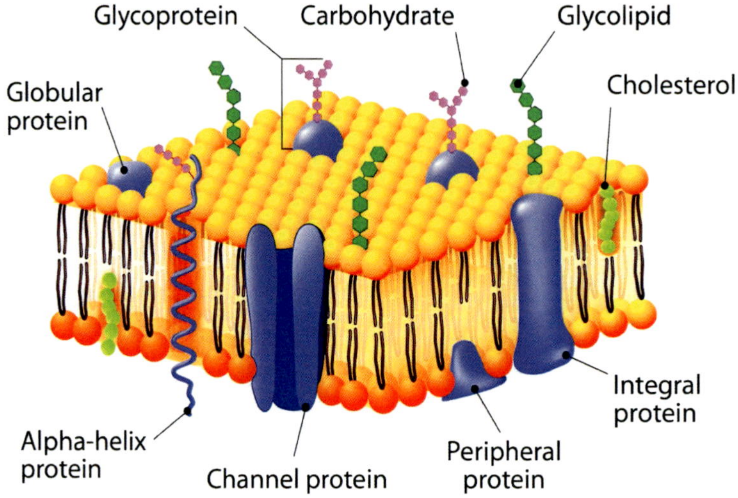

Figure 1.1. *Fluid mosaic model of the plasma membrane.*

Source: https://search-static.byjusweb.com/question images/toppr_ext/questions/947817_1021284_ans_b76bfe5fabe9461b8cdef9296644b59f.jpg.

Integral membrane proteins are securely inserted into the lipid bilayer and cannot be extracted. Transmembrane proteins, which are a type of integral proteins, extend across the entire width of the plasmalemma and protrude from both surfaces. This integral protein consists of three components: a domain facing the outer side of the cell, a domain traversing the lipid bilayer, and a domain facing the inner side of the cell (Bousquet et al., 2000). This particular integral protein is composed of amino acids that are arranged in an α-helix structure. It is classified as a tripartite single-pass integral membrane protein. Not all transmembrane proteins conform to this category. Multipass transmembrane proteins, which traverse the plasmalemma multiple times, are also present. The majority of identified transporters and ion channels are of this type. Transmembrane proteins are found in specific regions of the plasmalemma that are specialized for binding to other cells or the extracellular matrix. These molecules traverse the lipid bilayer and serve to connect cells or attach the cell to the extracellular matrix. Some integral proteins are not transmembrane proteins. Peripheral membrane proteins are proteins that can be extracted from the plasmalemma without causing any disruption to the lipid bilayer (Bousquet et al., 1996). Peripheral membrane proteins are typically bound to the plasmalemma, usually on its inner surface, and play a role in maintaining its stability. Peripheral membrane proteins can attach to the plasmalemma surface through ionic interactions with integral proteins, other peripheral proteins, or by binding to the polar head groups of the phospholipids (Brenmoehl et al., 2009). Two examples of peripheral membrane proteins are spectrin and ankyrin. These proteins are located on the cytoplasmic surface of the erythrocyte plasmalemma. Both serve to attach components of the cytoskeleton to the inner side of the cell membrane. Peripheral membrane proteins with similar characteristics can be found in the majority of other cells. Peripheral membrane proteins also serve to maintain the cohesion of plasmalemma molecules and prevent the cell membrane from rupturing. Proteoglycans are a type of membrane protein. The protein core of this molecule extends across the lipid bilayer, while the part of the long molecule that carries the carbohydrate side chains protrudes from the outer surface of the cell membrane. The carbohydrate portion of these molecules, along with glycoproteins and glycolipids, contribute to the formation of the glycocalyx, which is the fuzzy coat observed through electron microscopy. The coat, known as glycocalyx, is found on every cell and is characterized by the presence of ionized carboxyl and sulfate groups in the polysaccharide units. These groups contribute to the cell's external surface having a significant negative charge (Brown et al., 1997).

The glycocalyx also has a significant impact on the immunologic characteristics of the cell and its connections and interactions with other cells. Carbohydrates provide a significantly wider range of structural variations for recognition compared to proteins. The vast array of molecular arrangements of the subunits of the extensive polysaccharides that protrude from the plasmalemma is responsible for cell recognition. Integral membrane proteins can be composed of a polypeptide chain connected to a carbohydrate, specifically sialic acid. These proteins serve as adhesion molecules and are referred to as cell-adhesion molecules or CAMs. Multiple cell adhesion molecules (CAMs) have been discovered, including those specific to neurons, hepatocytes, muscle cells, glial cell-neuron adhesion, and various others. The plasmalemma is a membrane that allows selective passage of ions and small water-soluble molecules, such as amino acids and glucose. These molecules need to be transported through protein-lined channels that cross the plasmalemma to enter the cell interior. The predominant types of receptor proteins associated with ion channels include voltage-gated ion channels, which necessitate a transmembrane potential to initiate opening; mechanically-gated ion channels, which detect movement in the plasmalemma and are stimulated to open as a result; and neurotransmitter-gated ion channels. Neurotransmitter-gated ion channels are receptors that specifically bind neurotransmitters and facilitate the movement of ions. The receptors mentioned are the glycine receptor, the N-methyl-D-aspartate receptor, the nicotinic acetylcholine receptor, the 5-hydroxytrptamine serotonin receptor, and the γ-aminobutyric acid receptor. Channel proteins experience an allosteric modification that results in the opening of the channel when stimulated. Therefore, the transfer of solutes across the cell membrane relies on the functioning of particular transmembrane transport proteins (Burgess et al., 2003).

The process of a solitary solute (molecule) being transported across a membrane by specialized proteins is known as a uniport mechanism. The simultaneous movement of two or more solutes in the same direction across the plasmalemma is facilitated by a symport or cotransport mechanism. The process of coupled transport, where two or more solutes move in opposite directions across a cell membrane, is known as countertransport or antiport mechanism. G-protein-linked receptors are transmembrane proteins that extend across the plasma membrane and are associated with trimeric GTP-binding proteins known as G proteins. The dopamine receptor, glucagon receptor, α- and β-adrenergic receptors, and muscarinic acetylcholine receptor are all significant G-protein-linked receptors. These receptors initiate a series of cellular processes either via a calcium ion pathway or a cyclic adenosine monophosphate (cAMP) pathway. The latter pathway modulates c-AMP levels through the activation or inhibition of adenylate cyclase. The calcium ion pathway triggers the activation of phospholipase C, an enzyme that cleaves phosphatidylinositol biphosphate into inositol triphosphate and diacetylglycerol. Inositol triphosphate stimulates the liberation of calcium ions from the endoplasmic reticulum, leading to the activation of calcium ion/calmodulin-dependent protein kinase (Cam-kinase). Diacylglycerol triggers the activation of protein kinase C. Enzyme-linked receptors are membrane proteins that are connected to an enzyme. When the specific signal attaches to the receptor, a series of cellular processes is initiated that can potentially impact gene transcription in the nucleus. Notable enzyme-linked receptors include the fibroblast growth factor (FGF) receptor, the insulin receptor, and the epidermal growth factor (EGF) receptor (Busse and Sedgwick, 1992).

Aquaporins are integral membrane proteins that form channels and selectively facilitate the transport of water across the plasmalemma of various cell types in different organs. Currently, 10 distinct categories of aquaporins have been discovered in mammalian tissues. The plasmalemma is actively involved in the process of endocytosis, which is the uptake of macromolecular materials into the cell, as well as exocytosis, which is the release of materials from the cell. Phagocytosis is a type of endocytosis where a cell engulfs and internalizes solid particles (Carr et al., 2016). During the attachment phase, particles adhere to receptors on the cell membrane, while during the ingestion phase, the cytoplasm extends pseudopods that surround the particles, engulf them, and transport them into the cell's interior within vacuoles enclosed by membranes. Similarly, fluid can be introduced into the cell through small cytoplasmic vesicles via a process known as pinocytosis. Phagocytosis and pinocytosis are observable through light microscopy. Certain substances can be transported into the cell through tiny vesicles that are created by small invaginations of the plasmalemma. The process known as micropinocytosis can only be observed using an electron microscope. Both nonselective fluid-phase and selective adsorptive forms of micropinocytosis have been identified. Fluid-phase micropinocytosis typically takes place in cells, where small vesicles or caveolae are formed from the plasmalemma. The caveolae, which house fluid and its dispersed substances, traverse the cytoplasm towards the opposite side of the cell, merge with the plasmalemma, and release their contents (Carroll et al., 2000).

Transcytosis is the term used to describe the process of moving material across a cellular barrier to the extracellular spaces. This mechanism is particularly important in certain cells, such as endothelial cells. Caveolins, which are specific proteins, cover the outer surface of caveolae and enable the transportation across the cytoplasm of endothelial cells to the plasmalemma on the opposite side of the cell without any hindrance. Caveolae can also originate from the plasmalemma of various cell types and play a role in the targeted transportation of specific molecules. Three distinct caveolin proteins have been identified and are presently being investigated (Chan et al., 2006). Coatomer proteins, in addition to their role in coating cytoplasmic transport vesicles, facilitate the movement of materials between organelles, including transport to the plasmalemma (Cockcroft and Davis, 2006) (**Figure 1.2**).

Adsorptive (clathrin-mediated) micropinocytosis refers to the targeted internalization of particular macromolecules at specific receptor-binding sites on the cell membrane (Desmouliere et al., 1993). This type of micropinocytosis plays a crucial role in the uptake of nutrients, growth factors, antigens, recycling receptors, and pathogens. On the cytoplasmic surface, there may be small, stiff projections that resemble bristles. These projections can create coated pits, which then give rise to coated vesicles. The vesicles' cytoplasmic surfaces are covered with clathrin, a protein that forms radiating spikes, resulting in a fuzzy appearance (Doeing and Solway, 2013). Clathrin can inhibit the fusion of coated vesicles with membranous organelles, as shown in **Figure 1.3**.

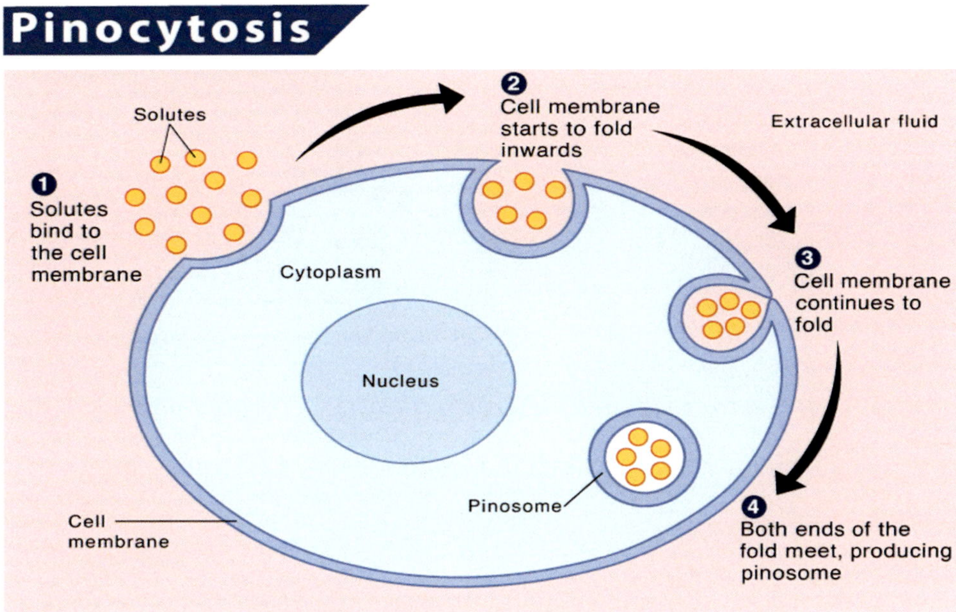

Figure 1.2. *Diagrammatic representation of fluid-phase micropinocytosis.*

Source: https://www.sciencefacts.net/wp-content/uploads/2021/06/Pinocytosis.jpg.

After the coated vesicle is formed, the clathrin coat is removed and the vesicles merge with preexisting vacuoles to create structures known as endosomes. When the molecules being transported are released from these early endosomes into the cytosol, sections of the endosome membrane that have receptors not being used form small vesicles. These vesicles then go back to the plasmalemma and merge with it (Dunnill et al., 1969). Therefore, certain receptors undergo recycling. Late endosomes can undergo fusion with lysosomes, resulting in the degradation of their contents. Exocytosis is the process by which materials like secretory granules are released from the cell. During this process, SNARE proteins in the limiting membranes of the granules identify and merge with the plasmalemma before releasing their contents. By following this approach, the occurrence of a breach in the restricting plasmalemma is prevented (Enilari and Sinha, 2019). Endocytosis removes the surplus membrane added to the plasmalemma during exocytosis. There are two distinct forms of exocytosis: regulated and constitutive. Regulated exocytosis is contingent upon external stimuli and takes place in cells that are specifically designed for the discharge of a substantial amount of secretory material, such as pancreatic acinar cells. Constitutive exocytosis takes place in cells where the secretory product is released continuously in small vesicles.

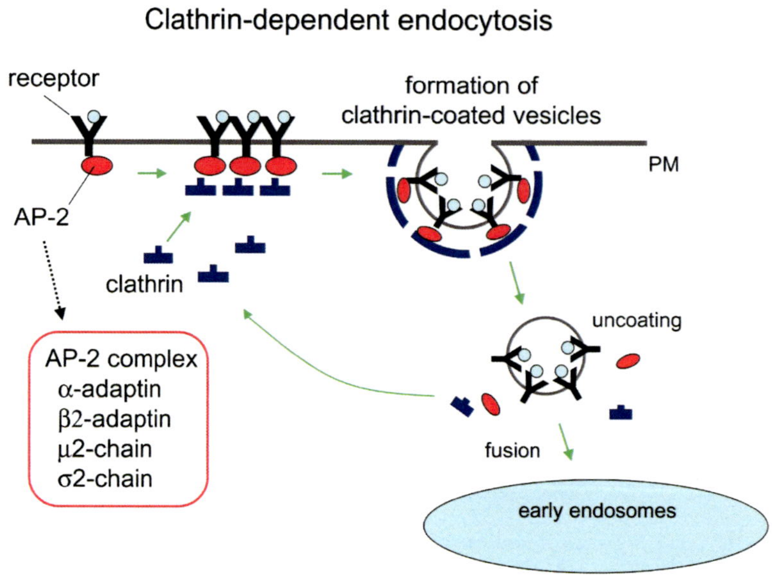

Figure 1.3. *Adsorptive (receptor-mediated) micropinocytosis via coated vesicles.*

Source: https://upload.wikimedia.org/wikipedia/commons/4/47/Itrafig2.jpg.

1.2.2. Ribosomes

Ribosomes are tiny, evenly sized particles made up of ribonucleoprotein, measuring 12 to 15 nm in diameter. They consist of both large and small subunits (Erjefält et al., 2000). Ribosomes can either be bound to the membranes of the endoplasmic reticulum or exist as free ribosomes in the cytosol, not connected to any membranes. Free ribosomes frequently form clusters known as polyribosomes or polysomes, where individual ribosomes are connected by a strand of messenger RNA (mRNA). Free ribosomes are locations where protein synthesis occurs, with the resulting proteins being utilized by the cell internally rather than being released. Ribosomes that are not attached to any membrane synthesize proteins that are found in the cytoplasm, proteins that are located on the outer surface of membranes, and proteins that are meant to be used by mitochondria, peroxisomes, and the nucleus. Isolated, free ribosomes are inactive; they only become active in protein synthesis when they bind to mRNA and form polyribosomes. Likewise, ribosomes located on the endoplasmic reticulum need to be connected to mRNA prior to participating in protein synthesis (Gizycki et al., 1997).

Messenger RNA is synthesized within the nucleus using a template of uncoiled deoxyribonucleic acid (DNA).

The message is encoded in sets of three nucleotides, known as codons, which determine the order in which amino acids are added to create a new protein. During the process of synthesis, messenger RNA (mRNA) is transported from the nucleus to the cytoplasm. It then binds to ribosomes, which travel along the mRNA molecule, decoding the genetic information and arranging amino acids in the correct sequence. Upon reaching the termination codon on the mRNA, ribosomes disengage and concomitantly liberate the recently formed protein molecule. Transfer RNA (tRNA), a type of ribonucleoprotein, transports amino acids to the ribosomes for their inclusion in the protein.

Each amino acid has a corresponding specific tRNA. Ribosomal and transfer RNA are synthesized through the process of transcribing specific segments of the DNA molecule. Therefore, in contrast to mRNA, the production of ribosomal RNA is guided by a distinct section of a chromosome (Gosens et al., 2006).

1.2.3. Endoplasmic Reticulum

The endoplasmic reticulum, a network of membrane-bound channels, is present in the cytoplasm of nearly all cells. Usually, this cellular structure is observed as interconnected tubules, but the membranes can also take the shape of parallel, flattened sacs known as cisternae. Unattached small transport vesicles, which are not connected to tubules or cisternae, may also be present and are considered to be a component of the endoplasmic reticulum (Halayko et al., 1999). Differentiating between smooth and granular forms of endoplasmic reticulum is possible. The granular endoplasmic reticulum (GER) typically comprises a series of flattened cisternae enclosed by a membrane. The external surface is adorned with a multitude of ribosomes.

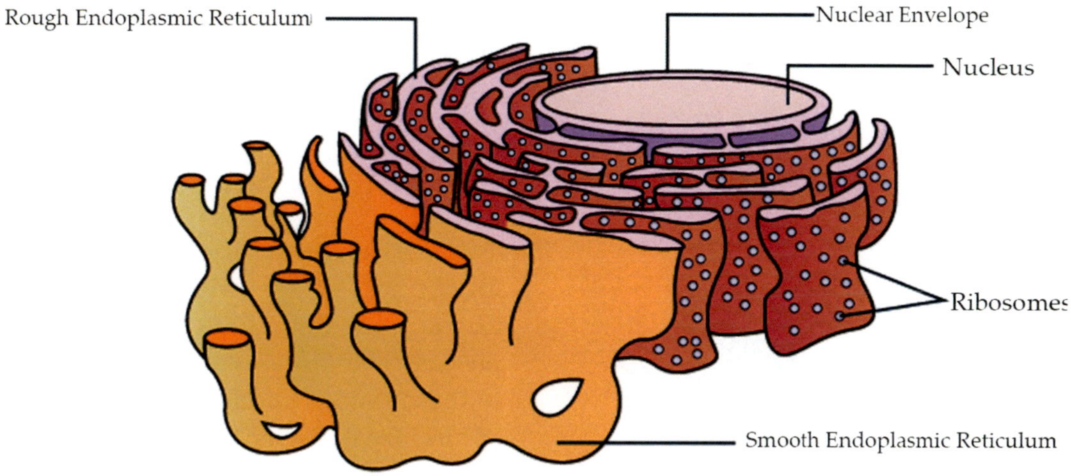

Figure 1.4. *Diagrammatic representation of endoplasmic reticulum.*

The GER is responsible for synthesizing secretory proteins, lysosomal enzymes, and plasmalemmal proteins (receptors). Proteins are produced by ribosomes located on the outer surface of the Golgi endoplasmic reticulum (GER). They subsequently enter the interior space of the endoplasmic reticulum, where they are separated from the surrounding cytoplasm. Proteins that are intended to be secreted, targeted to organelles, or incorporated into certain membranes possess an NH_2-terminal signal sequence, also known as a leader sequence. This signal sequence is identified by a signal-recognition particle in the cytosol while the protein is being synthesized from mRNA (Halayko et al., 1996). The signal-recognition particle (SRP) attaches to both the signal peptide and the ribosome, causing the translation process to halt. The signal recognition particle (SRP), ribosome, and the nascent NH_2 terminus of the polypeptide being synthesized, all associate with an integral membrane-docking protein known as a signal recognition receptor (ribosome receptor protein) located in the endoplasmic reticulum membrane (Hardy et al., 1996). Following docking, translation recommences, and the signal peptide, along with the developing polypeptide, enters a transmembrane channel (pore) to enter the cisternal lumen of the GER. Upon entering the lumen of the endoplasmic reticulum, the signal sequence of the polypeptide is cleaved by a signal peptidase situated on the inner membrane surface of the rough endoplasmic reticulum (Hinz et al., 2003). After the message is translated and the secretory polypeptide is synthesized, the ribosome is released from the endoplasmic reticulum. The transmembrane channel is then closed by the sideward movement of phospholipid molecules in the endoplasmic reticulum membrane. Once inside the cisternal lumen, these polypeptides and forming proteins are kept separate from the rest of the cytosol. At this stage, the newly formed proteins undergo a process called folding, which results in the formation of a three-dimensional structure. The majority of proteins produced by the GER undergo glycosylation once they enter the cisternal lumen, a process that is finalized in the Golgi complex (Hinz et al., 2007) (**Figure 1.4**).

The smooth endoplasmic reticulum (SER) is devoid of ribosomes and is primarily composed of a network of interconnected tubules, without the presence of cisternae. Typically, a specific type of endoplasmic reticulum is more abundant in the majority of cells (Hough et al., 2020). Protein-secreting cells, such as pancreatic acinar cells or plasma cells, have a large amount of rough endoplasmic reticulum (GER), while cells that secrete steroid hormones mainly have smooth endoplasmic reticulum. In certain cells, such as liver cells, both forms of endoplasmic reticulum are present in approximately equal quantities and may be connected. The GER is recognized for its involvement in protein synthesis, although the specific function of the SER can differ among different cells. It plays a role in the production of steroid hormones in specific endocrine cells, the production of membrane phospholipids, cholesterol, ceramide, and glycogen, the breakdown of drugs using cytochrome P450, and the extension of fatty acids. The smooth endoplasmic reticulum is involved in the release and reuptake of calcium ions during the contraction and relaxation of striated muscle.

1.2.4. Golgi Complex

The Golgi complex, also known as the Golgi apparatus, is not detectable in regular histologic preparations and is not visible in living cells. However, it may occasionally be observed as a negative image, appearing as a nonstaining region in the cytoplasm, typically located near the nucleus (Ihrie et al., 2019). The morphology of the Golgi complex exhibits variability depending on the cell's type and level of activity, ranging from a diminutive and condensed structure to a substantial and reticular one. Certain cells possess multiple Golgi complexes. Electron micrographs reveal that the Golgi complex is composed of multiple flattened saccules, known as cisternae, which are each surrounded by a smooth membrane. The saccules are discoidal, slightly arched, and frequently exhibit compression towards the center and dilation towards the periphery (Janulaityte et al., 2020).

The saccules are organized in vertical formations and are divided by gaps that measure 20 to 30 nm in width. The Golgi complex possesses both convex and concave faces due to the curvature of the saccules. The convex side of the organelle is typically oriented towards the nucleus and is referred to as the forming or cis-face. On the other hand, the concave side, known as the maturing or trans-face, is directed towards the cell membrane. The forming face is characterized by a multitude of small transport vesicles, and at this face, the outer saccule is penetrated by numerous small openings. The saccules on the maturing face exhibit greater dilation compared to those on the convex face. The Golgi complex contains concentrated secretory products, and its size changes depending on the cell's level of activity. Peptides initially gather in the lumen of the endoplasmic reticulum (ER) in cells that secrete proteins (Januskevicius et al., 2019). They are then carried to the Golgi complex in small transport vesicles. These vesicles are created by protrusions from regions of the ER that are free of ribosomes and are located next to the Golgi complex. The transport vesicles coated with coatomers transport small amounts of protein to the Golgi complex. At the forming face, these vesicles merge with and provide a membrane to the developing outer saccule. Proteins amass within the cisternae of the Golgi membranes and undergo modifications as they traverse the Golgi complex. During the maturation process, the saccules enlarge and separate to create membranes that enclose the protein within structures known as condensing vacuoles.

The addition of a new membrane to the side that is being formed compensates for the loss of membrane from the side that is maturing. The secretory materials contained in the vacuoles undergo an increase in concentration, leading to the maturation of the condensing vacuoles into secretory granules. It has been discovered that this simplified version of the Golgi function is significantly more intricate. The GER and SER are responsible for the production of numerous proteins and lipids, respectively. Some molecules are exported as secretory products, while others are intended to be integrated into the structural components of the cell. The Golgi complex is responsible for the post-translational modification, packaging, and sorting of proteins and lipids that are synthesized by the endoplasmic reticulum. It is also implicated in the process of membrane recycling. The luminal side of the endoplasmic reticulum and Golgi membrane cisternae contain crucial enzymes that are involved in glycosylation and other functions.

The Golgi complex can be divided into functional compartments based on the enzymes found in its cisternae, leading to different subdivisions. The cis-compartment of the forming face receives transport vesicles that have originated from the transitional elements of the endoplasmic reticulum (Jeffery, 2001). This compartment exhibits a high degree of fenestration, presenting itself as a complex network of interconnected tubules and vesicles. After undergoing modification of the proteins and lipids obtained from the endoplasmic reticulum, vesicles separate from the cisternae of this compartment and merge with the cisternae of a medial compartment. Once the lipids and proteins are processed by enzymes in this area, vesicles are formed again to transport these molecules to the cisternae of the trans-compartment located at the maturing face of the Golgi complex. The terminal cisternae in this area exhibit extensive fenestration and create a complex network of interconnected tubules and vesicles. The specific area within the Golgi complex that is being referred to is known as the trans-Golgi network (Jiang et al., 1992).

The sorting of proteins, glycoproteins, and lipids into distinct transport vesicles occurs within the trans-Golgi network. The addition of distinct chemical groups to proteins in the endoplasmic reticulum, followed by subsequent modifications in different compartments of the Golgi complex, determines the precise intracellular destinations of specific proteins. Sorting occurs at the maturing face of the trans-Golgi network, where specific proteins are selected to be packaged into larger secretory granules, some are enclosed in small, smooth-surfaced vesicles, and others are placed in clathrin-coated vesicles. The larger secretory granules, which are enclosed by a membrane, are typically intended for regulated exocytosis, which refers to stimulated secretion (Johnson et al., 2001). The products contained within small, smooth-surfaced vesicles are primarily involved in constitutive exocytosis and the transportation of membranes to other organelles. The mechanism involves the insertion of receptor proteins, which are cell membrane proteins, into the plasmalemma through nonclathrin-coated vesicles. Coated vesicles, which are small in size, transport acid hydrolase enzymes and specifically merge with endosomes to create developing lysosomes, also known as primary lysosomes. During the process of releasing secretory granules, the membranes of these granules only merge with the plasmalemma and become part of the cell membrane. The secretory granules are enclosed by membranes that contain specific proteins called vSNAREs. These vSNAREs have the ability to specifically recognize and bind with particular plasmalemmal proteins known as tSNAREs. Importantly, vSNAREs do not interact with the membranes of other organelles (Johnson et al., 2000).

Both these proteins are essential for the fusion of the phospholipid bilayer in both membranes, which allows the granule membrane to merge with the plasmalemma. As a result, the contents of the granule are released outside the cell. Therefore, the Golgi complex's membranous packaging grants the vacuoles/vesicles at the maturing face distinct characteristics. The membranes of the secretory granules can only recognize and fuse with the apical plasmalemma to release their contents during regulated exocytosis. Additional Golgi vesicles specifically identify and merge exclusively with the basolateral plasmalemma during constitutive exocytosis. However, some vesicles undergo fusion with particular organelles or endosomes, rather than being expelled from the cell as occurs in the creation of primary lysosomes. The membrane undergoes a continuous movement within the cell, starting from the endoplasmic reticulum and progressing through transport vesicles, the Golgi complex, secretory granules, and finally reaching the plasmalemma. The process of incorporating the cell membrane into the interior of the cell takes place through phagocytosis, pinocytosis, and micropinocytosis. Proteins that are connected to the membrane surrounding these vesicles, regardless of their specific type, are believed to assist in directing the vesicles to their intended location and subsequently identify matching proteins within the membranes of the target organelles (Johnson and Burgess, 2004).

1.2.5. Lysosomes Are Organelles

Lysosomes are tiny organelles enclosed by a membrane, characterized by their high density and measuring between 0.2 to 0.55 µm in diameter. Lysosomes contain over 50 identified enzymes. Lysosomal enzymes are commonly known as acid hydrolases because they exhibit activity in an acidic pH environment. The lysosomes' limiting membrane shields the rest of the cell from the potential harm caused by the enclosed enzymes (Kalinauskaite-Zukauske et al., 2019). If these enzymes were to be released into the cytosol, they would break down or rupture the cell. The phenomenon described is known as autolysis, which is believed to occur naturally in various situations such as the regression of the mesonephros during kidney development and the regression of mammary tissue after lactation has stopped. Lysosomal activity is heightened during the regression of certain tumors. The morphology of lysosomes is contingent upon their level of activity and their interaction with cellular structures or internalized material (Kalinauskaite-Zukauske et al., 2019). To positively identify lysosomes, a histochemical test must be conducted to detect the presence of at least two acid hydrolases, as lysosomes can display a wide range of morphological characteristics. Primary lysosomes are recently formed at the Golgi complex and have not yet participated in any digestive processes. The enzymes of the primary lysosomes are produced in the endoplasmic reticulum (GER) and then transferred to the Golgi complex (Kalinauskaite-Zukauske et al., 2019). Enzymes that are meant to go to lysosomes have their mannose components phosphorylated while they are in the Golgi cisternae. As these enzymes progress through the Golgi complex, they become attached to a transmembrane glycoprotein called the mannose-6-phosphate receptor, which is located on the inner side of the membranes that make up the trans-Golgi network. Subsequently, these receptor-enzyme complexes are sorted to specific areas of the trans-Golgi network, where they give rise to small vesicles covered with the protein clathrin. Vesicles covered with a layer of clathrin, which contain acid hydrolases bound to receptors, emerge from the trans-Golgi network. Shortly after their formation, these vesicles shed their clathrin coat. The diminutive transport vesicles, brimming with dormant acid hydrolases, subsequently merge with a tardy endosome originating from the plasmalemma, which harbors H+-ATPase (Kato and Schleimer, 1994). This enzyme generates an acidic milieu with a pH of 5.0, which triggers the activation of acid hydrolases in the developing primary lysosome.

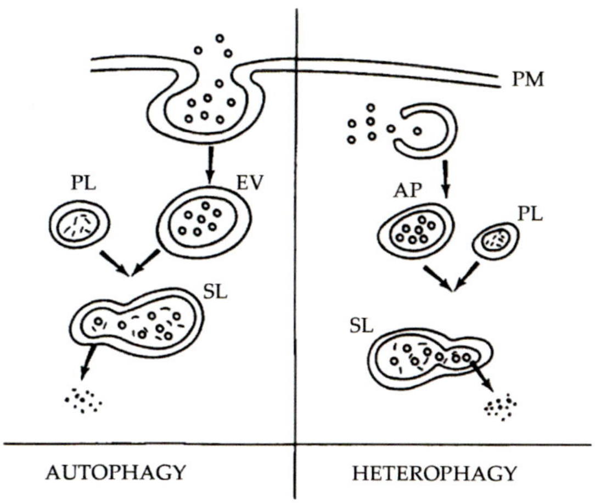

Figure 1.5. *Schematic representation of heterophagy and autophagy.*

Source: https://ars.els-cdn.com/content/image/3-s2.0-B9780433228806500242-f17-01-9780433228806.jpg.

Typically, primary lysosomes are retained within the cell and not released. Nevertheless, certain cells, such as neutrophils and osteoclasts, secrete primary lysosomes into the extracellular milieu. Secondary lysosomes are vacuolar structures that serve as locations where lysosomal activity has occurred or is currently occurring. They encompass heterophagic vacuoles, residual bodies, and cytolysosomes. For a better understanding of the relationships between these structures, it is most effective to examine the processes associated with phagocytosis. Certain cells, such as macrophages and certain granular leukocytes in the blood, possess a unique ability to engulf and eliminate extracellular substances.

Heterophagy refers to the cellular process of taking in substances from the external environment and breaking them down through lysosomal activity. The process entails the folding inward of the cell membrane and the confinement of the material within a vacuole that is surrounded by a membrane. Therefore, the extracellular material that is engulfed by the cell is enclosed within a vacuole known as a phagosome and remains separate from the cytoplasm (Kendall and Feghali-Bostwick, 2014). While traversing the cytoplasm of the cell, the phagosome comes across a primary lysosome. The membranes of the two structures merge and the enzymes of the lysosome are released into the phagosome. A heterophagic vacuole, which is a type of secondary lysosome, refers to the combined primary lysosome and phagosome.

The lysosomal enzymes digest the material inside the heterophagic vacuole, and any valuable substances are transported into the cytosol for cellular utilization. Non-biodegradable substances, such as certain dye particles, asbestos fibers, silica, or carbon, can persist within the vacuole, which is now referred to as a residual body. A residual body is a type of secondary lysosome that is believed by certain researchers to be expelled from the cell through exocytosis. Nevertheless, residual bodies tend to accumulate and persist for extended durations in numerous cells (Kohan et al., 2010) (**Figure 1.5**).

Autophagy is the process by which cytoplasmic organelles are broken down in normal, viable cells through lysosomal degradation. The lysosomal system plays a role in the degradation of surplus or impaired organelles and in the restructuring of the cytoplasm. During the process, a segment of the cytoplasm that contains an excessive amount, or damaged organelles is enveloped by a membrane, resulting in the formation of an autophagic vacuole. The membrane is believed to originate from the smooth endoplasmic reticulum (SER). A fusion occurs between the vacuole and a primary lysosome, resulting in the formation of a different type of lysosome known as a cytolysosome (Liang et al., 2007).

The destiny of the substances contained within the autophagic vacuoles, which could include the cell's own mitochondria, ribosomes, endoplasmic reticulum, and other components, is identical to that of heterophagic vacuoles. This process ultimately leads to the creation of residual bodies. Lipofuscin pigment, a brownish material, accumulates in the autophagic vacuoles of numerous cells, and its quantity rises as individuals age. Furthermore, lysosomes serve as an intracellular digestive system, capable of engulfing and decomposing most surplus molecules generated by cells. When a particular lysosomal enzyme is missing, its usual substance builds up inside the lysosome. Excessive build-up of material in lysosomes significantly impairs their function and is the underlying cause of various lysosomal storage disorders, such as Tay-Sachs and Gaucher's diseases. The multivesicular body is an alternative type of lysosome, characterized by a vacuolar structure enclosed by a membrane. It has a diameter of 0.5 to 0.8 μm and contains multiple small, transparent vesicles. The origin, function, and precise relationship of this lysosome to other lysosomes are unclear (Ma et al., 2002).

1.2.6. Peroxisomes

Peroxisomes, also known as microbodies, are a distinct category of organelles that are enclosed by a membrane (Ma et al., 1998). Typically, larger than lysosomes, vacuoles exhibit diverse internal structures that can be either crystalline or dense. The term "nucleoids" refers to the crystalline structures. Peroxisomes are devoid of acid hydrolases, but they do possess up to 40 other enzymes. Peroxisomes house enzymes such as amino acid oxidase and hydroxy acid oxidase, which produce a significant quantity of hydrogen peroxide (H_2O_2). When present in excessive amounts, hydrogen peroxide can be fatal to cells (Manuyakorn, 2014). Peroxisomes also possess a substantial quantity of the enzyme catalase, which can constitute up to 40% of the overall peroxisomal enzyme content. The surplus hydrogen peroxide generated by this cellular structure is transformed into oxygen and water through the action of catalase and other peroxidases. Peroxisomes play a crucial role in the process of oxidizing various substances, specifically very long-chain fatty acids, through the action of fatty acid β-oxidation enzymes. Peroxisomal oxidases also serve to counteract the harmful effects of free radicals, which are natural byproducts of cellular metabolism and can be detrimental to the cell if they build up. The Golgi complex does not seem to be involved in the formation of peroxisomes. Peroxisomes are believed to originate from the enlargement and division of pre-existing peroxisomes, as well as the importation of their contents (such as proteins, phospholipids, and membrane lipids) from the cytosol. Peroxisomes are highly prevalent in cells that are metabolically active, such as hepatocytes (liver cells) and proximal tubular cells in the kidney (McBrien and Menzies-Gow, 2017).

1.2.7. Mitochondria

Mitochondria are organelles enclosed by membranes that have a crucial function in generating the energy necessary for cells. These entities can be observed in living cells using phase contrast microscopy and can alter their shape while moving slowly within the cytosol. Appropriately fixed tissues can be stained to reveal the presence of mitochondria, which are observed as rod-shaped or filamentous structures. Typically, they are not observable in regular tissue samples due to the lipid solvents employed in tissue preparation. Mitochondria exhibit diverse shapes and sizes at the ultrastructural level, yet they are consistently surrounded by two membranes, both of which possess the characteristic trilaminar substructure. Nevertheless, there are significant differences in the chemical composition and physiological properties between the inner and outer mitochondrial membranes. The outer mitochondrial membrane is a uniform and unbroken structure that fully surrounds the organelle. Porins, which are specialized transmembrane transport proteins, enable the passage of specific metabolic substrates, by increasing permeability (McMillan et al., 2005).

The inner mitochondrial membrane is positioned parallel to the outer membrane and is characterized by multiple folds called cristae, which protrude into the interior of the mitochondrion. Cristae significantly enhances the surface area of the inner mitochondrial membrane and can have either a shelf-like or tubular structure; the tubular shape is predominantly observed in cells that participate in steroid synthesis. The inner mitochondrial membrane is adorned with club-shaped structures known as elementary particles. Each component is comprised of a spherical head and a slender stalk. The inner mitochondrial membrane serves as the location for numerous enzymatic reactions. The inner mitochondrial membrane houses enzymes involved in the electron transport chain, such as NADH dehydrogenase, succinate dehydrogenase, ubiquinone-cytochrome c oxidoreductase, and cytochrome oxidase. It also contains ATP synthase, which is restricted to elementary particles, and the ATP-ADP translocator. The ATP-ADP translocator transports ADP from outside the mitochondrial matrix into the matrix, while simultaneously exporting ATP out of the mitochondrial matrix. The intermembrane space, which is the narrow gap between the inner and outer membranes, is connected to the intracristal space found within each crista (Melzer et al., 2017). The intermembrane space is abundant in hydrogen ions.

The inner mitochondrial membrane encloses the intercristal space, which contains a denser substance known as the mitochondrial matrix (**Figure 1.6**). The enzymes involved in the tricarboxylic acid cycle (TAC), fatty acid β-oxidation, amino acid oxidation, carbamoyl phosphate synthetase I, ornithine transcarbamoylase, and pyruvate dehydrogenase are located in the mitochondrial matrix (Michalik et al., 2018). Substrates that undergo metabolism in the matrix generate acetyl CoA, which is then oxidized by the tricarboxylic acid cycle to form carbon dioxide. Nicotinamide adenine dinucleotide (NADH) and flavin adenine dinucleotide (FADH2) capture the energy produced from this oxidation process. When these nucleotides undergo oxidation, they generate hydrogen ions and electrons. Electrons are conveyed through the electron transport chain, while hydrogen ions migrate into the intermembrane space. Hydrogen ions subsequently move from the space within the membrane, passing through transmembrane hydrogen ion pores, and entering the matrix. ATP synthase catalyzes the conversion of adenosine diphosphate (ADP) to adenosine triphosphate (ATP) within the matrix (Miller et al., 2006).

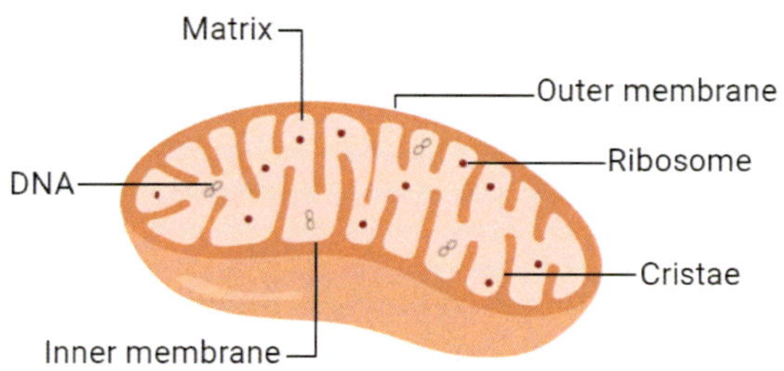

Figure 1.6. *Structure of a mitochondrion.*

Source: https://1.bp.blogspot.com/WDGLJaUbXlc/X4mTNl9KeTI/AAAAAAAAAMk/pWHeJBRpZC4Azk04nV1__ep4mlSvIDkpACLcBGAsYHQ/s720/structure%2Band%2Bfunction%2Bof%2Bmitochonria.PNG.

Mitochondria are unique among cellular structures because they have their own DNA and can self-replicate. Mitochondrial DNA is distinct from nuclear DNA due to its reduced molecular weight and unique structure, which consists of circular arrangements of varying thickness. Mitochondrial DNA makes up less than 1% of the cell's total DNA content. The human mitochondrial genome consists of 16,569 nucleotides (Muniz et al., 2012). These nucleotides represent 13 protein subunits that play a role in electron transport and oxidative phosphorylation. Consequently, mitochondria are required to import most of their proteins from the cytosol. The mitochondrial matrix also contains small particles of ribonucleoprotein that are 12 nm in diameter and are similar in structure and function to cytoplasmic ribosomes. Mitochondria have been found to contain both messenger RNA and transfer RNA (Ngo et al., 2006). The mitochondrial matrix contains scattered matrix granules, which have a diameter ranging from 30 to 50 nm. These granules contain calcium and magnesium ions and are believed to control the internal ionic composition of the mitochondrion. Therefore, mitochondria play a role in oxidative phosphorylation, a process that generates ATP through the transfer of electrons to oxygen. Additionally, mitochondria are involved in fatty acid oxidation, amino acid oxidation, and the production of acetyl coenzyme A (CoA). Adenosine triphosphate (ATP) serves as the main reservoir of energy for cellular processes (Ozier et al., 2011).

1.2.8. Annulate Lamellae

The annulate lamellae are organelles composed of parallel cisternae organized in stacks, with a membranous structure. The cisternae display multiple small pores at regular intervals, which seem to be sealed by thin, electron-dense diaphragms. Due to the presence of pores, they display a morphological resemblance to the nuclear envelope. The cisternae are evenly distributed throughout the stack, and the pores in consecutive cisternae may be arranged in a straight line. Annulate lamellae frequently reside near the nucleus and may be connected to components of the Golgi endoplasmic reticulum. They have been observed in germ cells, various somatic cells, and tumor cells, although they are relatively infrequent. The functional importance of the annulate lamellae remains uncertain (Pepe et al., 2005).

1.2.9. Centrioles

When observed using a light microscope, centrioles can be seen as small rods or granules that are typically found near the nucleus in a specific area of the cytoplasm known as the centrosome. Centrioles are positioned in certain cells between the nucleus and the free surface of the cell, at a specific distance from the nucleus (Prakash, 2013). The diplosome is typically composed of two centrioles found in the nondividing cell. As observed in electron micrographs, the two centrioles comprising the diplosome are oriented at a right angle to each other. Each centriole is composed of a wall comprising nine subunits, with each subunit consisting of three fused microtubules. These subunits are commonly known as triplets.

The nine sets of triplets are positioned in the centriolar wall in a manner that gives the appearance of a pinwheel when observed from a cross-sectional view. The microtubules within each triplet are designated as A, B, and C microtubules, with the A microtubule being the innermost, the B microtubule being the central tubule, and the C microtubule being the most peripheral tubule. The central region of the centriole is clear and contains a slender filament that coils in a spiral shape right next to the inner layer of the centriolar wall (Raeburn and Webber, 1994). Cells with multiple nuclei possess multiple centrioles. Centrioles are organelles that undergo self-replication immediately prior to cell division. A novel centriole, known as a procentriole, emerges perpendicular to each of the existing centrioles. At first, the wall of the procentriole is composed of a circular structure made of shapeless material that lacks microtubules. As the procentriole extends through the addition of material at its far end, microtubules form in the wall, and the newly formed structure takes on the same shape as the original centriole. Following duplication, both the parent centriole and the newly formed daughter centriole promptly move to opposite ends of the cell (Redhu et al., 2013). Once there, they play a crucial role in the formation of the mitotic spindle. The centriolar satellites, which are compact and small, are connected to the centrioles and play a crucial role in initiating the growth and formation of microtubules during the development of the mitotic spindle. Centrioles in certain cells migrate towards the surface and form basal bodies, which give rise to cilia or flagella. These structures also contain microtubules. During ciliogenesis, dense spherical bodies, known as procentriole organizers emerge in the cytoplasm, and multiple procentrioles are formed around each of them (Rolfe et al., 1992). Several recently formed centrioles move to locations directly below the cell membrane and align themselves perpendicular to it. The centriolar triplets' two innermost microtubules (A and B) initiate a swift tubulin polymerization process and act as blueprints for the formation of the axoneme's microtubules. The elongation of the cilium typically reaches full completion within a time frame of 60 minutes (Saito et al., 2004).

1.3. Cytoskeleton

The cytoskeleton provides structural reinforcement to the cytoplasm and is composed of microfilaments, intermediate filaments, microtubules, and a microtrabecular lattice. The interaction between the cytoskeleton and the plasmalemma is crucial for various cellular processes, including cell movement, intracellular transport, endocytosis, focal mobility of the plasmalemma, maintenance of cell shape, stabilization of cell junctions, and spatial orientation of enzymes and other molecules in the cytosol (Sakota et al., 2014).

1.3.1. Microfilaments

Cytoplasmic filaments exhibit contractility, a characteristic observed in nearly all cells to varying extents. The development of filaments is most optimal in muscle cells, specifically in the presence of the proteins, actin and myosin II. These proteins form two distinct types of filaments, which play a crucial role in the contraction of muscle cells. Microfilaments typically have a diameter of 7 nm and are commonly found directly beneath the plasmalemma (Salter et al., 2017). Actin exhibits identical dimensions to microfilaments and has been chemically detected within microfilaments. Actin is a crucial constituent of the cytoskeleton and exists in two molecular forms: G-actin, which is composed of spherical actin monomers, and F-actin, the polymerized form that consists of two identical strands coiled around each other in a helical manner. Actin filaments can be arranged into parallel bundles or dispersed randomly to create a complex, interconnected network. Actin-binding proteins, like filamin, connect actin filaments together in specific circumstances, creating a rigid and supportive structure for the plasmalemma. Actin can also form connections with transmembrane proteins in specific areas of the cell membrane called junctional complexes, thereby enhancing the cytoskeleton of individual cells. Several actin-binding proteins exist that interact with either G-actin monomers or F-actin filaments and impact the distribution and function of actin in the cytoplasm. Actin filaments participate in various cellular processes, including cell locomotion, ruffling of the cell membrane, invagination of the plasmalemma during endocytosis, and formation of the contraction ring during cell division. Here, a slender layer of actin filaments positioned along the cytoplasmic side of the cell membrane may engage with myosin (Sanz et al., 1997). Myosin is a protein that uses ATP to generate force and is activated by actin. It can exist in multiple forms as individual molecules. Myosins are a heterogeneous protein family comprising 18 distinct subtypes, with myosin II of muscle being the most extensively studied. Myosin V is found in the majority of cells and binds to actin filaments to produce motion of intracellular vesicles and organelles (Sapienza et al., 1991).

1.3.2. Intermediate Filaments

The intermediate filaments with a larger diameter of 9 to 12 nm form a varied group of filaments, which can exist as individual strands or loose bundles. Intermediate filaments frequently connect to the inner surface of the plasmalemma at cell junctions and play a role in the cell's cytoskeleton, offering structural support. Microfilaments and intermediate filaments can coexist within a single cell. Using immunocytochemical techniques, researchers have been able to identify five distinct types of intermediate filaments, despite their similar structural characteristics (Sapudom et al., 2015). The majority of cells consist of a singular type, although on rare occasions, a cell type may be of two types. Epithelial cells contain keratin filaments which organize into bundles that terminate in cellular attachments. This arrangement facilitates the connection of individual cells into cohesive structural units. They are most prevalent in the stratified squamous epithelia, particularly in the skin. Vimentin filaments are present in fibroblasts and other cells that originate from mesenchyme. Desmin filaments are located in skeletal, cardiac, and smooth muscle cells and facilitate the mechanical integration of the contractile proteins, actin, and myosin. Neurofilaments are exclusively found in nerve cell bodies and their processes, often forming bundles. Glial filaments are exclusively found in the glial cells of the central nervous system and are composed of glial fibrillary acidic protein. Glial filaments and neurofilaments offer structural support within their specific cell types. Familiarity with this limited distribution is frequently beneficial for evaluating malignant tumors to ascertain their point of origin (Schaafsma et al., 2004).

1.3.3. Microtubules

Microtubules are elongated cylindrical structures that are either straight or slightly curved. They have a uniform diameter of 21 to 25 nanometers and can reach lengths of several micrometers. The walls of the structure are approximately 6 nm in thickness and are composed of 13 protein filaments arranged in a helical pattern. Each filament has a diameter ranging from 4 to 5 nm. The central zone is electron-lucent, giving the structure the appearance of being hollow. Microtubules consist mainly of the protein tubulin, which exists in alpha and beta forms (Schaafsma et al., 2007). The quantity of microtubules in the cytoplasm differs among different cell types and can also vary over time within the same cell. Microtubules exhibit dynamic behavior, undergoing rapid assembly or disassembly in response to cellular activity. Microtubules maintain a state of dynamic equilibrium with a substantial supply of soluble tubulin in the cytoplasm. After their formation, microtubules undergo elongation by adding subunits at one end and typically depolymerize at the opposite end, thus recycling subunits back into the cytoplasm. Microtubule-associated proteins (MAPs), which are high-molecular-weight proteins, have been found in small amounts and are believed to be associated with the thin, sideways filamentous extensions of the microtubules. There are four distinct categories of microtubule-associated proteins (MAPs) that have been recognized: kinesin, dynein, dynamin, and axonemal dynein. Kinesin connects transport vesicles to microtubules and, through a cyclic interaction, propels the vesicle towards the growing end of the microtubule. Dynein is responsible for connecting transport vesicles to microtubules, specifically those that are intended to move towards the end of the microtubule where depolymerization takes place (Scharenberg et al., 2014).

This allows for bidirectional movement within a cell. Dynamin connects adjacent microtubules to form bundles, while axonemal dynein drives the movement of microtubules within cilia and flagella, causing them to beat. Microtubules are typically limited in resting cells but abundant in dividing cells, where they form the mitotic spindle. Following cell division, most microtubules disappear. Microtubules are significant elements of centrioles, cilia, and flagella in interphase cells, and they also play a role in the cytoskeleton of certain cells. Microtubules within platelets serve as rigid structures that contribute to the maintenance of their shape. Microtubules play a crucial role in the intracellular transport of materials within nerve cells (Serban et al., 2016). Nondividing cells undergo a temporary increase in the quantity of microtubules during cell movement and differentiation, which leads to changes in cell shape. There is a suggestion that a three-dimensional molecular framework, known as a microtrabecular lattice, exists in the cytoplasmic matrix. This lattice connects the cell organelles and cytoskeleton, allowing them to work together as a coordinated functional unit during cell movement and other activities (Shaifta et al., 2018).

1.3.4. Cytoplasmic Inclusions

Inclusions are inanimate components present in the cytoplasm and encompass a wide range of substances, including pigment granules, glycogen, lipid droplets, and crystals. Non-essential to the cell's life or functioning, they are metabolic byproducts, storage materials, or foreign substances absorbed from the environment (Singh et al., 2016).

1.3.5. Pigment Granules

Human cells contain naturally occurring pigments such as melanin, hemosiderin, and lipofuscin, each possessing its own distinct color. Melanin is present in melanosomes, which are granules enclosed by a membrane. These granules are produced and located in melanocytes and occasionally deposited in other specific cells. They are particularly noticeable at the junction between the skin's dermis and epidermis, playing a role in determining skin color. Melanin is present in the pigment epithelium of the retina and iris, as well as in specific cells of the brain. Hemosiderin is a chromatic substance with a golden-brown hue that originates from the degradation of hemoglobin found in erythrocytes. The liver, bone marrow, and spleen typically house phagocytic cells that possess this particular pigment. Lipofuscin is present in numerous cells throughout the body, especially in individuals of advanced age. Lipofuscin, also known as the "wear and tear" pigment, is a light brown substance that accumulates with age. It is the final result of lysosomal activity (Sukkar et al., 2004). Lipofuscin pigment serves as a marker for oxidative stress and is composed of phospholipids bound to proteins. Neurons, hepatocytes, and skeletal muscle cells typically possess this particular pigment.

1.3.6. Glycogen

Glycogen is a complex carbohydrate made up of many glucose molecules and serves as a storage form of glucose. The glucose units are connected by α1, 4 glycosidic bonds. Glycogen synthesis is facilitated by the enzyme glycogen synthase, while glycogen breakdown into glucose is facilitated by the enzyme glycogen phosphorylase. Glycogen is not visible in typical tissue preparations unless it is specifically stained. Hepatocytes, which are liver cells and skeletal muscle cells, possess the most substantial glycogen reserves among all the cells in the body. Although the liver has the highest glycogen content per gram of tissue, the total amount of glycogen stored in skeletal muscle is greater (Tanaka et al., 1995). Glycogen can be observed at the ultrastructural level in two forms: beta particles or glycosomes, which are small, dense particles measuring 15 to 45 nm in diameter and have an irregular shape, or alpha particles, which are larger with a diameter of 90 to 95 nm and are composed of several smaller beta particles of glycogen arranged in rosette-like structures.

1.3.7. Lipid

Adipocytes are the primary reservoirs for lipid storage, although numerous other cell types also store lipid droplets of different sizes. The cell synthesizes lipids that gather in cytoplasmic droplets without a surrounding membrane. Intracellular functions of lipids as energy **source** and provides short-chain carbon molecules for cellular synthesis. When preparing routine tissue sections, lipid is typically removed, and areas where lipid is stored are visible as empty spaces called vacuoles (Tobler et al., 1992). Preserved lipid droplets in electron micrographs exhibit a uniform spherical shape with varying densities.

1.3.8. Crystals

Crystalline inclusions are commonly found in various types of cells and can exist either freely in the cytoplasm or enclosed within secretory granules, mitochondria, endoplasmic reticulum, the Golgi complex, or even the nucleus. It is widely believed that the intracellular crystals that have been observed serve as a means of storing protein (Tomasek et al., 2002).

1.4. Nucleus

The nucleus is a vital organelle found in all fully developed "true" cells. Mature erythrocytes and blood platelets are the only cytoplasmic structures that lack nuclei. It is important to note that these structures should not be considered genuine cells. Typically, cells contain only one nucleus, but certain types of cells, like the parietal cells in the stomach, cardiac muscle cells, and liver cells, may have two nuclei. Some types of cells, like osteoclasts in bone, megakaryocytes in marrow, and skeletal muscle cells, can possess multiple nuclei. The nucleus can have different shapes, such as spherical, ovoid, or elongated, which correspond to the shape of the cell. Alternatively, it may be lobulated, as seen in the granular leukocytes found in the blood. The nucleus houses all the requisite information to commence and regulate the differentiation, maturation, and metabolic functions of every cell. The nucleus that does not undergo cell division is surrounded by a nuclear envelope and contains chromatin material and one or two nucleoli. These are held in suspension within a nuclear ground substance known as the karyolymph or nuclear matrix (Walford and Doherty, 2014).

1.4.1. Chromatin and Chromosomes

The genetic information is encoded within the DNA molecules that comprise the chromosomes. Every chromosome contains a solitary elongated DNA molecule composed of two linear polymers of nucleotide subunits. Each subunit is comprised of a phosphate group, a pentose sugar (deoxyribose), and four organic bases (adenosine, cytosine, guanine, thymidine). The bases extend and attach to complementary bases of the neighboring polymer. The two polynucleotide chains combine and create the antiparallel double helix structure of the DNA molecule. The genetic information contained within DNA molecules is encoded by the specific sequence of bases. A gene is a hereditary unit that contains a sequence of bases required for the production of a protein or nucleic acid. The human genome is believed to comprise approximately 20,000 to 25,000 genes. During interphase, when the cell's nucleus is not dividing, the chromosomes are mostly relaxed and spread out. However, certain parts of the chromosomes stay tightly packed, which makes them appear darker and visible under a light microscope. These condensed regions are known as chromatin. Chromatin is formed by a diverse array of proteins that are linked to nuclear DNA. The proteins can be classified into two broad categories: histones and nonhistone proteins (Webb, 2003). The latter category encompasses structural proteins, regulatory proteins, and the enzymes essential for nuclear function, such as DNA and RNA polymerases. Histones are highly prevalent proteins found in the nucleus that make up the central part of a DNA-protein complex known as a nucleosome. The nucleosome serves as the fundamental component of the chromatin fiber.

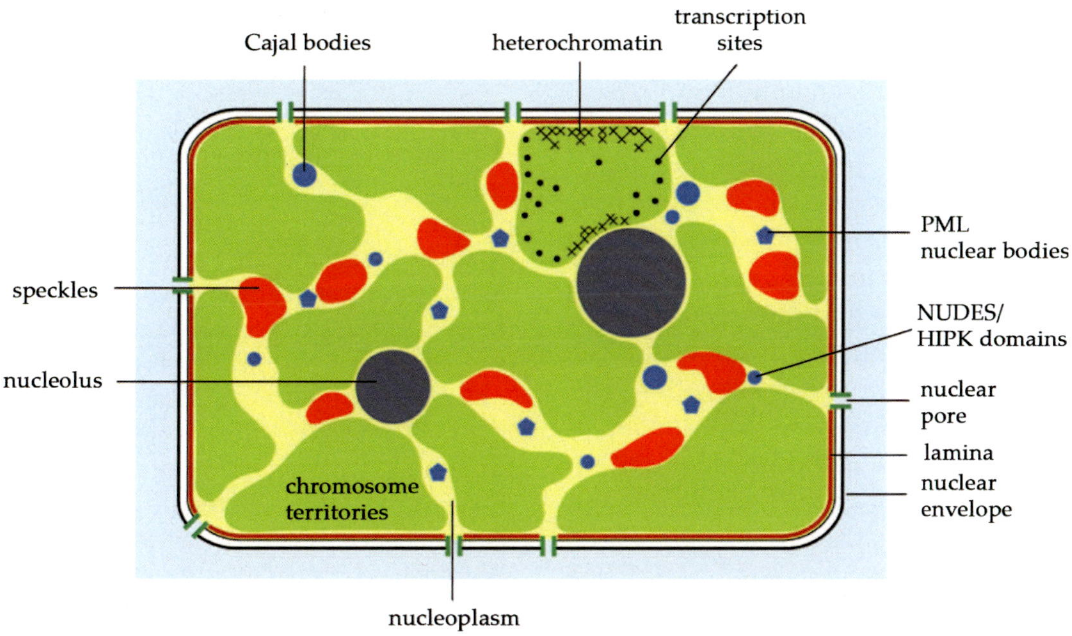

Figure 1.7. *Diagrammatic representation of nuclear structures.*

Source: https://www.researchgate.net/profile/CaroleBassett/publication/254218758/figure/fig2/AS:298096299921411@1448083104580/Nuclear-architecture-Diagrammatic-representation-of-nuclear-structures-Major-nuclear.png.

The nucleosome exhibits a linear arrangement of spherical particles and serves as the fundamental architectural component of chromatin. Every fiber is composed of a pair of intertwined DNA strands coiled around a central structure made of histones. Karyosomes refer to the individual masses of chromatin. While not completely consistent, the chromatin masses generally exhibit distinct sizes, patterns, and quantities that are specific to each cell type. The karyosomes, when combined, make up the heterochromatin of the nucleus. They are coiled sections of the chromosomes

(Figure 1.7). Heterochromatin is thought to be associated with histones and is considered to be transcriptionally inactive. Histones are basic proteins that consist mainly of basic amino acids. The chromatin region that is spread out stains faintly and forms euchromatin, which is responsible for actively regulating the metabolic processes of the cell. During cell division, the differentiation between heterochromatin and euchromatin is no longer apparent as all the chromatin condenses and becomes metabolically inactive (Weitoft et al., 2014).

Chromosomes are constant structures within the cell. They are present throughout all stages of the cell cycle. However, their appearance can vary depending on the physiological condition of the cell. During interphase, the chromosomes appear as loosely organized and thread-like. It is only during cell division that they take on the form of distinct, solid, rod-shaped structures. The most convenient way to analyze and study chromosomes is by examining dividing cells that have been stopped in metaphase. Alkaloids, such as the Vinca drugs and colchicine, disrupt the formation of spindles and allow for the buildup of metaphase chromosomes within cells, facilitating their examination. The number of chromosomes is typically consistent within a species but can vary significantly between different species (Wenstrup et al., 2004). The chromosome number in humans is 46. Germ cells, which include ova and sperm, possess half the number of chromosomes, and are referred to as haploid. Somatic cells contain two sets of chromosomes, one inherited from each parent. Homologous chromosomes are referred to as chromosomes that are similar in the male and female sets. In numerous higher animals with diploid set of chromosomes, a specific pair of sex chromosomes is dedicated to and actively involved in the process of determining an individual's sex; all remaining chromosomes are referred to as autosomes. Humans have a total of 44 autosomes and a pair of sex chromosomes (White, 2015). The sex chromosomes are homologous (XX) in females and heterologous (XY) in males. Homologous chromosomes can be identified during metaphase and are organized into groups that represent the karyotype of a particular species. Chromosomes can frequently be distinguished by the length of their arms and the position of the centromere. A chromosome is considered metacentric when its centromere is located in the middle, and its arms (telomeres) are of equal length. A chromosome is classified as acrocentric if its centromere is located near one end, and as submetacentric if the centromere is positioned between the midpoint and the end (Wong et al., 2007).

1.4.2. Nuclear Envelope

The nuclear envelope consists of two concentric unit membranes, each measuring 7.5 nm in thickness, with a perinuclear space between them that has a width ranging from 40 to 70 nm. The inner membrane is devoid of ribosomes and has a smooth surface, while the outer membrane is connected to the endoplasmic reticulum and frequently has multiple ribosomes on its cytoplasmic side. Nuclear pores, small octagonal openings, are formed when the inner and outer membranes of the envelope around the nucleus connect at irregular intervals. The diameter of the pores is approximately 10 nm, and they are sealed by a nuclear pore complex comprising two rings, one of which is oriented towards the cytoplasm. There are eight radial spokes that stretch from the rings towards a central granule. The quantity and arrangement of nuclear pores are contingent upon the specific cell type and its level of activity. The nuclear envelope facilitates the organization of chromatin and regulates the bidirectional movement of ions and molecules between the nucleus and cytoplasm. Molecules with a diameter of less than 10 nm can pass through the nuclear pore complex through passive diffusion. On the other hand, larger molecules, such as newly synthesized proteins and exiting ribonucleoproteins, require an energy-dependent transport mechanism. The prevailing belief is that a sequence of amino acids, known as a signal sequence, guides them to the nuclear envelope. Once the signal sequence binds to a receptor in the nuclear pore complex, the nuclear pore opens, resembling the action of an iris diaphragm in a camera, allowing larger molecules to pass through. The nuclear lamina is composed of three polypeptides and is a delicate network of filaments known as Lamins. It is located on the inner side of the nuclear membrane. The Lamins exhibit structural similarity to intermediate filaments and are categorized into types A, B, and C based on their positional and chemical characteristics. Type B Lamins are located closer to the outer surface of the nuclear lamina and they interact with specific integral proteins of the inner nuclear membrane (Wright et al., 2013). Lamins of types A and C are positioned on the inner surface of the nuclear lamina and connect the membrane-bound Lamin B to chromatin (Xu et al., 2017). The three Lamins are believed to play a role in the creation and upkeep of the nuclear envelope in cells during interphase. Additionally, they can assist in preserving the structure of the nucleus.

1.4.3. Nucleolus

The nucleolus is a compact and clearly defined structure, measuring 1 to 3 μm in diameter, found within the nucleus. Nucleoli are locations where the process of ribosomal RNA (rRNA) synthesis takes place. Due to their presence on five distinct chromosomes, it is possible for a single cell to have multiple nucleoli (Yamauchi et al., 2008). Typically, there are only one or two prominent nucleoli present due to the tendency of nucleolus-organizing regions to come together, causing the RNA produced in these regions to form larger clusters. Electron micrographs reveal that nucleoli are located within the nucleus and are not enclosed by a membrane. The image displays two distinct areas, each linked to a specific type of ribonucleoprotein. The main area, known as the pars granulosa (nucleolonema), comprises a network of compact granules containing RNA that measure 13 to 15 nm in diameter (Zagai et al., 2009). The second region, known as the pars fibrosa, is typically located in the center and is composed of compact clusters of filaments measuring 5 nm in diameter (Zhang et al., 2019). Deoxyribonucleoprotein is also found in the nucleolus and is present in chromatin filaments that encircle or protrude into the nucleolus. The chromatin that forms the nucleolus-associated chromatin is responsible for providing the DNA template for the synthesis of rRNA. Clusters of DNA segments near the tips of chromosomes 13, 14, 15, 21, and 22 in humans are where rRNA genes are found. RNA polymerase I facilitates the synthesis of ribosomal RNA. In other parts of the nucleus, RNA polymerase II facilitates the synthesis of messenger RNA (mRNA), while RNA polymerase III facilitates the synthesis of transfer RNA (tRNA). Ribosomal gene transcription takes place in the fibrillar region of the nucleolus. After transcription, the ribosomal RNAs (rRNAs) undergo processing and are subsequently assembled in the pars granulosa. After the small ribosomal subunit is added, ribosomes are transported to the cytoplasm via nuclear pores. Nucleoli are exclusively present in interphase nuclei and are particularly conspicuous in cells that are actively engaged in protein synthesis. They disperse during cell division but reassemble at the nucleolus-organizing regions during the reformation of the daughter nuclei after cell division (Zuyderduyn et al., 2008).

A Closer Look

Microtubules:

Microtubules are dynamic, cylindrical structures composed of tubulin protein subunits, playing crucial roles in various cellular processes. As one of the three primary components of the cytoskeleton—alongside microfilaments and intermediate filaments—microtubules provide structural support, facilitate intracellular transport, and are essential for cell division and motility.

Structure of Microtubules

Microtubules are typically about 25 nanometers in diameter and can vary in length from micrometers to several centimeters, depending on their cellular context. They are formed by the polymerization of α- and β-tubulin dimers, which stack together in a head-to-tail fashion to create protofilaments. Typically, 13 protofilaments align in a circular arrangement to form a hollow tube. The structure is not static; microtubules undergo constant growth and shrinkage in a process known as dynamic instability, where they rapidly switch between polymerization and depolymerization.

The dynamic nature of microtubules is crucial for their functions. GTP (guanosine triphosphate) binds to β-tubulin, promoting the stabilization of the microtubule. When GTP is hydrolyzed to GDP, the affinity of tubulin dimers for one another decreases, leading to disassembly. This dynamic behavior allows cells to respond rapidly to changing conditions, such as during mitosis when microtubules reorganize to form the mitotic spindle.

Functions of Microtubules

- **Cell Shape and Structural Support**: Microtubules contribute significantly to the cell's mechanical strength and shape. They form a network that maintains cellular integrity, providing a scaffold that resists compression and bending forces.
- **Intracellular Transport**: Microtubules serve as tracks for the movement of organelles and vesicles within cells. Motor proteins, such as kinesins and dyneins, travel along microtubules, carrying cellular cargo. Kinesins typically move towards the plus end (the growing end), while dyneins transport materials toward the minus end (the shrinking end). This directional transport is vital for cellular organization, particularly in neurons, where long distances must be traversed.
- **Cell Division**: During mitosis, microtubules play a critical role in forming the mitotic spindle, which segregates chromosomes into daughter cells. Spindle fibers, composed of microtubules, attach to the kinetochores of chromosomes and pull them apart during anaphase. Proper microtubule function during this process is essential to ensure that each daughter cell receives the correct number of chromosomes, and errors can lead to aneuploidy.

- **Cell Motility**: Microtubules are integral to the structure and function of cilia and flagella, organelles that enable cell movement. In cilia, microtubules are arranged in a "9+2" configuration—nine doublet microtubules surrounding two central microtubules. The coordinated beating of these structures propels cells through fluid environments, such as sperm cells in reproductive systems or respiratory cells clearing mucus.
- **Cell Signaling**: Microtubules are involved in various signaling pathways, serving as scaffolds for signaling molecules and contributing to signal transduction processes. They can influence the localization of signaling proteins, thereby affecting cellular responses to external stimuli.

Regulation of Microtubule Dynamics

Microtubule dynamics are tightly regulated by various proteins. Stabilizing proteins, such as tau and MAPs (microtubule-associated proteins), promote microtubule stability, while destabilizing proteins, like stathmin, facilitate depolymerization. The balance between these activities is crucial for maintaining proper microtubule organization and function.

Additionally, post-translational modifications of tubulin can affect microtubule properties. For instance, acetylation can stabilize microtubules and is often associated with non-dividing cells, while detyrosination can signal microtubule age and function.

Microtubules in Disease

Dysregulation of microtubule dynamics and function has been implicated in various diseases. In cancer, altered expression of tubulin and microtubule-associated proteins can lead to abnormal cell division and tumor growth. Drugs targeting microtubules, such as paclitaxel (Taxol) and vincristine, are commonly used in cancer therapy, as they disrupt microtubule dynamics and inhibit mitosis.

Neurodegenerative diseases, such as Alzheimer's disease, are also linked to microtubule dysfunction. Abnormal hyperphosphorylation of the tau protein leads to the formation of neurofibrillary tangles, disrupting microtubule stability and contributing to neuronal degeneration.

Microtubules are fundamental components of cellular architecture, with diverse roles that extend beyond structural support. Their ability to rapidly assemble and disassemble allows cells to adapt to various physiological demands, from maintaining shape and facilitating transport to ensuring accurate cell division. Understanding microtubule dynamics and regulation is essential for unraveling the complexities of cellular processes and their implications in health and disease. Continued research into microtubules will enhance our knowledge of their functions and potential therapeutic targets for diseases associated with microtubule dysfunction.

Summary

- Cells are the fundamental units of life, serving as the basic building blocks for all living organisms. They can be broadly categorized into two types: prokaryotic and eukaryotic cells. Prokaryotic cells, which include bacteria and archaea, lack a nucleus and membrane-bound organelles, making them generally simpler in structure. In contrast, eukaryotic cells, found in animals, plants, fungi, and protists, possess a defined nucleus and various organelles, allowing for more complex functions and higher levels of organization.
- The organization of eukaryotic cells is characterized by compartmentalization, where different cellular processes occur in specialized organelles. Key organelles include the nucleus (which houses genetic material), mitochondria (the energy producers), endoplasmic reticulum (involved in protein and lipid synthesis), and Golgi apparatus (which modifies and packages proteins). Plant cells also contain chloroplasts for photosynthesis and a rigid cell wall for structural support. This compartmentalization allows cells to maintain distinct environments and efficiently carry out various biochemical reactions.
- Additionally, the structure of cells is closely linked to their functions. For instance, muscle cells have a high density of mitochondria to meet their energy demands, while neurons have elongated structures to facilitate communication. The cell membrane, composed of a lipid bilayer with embedded proteins, regulates the movement of substances in and out of the cell, maintaining homeostasis. Overall, the organization and structure of cells are crucial for their diverse functions and the overall functionality of living organisms.

References

1. Akhtar F, Bokhari SRA. StatPearls [Internet]. StatPearls Publishing; Treasure Island (FL): Apr 30, 2024. Apoptosis.
2. Ballabio A. The awesome lysosome. EMBO Mol Med. 2016 Feb 01;8(2):73-6.
3. Bianconi E, Piovesan A, Facchin F, Beraudi A, Casadei R, Frabetti F, Vitale L, Pelleri MC, Tassani S, Piva F, Perez-Amodio S, Strippoli P, Canaider S. An estimation of the number of cells in the human body. Ann Hum Biol. 2013 Nov-Dec;40(6):463-71.
4. Costello LC, Franklin RB, Reynolds MA. The Important Role and Implications of Citrate in the Composition, Structure, and Function of Oral/Periodontal/Craniofacial Tissues. Madridge J Dent Oral Surg. 2018;3(1):85-90.
5. Fletcher DA, Mullins RD. Cell mechanics and the cytoskeleton. Nature. 2010 Jan 28;463(7280):485-92.
6. Hatano A, Chiba H, Moesa HA, Taniguchi T, Nagaie S, Yamanegi K, Takai-Igarashi T, Tanaka H, Fujibuchi W. CELLPEDIA: a repository for human cell information for cell studies and differentiation analyses. Database (Oxford). 2011;2011:bar046.
7. Jäkel S, Dimou L. Glial Cells and Their Function in the Adult Brain: A Journey through the History of Their Ablation. Front Cell Neurosci. 2017;11:24.
8. Lee DC, Chen JH, Hsu TY, Chang LH, Chang H, Chi YH, Chiu IM. Neural stem cells promote nerve regeneration through IL12-induced Schwann cell differentiation. Mol Cell Neurosci. 2017 Mar;79:1-

9. Lombardi ML, Lammerding J. Altered mechanical properties of the nucleus in disease. Methods Cell Biol. 2010;98:121-41.
10. Luby-Phelps K. The physical chemistry of cytoplasm and its influence on cell function: an update. Mol Biol Cell. 2013 Sep;24(17):2593-6.
11. Lui JC, Baron J. Mechanisms limiting body growth in mammals. Endocr Rev. 2011 Jun;32(3):422-40.
12. Mattes B, Scholpp S. Emerging role of contact-mediated cell communication in tissue development and diseases. Histochem Cell Biol. 2018 Nov;150(5):431-442.
13. Ozcan L, Tabas I. Role of endoplasmic reticulum stress in metabolic disease and other disorders. Annu Rev Med. 2012;63:317-28.
14. Schwarz DS, Blower MD. The endoplasmic reticulum: structure, function and response to cellular signaling. Cell Mol Life Sci. 2016 Jan;73(1):79-94.
15. Slaoui M, Bauchet AL, Fiette L. Tissue Sampling and Processing for Histopathology Evaluation. Methods Mol Biol. 2017;1641:101-114.
16. von Bartheld CS, Bahney J, Herculano-Houzel S. The search for true numbers of neurons and glial cells in the human brain: A review of 150 years of cell counting. J Comp Neurol. 2016 Dec 15;524(18):3865-3895.
17. Webster M, Witkin KL, Cohen-Fix O. Sizing up the nucleus: nuclear shape, size and nuclear-envelope assembly. J Cell Sci. 2009 May 15;122(Pt 10):1477-86.
18. Wong RS. Apoptosis in cancer: from pathogenesis to treatment. J Exp Clin Cancer Res. 2011 Sep 26;30(1):87.
19. Xu H, Ren D. Lysosomal physiology. Annu Rev Physiol. 2015;77:57-80.
20. Zhu J, Thompson CB. Metabolic regulation of cell growth and proliferation. Nat Rev Mol Cell Biol. 2019 Jul;20(7):436-450.

Chapter

2

EPITHELIUM AND GENERAL CONNECTIVE TISSUES

Contents

Introduction

Epithelial tissues and general connective tissues are fundamental components of the body, serving diverse and essential functions. Epithelial tissues form barriers that protect underlying tissues, facilitate selective transport, and participate in sensation. These tissues line body surfaces, cavities, and glands, exhibiting remarkable structural and functional diversity to suit their respective roles. General connective tissues provide structural support, binding and anchoring organs, and facilitating communication between tissues. They are characterized by a matrix containing various fibers, cells, and ground substances. This matrix composition varies, resulting in the classification of connective tissues into subtypes like loose, dense, and specialized connective tissues, each with unique properties and functions (Almuntashiri et al., 2020). Understanding the structure and function of epithelial and connective tissues is crucial for comprehending organ function and health. This chapter explores the characteristics, roles, and interplay of these tissues in maintaining homeostasis and responding to physiological challenges. Through a comprehensive examination of their features and functions, we aim to elucidate the relationship between epithelial and connective tissues in the human body.

Orientation and Directional Terms

Term	Definition	
Epithelium	A tissue composed of closely packed cells that line the surfaces of organs, cavities, and structures throughout the body, serving functions such as protection, absorption, and secretion.	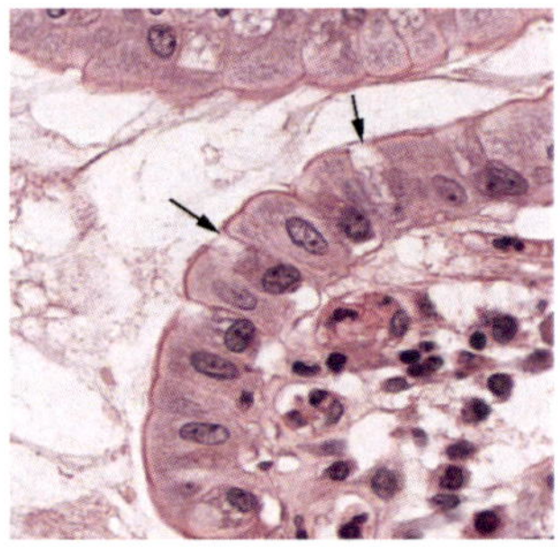
General Connective Tissue	A diverse group of tissues that provide support, binding, and protection to other tissues and organs; includes types like loose connective tissue, dense connective tissue, adipose tissue, and blood.	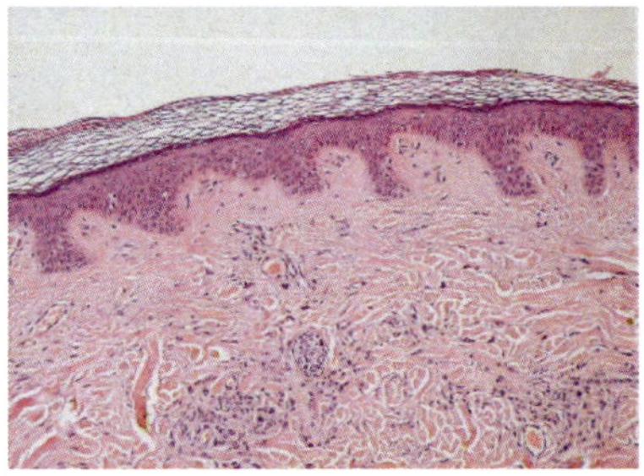
Epithelial Membranes	Thin layers of tissue that cover surfaces, line cavities, and form protective barriers; primarily consist of epithelium and underlying connective tissue, such as mucous membranes and serous membranes.	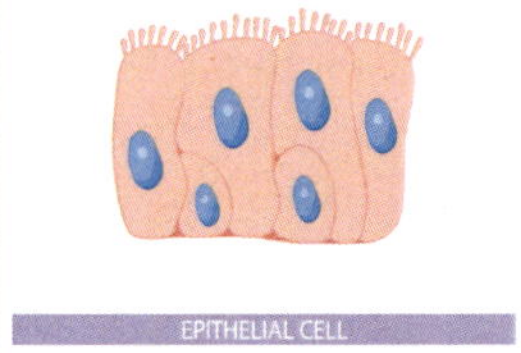
Glandular Epithelium	A specialized type of epithelium that forms the secretory units of glands, responsible for producing and releasing substances such as hormones, enzymes, and sweat.	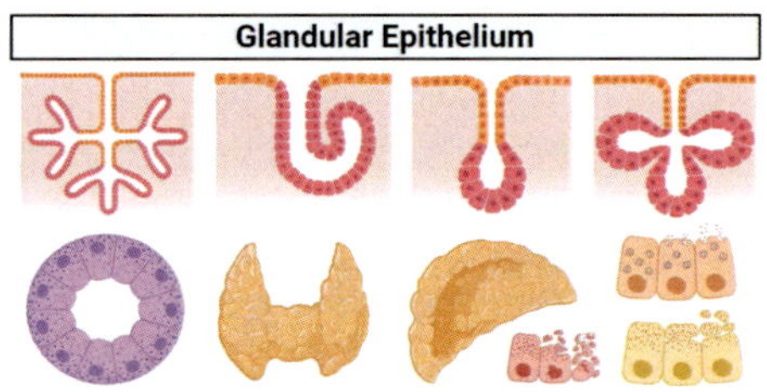
Transitional epithelium	Transitional epithelium is a type of tissue that lines the urinary tract and allows the bladder to expand. It's also known as urothelium.	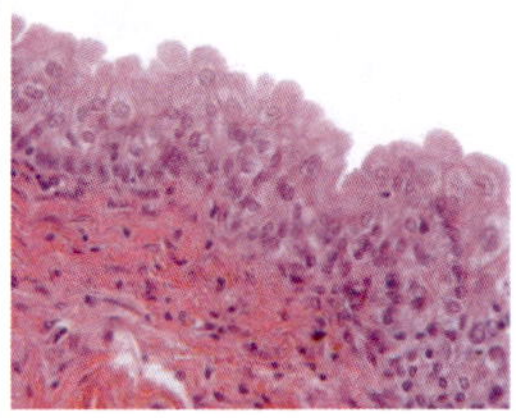

2.1. Epithelium

Epithelium is one of the four fundamental tissues, alongside connective, muscle, and nerve tissue. A fundamental tissue is a group of cells of the same kind that, along with their associated extracellular substances, are specialized to carry out a shared function or functions. Every fundamental tissue is present in varying amounts in all organs. The different types of epithelia are composed of closely packed cells with very little intercellular material between them (Arsalane et al., 2000).

2.1.1. Sheet/Barrier Epithelium

This particular type of epithelium consists of cells that are arranged in sheets or layers, creating barriers that protect the outer surface of the body and line various systems such as the digestive, respiratory, cardiovascular, and urogenital systems, as well as the main body cavities. Therefore, any substances that enter or exit the body must traverse an epithelial barrier. Epithelial cells are tightly interconnected and exhibit strong resistance against forces that attempt to dislodge them. The intercellular space between adjacent epithelial cells is narrow, measuring approximately 20 nm. It contains a small quantity of proteoglycan, which is primarily composed of calcium cations. Integral transmembrane glycoproteins, known as glycoproteins, serve as specialized adhesion molecules that facilitate the close proximity of adjacent epithelial cell membranes. Epithelial cells are situated on a basal lamina, which acts as supporting and anchoring structure. The basal lamina is composed of two layers: the electron-lucid lamina lucida, which is located directly next to the epithelium, and the denser layer called the lamina Densa, which is situated next to the underlying connective tissue. The basal lamina is primarily composed of two main components: laminin, a glycoprotein found mainly in the lamina lucida; and a proteoglycan rich in heparan sulfate, fibronectin, and type IV collagen, which is mainly found in the lamina Densa. These components are primarily produced by the epithelial cells. The connective tissue side is strengthened by a layer of reticular fibers that are embedded in proteoglycan. The basal lamina functions to provide structural support and a substrate for the adhesion of the epithelium above it. The epithelial basement membrane, which is observable under a light microscope, consists of the basal lamina and the reticular lamina, which form the interface with the underlying connective tissue. The basement membrane is further reinforced by anchoring fibers made of type VII collagen. These fibers extend from the basal lamina and form loops around collagen fibers (type I) in the underlying connective tissue. They ultimately end in anchoring plaques. Filamin, a glycoprotein, connects the basal lamina to elastic fibers in the connective tissue beneath it. The epithelium is generally lacking in blood vessels and relies on the diffusion of substances through the basement membrane for its nourishment, with only a few exceptions. Nevertheless, epithelium is supplied with nerves. Epithelial cells can also undergo specialization to secrete different substances and make up the cellular constituents of glands. Epithelial cells typically possess a significant ability to regenerate (Biscardi et al., 2004).

2.1.2. Classification of Epithelia

Epithelial linings or coverings can be composed of either a single layer of cells, known as simple epithelium, or multiple layers of cells, known as stratified epithelium. The epithelial cells can be classified into three categories based on their geometric shapes: squamous (thin, platelike cells), cuboidal (cells with approximately equal height and width), and columnar (cells with greater height than width). Cells that are intermediate in height between cuboidal and columnar are often referred to as low columnar (Braido et al., 2007).

2.1.2.1. Simple Epithelia

Epithelium, composed of a solitary layer of cells, can be categorized as simple squamous, simple cuboidal, or simple columnar, based on the morphology of the constituent cells. The pseudostratified columnar epithelium is a type of simple epithelium that consists of multiple cell types with nuclei at different levels, creating the false appearance of multiple layers. Although every cell in this particular type of epithelium is in direct contact with the basement membrane, not all of them reach the surface. The cells within an epithelial sheet exhibit distinct orientations on their surfaces. The apical surface is unobstructed, while the basal surface is oriented towards the underlying basement membrane, and the lateral surfaces are oriented towards neighboring epithelial cells. Cell function and morphology are influenced by variations in the orientation of the plasmalemma, specifically in the apical and basolateral regions. Organelles, such as the nucleus, often occupy specific positions within the cell, indicating that the cell exhibits polarity. Epithelial cells can exhibit apical or basal polarization in terms of the arrangement of their organelles, which is determined by the cell's functional state. Similarly, the outer membrane of the apex contains receptors, ion channels, and transporter proteins that have distinct functions compared to those found in the inner membrane (Broeckaert and Bernard, 2000).

Mesothelium refers to the specific type of simple squamous epithelia that forms the lining of the pleural, pericardial, and peritoneal cavities. The endothelium is a simple squamous epithelium that lines the cardiovascular and lymph vascular systems.

2.1.2.2. Stratified Epithelia

Stratified epithelia are categorized based on the morphology of the outermost cells, without considering the shapes of the cells in the inner layers. Except for cells in the basal layer, the cells of stratified epithelia do not touch the basement membrane. Only the outermost cells have a surface that is not attached to anything (Chen et al., 2023). In stratified types with a greater thickness, the cells located at deeper levels frequently exhibit irregular shapes. The stratified epithelia can be classified into three types: stratified squamous, stratified cuboidal, and stratified columnar. Stratified squamous epithelium is the most prevalent type of stratified epithelium, while stratified cuboidal and columnar epithelia are less common.

In areas where the surface is arid or prone to physical wear, such as the epidermis, the outer layers of cells undergo a conversion process and become saturated with a protein known as keratin. Keratin is an exceptionally durable protein. The cells in this layer are resilient to physical damage and are relatively impermeable to bacterial infiltration or dehydration. When this change takes place, this stratified epithelium is known as keratinized stratified squamous epithelium. The outer layer of cells, which has become hardened with keratin, is continuously being shed and renewed. Stratified squamous epithelium is present in moist regions of the body, where intact cells are shed from the surface instead of flat, keratin-filled cells. This epithelium is referred to as a wet or nonkeratinized stratified squamous epithelium. Transitional and germinal epithelia are not categorized based on the cells present in the outermost layer (Chowdhury et al., 2000).

Transitional epithelium, also known as uroepithelium, is found exclusively in the urinary passages. It spans from the minor calyces of the kidneys to the urethra. The tissue is a stratified epithelium with a thick structure, composed of large, rounded cells that have varying appearances depending on the level of distension they experience. The epithelial cells on the surface of a non-distended organ, such as the urinary bladder, have a rounded or dome-shaped appearance and often have a protruding convex border that extends into the inner cavity. The superficial cells in the distended organ can exhibit a range of shapes, from squamous to cuboidal. The germinal epithelium is exclusively found in the seminiferous tubules of the testes. The structure is a stratified epithelium with a complex composition of supporting cells and spermatogenic cells. This particular form of stratified epithelium is found in the male reproductive system.

2.1.3. Cell Attachments

Aside from the intercellular matrix, multiple attachment points or junctions exist between adjacent epithelial cells, facilitating the proximity of their cell membranes. Additionally, they function as sites where microfilaments and intermediate filaments of the cytoskeleton can anchor, thereby aiding in the stabilization of cell shape (Chu et al., 2005).

2.1.4. Junctional Complexes

Terminal bars are present at the apical and lateral interfaces of simple cuboidal and columnar epithelial cells that border luminal surfaces. Under the light microscope, they appear as compact, abbreviated lines. Electron micrographs reveal the presence of a terminal bar, which forms a specialized area known as the junctional complex. This complex is composed of three distinct regions. Near to the surface, the outer layer of neighboring cell membranes merge, resulting in the elimination of the space between the cells. The zonula occludens, also known as the tight junction, is a specialized area that encircles the outer edge of each cell. Its purpose is to create a tight seal between the uppermost parts of neighboring epithelial cells. Consequently, substances that traverse the epithelial layer must traverse the cell membranes and typically cannot traverse between cells via the intercellular spaces. The zonula occludens plays a crucial role in maintaining the separation between the apical and basolateral cell membrane domains. It achieves this by preventing the sideways movement of specific transmembrane proteins (such as receptors and ion transport proteins) in the cell membrane. Typically, membrane proteins in the apical plasmalemma exhibit distinct functions compared to those found in the basolateral regions (Elkhal et al., 2015). The apical domain's plasmalemma is abundant in cholesterol and glycolipids and comprises ion channels, transporter proteins, hydrolytic enzymes, and hydrogen-ATPase. Regulated secretory products are discharged from this region through exocytosis. On the other hand, the plasmalemma of the basolateral domain is distinguished by the presence of hormone receptors, anion channels, and sodium-potassium ATPase. This is the primary site for constitutive secretion. The distribution of the plasmalemma in epithelial cells enables it to control the movement of ions and solutes between external environments and body fluids, as well as between different compartments within the body (Facchiano et al., 1991).

Tight junctions are also present between simple squamous epithelial cells, which can form either an endothelium or a mesothelium. The zonula occludens can undergo rapid disassembly and reformation, as observed during the migration of leukocytes across an endothelial barrier. While the zonula occludens typically acts as a barrier to prevent the movement of substances between cells in an epithelial layer (known as the paracellular pathway), certain epithelia are categorized as either tight or leaky depending on the permeability of the zonula occludens. The presence of leaky zonula occludens permits the passage of specific ions across the epithelial barrier through the paracellular pathway (Guerra et al., 2015). The zonula adherens, which is the second component of the junctional complex, creates a belt or zone that encircles the top part of an epithelial cell, positioned directly below the zonula occludens. The cell membranes that are next to each other are divided by a 15 to 20 nm wide space. In this area, there are structures called plaques on the inside layer of the cell membranes, which are connected to a network of actin filaments. The plaques consist of α-actinin and vinculin, which are two proteins that bind to actin. Actin is associated with a transmembrane glycoprotein known as E-cadherin (also called adherens cell adhesion molecule or A-CAM), which binds cells together in this area when calcium ions are present (Guerra et al., 2016) (**Figure 2.1**).

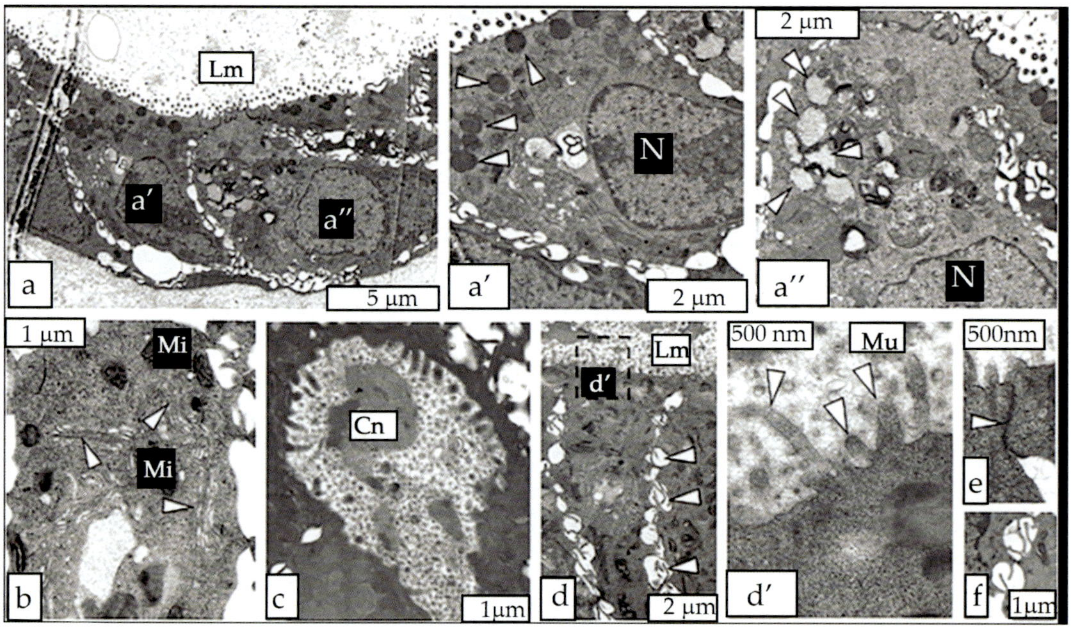

Figure 2.1. *Transmission electron microscopy of human gastric epithelial spheroids. A cross-section of a gastric spheroid shows a simple cuboidal to columnar microvillated epithelium with vacuolated secretory cells and basal nuclei. Lm lumen; bar 5 μm. a′ Epithelial cell from (a) with large, electron-dense vacuoles (arrowheads). N nucleus; bar 2 μm. a″ Epithelial cell from (a) with large, electron-lucent vacuoles (arrowheads). N nucleus; bar 2 μm. (b) Epithelial cell with copious amounts of rough endoplasmic reticulum (arrowheads) and multiple large mitochondria (Mi); bar 1 μm. (c) Large microvillated intracellular canaliculus (Cn) in a gastric epithelial cell. Bar 1 μm. (d) Columnar epithelial cells with luminal microvilli and lateral interdigitating intercellular leaflets (arrowheads)b bar 2 μm. d′ Enlarged image from (d, dashed box) shows luminal microvilli (arrowheads) and mucus (Mu); bar 500 nm. (e) Luminal-junctional complex (arrowhead) between two epithelial cells; bar 500 nm. (f) Lateral interdigitating intercellular leaflets; bar 1 μm.*

Source: https://www.researchgate.net/figure/Transmission-electron-microscopy-of-human-gastric-epithelial-spheroids-a-Cross-section_fig2_321291642.

The macula adherens, also known as the desmosome, is the third component of the junction complex. These small, elliptical discs serve as focal adhesions that connect the intermediate filament network of neighboring cells (Han et al., 2020). The attachment plaque, an amorphous material, causes the internal leaflet of the adjacent cell membranes to appear dense and thick. Desmoplakin I and II are situated within the plaque. Cytokeratin, typically intermediate filaments, extend into the plaque and seem to create hairpin loops. A thin and moderately dense layer is frequently observed in the space between cells in each desmosome. These structures consist of transmembrane glycoproteins (desmoglein I and desmocollin I and II) that bind to calcium and facilitate the adhesion of cells by bringing their membranes close together. Desmosomes are distributed randomly along the sides of epithelial cells and are not limited to areas where tight junctions are present. They are particularly plentiful in stratified squamous epithelia, where they are connected to numerous intermediate filaments of the keratin type (He et al., 2016). Epithelial cells can form desmosome-like junctions that do not have attachment plaques or associated keratin filaments. This particular form of cellular junction is commonly referred to as a punctum adherens (Hermans and Bernard, 1996) (**Figure 2.2**).

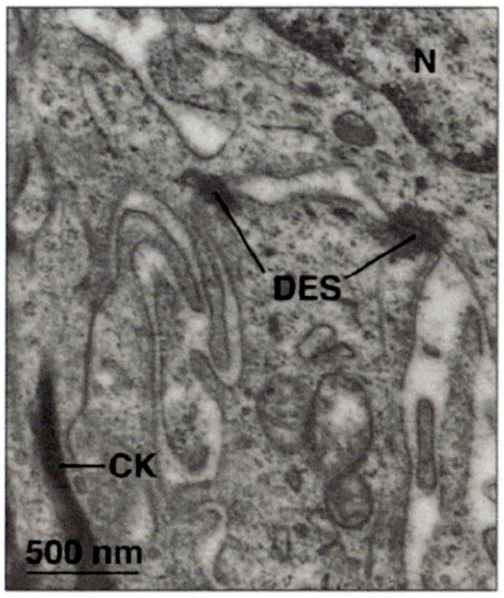

Figure 2.2. *Transmission electron micrograph showing desmosomes, also known as maculae adherens, located between two adjacent human intestinal epithelial cells.*

Source: https://www.researchgate.net/profile/Dieter-Bosshardt/publication/8114400/figure/fig3/AS:277852898512897@1443256701418/Transmission-electron-micrograph-illustrating-desmosomes-DES-and-cytokeratin-filaments.png.

Although the basal cell membrane is not directly adjacent to another cell, it exhibits an attachment known as the hemidesmosome, which closely resembles half of a desmosome. Hemidesmosomes serve as sites of attachment between the basal plasma membrane and the underlying basal lamina (Hong, 2012). They connect the intermediate keratin filament network of the epithelial cells to the extracellular matrix through transmembrane anchoring glycoproteins. These transmembrane glycoproteins function as receptors for laminin and specifically bind to laminin, a glycoprotein located in the lamina lucida of the basal lamina.

Focal adherens junctions are also present on the basal plasmalemma and connect actin filaments to the extracellular matrix. α-actinin, vinculin, and Talin are intracellular attachment proteins that connect actin filaments to integrin, a transmembrane glycoprotein that acts as a receptor for fibronectin (Iannuzo et al., 2022). The latter molecule forms a connection with fibronectin, a versatile extracellular glycoprotein found in the basal lamina. Fibronectin interacts with different types of collagens and proteoglycans in the extracellular matrix. Epithelial cells are tightly connected and firmly attached to the extracellular matrix through a group of transmembrane glycoproteins known as cellular adhesion molecules (CAMs) or integrins (Jiang et al., 2021). Desmosomes and hemidesmosomes function as robust attachment points for intermediate (keratin) filaments of the cytoskeleton. Furthermore, desmosomes serve to connect the keratin filament network between neighboring cells, while hemidesmosomes establish a connection between this network and the extracellular matrix. The arrangement of interconnected intermediate filaments provides mechanical stability to a group of cells, allowing them to maintain a specific three-dimensional shape and function as a cohesive unit. Similarly, actin microfilaments are connected not only to the cell membrane at zonula adherens and focal adherens junctions but also to the actin filaments of neighboring cells through these attachment points, as well as to components of the extracellular matrix. This configuration grants epithelial cells a certain level of motility, especially crucial for migrating epithelial cells (such as those found in the gastric and intestinal linings) that constantly traverse the basal lamina. The presence of calcium ions seems to be crucial for maintaining the integrity of desmosomes and hemidesmosomes. The basal lamina is endowed with a robust negative charge due to the presence of heparan sulfate-rich proteoglycans. This negative charge, in conjunction with calcium ions, facilitates the binding of transmembrane linker glycoproteins to components in the extracellular matrix (Johnson et al., 2021).

2.1.4.1. Nexus Junction

The nexus, also known as a gap junction, functions as a sturdy connection point between neighboring cells, similar to tight junctions and desmosomes. At a junction point, the cell membranes are positioned apart by a distance of 2 nanometers, and this gap is filled by particles that have a diameter of 8 nanometers. The connexons, which are primarily composed of the protein connexin, constitute these particles. A connexon unit is composed of six identical transmembrane connexin proteins that are organized in a circular formation around a small aqueous channel or pore. Connexon units traverse the plasmalemma and span the intercellular gap to connect with a corresponding unit from the adjacent cell membrane. The aqueous channel located in the core of each connexon allows for the transfer of ions, amino acids, and other small molecules between cells (Jung et al., 2023).

The nexus also serves as a conduit through which cyclic adenosine monophosphate (cAMP), released by one cell, can be transmitted to neighboring cells. The regulation of the central pore's opening and closing seems to be dependent on the intracellular concentration of calcium. Epithelial cells are interconnected both electrically and metabolically, allowing for coordinated responses among multiple cells in an epithelial sheet when exposed to a particular stimulus. Nexus junctions, also known as communication junctions, serve as communication sites between epithelial cells. Furthermore, nexus junctions can transition from a state of low resistance to high resistance, effectively impeding cellular communication.

Gap junctions are also present between cardiac and smooth muscle cells, osteocytes, astrocytes, and certain endocrine cells. Curiously, the presence of gap junctions between cancer cells has not been detected. The adjacent lateral cell membranes of epithelial cells frequently exhibit interdigitations rather than running parallel to each other. The interlocking of cell membranes is believed to contribute to the maintenance of cell-to-cell adhesion and stability in an epithelial sheet (Kraft et al., 2008).

2.1.5. Specializations of Epithelial Membranes

Epithelial cells frequently exhibit specialized modifications on their apical or basolateral surfaces, which serve to enhance the surface area of the cell or facilitate the movement of substances across the surface (Kraft et al., 2018). The surface adaptations consist of microvilli, cilia, and basal-lateral infoldings.

2.1.5.1. Microvilli

Microvilli are small, finger-like protrusions of the outermost cell membrane that contain cytoplasm inside. Scattered microvilli are present on the surfaces of the majority of cells in simple epithelia. However, they are typically too minuscule to be visible under a light microscope (Laucho-Contreras et al., 2015). In certain types of epithelial tissue, such as the lining of the small intestine, microvilli are present in large numbers, are uniform in shape, and are closely arranged. This arrangement is so dense that it creates a visible striated border when observed under a microscope (Laucho-Contreras et al., 2018) (**Figure 2.3**).

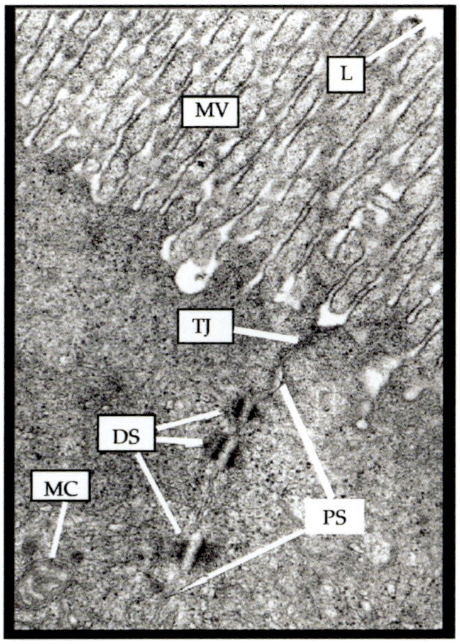

Figure 2.3. *Transmission electron micrograph (TEM) of the anterior intestinal brush border membrane from rainbow trout (Oncorhynchus mykiss). L, lumen; MV, microvilli; TJ, tight junctions; DS, desmosomes; PS, paracellular space; MC, mitochondria. Courtesy of Prof. Kristina Sundell.*

Source: https://www.researchgate.net/figure/Transmission-electron-micrograph-TEM-of-the-anterior-intestinal-brush-border-membrane_fig4_234102731.

Microvilli are abundant in cells that make up the proximal convoluted tubules of the kidney. In this location, they are slightly longer and less consistent compared to those in the small intestine, and they appear as clusters on the top of the cells. The term "brush border" is used to describe the appearance of these structures resembling paint-brush tips. Microvilli greatly enlarge the surface area, thereby improving the ability of epithelial cells to absorb substances (Ledford et al., 2018). The consistent structure of microvilli, which create the striated and brush borders, is upheld by a cluster of 25 to 40 actin filaments that are connected by the actin-binding proteins villin, fimbrin, and fascin. Minimyosin molecules connect the actin filament bundle in the microvillus core to the inner surface of the plasmalemma. The actin filaments span from the tips of the microvilli to the apical cytoplasm. Just below the cell surface, they connect to a region abundant in actin filaments known as the terminal web. The epithelial cells lining the epididymis exhibit elongated, slender, and branching microvilli, which are referred to as stereocilia. Contrary to popular belief, stereocilia are not cilia, but rather they are genuine microvilli. Their primary function is to enhance the surface area of a cell (Levin et al., 1986).

2.1.5.2. Cilia

Cilia, like microvilli, are extensions of the apical cell membrane. However, cilia are larger in size and frequently exhibit movement. They can exist as individual entities or appear in abundant quantities, and they are easily observable using a light microscope. The outer membrane of the cilium is connected to the cell's membrane and surrounds a central region of cytoplasm that contains 20 microtubules (Li et al., 2023).

The cilium is encircled by a ring comprising nine fused microtubule pairs, known as doublets, which enclose a central pair of individual microtubules. The configuration depicted in **Figure 2.4** is commonly referred to as the (9 + 2) arrangement. The microtubules within each doublet are designated as the A and B microtubules. Microtubule A possesses two briefs, diverging appendages that extend towards microtubule B of the neighboring doublet. The arms are composed of the protein dynein, which possesses adenosinetriphosphatase (ATPase) activity that hydrolyzes ATP to generate energy for ciliary motion. The radial spokes extend from the doublets to the central pair of microtubules (Lin et al., 2020).

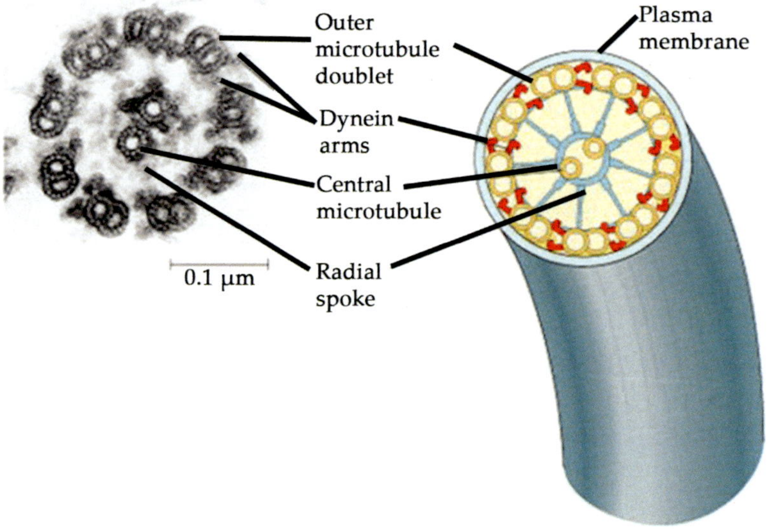

Figure 2.4. *4: 9+2 structure of a cilium. The electron microscopic picture of the cross-section of a cilium showing the microtubules and the dynein arms. On the right, a schematic of all the components of a cilium is drawn.*

Source: https://www.researchgate.net/profile/Karine_Guevorkian/publication/252261560/figure/fig7/AS:669549699543044@1536644496233/9-2-structure-of-a-cilium-The-EM-picture-of-the-cross-section-of-a-cilium-showing-the.ppm.

Cilia microtubules are derived from a basal body located in the apical cytoplasm of the cell. The basal body shares a similar structure with the centriole, appearing as a hollow cylinder with a wall composed of nine triplet microtubules. The absence of central microtubules in a basal body result in a microtubule arrangement. Each of the nine pairs of microtubules in the cilium is directly connected to the two innermost microtubules of the triplets in the basal body. The two central microtubules of the ciliary shaft end at the basal body without merging with it (Mango et al., 1998). Ciliary motion is believed to be driven by a mechanism in which microtubules slide past each other.

This mechanism relies on the dynein protein arms, which generate energy through their ATPase-like activity. Cilia are abundant in the epithelial cells that cover a significant portion of the respiratory tract and certain sections of the female reproductive tract. Cilia groups exhibit synchronized, rhythmic movements to propel a thin layer of fluid unidirectionally across the epithelial surface. In certain areas of the body, such as the distal tubules of the kidney or the olfactory epithelium, cilia are present on cells either individually or in small clusters. These cilia are not capable of movement and are thought to function as chemoreceptors. Cilia are also present in the maculae and cristae of the inner ear, where they function as mechanoreceptors. The outer segments of the rods and cones in the retina exhibit the most drastic alteration of cilia, which function as photoreceptors in this modified form. The presence of cilia is a determining factor in the classification of epithelia. The term "cilia" is included in the nomenclature when it is present (Miele et al., 1988). Hence, the lining of the oviduct, which consists of a single layer of tall cells with cilia on their surface, is known as a ciliated simple columnar epithelium. When cilia are present in conjunction with pseudostratified columnar epithelium, such as in the trachea, the epithelium is categorized as ciliated pseudostratified columnar epithelium. Kartagener's syndrome is a rare form of immotile cilia syndrome characterized by the absence of dynein arms. Individuals with this innate condition are prone to respiratory infections because the removal of substances from the lungs is hindered because of the lack of synchronized movement of cilia in the respiratory system. Individuals afflicted with this syndrome typically experience infertility due to the presence of defective axonemes in the flagella of their sperm. Curiously, women with Kartagener's syndrome may or may not experience infertility, despite having defective cilia in the oviducts' epithelium lining (Mukherjee et al., 1999).

2.1.5.3. Basolateral Infoldings

Some epithelial cells exhibit complex infoldings of the basolateral plasmalemma, in addition to their apical specializations. The structures referred to as basolateral infoldings are typically well-developed in epithelial cells that are involved in the transport of fluid and ions. This includes cells that make up the proximal and distal convoluted tubules of the kidneys, as well as cells that line the ducts of salivary glands. Like microvilli, they significantly enhance the surface area of the cell membrane.

The plasmalemma in these areas contains a high concentration of ion channel proteins, specifically sodium-potassium-ATPase. Mitochondria, which are frequently abundant in this region of the cell, typically align parallel to the invaginations of the plasma membrane and generate ATP from substrates. Due to this connection, the infoldings can be observed using a light microscope and appear as basal striations (Mukherjee et al., 2007).

2.1.6. Glandular Epithelium

Epithelial cells not only carry out functions like protection and absorption, but they also have the ability to secrete materials. Glands are composed of epithelial cells that have been specifically adapted for secretion. It is important to note that most intricate glands develop from an epithelial surface and extend outward from this layer. Exocrine glands are referred to as those that maintain a connection with the epithelial surface of origin through ducts. Endocrine glands are those that have lost the ductal connection to their point of origin (Nisar et al., 2007).

2.1.6.1. Classification of Glands

Glands can be categorized based on their histologic structure, presence of ducts, type of secreted material, and method of secretion. Unicellular glands are composed of a single cell, while multicellular glands are made up of groups of cells that secrete substances. These cells can be categorized as exocrine or endocrine-based on whether they release their secretions onto a surface or into a ductal system (exocrine) or directly into the tissue fluid of the intercellular space (endocrine). Complex exocrine glands can be further classified based on the branching pattern of their ducts, the structure of the secretory end piece, and the type and method of secretion (Nomori et al., 1995).

2.1.6.1.1. Unicellular Glands

An exemplary instance of a single-celled, exocrine gland is the goblet cell, which is dispersed throughout the epithelial cells that line the trachea, small intestine, and colon. The cell possesses a slender base and an enlarged apex that is replete with secretory granules. Goblet cells secrete mucin, which, when hydrated, forms a thick lubricating fluid known as mucus. Mucin is excreted onto an epithelial surface. Therefore, a goblet cell is categorized as a unicellular exocrine gland. There are also unicellular endocrine cells, which are glands (Pang et al., 2018). These cells are abundant in the epithelium that lines the gastrointestinal tract and they secrete various peptide hormones and/or amines. Additionally, they can be located within the epithelium that lines the respiratory system. These cells secrete their product into the extracellular space, which can then enter the nearby blood vessels (Pang et al., 2017).

2.1.6.1.2. Multicellular Glands

The most basic type of multicellular exocrine gland is the secretory sheet, as seen in the gastric lining epithelium. In this type of gland, the cells that secrete substances form a continuous layer of epithelial cells. Intraepithelial glands are compact aggregations of exocrine cells that are completely enclosed within an epithelial layer, arranged around a small central cavity. Both types of gland cells release their product onto the epithelial surface.

2.1.6.1.3. Complex Exocrine Glands

Exocrine glands release their secretions onto the surface of epithelial cells, either directly through secretory sheets and intraepithelial glands or through a system of ducts.

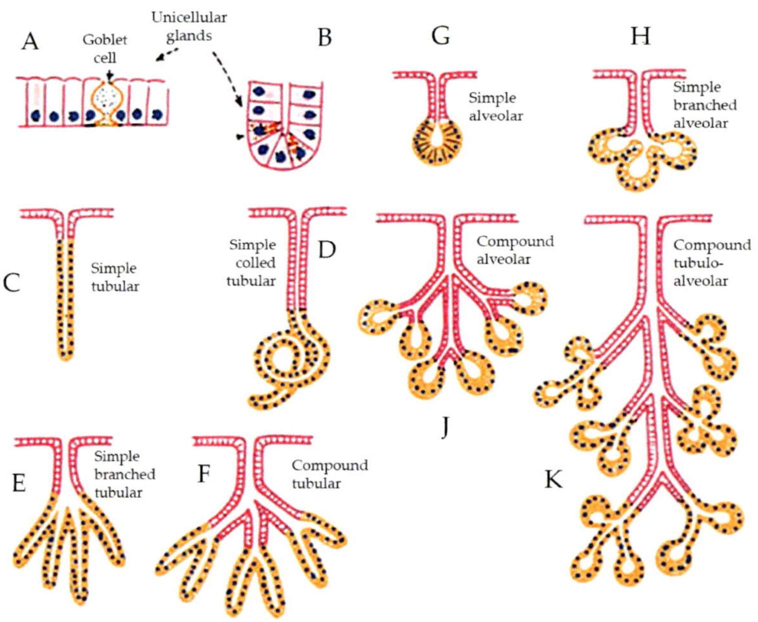

Figure 2.5. *Schematic illustration of several glandular forms.*

Source: https://d45jl3w9libvn.cloudfront.net/jaypee/static/books/9788180618093/Chapters/images/55-1.jpg.

A gland is considered compound if its duct system branches, while a gland is classified as simple if its duct system does not branch. The secretory cells can be arranged in tubules, acini, alveoli (resembling berries), or saccules (enlarged, flask-shaped end pieces). Glands can be classified as simple or compound based on the morphology of their secretory portion. Therefore, simple glands can be categorized as either simple tubular, simple coiled tubular, simple branched tubular, or simple branched acinar (Paulsson et al., 2019). Compound glands can be further categorized into compound tubular, compound saccular, and compound tubuloacinar (tubuloalveolar) glands. The initial categorization into simple and compound is based on whether or not the ducts bifurcate. The subsequent categorization depends on the form and arrangement of the excreting segment, known as the secretory unit. It is important to note that the epithelial cells that make up the tightly packed tubular structures of complex glands maintain a single-layer arrangement, even though the overall glandular structure may appear complex. This approach allows for the optimal arrangement of a maximum number of secretory cells within the smallest possible area (Periayah et al., 2017) (**Figure 2.5**).

2.1.6.1.4. Endocrine Glands

Similar to exocrine glands, complex endocrine glands originate from an epithelial sheet. However, during their development, endocrine glands disconnect from the surface and consequently do not possess ducts. Endocrine gland cells release hormones directly into the extracellular space. Hormones can act on the releasing cell itself (autocrine secretion), nearby cells (paracrine secretion) or travel through the bloodstream to affect target cells in distant organs. Endocrine cells are found sporadically and individually in the gastrointestinal tract and along the conducting part of the respiratory tract. The complex endocrine glands possess such a wide range of structures that they are not easily categorized using histologic classification. Nevertheless, it is possible to discern certain general structural patterns, and the cells can be organized in clusters, strands, or empty spherical formations known as follicles. These will be specifically addressed in the discussion on Endocrine Glands (Plopper et al., 2006).

2.1.6.1.5. Type and Mode of Secretion

Glands can be categorized as mucous, serous, or mixed based on the specific substance they secrete. The cytoplasm of mucous gland cells appears pale and contains vacuoles, while their nuclei are flattened and dense, positioned towards the base of the cell. The serous cells exhibit spherical nuclei encased in a basophilic cytoplasm, which contains distinct secretory granules (Prince et al., 2018).

Mixed glands consist of varying proportions of serous and mucous cells. There are two distinct types of glands that can be differentiated based on their method of secretion. Merocrine secretion is the process by which the product is released through the fusion of secretory vesicles with the apical plasmalemma. Exocytosis is the process by which this type of secretion is regulated and stimulated, and it is the primary mechanism for most exocrine secretions. Holocrine secretion is a process where either complete cell, like sperm from the testes, are released, or an entire cell is broken down to form the secretion, such as sebum in sebaceous glands. Apocrine secretion is a type of secretion where both the secretory material and a portion of the apical cytoplasm are lost. Electron microscopy has not provided conclusive evidence to support this method of secretion, except possibly in the case of mammary glands during lactation. Even in this context, the presence of an apocrine secretion is uncertain (Rava et al., 2013).

2.1.6.1.6. Myoepithelial Cells

Myoepithelial cells, specialized cells positioned between the glandular epithelial cells and the basal lamina, are connected to the secretory units of certain glands. These cells are capable of contraction and their cytoplasm contains the contractile proteins actin and myosin, which are arranged in a similar manner to those found in smooth muscle cells. Furthermore, these cells are equipped with the intermediate filament, desmin. The cell-body is connected to the secretory unit by long cytoplasmic processes. The contraction of the processes facilitates the movement of products from the secretory units into the ductal system. Myoepithelial cells are present in sweat, mammary, and salivary glands, as well as in glands located along the bronchi and esophagus (Rojas-Quintero et al., 2023).

2.1.7. Histogenesis

Epithelium can originate from ectoderm, endoderm, or mesoderm. Layers of epithelium originating from the germ layers envelop the surface of the developing embryo and form linings for the emerging body cavities and tubular structures. Glands are created when epithelial sheets form outpockets, which then develop into ductal systems and secretory units as the ductal outgrowth expands (Shrine et al., 2019). An exocrine gland is formed when the ductal connections are preserved with the original epithelial sheet. In the event of a lost connection, the consequence is the formation of an endocrine gland (**Figure 2.6**).

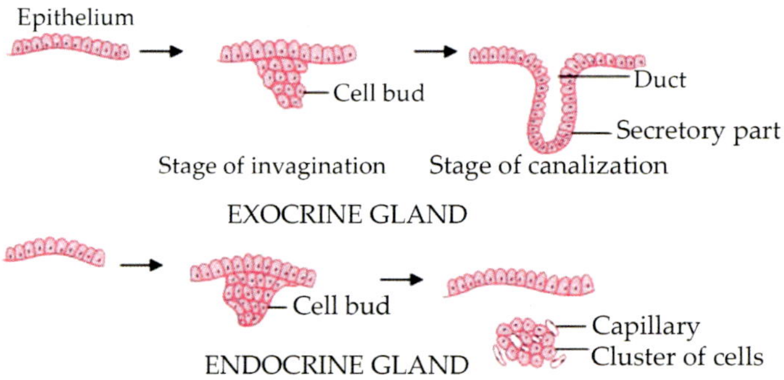

Figure 2.6. *Development of exocrine and endocrine glands. Glands develop by forming an inward growth from a layer of epithelial cells. Exocrine glands are classified as glands that maintain a connection (duct) to the original epithelial sheet. The glands that lose their connection are referred to as endocrine glands and typically secrete their products into the bloodstream.*

Source: https://d45jl3w9libvn.cloudfront.net/jaypee/static/books/9789385999321/Chapters/images/40-3.jpg.

2.2. General Connective Tissue

Connective tissues are a varied group of tissues that originate from mesenchyme and serve various functions due to their diverse types. Connective tissues fulfill various functions such as providing structural support, serving as a foundation for organ support, acting as a filler for empty spaces, functioning as an insulating layer (fat) that also serves as an energy storage, and playing a crucial role in the body's defense mechanisms and repair processes following injury (Silva et al., 2004).

Some functions are attributed to regular (common) connective tissues, while others are attributed to specialized connective tissues. The stroma of organs is composed of connective tissues, while the parenchyma consists of epithelial (cellular) components.

2.2.1. Organization

Connective tissues, like other fundamental tissues, consist of cells and intercellular substances. The latter comprises fibers, extracellular matrix, and interstitial fluid. Unlike epithelium, where cells are closely packed with minimal intercellular material, connective tissue cells are widely dispersed within a matrix of fibers and ground substance.

The fibers and ground substance combine to create the matrix of connective tissue. Connective tissue is typically highly vascularized, with a few exceptions.

2.2.2. Classification

The classification of connective tissues into different subgroups primarily focuses on describing the characteristics of the extracellular materials rather than the cellular components. There are two primary classifications – general and special – from which additional divisions are derived. Connective tissues are classified as either loose or dense based on the degree of fiber packing.

Loose connective tissues can be classified based on specific characteristics of their components, including adipose (fatty) tissue, reticular tissue, and others. Dense connective tissues can be classified based on the distribution of fibers, which can either be randomly dispersed or arranged in an organized manner. Therefore, dense connective tissues are categorized as either dense irregular or dense regular connective tissues.

2.2.2.1. Loose Connective Tissue

Loose connective tissue is a prevalent and uncomplicated type of connective tissue that serves as the standard example of connective tissue. Basically, all other types of connective tissues are variations of loose connective tissue where certain components have been emphasized to fulfill specific functions (Terada et al., 2004).

2.2.2.2. Fibers of Connective Tissue

The connective tissue is primarily composed of collagenous, reticular, and elastic fibers, which form fibrous intercellular substances.

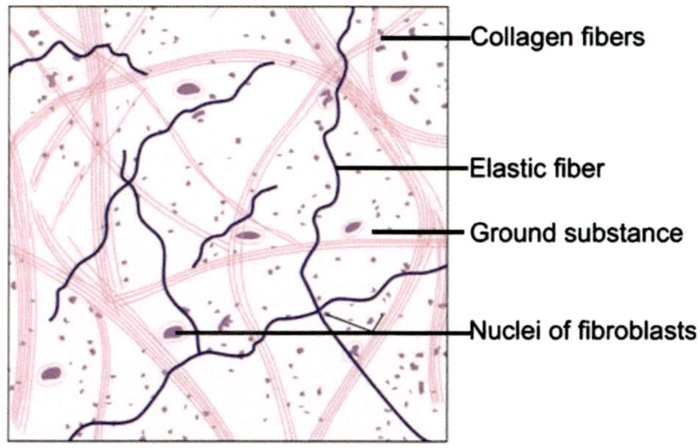

Figure 2.7. *The transmission electron microscope reveals the presence of elastic and collagen fibers in the connective tissue component of the pleura.*

Source: https://d45jl3w9libvn.cloudfront.net/jaypee/static/books/9789385999321/Chapters/images/41–1.jpg.

Collagen fibers are found in every connective tissue and have a non-uniform path with extensive branching. The fibers exhibit a range of thicknesses, ranging from 1 to 10 μm, and their length is not specified. Collagenous fibers possess exceptional tensile strength and flexibility. At the ultrastructural level, the fibers are composed of parallel fibrils, with each fibril serving as a structural unit. The fibrils exhibit regular transverse bands, spaced 64 nm apart.

These fibrils are made up of tropocollagen macromolecules, which are approximately 260 nm in length and 1.5 nm in width (**Figure 2.7**).

The tropocollagen molecules are oriented in a parallel manner, with each molecule overlapping approximately one-fourth of its length. This overlapping is the cause of the observed banding pattern. Tropocollagen is composed of three alpha units, which are polypeptide chains arranged in a helical structure and connected by hydrogen bonds. The polypeptides are abundant in glycine and proline, and they also consist of hydroxyproline and hydroxylysine. Nevertheless, alpha units derived from collagens obtained from various locations exhibit slight differences in the composition and order of amino acids. Multiple discrete molecular forms of collagen have been discovered, each composed of three alpha units organized in a helical structure and primarily varying in the amino acid composition of the alpha chain. Not all individual fibrils of the different types of collagens exhibit a striped, fibrous appearance, nor are they organized in a similar manner. Collagen is a group of more than 12 closely related proteins that are genetically distinct from each other. Tropocollagen has been extracted from the ground substance as well, although its histological demonstration is not possible. Collagen can be produced by cells other than fibroblasts, such as chondroblasts, odontoblasts, epithelial cells, endothelial cells, and smooth muscle cells (Waites and Talkington, 2004). Collagen molecules play a crucial role in the composition of basement membranes. Reticular fibers do not aggregate into substantial bundles like collagenous fibers, but instead, they tend to create intricate networks. These structures are not visible in regularly prepared sections, but they can be revealed using silver stains or the periodic acid-Schiff (PAS) reagent. The PAS reagent reacts with proteoglycans that bind reticular unit fibrils together. The unit fibrils of reticular fibers exhibit an identical banding pattern to that of type I collagen fibers in electron micrographs. Structurally, they vary in terms of their number, diameter, and the organization of the individual fibrils. Reticular fibers are composed of type III collagen unit fibrils (Waites et al., 2017).

Elastic fibers are observed as slender, consistent strands that exhibit a greater degree of uniformity in size compared to collagen fibers. They are not easily distinguishable in regular H&E sections and necessitate special stains to enhance their visibility. Electron micrographs reveal that elastic fibers are composed of clusters of microfibrils that are encased within an amorphous substance known as elastin. The diameter of the microfibrils is approximately 11 nm and they do not exhibit cross-banding. During the process of elastic fiber formation, microfibrils are initially deposited, followed by the subsequent addition of elastin, which eventually becomes the main component of the fiber. Cells release a precursor molecule called tropoelastin, which then undergoes extracellular polymerization to form elastin. The microfibrillar component is typically found at the outer edges of the fiber. Elastin, like collagen, comprises glycine and proline amino acids, with minimal hydroxyproline and absence of hydroxylysine (**Table 2.1**).

It possesses a significant amount of valine and includes two amino acids, desmosine, and isodesmosine, which are exclusive to elastin. Fibrillin is a nonsulfated glycoprotein that makes up microfibrils. There are also microfibrils that are associated with the basal lamina of epithelia. Fibrillin facilitates the attachment of elastin to the other constituents of the extracellular matrix. Elastic fibers can stretch beyond 130% of their original length. Their presence allows connective tissues to undergo significant expansion or stretching and then return to their original shape or size once the deforming force is no longer applied. Elastin can be found in the walls of blood vessels, where it forms fibers and exists in fenestrated sheets or layers known as elastic laminae (Wang et al., 2003).

Table 2.1. Types of Collagen

Type	Morphological Features	Distribution
I	Broad, banded unit fibrils	Widespread; tendon, bone, dermis, dentin, fascia
II	Small-diameter, banded unit fibrils	Hyaline cartilage, vitreous body, nucleus pulposus, notochord
III	Small-diameter, banded unit fibrils	Corresponds to reticular fibers; prominent in organs with a major smooth muscle component; forms the supporting framework for the parenchyma of most glands and organs, fat, lymphoid tissue, uterus, and blood vessels
IV	Feltwork of non-banded unit fibrils	Basal laminae of epithelial cells, glomerular epithelium; lens capsule; external laminae
V	Thick non-banded unit fibrils	Widespread; pericellular laminae of smooth and striated muscle cells, tendon sheaths
VI	Thin, banded unit fibrils	Make up about 25% of collagen in cornea; small amounts where types I and III are found
VII	Small-diameter, banded unit fibrils	Form anchoring fibrils that link the basal lamina of many epithelia to the underlying connective tissue
VIII	Unknown	A major component of Descemet's membrane; associated with and produced by endothelial cells
IX	Unknown	Found mainly in cartilage; links type II collagen in three-dimensional arrangement
X	Unknown	Cartilage matrix surrounding hypertrophic chondrocytes during endochondral bone formation

Source: Adapted from Alberts B, Johnson A, Lewis J, et al., (2002). Molecular Biology of the Cell. 4th edition. New York: Garland Science.

Table 2.2. Types of Glycosaminoglycans

Type of Glycosaminoglycan	Some Locations
Hyaluronic acid	Umbilical cord, vitreous humor, synovial fluid, loose connective tissue
Chondroitin	Cornea
Chondroitin-4-sulfate	Aorta, bone, cartilage, cornea
Chondroitin-6-sulfate	Cartilage, nucleus pulposus, sclera, tendon, umbilical cord
Dermatan sulfate	Aorta, heart valves, ligamentum nuchae, sclera, skin, tendon
Keratan sulfate	Bone, cartilage, cornea, nucleus pulposus

Source: Berdiaki et al., 2021

- **Ground Substance:** The fibers and cells of connective tissue are enclosed within an amorphous substance known as ground substance, which exists as a transparent gel with varying viscosity. The ground substance of connective tissues is composed of proteoglycans, glycosaminoglycans, and glycoproteins. The composition of these substances varies in different connective tissues, as shown in **Table 2.2**.

Proteoglycans have a structure resembling a bottle brush, with a protein core and attached glycosaminoglycan side chains. Glycosaminoglycans are unbranched macromolecules composed of repetitive disaccharide units, which consist of hexosamine (N-acetylglucosamine, N-acetyl galactosamine), D-glucosamine, D-galactosamine, or uronic (glucuronic) acid, which is their most consistent characteristic. The macromolecules of the ground substance commonly contain sulfate groups (SO_3–) or carboxyl groups (COO–) from uronic acid, which give the molecule a negative charge. Consequently, these molecules exhibit a pronounced hydrophilic nature and play a crucial role in retaining positive ions (Na^+) along with water in the extracellular matrix. Therefore, these substantial, negatively charged molecules create and sustain a significant hydration area (an extracellular fluid compartment) in the extracellular matrix. Due to the presence of these molecules, the ground substance contains a significant amount of water, which is attached to long-chain carbohydrates and proteoglycans. Most of the fluid outside the blood vessels (tissue fluid) exists in this form (Yuliani et al., 2022). The bound water serves as a conduit for the exchange of nutrients, gases, and metabolites between the blood and tissue cells. Hyaluronic acid is the primary glycosaminoglycan found in loose connective tissue. Its main function is to bind water, which leads to alterations in the permeability and viscosity of the tissue. Furthermore, proteoglycans have a crucial function in preserving the structural arrangement of the fibrous components in the matrix and basal laminae. They also assist in inhibiting or slowing down the dissemination of microorganisms and their harmful substances from the location of an infection.

The main glycoproteins found in the matrix are fibronectin, laminin, and thrombospondin. These glycoproteins serve the purpose of connecting cell membranes of different cell types to components of the extracellular matrix. Laminin is the largest glycoprotein involved in adhesion. It is primarily found in the lamina lucida of epithelial basal laminae and in the external laminae of muscle cells. The plasmalemma is connected to type IV collagen and proteoglycans (specifically heparan sulfate) in the neighboring matrix through a transmembrane glycoprotein called laminin receptor. This binding occurs in both epithelial and muscle cells. Fibronectin is a sizable and adaptable glycoprotein found in the extracellular matrix. It is produced by fibroblasts and certain epithelial cells. It is also present in the outer layers of muscle cells and Schwann cells, as well as on the surfaces of other types of cells. Fibronectin facilitates the attachment of cells to each other and to the surrounding matrix. The protein possesses multiple receptor-binding domains and connects the plasma membrane of epithelial cells to collagen fibers and glycosaminoglycans. Fibronectin connects actin filaments in the cytoplasm of basal epithelial cells to elements of the extracellular matrix through fibronectin receptors called integrins. Fibronectin is believed aid in the process of cell spreading and mobility. Thrombospondin is an additional adhesive glycoprotein that attaches to collagen and certain proteoglycans. The production of this substance is carried out by fibroblasts, smooth muscle cells, and epithelial cells. It then attaches to the plasmalemma of these cell types and connects them to the extracellular matrix (Zhai et al., 2022).

2.2.2.3. Cells of Connective Tissue

Connective tissue comprises a variety of cellular components. Some microorganisms naturally inhabit the tissues, while others are temporary residents that come from the bloodstream. Fibroblasts are the most prevalent type of connective tissue cells. They are large, flattened cells with elliptical nuclei that typically have one or two nucleoli. The cellular morphology is irregular and frequently exhibits a stellate appearance, characterized by elongated cytoplasmic processes that extend along the connective tissue fibers. The cell boundaries are typically imperceptible in the majority of preparations, and the morphology of the cell varies depending on its level of activity. The nuclei of active cells exhibit a plump morphology and light staining, while the nuclei of inactive cells display a slender shape and a dense staining. Active cells exhibit higher quantities of granular endoplasmic reticulum (GER) at the ultrastructural level. Fibroblasts synthesize the precursor molecules of collagen, reticular, and elastic fibers, generate the ground substance, and preserve these extracellular components, which undergo continuous remodeling and renewal. This fact elucidates the relationship between conditions such as scurvy and a lack of vitamin C in one's diet. Vitamin C is essential for the appropriate formation of cross-links between the molecules constituting collagen fibers. Insufficient intake of vitamin C leads to the weakening of collagen and connective tissue in the entire body. Collagen peptides are synthesized on the ribosomes of the GER and then transported to the Golgi complex. Procollagen, a molecular variant of collagen, is secreted from the maturing side of the Golgi complex through secretory vesicles into the adjacent cytoplasm, and subsequently expelled from the cell via exocytosis. Procollagen peptidase, an enzyme found outside of cells, transforms procollagen molecules into tropocollagen. Tropocollagen subsequently undergoes extracellular polymerization, resulting in the formation of collagen fibrils (Figure 2.8).

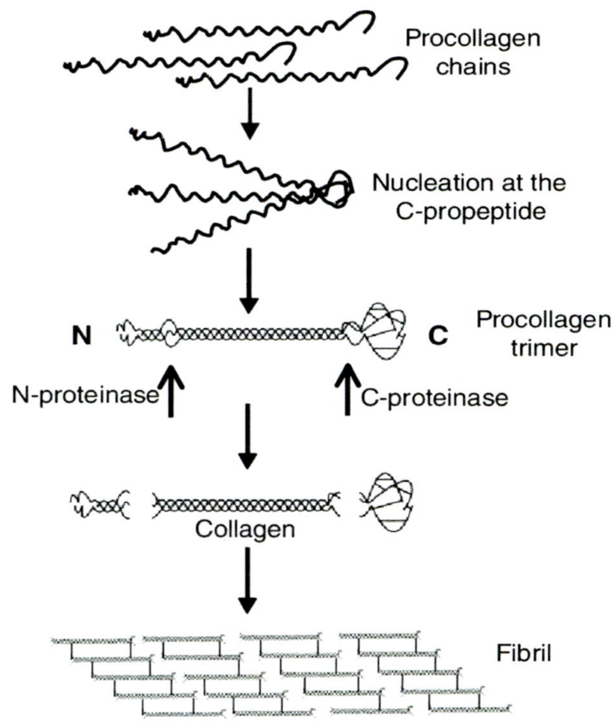

Figure 2.8. *Overview of the steps involved in the production of collagen fibrils by fibroblasts.*

Source: https://www.researchgate.net/profile/Elizabeth-CantyLaird/publication/7946543/figure/fig2/AS:394529128632335@1471074482953/Overview-of-the-steps-involved-in-the-production-of-collagen-fibrils-by-fibroblasts.png.

Myofibroblasts are similar to fibroblasts, but they have clusters of contractile microfilaments, specifically actin and myosin. Unlike smooth muscle cells, myofibroblasts do not have an external lamina surrounding them. Typically present in limited quantities, their numbers rise in response to tissue damage. Myofibroblasts are responsible for the production of collagen, and their ability to contract helps in the reduction and shrinking of newly formed scar tissue (Zhai et al., 2019). Macrophages, also known as histiocytes, are present in areolar connective tissue in nearly equal numbers to fibroblasts. They exhibit active phagocytosis, consuming a wide range of substances including particulate matter, bacteria, tissue debris, and dead cells. The ingested material undergoes degradation through lysosomal digestion. Macrophages undergo activation in response to lipopolysaccharides, which are a surface component of gram-negative bacteria, as well as interferon-γ. Macrophages become more effective when complement and antibodies bind to the surface of bacteria, a process known as opsonization. Phagocytosis is more effective against opsonized bacteria. The complement system is a collection of proteins that circulate in the blood plasma and are produced and secreted by the liver. The C3 receptors, part of the complement system, and the Fc antibody receptors on the macrophage cell membrane bind to material that has been coated, and then engulf and digest it in the lysosomes through phagocytosis. Certain invasive substances, such as asbestos, tuberculosis bacilli, and toxoplasma, are resistant to lysosomal digestion. As a result, macrophages merge to create giant foreign body cells. Macrophages engage in interactions with lymphocytes through the release of interleukin-6, which promotes the transformation of B lymphocytes into plasma cells, and interleukin-1, which stimulates the division of T lymphocytes. These interactions serve to combat infections (Zhang et al., 2021).

Macrophages can produce and release various substances, including pyrogens (which cause fevers), granulocyte-macrophage colony-stimulating factor, fibroblast growth factor, transforming growth factor, and tumor necrosis factor. They can also produce connective tissue enzymes like collagenase and elastase. Macrophages are typically characterized as cells with irregular shapes, blunt cytoplasmic extensions, and oval or indented nuclei that are smaller and more intensely stained compared to fibroblasts. Macrophages can be challenging to differentiate morphologically from fibroblasts, particularly when the fibroblasts are active unless the macrophages exhibit signs of phagocytosis. The macrophages found in loose connective tissue are a component of a widespread network of mononuclear phagocytes, which also includes phagocytes in the liver (known as Kupffer cells), lungs (alveolar macrophages), serous cavities (pleural and peritoneal macrophages), nervous system (microglia), lymphatic tissue, and bone marrow. Macrophages, regardless of their location, all begin as precursor cells in the bone marrow. The monocytes in the circulation are an intermediate stage of immature macrophages.

Mast cells are found in varying quantities within loose connective tissue and tend to aggregate around small blood vessels. These cells are characterized by their large, oval shape, measuring 20 to 30 μm in diameter, and their cytoplasm filled with abundant granules. There are two distinct populations of mast cells: connective tissue mast cells and mucosal mast cells. In humans, the granules of mast cells in connective tissue are enclosed by a membrane and exhibit a distinctive tubular pattern when observed under an electron microscope. The granules consist of heparin, a powerful anticoagulant; histamine, a substance that induces contraction of smooth muscles in the bronchi and increased permeability of blood vessels; leukotriene C4 and D4, which enhances blood vessel permeability, promotes vasodilation, and cause contraction of smooth muscles in the bronchi; and eosinophil chemotactic factor. This factor serves as an attraction for eosinophils, drawing them towards the site of inflammation. Mucosal mast cells contain chondroitin sulfate in their granules, instead of heparin. Mast cells possess highly specialized membrane receptors that specifically bind to the Fc portion of IgE antibodies, which are generated in response to allergens. Both mast cell types originate from hematopoietic stem cells in bone marrow. Mast cells are particularly abundant adjacent to small blood vessels and beneath the epithelial layers of the gastrointestinal tract and respiratory system. These cells identify the presence of foreign proteins and promptly release their secretory granules to initiate a localized inflammatory response. The expulsion of granules is distinct, in that, multiple granules amalgamate and simultaneously release their contents. Mast cells can also facilitate immediate hypersensitivity reactions such as hay fever, asthma, and anaphylaxis by releasing secretory granules that function as chemical mediators. Adipocytes are specialized for the process of lipid synthesis and storage.

Adipose tissue can be formed when fat cells accumulate to the point where they crowd out other cells, either by being scattered throughout loose connective tissue or by clustering together. Every adipocyte accumulates such a significant amount of lipid that the nucleus becomes compressed to one side of the cell, while the cytoplasm forms a narrow border around a sizable central droplet of lipid. In conventional H&E sections, adipocytes appear devoid of lipid content because of lipid depletion during tissue processing, and clusters of adipocytes exhibit a honeycomb-like structure. Plasma cells are infrequent in most connective tissues, but they can be abundant in the lamina propria of the gastrointestinal tract and are found in lymphatic tissues. Plasma cells have an ovoid shape and contain small nuclei that are positioned off-center. The heterochromatin in the nuclei is organized into coarse blocks, creating a pattern resembling a "clock face." The cytoplasm appears basophilic because it contains a large amount of GER. The negative Golgi image, which is a lightly stained region of cytoplasm, typically appears next to one side of the nucleus and corresponds to the location of the Golgi complex. Plasma cells generate immunoglobulins, also known as antibodies, which play a crucial role in defending the body against infections. Several acidophilic inclusions can be observed in the cytoplasm of certain plasma cells. Plasma cells are a specialized variant of the B-lymphocyte. Leukocytes migrate into connective tissues from the blood in varying numbers through a process called diapedesis. Neutrophils are a specific type of white blood cell that can be identified by their nucleus, which is divided into lobes. In this cellular subtype, the granules are described as neutrophilic, although they appear faintly pink when stained in sections (i.e., acidophilic). The cells exhibit a strong tendency to engulf small particles and bacteria and are particularly abundant at locations where infection is present. Neutrophils possess antioxidants capable of eliminating potentially harmful peroxides produced during lysosomal activity. Upon activation in tissues, neutrophils have a short lifespan and undergo cell death. They constitute the primary cellular constituent of the substance known as pus.

Eosinophils possess lobed nuclei and exhibit larger, more spherical, and more distinct cytoplasmic granules compared to neutrophils. The granules exhibit a strong affinity for acid dyes, such as eosin, resulting in intense staining. Every eosinophil possesses surface receptors for IgE. These cells possess the ability to engulf specific molecules and exhibit a particular attraction towards antigen-antibody complexes. Their population grows due to allergic or parasitic diseases. Eosinophils are drawn to the locations where histamine is released by the eosinophilic chemotactic factor of anaphylaxis (ECF-A), and their cytoplasmic granules contain enzymes that can degrade histamine. Eosinophils also secrete major basic protein, which amplifies the antibody-mediated eradication of the larvae of certain helminthic parasites. Lymphocytes are a type of mononuclear leukocytes, which are characterized by having a single, round, nonlobed nucleus. These cells are the tiniest among those that move into connective tissues and have a diameter of approximately 7 μm. These cells are a component of the immune defense system and have the ability to generate B lymphocytes, which produce antibodies, or T lymphocytes, which release nonspecific factors that eliminate foreign cells. B and T lymphocytes cannot be differentiated based on their appearance using standard H&E preparations. In normal connective tissue, their population is limited, but they significantly multiply in regions with chronic inflammation. Monocytes are the precursors of tissue macrophages present in the bloodstream. Once these cells have migrated into connective tissue, it becomes challenging, if not impossible, to differentiate them from macrophages (Zheng et al., 2019).

Upon exiting the blood vessels and transforming into macrophages, monocytes undergo specific molecular programming that is influenced by the particular microenvironment (such as the spleen, lung, or brain) in which they are located. Certain macrophages possess antigen-presenting capabilities, and these specialized macrophages constitute a group of cells known as antigen-presenting cells.

These macrophages engulf antigens that originate from within the body and break them down into smaller fragments called antigen peptides. Subsequently, these fragments are displayed on the surface of the macrophage along with class II major histocompatibility complex (MHC). $CD4^{+}$ helper T lymphocytes recognize the presented antigen peptide fragment and subsequently stimulate B lymphocyte differentiation.

2.2.3. Subtypes of Loose Connective Tissue

Mesenchyme, a pliable and porous tissue, functions as a filler between developing structures of the embryo. It is composed of dispersed star-shaped and elongated cells surrounded by shapeless material with thin, scattered fibers. These cells possess diverse developmental capacities and can generate any connective tissue type. While the existence of mesenchymal cells in adults has been suggested to explain adult connective tissue growth, fibroblasts, with their ability for consecutive cell divisions, may also serve this function (Zheng et al., 2019).

Mucoid tissue, similar in cellular composition to mesenchyme, is found in various regions of the embryo, notably in Wharton's jelly of the umbilical cord. It consists of stellate fibroblasts with elongated processes connecting adjacent cells, embedded in a soft, gelatinous intercellular substance containing delicate collagen fibers. The fiber content increases with fetal age. Unlike mesenchyme, mucoid tissue lacks developmental capacity.

Areolar connective tissue, sparsely organized and widely distributed, consists of collagen, reticular, and elastic fibers embedded in a thin, almost liquid-like matrix. It forms the stroma, uniting organs and their components, and coils around the elongated axes of flexible tubular structures like gland ducts, the digestive system, and blood vessels.

2.2.3.1. Adipose Tissue

Adipose tissue distinguishes itself from other connective tissue in two ways: fat cells are the main component, rather than intercellular substances, and unlike other connective tissue cells, each fat cell is enclosed by its own basal lamina. The reticular and collagenous fibers surround each fat cell, creating a delicate framework that houses multiple capillaries.

Adipose tissue can be classified into two types: white fat and brown fat. White adipose tissue is the predominant type of fat and is primarily located in the subcutaneous tissue (where it forms the panniculus adiposus), omenta, mesenteries, pararenal tissue, and bone marrow. White fat is a highly vascularized tissue that also harbors numerous nerve fibers originating from the autonomic nervous system. White fat cells contain a single, large lipid droplet, which is why it is commonly known as unilocular fat. The lipid droplet consists of glycerol esters and fatty acids. The constituents of the fat droplet undergo continuous change and are not enduring entities. Adipocytes possess receptors for insulin, thyroid hormone, glucocorticoids, and norepinephrine, which regulate the release and absorption of lipids. White adipose tissue functions as a reservoir for surplus calories that exceed the body's energy requirements. It can be utilized to generate energy when needed or serve as a **source** of raw materials, such as for the synthesis of steroid hormones. Additionally, it serves as an insulating barrier to retain body heat, functions as a packing material, and creates shock-absorbing cushions in the palms, soles, and around the eyes. Adipocytes release a hormone known as leptin, which functions to suppress appetite. The mechanism behind this action is believed to be facilitated by satiety centers located in the hypothalamic region of the brain, where leptin receptors are present. Brown adipose tissue is found in various species and is particularly abundant in hibernating animals and newborn humans. Brown adipose tissue exhibits a limited distribution, primarily found in the interscapular and inguinal regions. The presence of a significant amount of cytochrome enzymes is responsible for the brown or tan color. The cells exhibit spherical nuclei, and the cytoplasm contains numerous tiny lipid droplets, hence, the term multilocular fat. The mitochondria in these cells are more abundant and larger compared to the mitochondria found in white fat cells. Every individual brown fat cell is directly innervated by the sympathetic nervous system. Upon emerging from hibernation in animals or after birth in the case of humans, the lipid stored in brown fat undergoes rapid oxidation, generating heat and releasing substances like glycerol that are utilized by other tissues. The energy generated by mitochondria in brown adipose tissue is dissipated as thermal energy instead of being stored as adenosine triphosphate (ATP). Due to its higher vascularity compared to white fat, brown fat generates heat that raises the blood temperature significantly, resulting in an overall increase in body temperature.

2.2.3.2. Reticular Connective Tissue

Reticular connective tissue is distinguished by its cellular framework, which is observed in lymphatic tissues and bone marrow. Reticular cells have a star-like shape, and their processes extend along the reticular fibers to establish contact with nearby cells. The cytoplasm appears pale and diminished in intensity, while the large nucleus exhibits a low staining intensity. The reticular cell functions analogously to the fibroblast found in other types of connective tissues. Its primary role is to generate and sustain the reticular fibers, which are indistinguishable from those present in loose connective tissue.

2.2.4. Dense Connective Tissue

Dense connective tissue is distinguished from loose connective tissue primarily by its higher fiber concentration and lower presence of cellular and amorphous components. There are two identified types: dense irregular and dense regular. Dense irregular connective tissue is composed of a large amount of thick collagenous bundles that are tightly interwoven into a compact network. Within the collagen fibers lies a vast network of elastic fibers. The dermis of the skin serves as an illustration of dense irregular connective tissue. Dense regular connective tissue is characterized by a high concentration of collagen fibers that are organized in bundles with a consistent and orderly pattern. The arrangement of the collagen fibers is a direct reflection of the mechanical requirements of the tissue. In structures such as tendons, aponeuroses, and ligaments, their alignment is parallel to the direction of force application. Fibroblasts are the predominant cells that are arranged in parallel rows alongside the collagen fiber bundles (Zhou et al., 2019).

A Closer Look

Glandular Epithelium

Glandular epithelium is a specialized type of epithelial tissue that plays a critical role in the secretion of various substances in the body. Composed of closely packed cells, this tissue forms the functional units of glands—structures responsible for producing and releasing hormones, enzymes, mucus, and other important secretions. Glandular epithelium can be categorized into two main types: endocrine and exocrine glands. Endocrine glands, such as the thyroid and adrenal glands, release their secretions directly into the bloodstream, affecting distant target organs. In contrast, exocrine glands, such as sweat and salivary glands, secrete their products onto epithelial surfaces through ducts. This distinction is crucial, as it underscores the varied roles that glandular epithelium plays in maintaining homeostasis and facilitating communication within the body.

Structural Characteristics

The structural characteristics of glandular epithelium are tailored to its function in secretion. The cells in this tissue type often exhibit a cuboidal or columnar shape, which enhances their secretory capacity. These cells possess numerous organelles, particularly the rough endoplasmic reticulum and Golgi apparatus, which are essential for synthesizing and packaging proteins—key components of many secretions. Additionally, glandular epithelial cells may have specialized modifications, such as microvilli or cilia, that facilitate absorption or transport. The basement membrane, a thin layer of extracellular matrix, supports the epithelium and provides a barrier that separates the glandular tissue from underlying connective tissue. This structural arrangement allows for efficient nutrient exchange while protecting the delicate glandular cells from mechanical stress and pathogens.

Functional Significance

The functional significance of glandular epithelium extends beyond mere secretion; it plays a vital role in regulating numerous physiological processes. Endocrine glands release hormones directly into the bloodstream, which serve as chemical messengers to regulate metabolism, growth, and development. For instance, the pancreas produces insulin and glucagon, hormones that are critical for glucose metabolism and energy balance. Similarly, the adrenal glands produce cortisol, which helps manage stress responses. On the other hand, exocrine glands, such as the pancreas (which functions as both endocrine and exocrine), secrete digestive enzymes into the gastrointestinal tract, facilitating the breakdown and absorption of nutrients. Furthermore, glands such as sweat and sebaceous glands help regulate body temperature and maintain skin health, demonstrating the multifaceted roles of glandular epithelium in maintaining homeostasis and overall health.

Pathological Considerations

Understanding glandular epithelium also involves recognizing its susceptibility to various pathological conditions. Abnormalities in glandular function can lead to a range of disorders, including hyperplasia, neoplasia, and autoimmune conditions. For example, hyperplasia of glandular epithelium may occur in response to hormonal stimulation, leading to conditions such as goiter, where the thyroid gland enlarges. Conversely, neoplastic changes can result in benign or malignant tumors, which may disrupt normal glandular function and lead to systemic effects. Autoimmune diseases, such as Graves' disease, can result in the immune system attacking glandular tissue, leading to dysfunction. Furthermore, environmental factors, such as exposure to toxins or endocrine disruptors, can adversely affect glandular epithelium, highlighting the need for ongoing research to understand these impacts. Overall, the study of glandular epithelium is crucial not only for its role in normal physiology but also for its implications in disease and health management.

Summary

The epithelium is a specialized tissue that lines the surfaces and cavities of organs and structures throughout the body. It plays a critical role in protection, secretion, absorption, and filtration. Epithelial cells are closely packed and can be classified based on their shape (squamous, cuboidal, columnar) and the number of layers (simple or stratified). This tissue serves as a barrier against mechanical injury, pathogens, and fluid loss while facilitating essential functions such as nutrient exchange and hormone secretion in glands.

General connective tissues, on the other hand, provide structural support, connect different tissues, and play a key role in tissue repair and immune responses. These tissues are characterized by a matrix consisting of fibers (collagen, elastic, and reticular) and a ground substance that varies in consistency. Connective tissue types include loose connective tissue, which provides cushioning and flexibility, and dense connective tissue, which offers strength and durability, particularly in tendons and ligaments. Specialized forms like adipose tissue store energy, and cartilage and bone provide rigidity and structure. Together, the epithelium and connective tissues form the foundational components of organs, enabling them to function properly. While the epithelium covers and protects, the underlying connective tissues provide strength, elasticity, and a medium for nutrient and waste exchange. Their coordination is essential for maintaining the structural integrity and physiological balance in tissues and organs.

References

1. Annese, T.; Tamma, R.; Bozza, M.; Zito, A.; Ribatti, D. Autocrine/paracrine loop between SCF+/c-Kit+ mast cells promotes cutaneous melanoma progression. Front. Immunol. 2022, 13, 794974.
2. Baccari, G.C.; Pinelli, C.; Santillo, A.; Menucci, S.; Rastogi, R.K. Mast cells in nonmammalian vertebrates: An overview. Int. Rev. Cell Mol. Biol. 2011, 290, 1–53. Boisset, J.C.; van Cappellen, W.; Andrieu-Soler, C.; Galjart, N.; Dzierzak, E.; Robin, C. In vivo imaging of haematopoietic cells emerging from the mouse aortic endothelium. Nature 2010, 464, 116–120.
3. Carmeliet, P. Angiogenesis in health and disease. Nat. Med. 2003, 9, 653–660.
4. Cavalcante, M.C.M.; Allodi, S.; Valente, A.P.; Straus, A.H.; Takahashi, H.K.; Mourao, P.A.S.; Pawao, M.S.G. Occurrence of heparin in the invertebrate Styela plicata (Tunicata) is restricted to cell layers facing the outside environment: An ancient role in defense? J. Biol. Chem. 2000, 275, 36189–36196.
5. Chia, S.L.; Kapoor, S.; Carvalho, C.; Bajenoff, M.; Gentek, R. Mast cell ontogeny: From fetal development to life-long health and disease. Immunol. Rev. 2023, 315, 31–53.
6. Crivellato, E.; Travan, L.; Ribatti, D. The phylogenetic profile of mast cells. Methods Med. Biol. 2015, 1220, 11–27.
7. Dahlin, J.S.; Maurer, M.; Metcalfe, D.D.; Pejler, G.; Sagi-Eisenberg, R.; Nilsson, G. The ingenious mast cell: Contemporary insights into mast cell behavior and function. Allergy 2022, 77, 83–99.
8. Dileepan, K.N.; Raveendran, V.V.; Sharma, R.; Abraham, H.; Barua, R.; Singh, V.; Sharma, R.; Sharma, M. Mast cell-mediated immune regulation in health and disease. Front. Med. 2023, 10, 1213320.

9. Dudeck, A.; Köberle, M.; Goldmann, O.; Meyer, N.; Dudeck, J.; Lemmens, S.; Rohde, M.; Roldan, N.G.; Dietze-Schwonberg, K.; Orinska, Z.; et al. Mast cells as protectors of health. J. Allergy Clin. Immunol. 2019, 144, S4–S18.

10. Dwyer, D.F.; Barrett, N.A.; Austen, K.F. Expression profiling of constitutive mast cells reveals a unique identity within the immune system. Nat. Immunol. 2016, 17, 878–887.

11. Galli, S.J.; Gaudenzio, N.; Tsai, M. Mast cells in inflammation and disease: Recent progress and ongoing concerns. Ann. Rev. Immunol. 2020, 38, 49–77.

12. Gentek, R.; Ghigo, C.; Hoeffel, G.; Bulle, M.J.; Msallam, R.; Gautier, G.; Launay, P.; Chen, J.; Ginhoux, F.; Bejenoff, M. Hemogenic endothelial fate mapping reveals dual developmental origin of mast cells. Immunity 2018, 48, 1160–1171.

13. Hellman, L.; Akula, S.; Fu, Z.; Wernersson, S. Mast cell and basophil granule proteases—In vivo targets and function. Front. Imunnol. 2022, 13, 918305.

14. Krystel-Whittemore, M.; Dileepan, K.N.; Wood, J.G. Mast cell: A multi-functional master cell. Front. Immunol. 2016, 6, 620.

15. Li, Z.; Liu, S.; Xu, J.; Zhang, X.; Han, D.; Liu, J.; Xia, M.; Yi, L.; Shen, Q.; Lu, L.; et al. Adult connective tissue-resident mast cells originate from late erythro-myeloid progenitors. Immunity 2018, 49, 640–653.

16. Marshall, J.S.; Jawdat, D.M. Mast cells in innate immunity. J. Allergy Clin. Immunol. 2004, 114, 21–27.

17. Maurer, M.; Köberle, M.; Metz, M.; Biedermann, T. Mast cells: Promoters of health and modulators of disease. J. Allergy Clin. Immunol. 2019, 144 (Suppl. S4), S1–S3.

18. Meyer, N.; Zenclussen, A.C. Mast cells—Good guys with a bad image? Am. J. Reprod. Immunol. 2018, 80, e13002.

19. Molderings, G.J.; Afrin, L.B. A survey of the currently known mast cell mediators with potential relevance for therapy of mast cell-induced symptoms. Naunyn Schmiedebergs Arch. Pharmacol. 2023, 396, 2881–2891.

20. Moon, T.C.; Befus, A.D.; Kulka, M. Mast cell mediators: Their differential release and the secretory pathways involved. Front. Immunol. 2014, 5, 569.

21. Norrby, K. Do mast cells contribute to the continued survival of vertebrates? APMIS 2022, 130, 618–624.

22. Tauber, M.; Basso, L.; Martin, J.; Bostan, L.; Pinto, M.M.; Thierry, G.R.; Houmadi, R.; Serhan, N.; Loste, A.; Blériot, C.; et al. Landscape of mast cell populations across organs in mice and humans. J. Exp. Med. 2023, 220, e20230570.

23. Weimerhaus, M.; Carvalho, C.; Rignault, R.; Waeckel-Enee, E.; Dussiot, M.; van Endert, P.; Maciel, T.T.; Hermine, O. Mast cell-mediated inflammation relies on insulin-regulated aminopeptidase controlling cytokine export from the Golgi. J. Allergy Clin. Immunol. 2023, 151, 1595–1608.

24. Weller, P.; Grabbe, J.; Gibbs, B.; Zauberbier, T.; Henz, B.M. Human mast cells produce and differentially express both soluble and membrane-bound stem cell factor. Scand. J. Immunol. 1999, 49, 495–500.

25. Wong, G.W.; Zhou, L.; Kimata, K.; Lam, B.K.; Satoh, N.; Stevens, R.L. Ancient origin of mast cells. Biochem. Biophys. Res. Commun. 2014, 451, 314–318.

Chapter 3

SPECIAL CONNECTIVE TISSUE

Contents

Introduction

Special connective tissues are a unique category within the broader class of connective tissues, distinguished by their specialized functions and unique histological characteristics. These tissues play crucial roles in supporting, connecting, and protecting various organs and structures in the body. Unlike other connective tissues, special connective tissues often have a more specific and defined organization, reflecting their specialized functions. Histologically, special connective tissues exhibit distinct features that set them apart from other connective tissue types. For example, they may contain specialized cells, such as chondrocytes in cartilage or osteocytes in bone, which are responsible for the tissue's unique properties. The extracellular matrix of special connective tissues is often highly organized and may include specific components such as collagen fibers, elastic fibers, and ground substances, all of which contribute to the tissue's specialized functions. Understanding the histology of special connective tissues is essential for appreciating their roles in the body and their contributions to overall health and function. This knowledge is particularly relevant in fields such as anatomy, physiology, and pathology, where an in-depth understanding of tissue structure and function is crucial (Alvarez-Nemegyei et al., 2016).

Orientation and Directional Terms

Term	Definition	Illustration
Cartilage	A flexible connective tissue that provides support and cushioning in joints, forms structures such as the nose and ears, and is involved in the growth and development of bones.	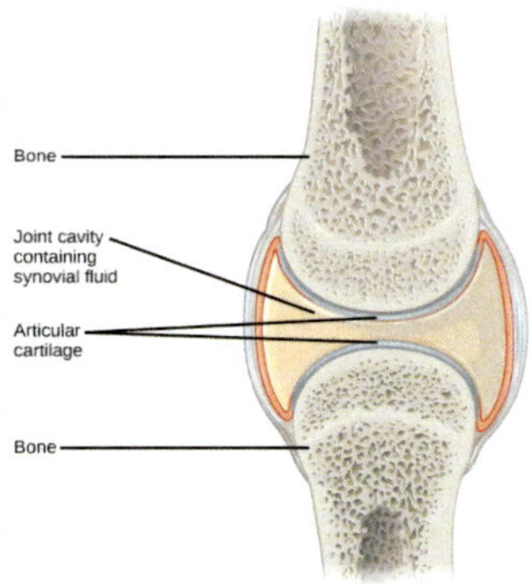
Erythrocytes	Also known as red blood cells, these are the most abundant cells in the blood, responsible for transporting oxygen from the lungs to the body tissues and carrying carbon dioxide back to the lungs.	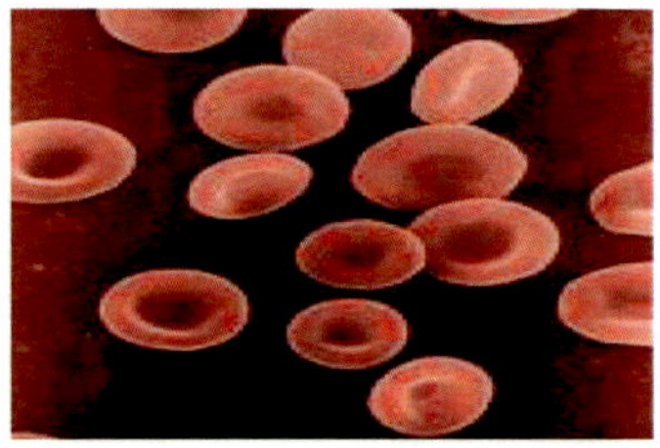
Leukocytes	Also known as white blood cells, these cells are part of the immune system and help defend the body against infections and foreign substances. There are various types, including neutrophils, lymphocytes, and monocytes.	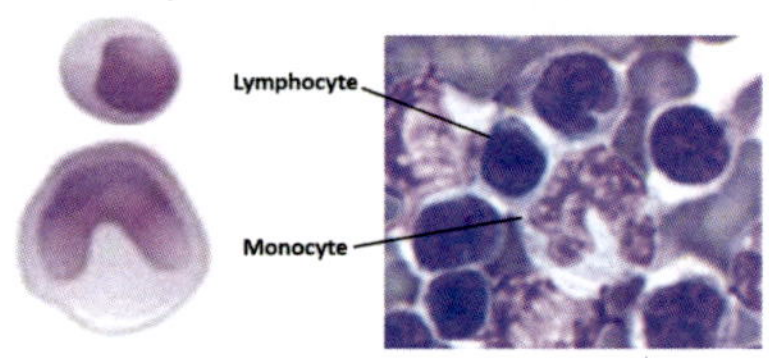
Bone Marrow	A soft, spongy tissue found in the center of bones, responsible for the production of blood cells, including erythrocytes, leukocytes, and platelets, as well as playing a role in the immune response.	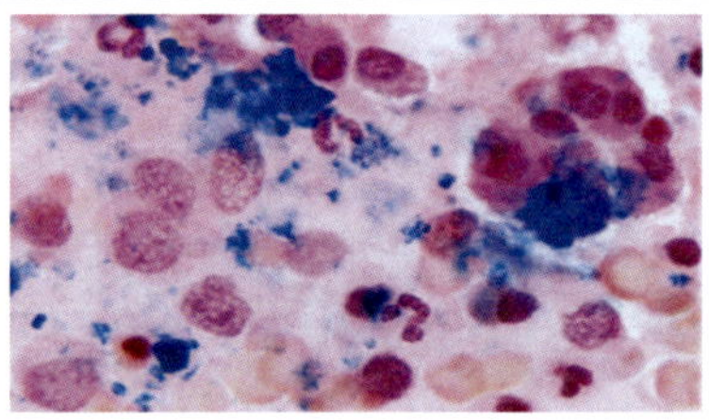
Monocytes	A type of white blood cell that is part of the immune system; they differentiate into macrophages and dendritic cells, which help engulf and digest pathogens and present antigens to T cells.	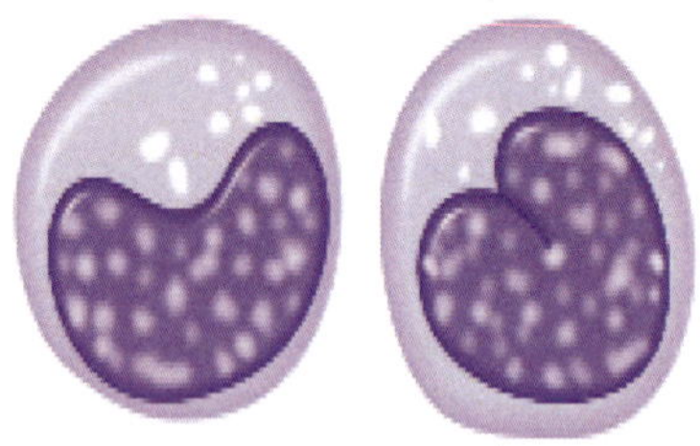

3.1. Cartilage, Bone, and Joints

3.1.1. Cartilage

Cartilage, despite its supportive function, consists solely of the typical components found in connective tissue, including cells, fibers, and ground substance. The firm consistency and ability of cartilage to withstand compression and shearing forces are attributed to the ground substance. The tensile strength and elasticity of the ground substance are enhanced by the presence of collagen and elastic fibers. The fibers and ground substance combine to create the matrix of cartilage. Cartilage is distinct from other types of connective tissues because it does not have nerves, blood vessels, or lymphatic vessels. Instead, it relies solely on the diffusion of materials from nearby blood vessels in adjacent tissues for nourishment. Despite its relative rigidity, the cartilage matrix contains a significant amount of water (approximately 75%) and is highly permeable, allowing even relatively large particles to pass through. The classification of cartilage into hyaline, elastic, and fibrous types is determined by variations in the quantity and composition of fibers present in the matrix.

3.1.1.1. Hyaline Cartilage

Hyaline cartilage is the predominant form of cartilage and is found in the costal cartilages, articular cartilages of joints, and cartilages of the nose, larynx, trachea, and bronchi. It is located in the distal ends of elongated bones. During fetal development, most of the skeletal structure is initially formed as hyaline cartilage. Chondrocytes, which are the cells of cartilage, are located in lacunae, which are small spaces distributed throughout the matrix. The cells typically adopt the shape of the lacunae in which they are enclosed. The cells and their lacunae within the cartilage typically have a rounded shape when observed deep within, while at the surface, they have an elliptical shape with the long axis aligned parallel to the surface. Chondrocytes frequently form compact clusters known as isogenous groups, which are comprised of the descendants of a single cell (Alvarez-Nemegyei et al., 2020).

During the typical preparations, the cells exhibit an asymmetrical contour and seem to have contracted and moved away from the walls of the lacunae. Electron microscopy demonstrates that every cell occupies the lacunar space entirely and extends brief processes into the adjacent matrix, while adjacent cells do not contact each other. The nucleus is typically spherical or ellipsoidal in shape and contains one or more nucleoli. The cytoplasm exhibits the typical organelles, along with lipid and glycogen inclusions. The Golgi complex and endoplasmic reticulum exhibit significant development in growing chondrocytes. The matrix in fresh cartilage and routine histologic sections appears homogeneous due to the matching refractive index of the ground substance and the collagen fibers. The collagen in hyaline cartilage is typically found in the form of a network of thin individual fibrils. The arrangement of these fibrils can have different periodicities or may even lack a distinct pattern. Type II collagen is classified as collagen in cartilage, and it seems to have a lower degree of polymerization compared to collagen in other tissues. The primary components of the ground substance are proteoglycans, with the specific glycosaminoglycans found in cartilage being chondroitin-4- and chondroitin-6-sulfate, keratan sulfate, and a small quantity of hyaluronic acid. Proteoglycans are accountable for the basophilic characteristics of the ground substance. Chondronectin, a glycoprotein found in the ground substance, facilitates the attachment of type II collagen to chondrocytes. Chondrocalcin, a glycoprotein that binds to calcium, has also been found in the ground substance of hyaline cartilage. The matrix surrounding each lacuna and isogenous group exhibits a greater affinity for staining compared to other areas, resulting in the formation of the territorial matrix. The areas between the stained regions have a lower density and are referred to as the interterritorial matrix. The perichondrium is a specialized connective tissue sheath that surrounds hyaline cartilage, except for its free surfaces found in articular cartilage. The outer layers of the perichondrium are composed of highly vascularized, dense, irregular connective tissue that contains elastic and collagen fibers as well as fibroblasts. The perichondrium, which is located adjacent to the cartilage, has a higher concentration of cells and smoothly transitions into the cartilage without being easily noticed. The thin collagen fibrils of the cartilage matrix merge with the broader, type I collagen fibrils of the perichondrium. The perichondrial cells located next to the cartilage have the ability to generate new cartilage (Alvarez-Nemegyei et al., 2020).

3.1.1.2. Elastic Cartilage

Elastic cartilage is a type of hyaline cartilage that is distinguished by the presence of branched elastic fibers within its matrix. Collagen fibers similar to those found in hyaline cartilage are also present, but they are concealed. The elastic fibers in the cartilage are densely packed and create a mesh that makes it difficult to see the ground substance. However, beneath the perichondrium, the fibers form a looser network and are connected to the fibers of the perichondrium. The chondrocytes resemble those found in hyaline cartilage and produce elastic and collagen fibers. Elastic cartilage is characterized by greater flexibility compared to hyaline cartilage. It is primarily located in the external ear, auditory tube, epiglottis, and certain smaller laryngeal cartilages.

3.1.1.3. Fibrous Cartilage

Fibrous cartilage, also known as fibrocartilage, serves as an intermediary between dense connective tissue and cartilage. The structure comprises of conventional cartilage cells surrounded by lacunae, with a limited quantity of ground substance found in close proximity to the cells. The chondrocytes are positioned individually, in pairs, or in small rows amidst bundles of tightly packed collagen fibers. These collagen fibers are composed of unit fibrils that exhibit the characteristic 64-nanometer banding pattern found in type I collagen. Fibrous cartilage is characterized by the absence of a perichondrium and its integration with hyaline cartilage, bone, or dense fibrous connective tissue. It is present in the intervertebral discs, certain articular cartilages, the symphysis pubis, and areas where certain tendons attach to bone.

3.1.2. Bone

Bone is a type of connective tissue that is specifically adapted for providing support. Nevertheless, within bone tissue, the matrix undergoes mineralization, resulting in the formation of a compact, rigid material that possesses exceptional tensile, weight-bearing, and compression strength. Although bone is strong and rigid, it is a dynamic and living tissue that undergoes constant turnover, renewal, and reforming throughout an individual's life.

3.1.2.1. Macroscopic Structure

The different types of bone, namely cancellous and compact, can be easily distinguished. Cancellous bone, also known as spongy bone, is composed of irregular bars or trabeculae of bone that branch and merge to create a three-dimensional, interwoven network of bony rods. This network forms a large system of interconnected spaces filled with bone marrow during life. The trabeculae of spongy bone in weight-bearing lower limb bones are not randomly arranged but rather follow a precisely organized pattern along lines of compression and tension stress. The arrangement of the trabeculae in a strut-like manner enhances the structural integrity of these bones. Compact bone is characterized by its dense structure, appearing as a solid and uninterrupted mass that lacks visible spaces when observed without magnification. The distinction between the two types of bone is not clearly defined, and they blend together. A long bone typically consists of a hollow cylinder of compact bone known as the shaft or diaphysis, which encloses a spacious central area called the marrow cavity. The epiphyses, which are located at the ends of the long bones, primarily comprise cancellous bone that is encased by a thin layer of compact bone. The small interconnected spaces within the spongy bone are directly connected to the marrow cavity of the shaft. The periosteum is a dense irregular fibroelastic connective tissue that covers bone, except for articular surfaces and areas where tendons and ligaments attach. The endosteum, which is thinner and less fibrous than the periosteum, lines the marrow cavity of the diaphysis, and the spaces within the spongy bone. Both the periosteum and endosteum possess the capacity to generate new bone when appropriately stimulated. Flat bones, such as those found in the skull, are composed of both compact and spongy bone tissue. The inner and outer plates, also known as tables, are composed of dense layers of cortical bone, while the gap between the plates is filled with trabecular bone known as the diploë (Amine et al., 2011).

3.1.2.2. Microscopic Structure

One essential feature of bone is the organization of its mineralized matrix into layers or plates known as lamellae. The lacunae, which are small and ovoid spaces, are evenly distributed within and between the lamellae. Each lacuna contains a single bone cell or osteocyte. Canaliculi, which are slender tubules, extend outward from each lacuna and penetrate the lamellae to connect with the canaliculi of neighboring lacunae. Therefore, gaps are connected by a vast network of narrow channels. The lamellae in compact bone exhibit three different configurations. Most of these units are organized in a concentric manner around a central longitudinal space, resulting in cylindrical structures that align parallel to the bone's long axis. Osteons, also known as Haversian systems, constitute the fundamental structural components of bone. Osteons exhibit size variation and are composed of 8 to 15 concentric lamellae encircling a spacious region containing blood vessels. Longitudinal sections of an osteon reveal bony matrix plates that are aligned parallel to the vascular channel's slitlike space. Compact bone consists of multiple osteons arranged parallel to each other throughout its thickness. Osteons exhibit a non-uniform trajectory along the length of the bone and have the potential to bifurcate. Additional lamellae manifest as angular and irregular clusters of lamellar bone, occupying the gaps between osteons. The term for these structures is interstitial lamellae. Osteons and interstitial lamellae are delineated by a refractile line known as the cement line, composed of a modified matrix. Canaliculi do not cross cement lines. Several lamellae encircle the entire bone just beneath the periosteum, which is the outer surface of the bone. A comparable yet less advanced arrangement of lamellae exists on the inner surface, positioned directly below the endosteum. The two systems of lamellae are the outer and inner circumferential lamellae, respectively. Figure 3.1 illustrates the lamellar organization of compact bone.

The Haversian canals are the longitudinally oriented channels found at the center of osteons. These structures establish communication through diagonal branches and transverse connections known as Volkmann's canals, which penetrate the bone from the inner and outer surfaces. Volkmann's canals lack the presence of concentric lamellae, unlike Haversian canals. Volkmann's canals connect the blood vessels in the Haversian canals with the vessels of the marrow cavity and periosteum. The nutritional requirements of compact bone are fulfilled by an extensive and uninterrupted network of vascular channels. The canaliculi that are next to a Haversian canal connect to the perivascular space, and the canalicular system allows all the lacunae within that osteon to communicate with the canal. Spongy bone exhibits a lamellar structure, similar to compact bone, but it typically lacks blood vessels passing through it (Bechtold et al., 2010). Thus, spongy bone, which consists of irregular rods of lamellar bone, generally has a scarcity or absence of osteons. there is a specific number of lamellae that represent a critical distance, beyond which the canalicular system is unable to support the survival of osteocytes. These requirements are fulfilled within trabeculae that are only a few lamellae wide, as the canalicular system is connected to the perivascular area of the marrow cavity that surrounds all trabeculae. Trabeculae that surpass this crucial distance, similar to compact bone, must possess Haversian systems in order to fulfill their nutritional requirements.

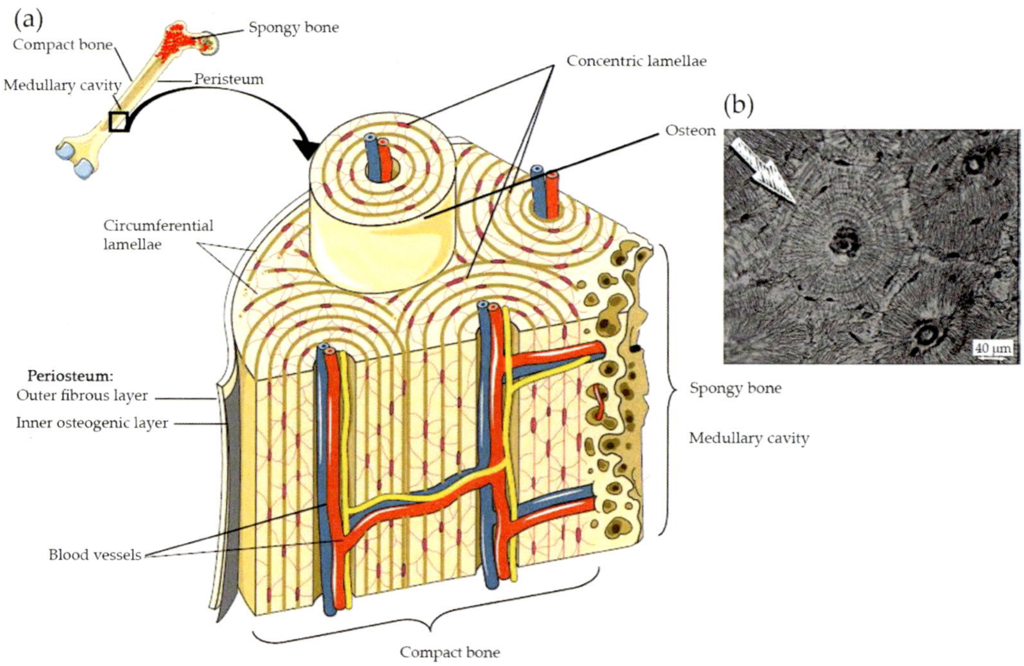

Figure 3.1. *Illustration depicting a cross-sectional view of compact bone.*

Source: *https://www.researchgate.net/profile/Bilal-Osta/publication/278382914/figure/fig1/AS:413937662218240@1475701838049/Structure-of-compact-bone-a-Cross-sectional-view-of-compact-bone-shows-the-basic.png.*

3.1.2.3. Periosteum and Endosteum

The outer layer of the periosteum is primarily composed of a dense irregular connective tissue that has a low number of cells. It contains a large amount of collagen fibers, a small number of elastic fibers, and a network of blood vessels. These blood vessels extend into Volkmann's canals. The innermost layers of the periosteum, which are in close proximity to the bone, are characterized by a higher number of cells with the ability to generate bone tissue. Additionally, these layers are composed of connective tissue that is more loosely organized. During the process of bone development, collagen fibers from the periosteum become trapped in the circumferential lamellae and create Sharpey's fibers. These fibers serve to attach the periosteum to the underlying bone. The endosteum covers all the internal cavities of the bone, such as the marrow spaces in the diaphysis and epiphysis, as well as the Haversian and Volkmann's canals. The structure is composed of a singular layer of flat to cube-shaped cells, accompanied by a limited and fluctuating amount of reinforcing reticular and collagen fibers. Like the cells in the inner layer of the periosteum, the cells in the endosteum also possess the ability to generate bone tissue.

3.1.2.4. Cells of Bone

Osteocytes are the predominant cells present in fully developed bone and assume the form of the lacunae in which they reside. Osteoblasts, which are cells that form bones, are distinct from them. Osteocytes do not exist in isolation within their lacunae, but instead maintain extensive communication with adjacent osteocytes. The cell bodies have delicate cytoplasmic processes that extend and connect with processes from neighboring cells through the canaliculi. The apposed cells create communicating junctions at their points of contact. An extremely thin layer of a non-mineralized matrix acts as a barrier between the cell and its processes and the walls of the lacunae and canaliculi. This layer facilitates the diffusion of materials throughout the bony matrix. Osteocytes possess the typical cellular organelles, although the Golgi apparatus is relatively inconspicuous, and there is a limited presence of ribosomes, mitochondria, and endoplasmic reticulum. While the osteocyte may not actively produce protein, it is not metabolically inactive. It is accountable for preserving bone, actively participates in controlling calcium levels in bodily fluids, and is involved in the breakdown of bone. Large multinucleate giant cells are found in regions where bone resorption is occurring (Bechtold and Roth, 2009). Osteoclasts are commonly found in shallow depressions on the surface of the bone, particularly on the endosteal surface. These hollow spaces are referred to as Howship's lacunae. Despite the presence of up to 30 nuclei, the individual nuclei within the cell do not exhibit any abnormal characteristics and are typically found in the region of the cell that is farthest from the bone. The cytoplasm, typically exhibiting a mild to moderate acidic nature, contains multiple Golgi complexes and pairs of centrioles, as well as numerous mitochondria and lysosomes. Osteoclasts possess a distinctive surface modification known as a ruffled border, which is located next to the bone. Osteoclasts that do not have a ruffled border do not engage in bone resorption. The ruffled border is made up of intricate creases and gaps that touch the surface of the bone. The plasmalemma of the ruffled border is covered by tiny, bristle-like projections. There is a distinct area next to the ruffled border that contains numerous actin filaments, and mitochondria tend to gather in close proximity. The outermost cell surface exhibits a sleek and even shape. The cytoplasm of active osteoclasts exhibits a foamy appearance as a result of the presence of numerous vacuoles that contain fragments of collagen and matrix crystals. The plasmalemma of the ruffled border contains a significant amount of sodium/potassium ATPase and carbonic anhydrase enzymes, which are responsible for the production of hydrogen ions. The space below the fringed edge is isolated by the osteoclast and an acidic environment is established to facilitate the breakdown of the mineral part of the bone structure. Furthermore, the osteoclasts secrete lysosomal enzymes, specifically β-glucuronidase and aryl sulfatase, to degrade the proteoglycans found in the bone matrix. Additionally, they utilize collagenase to break down type 1 collagen. Osteoclasts are formed through the fusion of monocytes that have migrated from the bloodstream. Osteoclast activity is indirectly enhanced by parathyroid hormone and vitamin D, which stimulate osteoblasts to secrete Interleukin-1.

This leads to an increase in bone resorption and a rise in blood calcium levels. Osteoclasts possess calcitonin receptors, and the presence of calcitonin diminishes their activity, resulting in a decrease in blood calcium levels (Bechtold and Roth, 2009).

3.1.2.5. Matrix of Bone

The primary composition of bone is the bone matrix, which is composed of collagen fibers, ground substance, and inorganic components. The ground substance contains proteoglycans that are like those found in cartilage, but they are present in lower quantities. The bone contains glycosaminoglycans such as chondroitin sulfate, keratin sulfate, and hyaluronic acid. Osteocalcin and osteopontin are glycoproteins found in bone that have the function of binding calcium salts to the collagenous part of the matrix. Osteonectin, a glycoprotein found in bone, assists in the attachment of bone cells to the matrix. Bone has a modest level of hydration, containing approximately 7% water.

The majority of the bone matrix is composed of approximately 90% type I collagen. When long bones, like the fibula, undergo demineralization, they maintain their original shape and size because of the significant presence of collagen. However, they become highly pliable or bendable. They can be knotted. The collagen unit fibrils create an intricate internal network that serves as a foundation for the deposition of bone minerals. In mature bone, collagen is deposited in a highly organized manner. Within each lamella, the individual fibrils are aligned parallel to each other and follow a helical path around the Haversian canal. The pitch of the helix varies between adjacent lamellae, causing the collagen unit fibrils of adjacent lamellae to be positioned perpendicular to each other. The strength of bone is derived from the highly organized arrangement of collagen unit fibrils. The inorganic component of bone, comprising calcium phosphate, citrate ions, and bicarbonate ions, along with trace amounts of calcium and magnesium fluoride, is responsible for its rigidity. The minerals are formed as hydroxyapatite crystals ($Ca_{10}(PO_4)_6(OH)_2$), which consist of calcium and phosphate hydroxides. These crystals are found both on and inside the osteoid collagen (type 1) at consistent intervals along the fibers.

3.1.3. Joints

Juxtaposed bones are fused together at articulations, which exhibit significant diversity in their anatomy and purpose. Certain joints exhibit such a high degree of interlocking between the articulating bones that they become incapable of movement, whereas other joints possess a joint structure that allows for a broad spectrum of motion. Joints can be categorized as fibrous, cartilaginous, or synovial based on their structure.

3.1.3.1. Fibrous Joints

Fibrous joints are created by dense fibrous connective tissue and allow minimal or no mobility. Sutures are non-movable fibrous joints exclusively located in the skull. The space between the bones that move against each other is occupied by a connective tissue that contains both fibers and blood vessels. The surfaces of this space are connected by a layer of tissue called periosteum. Sutures serve as locations where new bone tissue is formed and enable the expansion of the skull. These joints are temporary, as the fibrous connective tissue is gradually replaced by bone as we age, resulting in a permanent bony union known as synostosis. The adjacent edges of the bones are extremely uneven and interlock to form a strong connection. A syndesmosis, such as the one found at the inferior tibiofibular joint, has a higher amount of connective tissue compared to a suture, which allows for a slightly greater degree of movement. The gomphosis is a specific type of fibrous joint that is limited to the attachment of teeth to the alveolar bone in the jaws.

3.1.3.2. Cartilaginous Joints

Cartilaginous joints occur when bones are connected by a continuous layer of hyaline cartilage or a fibrocartilage disc. The hyaline cartilage of an epiphyseal plate serves as a transient articulation between the diaphysis and epiphysis of a long bone during its growth. A synchondrosis, which is a type of immovable joint, is occasionally categorized as a primary cartilaginous joint. Symphyses, which are permanent or secondary cartilaginous joints, consist of unions between structures such as the pubic bones (pubic symphysis) and the vertebral bodies. The articular surfaces are coated with thin layers of hyaline cartilage, which are connected to a central disc of fibrous cartilage. The bone, hyaline cartilage, and fibrous cartilage are closely fused together, forming a joint that permits only restricted movement (amphiarthrosis). The extent of mobility achievable is contingent upon the thickness of the fibrous cartilage. Within the fibrous cartilage of certain symphyses, a narrow cavity may be present, such as the symphysis pubis. However, the specialized surfaces that allow sliding movement in a synovial joint are not present. The intervertebral discs, composed of specialized fibrous cartilage, are the crucial connections between adjacent vertebral bodies in the spine. The outer region of the disc, known as the annulus fibrosus, is composed of a peripheral area containing collagen fibers and an inner area made up of fibrous cartilage, which is particularly abundant in collagen. The nucleus pulposus, which is the central region of the disc, starts off as a soft and gelatinous substance in young individuals. However, as one ages, it is progressively substituted by fibrous cartilage. The articular surfaces of each vertebra are coated with thin layers of hyaline cartilage. The annulus fibrosus is securely connected to the vertebral body through collagen fibers that penetrate the cartilaginous end-plates and enter the dense bone of the vertebral body as Sharpey's fibers (Bechtold and Simon, 2014).

3.1.3.3. Synovial Joints

Synovial joints, known as diarthroses, are intricate joints that allow for extensive and unrestricted movement. Most of the joints in the limbs belong to this category. The bones participating in the joint are enclosed and connected by a capsule made of dense irregular connective tissue, which is seamlessly connected to the periosteum covering the bones involved in the joint. Intra- and extracapsular ligaments, which are dense irregular connective tissue, can offer further stability. The articular cartilages on the opposing bony surfaces facilitate smooth movement by reducing friction. The free surface of the articular cartilage is not actually smooth but rather contains numerous undulations, troughs, and valleys that are not visible to the naked eye. The interior of the capsule is covered by a synovial membrane that produces the lubricating synovial fluid. An articular disc can be fully or partially positioned between the articular surfaces. When the disc is only partially present, it is referred to as a meniscus. Discs and menisci are composed of fibrous cartilage that contains a large number of collagen fibers. They are attached to the capsule at the outer edges. Figure 3.2 illustrates the overall arrangement of a synovial joint.

The articular cartilages of most joints are primarily composed of hyaline cartilage, which exhibits a higher concentration of collagen compared to typical cartilage (Bechtold and Simon, 2014). Fibrous cartilage is found in certain joints, such as the temporomandibular joint. Articular cartilage does not have a perichondrium, and the contact between joints occurs directly between the exposed surfaces of the opposing articular cartilages. The arrangement of collagen fibers in articular cartilage is distinct. On the surface, the fibers are arranged in compact clusters that typically intersect at right angles and align parallel to the surface. This creates the tangential region. The collagen fibers in the deeper transitional and radial zones are randomly arranged. The articular cartilage becomes calcified and fuses with the underlying bone, creating a calcified zone where the collagen fibers are perpendicular to the surface. The diameters of the collagen fibers gradually increase as they transition from the tangential zone to the calcified zone. The calcified layer's fibers infiltrate the subchondral bone, becoming deeply embedded similar to Sharpey's fibers. The lamina splendens, which is situated above the tangential zone, consists of fine fibrils that are randomly arranged. The interface between bone and calcified cartilage is characterized by an uneven surface with delicate ridges, grooves, and interlocking structures that facilitate the connection between the underlying bone and the cartilage covering it. In sections, the boundary between the calcified and radial zones is visible as a basophilic "tide line" that signifies the progression of the calcification process (Billiau et al., 2010).

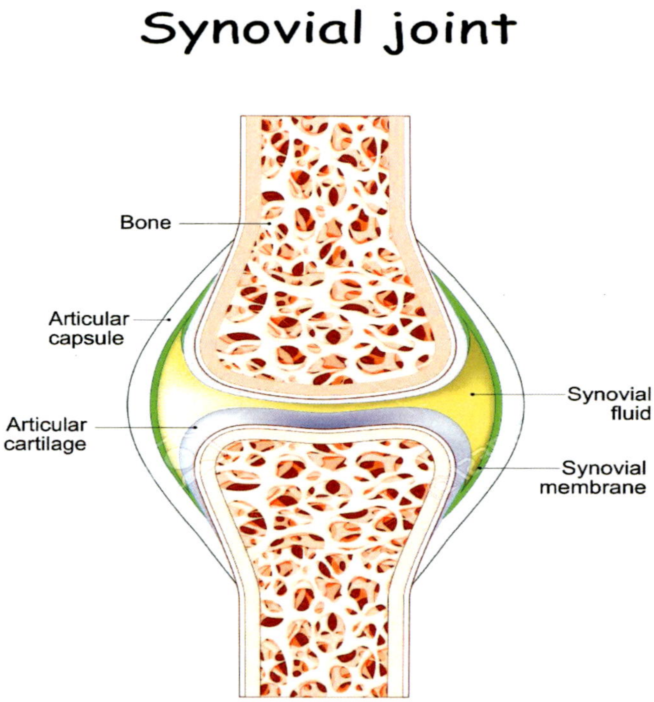

Figure 3.2. *Schematic depiction of the synovial joint.*

Source: https://t4.ftcdn.net/jpg/03/65/85/47/360_F_365854764_sPJtkUG85dRF6wH4ZNRVdLYJQMVHfRSN.jpg.

The articular cartilage cells exhibit zonal variations. The tangential zone consists of multiple layers of flattened cells that resemble fibroblasts. These cells are oriented parallel to the surface, similar to the alignment of collagen fibers. The nuclei of these cells are typically oval or elongated, with generallt smooth outlines. However, some nuclei may be irregular and exhibit various undulations, deep indentations, or clefts. The chromatin within the nuclei appears patchy and clumped, and it stains deeply. The cytoplasm consists of compact cisternae of granular endoplasmic reticulum

(GER), a diminutive Golgi complex, and small, spherical mitochondria. Lipids and glycogen are infrequent inclusions, while pinocytotic vesicles are abundant. Within the transitional zone, the cells exhibit a rounded shape and display numerous elongated cytoplasmic extensions that frequently split into two branches at their ends. The nuclei are typically round and often with an irregular shape. They contain chromatin that is finely granular and frequently have one or more nucleoli. The presence of GER is extensive, the Golgi apparatus is highly developed, and secretory granules are conspicuous. The cells are distributed haphazardly within the transitional zone. The cells in the radial zone exhibit a rounded shape and have a tendency to arrange themselves in short columns or isogenous groups. The endoplasmic reticulum exhibits reduced development, the Golgi complex is characterized by a scarcity of components, and the mitochondria display a compact and diminutive structure. The number of intracellular filaments is elevated, and lipid droplets and glycogen granules are frequently observed. The calcified zone is distinguished by compacted columns of enlarged, pale-stained cells that are in an advanced state of degeneration. The nuclei exhibit high density and pyknosis, with a fragmented nuclear envelope and absence of cytoplasmic organelles. The arrangement of chondrocytes in articular cartilage, organized into successive zones, bears resemblance to the cellular arrangement in an epiphyseal plate during the process of endochondral bone formation. Articular cartilage does function as a growth zone for the subchondral bone during the process of growth. Once epiphyseal growth reaches its full development, the inner layers of chondrocytes within the articular cartilage undergo a transformation into dense bone tissue and become part of the subchondral bone layer. Like other types of cartilage, articular cartilage lacks blood vessels and nerves. The central regions of the cartilage obtain their nourishment through the process of diffusion from the synovial fluid, which surrounds the cartilages, and to a lesser degree, from blood vessels in the subchondral bone. The articular cartilage receives ample nourishment from blood vessels located in the adjacent synovial membrane.

3.1.3.4. Synovial Membrane

The synovial membrane is a distinguishing characteristic of a synovial joint. The described tissue is a type of connective tissue that has a loose texture and is highly vascular. It covers the fibrous capsule and also extends to all surfaces within a joint, except for the ones that experience compression during joint movement. Therefore, synovial membranes do not envelop articular cartilages, articular discs, and menisci. The synovial membrane contains synovial villi and folds that extend into the joint cavity. The synovial membrane's free surface, also known as the synovial intima, is composed of flattened synovial cells arranged in one to three layers. These cells are embedded in a matrix that is granular and devoid of fibers. The surface cells are not contiguous, and in certain areas, adjacent cells are separated by gaps that allow communication between the synovial cavity and tissue spaces in the synovial membrane. The surfaces of the cells that come into contact with each other may be intricate and interlocked. Desmosomal junctions have been observed in synovial membranes of rats, however, their existence in humans has not been verified. At the ultrastructural level, two distinct types of synovial cells have been identified. A-cells are the most abundant and have a similar appearance to macrophages, which is why they are also called M-cells. The cell membrane displays multiple invaginations, filopodia, and micropinocytotic vesicles, while the cytoplasm contains prominent Golgi complexes and abundant mitochondria and lysosomes, but only a few profiles of the rough endoplasmic reticulum (GER). B-cells bear a resemblance to fibroblasts and are occasionally referred to as F-cells. Their contour is sleek and they are rich in GER and have dispersed free ribosomes. Both cell types have a significant amount of glycogen, but only a small number of lipid inclusions. The relationship between A- and B- cells is currently undetermined, however, the presence of intermediate forms (AB-cells) implies that the two may potentially be distinct functional variations of a singular type. The subintimal tissue within the same joint exhibits variations, and the synovial membrane is classified as areolar, adipose, or fibrous depending on its structure. The underlying tissue in areolar synovial membranes is characterized by a sparse distribution of collagen fibers and a plentiful matrix, consisting of loose connective tissue.

The cellular components comprise fibroblasts, mast cells, macrophages, and lymphocytes. The articular fat pads are lined by adipose synovial membranes, and the subintimal tissue primarily comprises adipocytes. Fibrous synovial membranes consist of a dense irregular connective tissue that is located in areas of the body that experience tension. In regions where the tension is particularly intense, fibrous cartilage may also be present. Synovial fluid is a transparent or slightly yellow thick fluid that covers the surfaces of the joints.

Typically, the amount of fluid is enough to create a thin layer that covers all the surfaces inside a joint. Synovial fluid is a plasma ultrafiltrate supplemented with mucin. Mucin is a substance produced by the surface synovial cells and is primarily composed of densely polymerized hyaluronic acid, which contributes to the thickness of the synovial fluid. Typical synovial fluid has a cell count of 50 to 100 cells per milliliter, which primarily includes macrophages, free synovial cells, and sporadic leukocytes. Amorphous particles and fragments of cells and fibrous tissue may be present, and it is hypothesized that they are the result of gradual erosion of the joint surface (Caetano et al., 2009).

3.1.4. Histogenesis

3.1.4.1. Cartilage

Cartilage originates exclusively from mesenchyme, and in areas where cartilage is intended to develop, the mesenchymal cells undergo a process of losing their extensions, assuming a rounded shape, multiplying, and compacting into a concentrated mass of chondrogenic cells known as a center of chondrification. The cells within the mass are chondroblasts, responsible for depositing fibers and ground substance. As the quantity of material between cells increases, the cells become separated into separate compartments (lacunae) and acquire the properties of chondrocytes. Additional chondroblasts are enlisted from the immature cells located towards the outer edges. The perichondrium originates from the condensation of the mesenchyme that envelops the developing cartilage. Additional growth is achieved through the expansion of the cartilage mass from within (interstitial growth) and the addition of new cartilage on the surface (appositional growth). Interstitial growth occurs when young chondrocytes undergo cell division and deposit a new matrix, leading to the internal expansion of cartilage. Such proliferation takes place exclusively in juvenile cartilage that possesses sufficient pliability to facilitate the separation of daughter cells following cell division. Appositional growth is the outcome of chondrogenic activity in the perichondrium. Chondrogenic cells are derived from the inner layer of the perichondrium. The cells in question arrange themselves into a layer, undergo division and specialization into chondroblasts, release a matrix around themselves, and contribute new cartilage to the outer layer. When these cells are trapped within their own matrix, they are correctly referred to as chondrocytes. The adult perichondrium has a limited ability to generate new cartilage due to its lack of blood vessels. The mitotic rate of adult cartilage is the lowest among all skeletal tissues. Elastic cartilage formation involves the initial production of fibers by chondroblasts, which possess neither elastic nor collagenous properties. These apathetic fibers eventually develop into elastic fibers. Fibrous cartilage forms similarly to regular connective tissue, but certain fibroblasts undergo a transformation into chondroblasts and produce a limited quantity of cartilage matrix around themselves.

3.1.4.2. Bone

Bone originates from mesenchyme and forms through the substitution of an existing tissue. Intramembranous ossification refers to the formation of bone directly within a primitive connective tissue, while endochondral ossification is the process of replacing a preformed cartilaginous model with bone. The fundamental process of bone formation is identical in both cases (Caetano et al., 2012).

3.1.4.3. Intramembranous Ossification

The cranial flat bones and a portion of the mandible are formed through the process of intramembranous ossification. These bones are commonly referred to as membrane bones. Vascularization of the mesenchyme occurs in the regions where bone will develop, leading to active cell proliferation. Osteoprogenitor cells are a type of cells that undergo changes which ultimately result in the formation of bone. Structurally, they bear a strong resemblance to the mesenchymal cells from which they originate, and their identification primarily relies on their proximity to developing bone.

Osteoprogenitor cells undergo enlargement and differentiation into osteoblasts, which deposit multiple layers of matrix. Osteoblasts possess receptors for parathyroid hormone and 1, 25-dihydroxyvitamin D3 on their plasmalemma, which can be activated by these molecules. The osteoblasts maintain communication with each other through elongated tapering extensions. As the matrix continues to be deposited, the cells and their extensions become trapped within the matrix. Subsequently, these cells are referred to as osteocytes. The cells and cell processes are ultimately fully contained within the matrix, resulting in the formation of lacunae and canaliculi. The initial matrix is composed of collagen fibers of type I that are immersed in a gel of glycosaminoglycan. This gel contains particular glycoproteins and is soft due to its lack of mineralization. During this phase, the matrix is referred to as osteoid. Following a brief delay, it undergoes mineralization to develop into actual bone. Osteoblasts produce osteocalcin and alkaline phosphatase, enzymes that break down substrates containing phosphate and calcium to release phosphate and calcium. Furthermore, osteoblasts secrete matrix vesicles that specifically accumulate calcium and phosphate as part of the mineralization process. Blood alkaline phosphatase levels serve as reliable indicators for assessing both osteogenesis and bone repair. As osteoblasts become ensnared in the recently formed matrix and transform into osteocytes, fresh osteoblasts are enlisted through the differentiation of osteoprogenitor cells. Intramembranous ossification involves the development of bone in multiple areas within the mesenchymal field. This process leads to the creation of scattered and irregular trabeculae, or small beams, of bone. These trabeculae grow larger by the addition of new bone to their surfaces. The resultant bone exhibits a spongy morphology. The initial bone formation consists of collagen fibers that are oriented in various directions. This type of bone is referred to as woven bone, characterized by osteocytes that are randomly distributed and the absence of a lamellar organization. Lamellar bone gradually replaces woven bone. In regions where compact bone forms, such as the inner and outer layers of the skull, the trabeculae continue to increase in thickness through appositional growth, resulting in the gradual elimination of the spaces between them. When bone invades the spaces where blood vessels are located, it forms layers of matrix in a non-uniform, concentric pattern. These layers surround the blood vessels and resemble osteons, although the collagen fibers in the lamellae are arranged randomly. These structures are referred to as primary osteons. The thickening of the trabeculae stops in the area where spongy bone is present between the plates of compact bone, and the connective tissue in between becomes the marrow responsible for producing blood cells (Cleary, 2004). The connective tissue that surrounds the developing bone undergoes condensation to create the periosteum. The osteoblasts located on the external surface of the bone acquire a fibroblast-like morphology and become part of the inner layer (cambium) of the periosteum, where they remain as cells with the ability to form bone. Likewise, osteoblasts located on the inner surface and those that cover the trabeculae of spongy bone become part of the endosteum and maintain their ability to generate bone.

3.1.4.4. Endochondral Bone Formation

The bones of the vertebral column, pelvis, extremities, face, and base of the skull are formed by the process of bone formation in a cartilage model or precursor. This cartilage must be removed before the bone can be deposited. Endochondral ossification entails the concurrent synthesis of the bone matrix and elimination of the cartilage template. Cartilage does not directly contribute to bone formation, and a significant portion of the intricate process of endochondral bone formation is focused on the elimination of cartilage. Ossification of a long bone begins in the central region of the cartilage model, specifically in the area that will develop into the shaft or diaphysis. Within this specific region, known as the primary ossification center, the chondrocytes undergo hypertrophy, resulting in the vacuolation of their cytoplasm. The lacunae expand, causing the surrounding matrix to shrink, and the cartilage between neighboring lacunae becomes thin and fenestrated. The matrix surrounding the enlarged chondrocytes undergoes calcification through the accumulation of calcium phosphate. The diffusion of nutrients through the calcified matrix is diminished, resulting in degenerative changes in the cells that ultimately cause their demise. During the occurrence of these events, the vascular perichondrium in the cartilage area takes on the role of generating bone tissue. The periosteal collar, a layer of bone, develops around the modified cartilage and acts as a splint, preserving the integrity of the shaft.

The osteoblasts involved in bone development originate from perichondrial cells located directly next to the cartilage. The perichondrium in the collarbone region has transformed into a periosteum. The periosteal bud is formed when blood vessels from the periosteum invade the modified cartilage. The blood vessels are accompanied by a connective tissue sheath that contains cells with osteogenic properties. When the chondrocytes die, there is no longer a way to keep the matrix intact, causing it to become soft. The invading blood vessels facilitate the erosion of the thin plates of matrix between lacunae. When the adjacent lacunar spaces are expanded, they create narrow tunnels that are divided by thin bars of calcified cartilage. Vascularization occurs within the tunnels, as blood vessels infiltrate and deliver osteogenic cells that align along the surface of the cartilaginous trabeculae. These cells then differentiate into osteoblasts and commence the production of bone matrix. Initially, the matrix is deposited as osteoid, but it rapidly undergoes mineralization to develop into authentic bone.

The initial trabeculae are composed of a central region of calcified cartilage that is enveloped by a layer of bone. The primitive trabeculae are eventually eliminated through the ongoing resorption of the calcified cartilage and the action of osteoclasts that emerge on the bony shell. A growing hollow space is created inside the developing shaft. The bone is supported by the extension of the periosteal collar, which also increases in thickness as the periosteum deposits new bone on the surface. This entire process is characterized by a systematic sequence of actions that extends in both directions along the growing bone. The cartilage can be divided into several distinct areas or zones of activity (Galíndez and Carmona, 2016). Beginning at the ends farthest from the primary ossification center, these are the following:

- **Zone of Reserve Cartilage**: This region is composed of hyaline cartilage and initially has a long length, but it becomes shorter as the process of ossification gradually replaces it. The cells and their lacunae exhibit a random distribution within the matrix, and there is gradual expansion in all dimensions.
- **Zone of Proliferation:** In this region the chondrocytes actively proliferate, and as the cells divide, the daughter cells become aligned in rows separated by a small amount of matrix. Within the rows, the cells are separated only by thin plates of matrix. Growth occurs mainly in the regions farthest from the reserve cartilage, and the length is increased more than the diameter.
- **Zone of Maturation and Hypertrophy**: Cell division ceases and the cells mature and enlarge, further increasing the length of the cartilage. Lacunae expand at the expense of the intervening matrix, and the cartilage between adjacent cells in the rows becomes even thinner.
- **Zone of Calcification and Cell Death**: The matrix between the rows of chondrocytes becomes calcified and the cells die, degenerate, and leave empty spaces. The thin plates between the cells break down, and the lacunar spaces are opened up to form irregular tunnels bounded by the remains of calcified cartilage that had been present between the rows of cells.
- **Zone of Ossification**: Vascular connective tissue invades the tunnel-like spaces and provides osteogenic cells that differentiate into osteoblasts. These gather on the surface of the calcified matrix and lay down bone.
- **Zone of Resorption**: Osteoclasts appear on the trabeculae and begin to resorb the bone. Ultimately all the calcified cartilages and their boney coverings are resorbed, and the marrow cavity increases in size.

During the process of cartilage changes, the periosteal collar grows in both length and thickness. It gradually extends towards the ends of the developing bone, creating a continuous splint that surrounds the area where the cartilage is undergoing transformation and becoming weaker. During the time of birth, new centers of ossification, known as epiphyseal or secondary ossification centers, emerge in the ends of long bones. The cartilage of the epiphyses undergoes the same sequences as in the diaphysis, but cartilage growth and subsequent ossification occur in all directions, leading to the formation of a spongy bone mass. In the end, all of the cartilage in the epiphysis is replaced by bone, except for the cartilage at the free end, which remains as articular cartilage. Cartilage remains present between the epiphysis and diaphysis, forming the epiphyseal plate. This plate's ongoing growth allows for additional bone elongation. Ossification takes place at the diaphyseal side, where new cartilage is formed and replaced by bone at an equal rate, resulting in a constant thickness of the epiphyseal plate. Ultimately, the growth in the plate stops, the cartilage is substituted with bone (epiphyseal plate closure), and any further elongation of the bone becomes impossible. The bone's diameter increases due to the deposition of bone on the outer surface caused by the periosteum's activity, while osteoclasts simultaneously resorb smaller amounts of bone on the endosteal surface. Consequently, the overall diameter of the bone is enlarged, and both the thickness of the dense bone and the size of the central cavity are augmented. The bone produced by the periosteum is classified as intramembranous bone, which leads to the formation of an intricate network of irregular bony trabeculae. The spaces between trabeculae are gradually filled, converting it into compact bone (George et al., 2017). Bone is deposited in indistinct layers, and when it encompasses blood vessels, the initial Haversian systems or primitive osteons are created, similar to their formation during the development of membranous bone. Collagen is deposited haphazardly in each lamella of the primitive osteons. Bone undergoes continuous remodeling and reconstruction throughout an individual's lifespan, where the original osteons are replaced by more developed osteons, which are then replaced by subsequent generations of osteons. The process of osteon replacement commences with the creation of tunnels within the compact bone, brought about by the osteolytic actions of osteocytes and osteoclasts. The Haversian canals have the ability to expand and grow to achieve significant lengths. Once osteolytic activity stops, osteoblasts are mobilized from osteoprogenitor cells in the endosteum and begin depositing bone on the cavity walls until it is completely filled, forming a definitive osteon. The process of resorption cavities formation and subsequent filling with third, fourth, and subsequent generations of osteons persists throughout an individual's lifetime. The resorption cavities may not always align with the osteon that is being replaced, resulting in the presence of fragments of older osteons known as interstitial lamellae. **Figure 3.3** illustrates the process of osteon replacement and bone remodeling.

Figure 3.4 provides a concise summary of the sequential modifications that take place during the development of a long bone. The cartilage model (A) is surrounded by a periosteal collar in the region that will develop into the shaft (B), and the cartilage matrix in this area undergoes calcification and degeneration (C). A vascular bud consisting of connective tissue and blood vessels invades the modified cartilage, leading to its absorption. The remaining cartilage fragments are then enveloped by bone, resulting in the formation of irregular trabeculae. Subsequently, these are rapidly absorbed, leading to the formation of a growing cavity filled with bone marrow as the process progresses towards both ends (D). Secondary ossification centers develop in the epiphyses and gradually increase in size in all directions (E). Cartilage remains present at the extremities of the bone and, temporarily, as the epiphyseal plate, which is responsible for all subsequent growth in length (F). The growth of cartilage in the epiphyseal plate comes to a halt and is substituted by bone. The marrow cavity subsequently extends uninterrupted along the entire length of the bone (G).

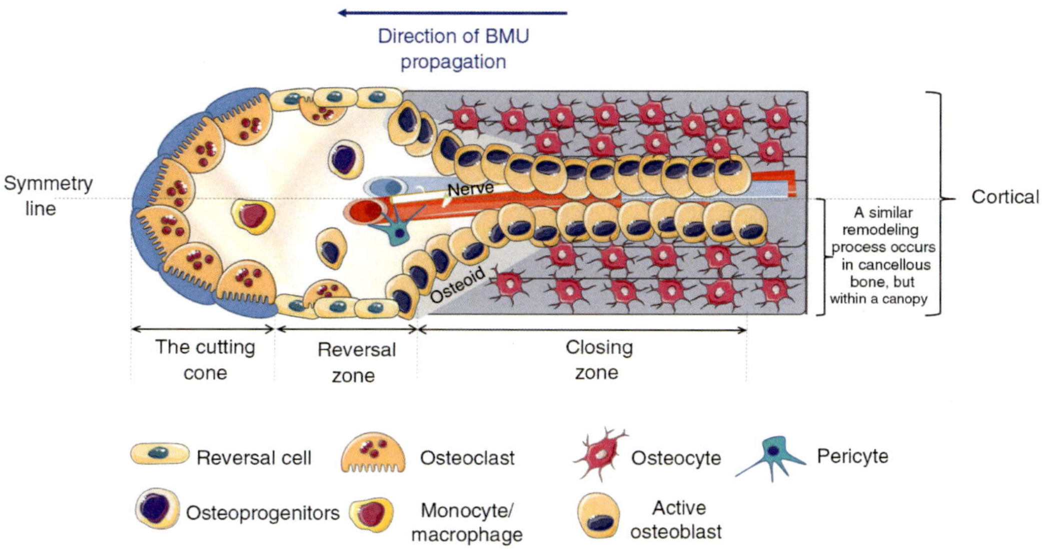

Figure 3.3. *Replacement of osteons during remodeling of compact bone.*

Source: https://media.springernature.com/full/springer-static/image/art%3A10.1038%2Fs41413-022-00219-8/MediaObjects/41413_2022_219_Fig1_HTML.png.

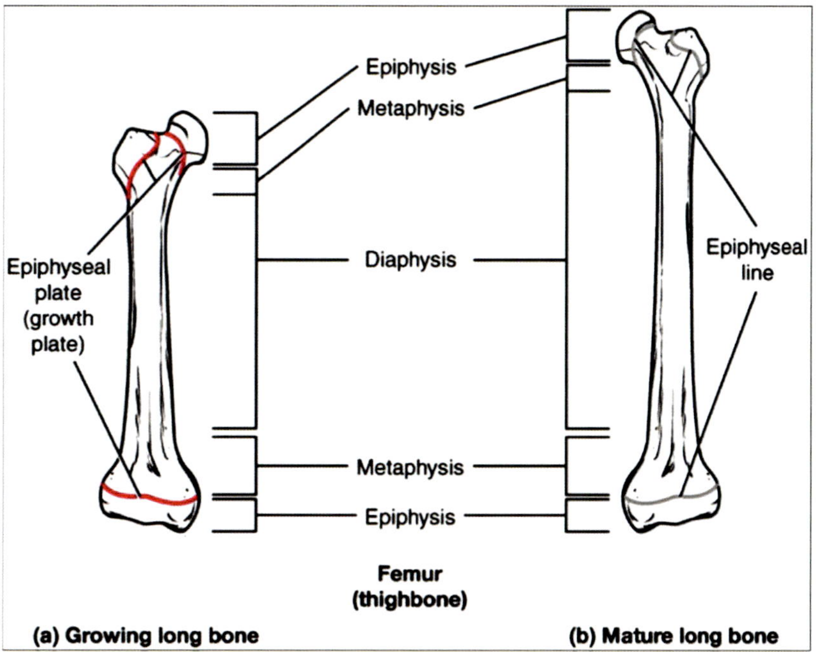

Figure 3.4. *Schematic illustration depicting the sequential alterations that occur during the maturation process of a lengthy skeletal structure.*

Source: https://usq.pressbooks.pub/app/uploads/sites/39/2021/01/progression.png.

Cartilage is the optimal rigid and lightweight tissue for the embryonic skeleton due to its ability to grow quickly, which allows it to keep up with the rapid growth of the fetus. Similarly, the expansion of the hyaline cartilage in the epiphyseal plate facilitates the swift development of long bones in the adolescent stage. In the end, the cartilage of the temporary skeleton, as well as the cartilage of the growth plate, is substituted with bone that grows at a slower rate (Gorska et al., 2014).

3.1.4.5. Joints

3.1.4.5.1. Fibrous Joints

Fibrous joints are created through the condensation and differentiation of the mesenchyme that remains between developing bones. This process leads to the formation of a dense irregular connective tissue that binds the bones together.

3.1.4.5.2. Cartilaginous Joints

During the initial phases of growth, a symphysis is depicted as a layer of mesenchyme situated between distinct cartilaginous structures of bone; the mesenchyme then undergoes differentiation into fibrous cartilage. After the neighboring cartilaginous bone models have turned into bone, small layers of hyaline cartilage remain unconverted and continue to exist as thin sheets of hyaline cartilage between the bone and fibrous cartilage. The nucleus pulposus of an intervertebral disc originates from the notochord.

During the early stages of embryonic development, cells known as notochordal cells located between future vertebrae undergo rapid proliferation. However, as development progresses, these cells undergo a process called mucoid degeneration, which results in the formation of the gelatinous nucleus pulposus. The fibrocartilage that surrounds the annulus fibrosus originates from the mesenchyme located between neighboring vertebrae (Grönlund et al., 2014).

3.1.4.5.3. Synovial Joints

The formation of appendicular bones is initiated by the development of cartilage in the central region of each future skeletal component. As the cartilage models grow larger, their ends move closer to each other, and the undifferentiated tissue in between becomes more compact, forming the interzonal mesenchyme or midzone, which will eventually develop into the joint. At the same time, the outer layer of mesenchyme condenses to create the initial joint capsule. This capsule is connected to the mesenchyme that formed the perichondrium around the nearby cartilage model. The mesenchyme surrounded by the primitive joint capsule is divided into three separate zones: a central layer of loosely arranged cells located between two dense layers where the cells are aligned parallel to the surface of the underlying cartilage. The compact regions generate the articular cartilage. The formation of the joint cavity initiates in the central area of the interzone, characterized by the emergence of small, fluid-filled gaps between the mesenchymal cells. The gaps merge and create a continuous hollow space that separates the dense layers of cartilage and extends along the edges of the cartilage structures. As the spaces come together, the basic joint capsule undergoes specialization and develops into two distinct layers. The outer layer of the joint capsule develops into the dense, uneven connective tissue, while the inner layer becomes cellular and gives rise to the synovial membrane. The menisci and articular discs originate from the mesenchyme that formed the fibrous joint capsule.

3.1.5. Repair of Cartilage and Bone

3.1.5.1. Cartilage

Due to its lack of blood vessels, mammalian cartilage has a restricted ability to regenerate itself following injury. Regions of cartilage that have been damaged undergo necrosis, after which they are subsequently repaired by connective tissue originating from the perichondrium. While a portion of the connective tissue may gradually transform into cartilage, the majority remains as dense irregular connective tissue, which has the potential to later undergo calcification or ossification.

3.1.5.2. Bone

The repair of a fractured bone is affected by the dimensions of the bone, the density of its cortical bone, and the intricacy of the fracture. Nevertheless, the fundamental process of repair remains unchanged and typically mirrors the occurrences of bone formation. A fracture causes the rupture of blood vessels in the marrow, periosteum, and the bone itself, resulting in significant bleeding. Due to the vascular damage, the bone, periosteum, and marrow all undergo necrosis for a certain distance from the site of the fracture. However, the latter (referring to the tissues) possess a more extensive blood supply compared to the bone tissue itself, resulting in a lesser extent of cell death in these tissues. The blood clot is eliminated through the processes of lysis and phagocytosis. In humans, the occurrence of fibrovascular invasion of the clot surrounding and within the fracture, as well as its transformation into fibroconnective tissue, is not a prominent phenomenon. Repair takes place through the activation of osteogenic cells in the viable endosteum and periosteum located near the site of the fracture. The cells undergo rapid multiplication and generate new networks of bone within the central cavity of the bone and underneath the outer layer of the bone. Regeneration taking place in the marrow cavity is crucial for healing human fractures. Medullary healing initiates with the development of concentrated areas of blood vessel and fibroblast growth in the living tissue surrounding the injured bone marrow. This is then followed by the formation of new bone through the process of bone cell production. In the end, a complex network of delicate bony trabeculae spans the marrow cavity from one side of the fracture to the other, and eventually bridges the fracture itself. This network acts as an internal framework, supporting the fractured ends until they can be successfully joined together. The formation of all this new bone occurs through intramembranous ossification and results in woven bone. Medullary bone healing is crucial for the fusion of fractures in spongy bones like the vertebral bodies and lower end of the radius, as well as fractures through the metaphysis of long bones. The repair process on the periosteal surface originates from the inner osteoblastic layer of the periosteum, specifically the osteogenetic layer, which starts a short distance away from the fracture zone. Periosteal proliferation occurs bilaterally around the fracture gap, leading to the formation of bony trabeculae collars that grow outward and inward, eventually merging to form a continuous arch that spans the gap. The newly formed trabeculae are securely adhered to the existing bone surface, encompassing even the necrotic bone tissue. The osteogenic cells in the midzone of the fracture site differentiate into chondroblasts instead of osteoblasts due to their faster growth compared to their vascular supply. As a result, they form a callus of hyaline cartilage (Guzik et al., 2006). This also connects the gap in the fracture to create a stabilizing splint around the fracture. Endochondral bone formation converts cartilage into bone, but this process is limited and results in the complete disappearance of cartilage. Unlike the epiphyseal plate, there is no continuous formation of new cartilage. Cartilage consistently forms during the process of long bone regeneration, while flat bones undergo healing without the formation of cartilage. The consolidation of the dense outer layer of the bone is achieved through the contribution of sources originating either from the central cavity or from the outer layer of the bone. Direct union of the fractured ends is extremely rare, if it occurs at all, because the ends of the bone at the fracture line are composed of dead bone. Sometimes, the gap is filled by the development of hyaline cartilage, which later undergoes endochondral ossification to achieve cortical union. Often, the bone that initially connects the fractured ends is a complex network of woven bone created through intramembranous bone formation. The final stage in the process of repair involves the absorption of surplus bone and the restructuring of both newly formed and deceased bone, which is then substituted with lamellar bone. Bone morphogenic proteins, classified within the TGF-β superfamily, play a role in the regulation of bone formation and repair. Bone morphogenic proteins play a crucial role in various stages of the process that leads to the formation of new bone. These stages include attracting progenitor cells towards the desired location, promoting cell division, facilitating the specialization and multiplication of chondrocytes and osteoblasts, encouraging the creation of the extracellular matrix, and binding to specific molecules within this matrix.

3.2. Special Connective Tissue: Blood

Blood is commonly described as a unique type of connective tissue, where the fluid component serves as the intercellular substance. Contrary to other types of connective tissues, the intercellular substance of blood does not contain any fibrous component. Additionally, the majority of the intercellular protein in blood is not produced by blood cells themselves, but rather by cells in other tissues, primarily the liver.

A significant portion of the cellular components of blood are composed of anucleate entities known as erythrocytes, as well as fragments of cytoplasm referred to as platelets. Leukocytes, also known as true cells, constitute a small portion of the formed elements in the blood. They are temporary residents that utilize the bloodstream to travel to various organs and tissues, where they perform their designated tasks. The formed elements in the blood do not typically undergo replication within the bloodstream. Instead, when these elements are lost, new ones are produced from specific blood-forming tissues located outside the circulation.

Therefore, blood can be regarded as the excretory output of various organs and tissues, rather than being classified as a distinct tissue. The overall volume of blood remains relatively consistent in relation to the body's mass. The volume in humans is approximately 5 liters, which corresponds to approximately 7.5% of their body weight.

3.2.1. Components of Blood

Blood is composed of various components, including red blood cells, platelets, white blood cells, and a fluid substance known as plasma. Centrifugation can be used to separate these elements, and when performed in calibrated tubes, the resulting hematocrit provides an estimation of the volume of the formed elements. The most weighty constituents, erythrocytes, constitute the lower layer and account for approximately 45% of the volume of blood. Platelets and leukocytes can be found in the buffy coat, which is a grayish white layer located directly above the erythrocytes. Together, they make up approximately 1% of the total volume of blood. The topmost layer is composed of plasma, a protein-rich solution, containing three primary protein types: albumin, globulin, and fibrinogen. Albumin, the predominant and smallest protein in the plasma, is responsible for maintaining blood colloidal osmotic (oncotic) pressure. It is synthesized in the liver, along with fibrinogen, a crucial factor in blood clotting. The globulins, namely alpha, beta, and gamma, consist of various proteins with distinct sizes. Globulins play a role in the transportation of hormones, ions, metals, and lipids. Gamma globulins are immunoglobulins, or antibodies, that are produced by cells in the lymphatic organs and tissues. The plasma also contains hormones derived from various endocrine organs, as well as metabolites, nutrients, and various other substances. **Table 3.1** presents a partial compilation of typical values for various substances detected in human blood (Guzman et al., 2017).

Table 3.1. A Partial list of Normal Values of Human Peripheral Blood

Parameter	**Reference Range**
pH (arterial)	7.35–7.45
Osmolality	280–296 mOsm/kg H_2O
O_2, saturated	96%-100%
CO_2	24–30 mEq/liter
PCO_2 (arterial)	35–45 mmHg
Total protein	6.0–8.4 g/100 ml
Albumin	3.5–5.0 g/100 ml
Globin	2.3–3.5 g/100 ml
Cholesterol	120–220 mg/100 ml
Triglycerides	40–150 mg/100 ml
Lactic acid	0.6–1.8 mEq/liter
Ascorbic acid	0.4–1.5 mg/100 ml
Uric acid	3.0–7.0 mg/100 ml
Glucose (fasting)	70–110 mg/100 ml
Sodium	135–145 mEq/liter
Potassium	3.5–5.0 mEq/liter
Chloride	100–106 mEq/liter
Calcium	8.5–10.5 mg/100 ml
Phosphorus	3.0–4.5 mg/100 ml
Magnesium	1.5–2.0 mEq/liter
Iron	50–150 µg/100 ml

Source: Adapted from various **sources**.

Plasma is derived from blood following the administration of an anticoagulant, and it encompasses all the constituents of the liquid part of blood. It constitutes approximately 55% of the total volume of blood. On the other hand, serum is acquired from blood that has clotted or had its fibrin removed, and it lacks fibrinogen. However, it does contain other substances produced during the blood clotting process.

3.2.2. Erythrocytes

During a state of rest, the typical human consumes approximately 250 ml of oxygen and generates nearly 200 ml of carbon dioxide every minute. Through engagement in physical or mental exertion, these quantities have the potential to multiply by a factor of 10 to 20. Erythrocytes efficiently transport oxygen and carbon dioxide. The exchange of gases takes place in the blood capillaries of the lung, where erythrocytes pass through in less than 1 second. However, the process of gaseous exchange is completed within the first third of this time.

3.2.2.1. Structure

In blood smears and tissue sections, erythrocytes are observed as anucleate, uniformly acidophilic entities lacking any internal structure. Hemoglobin, a pigment, comprises approximately 95% of the dry weight. Erythroplastid is a more accurate term to describe these elements, but due to tradition and widespread usage, the terms erythrocyte and red cell have become accepted as the correct terminology. Electron microscopy verifies that mature red cells lack organelles in their interior and are incapable of protein synthesis or renewal of their cell membrane constituents. The plasmalemma's cholesterol, which is crucial for cell flexibility, is regulated by the plasma cholesterol concentration rather than cell metabolism (Haarbo et al., 1991). The ABO blood-group system is determined by the presence of antigenic determinants found in carbohydrate chains that extend from glycoproteins and glycolipids of the erythrocyte plasmalemma. The cell membrane of erythrocytes in certain individuals may contain either antigen A (indicating type A blood), antigen B (indicating type B blood), or both antigens A and B (indicating type AB blood). Individuals with type O blood are classified as lacking both antigens on their erythrocytes. The majority of individuals possess antibodies in their blood plasma that target erythrocyte antigens, excluding their own. If a transfusion of a different blood type is administered, an immune response will ensue. Hence, it is crucial to ascertain the specific antigens found on the red blood cells of the blood donor and the antibodies present in the recipient's plasma prior to administering a transfusion.

3.2.2.2. Shape and Size

The human red blood cell is commonly characterized as a biconcave disc. When viewed from the front, the typical red blood cell appears as a smooth, rounded shape with a central indentation. Human erythrocytes have an average diameter of 7.6 μm in smears. In tissue sections, they are slightly smaller, ranging from 6.5 to 7.0 μm. In fresh blood, they are slightly larger, measuring about 8 μm. The red cell has a thickness of approximately 2 μm. Evidently, this thickness enables hemoglobin to sustain an ideal distance from the surface of the cell, which is crucial for its proper functioning. Red blood cells are surrounded by a standard cell membrane, which is flexible and elastic, enabling the red blood cell to pass through narrow capillaries. Within a living organism, red blood cells frequently adopt a concave shape while traversing narrow blood vessels. A network of spectrin protein located beneath the plasma membrane helps to preserve the biconcave shape of cells while also allowing for flexibility. Spectrin, connected by actin, seems to create a network directly below the plasmalemma and potentially functions as a cytoskeleton. The network is connected to the inner side of the cell membrane through the protein ankyrin, allowing the cytoskeleton and cell membrane to function as a single entity. Hemoglobin may also contribute to the maintenance of cell shape, as significant alterations in shape are linked to the atypical hemoglobin found in sickle cell anemia.

3.2.2.3. Number and Survival

There is a consistent disparity in the number of red blood cells between men and women, with women generally having lower values. The normal range for red blood cell count in men is between 4,500,000 and 6,000,000/mm^3, while in women it is between 3,800,000 and 5,000,000/mm^3. The lifespan of red blood cells is approximately 120 days. While red blood cells are typically eliminated as they age and deteriorate, there is also a degree of spontaneous destruction. Numerous red blood cells are destroyed within the bone marrow before they are even released. As red blood cells become older, they deplete a significant amount of the enzymes involved in adenosine triphosphate (ATP) and are incapable of sustaining themselves, producing protein, or regenerating their cell membranes. At the end of their lifespan, red blood cells become inflexible as a result of cholesterol loss from the cell membrane and the breakdown of protein, which then forms cross-links with calcium.

Phagocytes primarily in the spleen, as well as in the liver and bone marrow, capture and eliminate these old red blood cells. Approximately 1% of red blood cells in circulation are eliminated on a daily basis. The liver retrieves iron from hemoglobin, stores it, and then repurposes it for the production of new red blood cells (Haugen et al., 1992).

3.2.2.4. Reticulocytes

The majority of erythrocytes exhibit an orange-red color when stained with typical blood stains, while a small number display a bluish or slate gray hue. These polychromatophilic cells are immature erythrocytes that contain a small amount of ribonucleoprotein. When stained with brilliant cresyl blue or new methylene blue, this ribonucleoprotein precipitates as a network or web. The proper term for these cells is reticulocytes. Their presence in the bloodstream serves as a general measure of red blood cell generation. Typically, reticulocytes constitute a mere 1 to 2% of the red blood cells found in the peripheral blood.

3.2.2.5. Rouleaux

Erythrocytes have a tendency to adhere to one another by their wide surfaces, resulting in the formation of stacks known as rouleaux. Rouleaux formation is dependent on alterations in the blood plasma rather than the individual cells themselves. Any circumstance that augments the overall positive charge in the plasma leads to alterations in the surface charge of erythrocytes, enabling them to adhere to one another more easily. Rouleaux are transient occurrences that can happen within blood vessels and do not seem to cause any damage to red blood cells. An elevation in rouleaux formation is manifested by an augmentation in the velocity at which red blood cells precipitate or settle (Haugen et al., 2002).

3.2.2.6. Abnormalities

Deviation from the typical size, shape, or staining characteristics of red blood cells can serve as significant indicators of disease. However, to a lesser extent, some of these irregularities may also be present in healthy individuals. Anisocytosis refers to atypical deviations in the size of red blood cells, which can manifest as either macrocytes (larger than the average size) or microcytes (smaller than the average size). Macrocytes exhibit a less pronounced central pale area compared to normal cells, but there is no increase in the concentration of hemoglobin. Poikilocytosis refers to an irregularity in the shape of cells, which can manifest as blunt, pointed, or hook-shaped projections on their surfaces. Under different circumstances, red blood cells cultured outside of the body may undergo shrinkage and develop multiple projections on their surfaces. These cells are referred to as crenated and are specifically known as echinocytes. Crenated cells can be generated by exposing regular red cells to fatty acids, anionic compounds, high pH levels, or hypertonic solutions. The alterations are capable of being undone. Sickle cell anemia causes red blood cells to change shape dramatically, resulting in the appearance of crescents, holly leaves, or even tubes. Hypochromia refers to cells that have a reduced ability to stain due to a decrease in hemoglobin. It often occurs together with microcytosis. In its most severe manifestations, staining can be limited to a narrow band around the outer edge. Leptocytes, which are cells that are thinner than normal, frequently exhibit a target-like appearance with staining concentrated in a central disc and an outer band, with an unstained area in between. Howell-Jolly bodies are residual nuclear fragments derived from the nucleated precursors of red blood cells. They are visible as either one or two rounded or rod-shaped basophilic granules. Siderocytes consist of aggregations of diminutive, deeply pigmented granules that exhibit a positive response to iron. While they are infrequent in regular peripheral blood, they are abundant in bone marrow. Typically, the spleen eliminates the iron-containing granules without causing harm to the cell. Polychromatophilia is closely related to basophilic stippling, which manifests as blue-black dots. These dots can vary in size and are composed of ribonucleoprotein that has precipitated. It is sporadically detected in cases of leukemia and severe anemias, but it is particularly significant for diagnosing chronic lead poisoning. Under certain pathological circumstances, spherical red blood cells are generated instead of the normal bi-concave shape. The cells that are small, deeply stained, and have a sharp, distinct outline are known as spherocytes.

3.2.2.7. Hemoglobin

Erythrocytes contain both hemoglobin and the enzyme, carbonic anhydrase. Oxygen is not soluble, and transport is carried out by hemoglobin, an iron- containing respiratory pigment that gives the red color to human blood. In contrast, 90% of the carbon dioxide is transported as bicarbonate in plasma. Dissolved carbon dioxide (CO_2) enters the erythrocyte and reacts with water to form carbonic acid (H_2CO_3). *Carbonic anhydrase* within the erythrocyte immediately converts the formed carbonic acid to hydrogen ion (H^+) and bicarbonate (HC03–). Once formed the bicarbonate leaves the erythrocyte in exchange for chloride ion (Cl^-). On reaching the lung bicarbonate passes back into the erythrocyte, combines with hydrogen ion carried and buffered by the hemoglobin to form carbonic acid which is catalyzed by carbonic anhydrase back to carbon dioxide and water. The former then diffuses from the erythrocyte into the alveoli of the lung to be exhaled (Helgeland et al., 2000).

3.2.2.8. Structure

Hemoglobin is an iron-containing porphyrin group, called heme, that is attached to a protein called globin. It is part of a group of catalytic compounds. The heme group is composed of four pyrrole rings that are bonded to iron through their nitrogen groups. Hemoglobin is a symmetrical molecule that consists of two identical mirror-image halves. Each half molecule consists of two distinct peptide chains, each carrying a heme group around which the chain is coiled. The heme groups constitute the functional component, while the peptide chains comprise the globin portion of the molecule. The specific arrangement and types of amino acids in the globin protein determine the species specificity and the type of hemoglobin present in the molecule. Humans produce four distinct globin chains: alpha, beta, gamma, and delta. Approximately 95% of hemoglobin found in normal adults is hemoglobin A (HbA), composed of two alpha and two beta chains. HbA2, which is about 2% of total hemoglobin, consists of two alpha and two delta chains. Fetal hemoglobin (HbF) consists of two alpha and two gamma chains, forming the remaining portion. Fetal hemoglobin is the dominant type during fetal development, but it is replaced by the adult hemoglobin after birth. Fetal hemoglobin exhibits a greater affinity for oxygen compared to adult hemoglobin, enabling it to extract oxygen from maternal blood's red blood cells and transport it to the fetus during the prenatal period. Even slight alterations to the peptide chain can lead to significant alterations in the entire hemoglobin molecule, as demonstrated by the presence of sickle hemoglobin (HbS) in individuals with sickle cell anemia. In this particular state, the sole defect in the molecule occurs at the sixth position of the beta chain, where the glutamic acid found in normal hemoglobin is substituted with valine.

3.2.3. Platelets

Platelets are the second most abundant type of blood cells. Platelets are not cellular entities, but rather fragments of cytoplasm that originate from a larger precursor cell known as a megakaryocyte, which is found in the bone marrow.

3.2.3.1. Structure

Platelets are tiny, non-nucleated structures measuring 2 to 5 μm in diameter. Platelets in stained smears exhibit a distinct granular region called the granulomere, as well as a pale region devoid of granules known as the hyalomere. The granulomere, also known as chromomere, frequently occupies the central area of the platelet and can be densely packed, resembling a nucleus. The division into two zones is not observed in platelets that are circulating or in those that are immediately fixed by drawing blood into a fixative. Under these circumstances, the granulomere maintains a uniform distribution. Electron micrographs reveal that the granulomere is composed of lysosomes, mitochondria, dense-cored granules containing serotonin, adenosine diphosphate (ADP), ATP, calcium, alpha particles containing platelet-specific proteins, fibrinogen, and other clotting factors, actin, myosin, adenosinetriphosphatase (ATPase), and substances that enhance vascular permeability. Mitochondria are characterized by their small size, limited quantity, and a scarcity of cristae. There are varying amounts of glycogen granules present. The hyalomere is the cytoplasmic matrix and is characterized by its homogeneous and finely granular appearance. A network of actin and myosin filaments is located directly below the plasmalemma. The periphery of the zone is devoid of granulomere elements and contains a network of microtubules that constitutes the marginal bundle. This configuration has been characterized as a solitary, spiral microtubule that functions as a rigid component to uphold the discoid shape. Every platelet is enclosed by a standard cell membrane that confines the cytoplasm and connects to a complex network of channels.

3.2.3.3. Number

The quantity of platelets exhibits significant variation across different species and within individuals as well. The variations in platelet counts are a result of challenges in obtaining precise measurements due to physiological factors that impact the numbers, as well as inherent properties of platelets, such as their inclination to adhere to foreign surfaces or aggregate with each other to form clumps. Upon encountering a foreign surface, platelets undergo spreading to encompass an area that is several hundred times larger than their original surface. The normal range for platelet count in humans is typically reported as 250,000 to 400,000 platelets per cubic millimeter (mm^3) of blood, although some estimates suggest that the upper limit could be as high as 900,000/mm^3. Fluctuations in platelets that occur temporarily have been linked to changes in oxygen levels, exposure to cold temperatures, and consumption of food. Interestingly, foods that are heavily seasoned with spices have been found to cause a substantial decrease in the number of platelets in the bloodstream. Emotional states such as fear and rage lead to significantly increased counts. Women experience a gradual decline in platelet count in the two weeks leading up to menstruation, followed by a quick return to normal levels afterwards. Thrombocytopenia is the medical term used to describe a significant decrease in the quantity of platelets in the bloodstream (Henche et al., 2008).

3.2.4. Leukocytes

Leukocytes, also known as white blood cells (WBCs), are genuine cells with nuclei and cytoplasmic organelles. They possess the ability to undergo ameboid movement. They transition from the bloodstream to the body's tissues, where they carry out their designated tasks.

3.2.4.1. Classification

Leukocytes can be categorized as either granular or agranular based on the presence of cytoplasmic granules, or as polymorphonuclear or mononuclear based on the shape of the nucleus. Granular leukocytes possess nuclei with multiple lobes, therefore the terms granular leukocyte and polymorphonuclear leukocyte refer to the same category of cell. Granular leukocytes, also known as granulocytes, can be classified into neutrophils (heterophils), eosinophils, or basophils based on the color of their cytoplasmic granules when stained with standard blood stains. The term "heterophil granules" is used to refer to a specific type of granular leukocyte, regardless of the staining reaction or species, as these granules do not stain uniformly across different species. The term "neutrophil" is used to describe the heterophil of humans. Agranular leukocytes, namely lymphocytes and monocytes, lack visible granules and possess a solitary, non-lobed nucleus. Therefore, the terms mononuclear leukocytes and agranular leukocytes are synonymous and refer to the same category of cells. The differentiation between granular and agranular leukocytes is not completely distinct: monocytes often exhibit small, particle-like granules that are barely distinguishable under light microscopy, and lymphocytes occasionally display a few larger granules. The distinction is a longstanding one that relies on the outward characteristics of leukocytes, using less sophisticated dyes. However, it continues to be valuable due to the specific, distinct, and prominent granules found in granular leukocytes.

3.2.4.2. Neutrophil (Heterophil) Leukocytes

The diameter of the neutrophil granulocyte ranges from 12 to 15 μm. It is distinguished by the shape of its nucleus, which consists of small lobes connected by thin filaments. The nucleus exhibits intense staining, and the chromatin is condensed into clusters, creating a fragmented network. There is a lack of nucleoli. There is variation in the number of lobes, but typically, humans have two to four lobes. Band forms, which are granulocytes with a single elongated nucleus and no lobes, are observed in a limited quantity. These cells are indicative of recently released cells from the bone marrow. Some diseases or inherited anomalies in humans can result in excessive lobation. Furthermore, nuclear appendages resembling hooks, hand racquets, clubs, or drumsticks may also be observed, in addition to nuclear lobation. The drumstick is the sole significant indicator, symbolizing female sex chromatin, and typically appears in the terminal lobe of approximately 2 to 3% of neutrophils in women. Neutrophils contain three distinct types of granules within their cytoplasm. The specific granules, also known as secondary or type B granules, are the most abundant. They are small in size and have a pinkish color. The granules contain lysozyme, which is an enzyme complex that targets various components of bacterial cell walls. Additionally, the granules also contain alkaline phosphatase, collagenase, and lactoferrin, which are other substances that have antibacterial properties. There are several other basic proteins (phagocytins) that are not well characterized, but they also have antibacterial properties. Azurophil granules, also known as primary or type A granules, are not as abundant, but are larger in size and exhibit a reddish purple stain. They possess myeloperoxidase along with a range of acid hydrolases and are regarded as altered lysosomes. Azurophil granules are characterized by their large size and uniformity, while the smaller, less dense-specific granules may contain a crystalloid body. Myeloperoxidase forms complexes with peroxide to generate activated oxygen, which is a highly effective bactericide. Neutrophils secrete tertiary granules that facilitate cell adhesion. These factors may also play a role in the mechanics of phagocytosis. Cytokines stimulate both leukocytes and the endothelium to generate adhesion molecules, facilitating the firm attachment of leukocytes to the endothelium. Once activated, the white cells become mobile, traverse the endothelial cell barrier, and actively move through adjacent tissues using ameboid movement. Under normal conditions, approximately 40% of neutrophils in the peripheral circulation are estimated to be marginated, meaning they adhere to the endothelium of small blood vessels. Leukocytes migrate towards the area with the greatest concentration of chemotaxins. Diapedesis is the term used to describe the process of crossing the endothelial lining (Kotaniemi, 1997). The granules are dispersed throughout the cytoplasm of the neutrophil, with the exception of a small outer region. This outer region contains delicate filaments and microtubules that seem to play a role in the movement of the cell. The cell contains a compact Golgi complex and a set of centrioles positioned at the center. Additionally, there are limited quantities of endoplasmic reticulum, mitochondria, and ribosomes. Neutrophils generate a protein that transforms plasminogen into plasmin, the proteolytic enzyme accountable for fibrinolysis. While the release of granule-associated factors is linked to cell death, the release of plasminogen-activating substance is a secretory process that is directly connected to the survival of the cell. Neutrophils are the primary type of white blood cells in humans, comprising 55 to 70% of the total white blood cell count in the bloodstream. Neutrophils are in a quiescent state while they circulate. Upon activation, these entities have a brief lifespan and perish as a result of the release of their lysosomal enzymes, which also leads to the liquefaction of neighboring tissues. Neutrophils have the main role of phagocytosing and eliminating bacteria.

3.2.4.3. Eosinophil Leukocytes

Eosinophils constitute a minor fraction of the white blood cells and typically account for 1 to 3% of the total circulating leukocytes in humans. The quantity of eosinophils in the bloodstream is correlated with the functioning of the adrenal glands. During the alarm reaction, there is a reduction in eosinophil count. Their population proliferates during parasitic infestations. This relationship could explain the broad spectrum of values that have been documented. There are clear daily variations in activity cycles, with the highest numbers occurring in the morning and the lowest numbers reported in the afternoon. The eosinophil is approximately the same size as the neutrophil and is also distinguished by nuclear lobation. While eosinophils are typically characterized by a bilobed nucleus, it is not uncommon to find eosinophils with three or four lobes. Conditions that cause hypersegmentation in neutrophils also impact eosinophil granulocytes. Eosinophils are characterized by their densely packed, uniform, spherical granules that exhibit a vibrant red or orange-red color when stained. The granules are enclosed by a membrane and exhibit an internal structure known as a crystalloid, or internus. In humans, the crystalloid can take on different shapes and may exist in multiple forms. The crystalloid is immersed within a finely textured matrix. Eosinophil granules consist of lysosomes that contain the typical lysosomal enzymes. The myeloperoxidase content in them is higher compared to the azurophil granules of neutrophils, and they do not contain lysozyme and phagocytin. The granules also contain lipid and major basic protein (MBP), which is responsible for the presence of eosinophils in the body. Eosinophils exhibit chemotactic responses to bacterial products, complement components, and substances such as histamine and eosinophilic chemotactic factor of anaphylaxis released by mast cells. Eosinophils possess a unique attraction towards antigen-antibody complexes, which tend to attach to complement and trigger the destruction of cells. Phagocytosis of these complexes may prevent cell damage in healthy tissues. Eosinophils release histaminase, which degrades histamine and histamine-like substances released from mast cells and basophils, thereby reducing allergic responses (Lien et al., 2003). Eosinophils release prostaglandins E1 and E2, which can prevent mast cell secretion. Eosinophils play a significant role in regulating parasitic infections such as ascariosis, trichinosis, and schistosomiasis. They specifically interact with the larvae of certain parasites and harm them through oxidative mechanisms. The presence of the major basic protein (MBP) in the crystalloid core of the eosinophil granules improves the process of antibody-mediated destruction of parasites. Eosinophils possess surface receptors that specifically bind to IgE antibodies. Eosinophils primarily serve to suppress or halt allergic reactions and parasitic infections.

3.2.4.5. Basophil Leukocytes

Basophils constitute a mere 0.5% of the overall leukocyte population. Lymphocytes are marginally smaller than neutrophil granulocytes and have a diameter of 10 to 12 μm when observed in blood smears. The nuclear lobes in the neutrophil or eosinophil are more distinct compared to other cells, and it is uncommon to find nuclei with more than two or three lobes. The filaments connecting the lobes are typically of short and wide nature, and they seldom develop the slender thread-like structures observed in neutrophils. The chromatin exhibits a uniform composition and has a lower affinity for staining compared to the other types of granulocytes. There is a lack of nucleoli. Basophils have a cytoplasm that contains noticeable and rough granules. These granules can be stained in a deep violet color using standard blood stains, as well as metachromatically using toluidine blue or thionine. The granules that are well-preserved have a spherical and uniform shape. However, when they are dissolved in water or glycerin, they often appear irregular in size and shape in fixed preparations. The granules are distributed unevenly within the cytoplasm, frequently covering and obstructing the nucleus. They are less abundant and less densely packed compared to the granules found in eosinophil leukocytes. The granules exhibit an internal striated pattern as observed through electron microscopy. The granules consist of myeloperoxidase, glycosaminoglycans, leukotriene 3, eosinophilic chemotactic factors, prostaglandins, and a platelet-activating factor. The granules exhibit basophilia because of the presence of heparin. There is no empirical evidence to support the claim that the granules possess lysosomal activity. Basophils possess surface receptors that specifically bind to IgE antibodies, which are generated by the immune system in response to allergens. Basophil granules contain significant amounts of heparin, histamine, vasodilating agents, and slow-reacting substances (SRS). Histamine causes a rapid and temporary widening of blood vessels, while the widening caused by SRS is longer-lasting and happens after a delay. Both cause an increase in the permeability of blood vessels. Antigens that attach to locations on the basophil cell membrane induce degranulation, resulting in the release of substances that trigger contraction of smooth muscles, secretion of mucus, development of hives, itching, and inflammation of the nasal passages. Basophils are involved in immediate hypersensitivity reactions, such as anaphylactic reactions (hay fever), and certain types of asthma.

3.2.4.6. Lymphocytes

Lymphocytes are the predominant agranulocyte and in the adult human account for 20 to 35% of the circulating leukocytes.

3.2.4.7. Classification

Lymphocytes are a group of cells that vary in terms of their function, lifespan, origin, and size. They can be located in the bloodstream, lymphatic system, lymphatic tissues, and various organs. The predominant type is the small lymphocyte. When observed in blood smears, this cell typically measures 6 to 8 μm in diameter and appears to consist mainly of a nucleus encircled by a narrow, pale blue cytoplasmic rim. On one side of the cell, the cytoplasm may exhibit a slight expansion. The nucleus, which is either round or slightly indented, contains heterochromatin and exhibits a strong staining affinity. Nucleoli are typically not visible, except in living cells or electron micrographs. Lymphocytes are classified as mononuclear leukocytes due to their round nucleus. The electron micrographs show a diminutive Golgi complex and a limited number of mitochondria and lysosomes. There is a small quantity of smooth endoplasmic reticulum (SER), but the presence of rough endoplasmic reticulum (GER) is extremely rare. Lymphocytes, although categorized as agranular leukocytes, may contain a small number of nonspecific azurophil granules which are actually lysosomes. Small lymphocytes, although visually identical, can be classified into three main categories based on their distinct surface markers: B-lymphocytes, T-lymphocytes, and natural killer (NK) cells. B-lymphocytes, also known as B-cells, have a crucial function in humoral immunity. They are specialized cells that can undergo transformation into plasma cells and release antibodies in response to foreign antigens. The antibody exhibits a targeted response towards the antigen that triggered its development. The bone marrow seems to be the organ that conditions B-cells in mammals. B-cells in birds undergo maturation in the bursa of Fabricius, which is a lymphoreticular diverticulum located in the cloaca and has a structure similar to an appendix. B-cells constitute approximately 5 to 10% of the lymphocytes present in the bloodstream of humans (Lien et al., 2005).

T-lymphocytes, also known as T-cells, undergo maturation in the thymus, during which they acquire specific T-cell markers and develop immunological competence. Nevertheless, the immune system's abilities are not completely matured until the cells are transported to peripheral lymphatic organs, particularly the spleen. T-cells play a role in cell-mediated immunity and carry out various functions in the immune system. T-lymphocytes are typically classified into three distinct functional subtypes. When adequately stimulated, certain T-cells engage with activated B-cells and, in their role as T-helper cells, enhance the production of antibodies. In their capacity as T-suppressor cells, they reduce the formation of antibodies. Additionally, as cytotoxic T-cells, some possess the ability to eliminate target cells. T-cells are capable of producing lymphokines, which play crucial roles in the body's defense mechanisms. Among the numerous lymphokines that have been described, the most well-studied are substances that harm or eliminate foreign cells or disrupt their ability to reproduce. These include lymphotoxin, interleukin, interferon, and tumor necrosis factor. Additionally, there are substances like macrophage inhibitory factor (MIF) that prevent the migration of macrophages, causing them to accumulate at the site of an antigen. Macrophage-activating factor stimulates the activity of macrophages, while lymphocyte blastogenic factor (LBF) induces the transformation, growth, and differentiation of small lymphocytes. There are also chemotactic agents that attract neutrophil, eosinophil, or basophil granulocytes to antigen sites, as well as factors that increase vascular permeability. Lymphokines are a diverse group of substances produced by lymphocytes that play a role in regulating immune and inflammatory responses, as well as having cytotoxic effects.

Certain activated T-cells, specifically cytotoxic T-cells or killer (K) lymphocytes, engage in antibody-dependent, cell-to-cell interactions with foreign cells, leading to the destruction of the target cell through lysis. Only the target cells that possess antigens identical to those of the foreign cell that initially triggered the activation of cytotoxic cells are eliminated. The destruction of the foreign cell necessitates close interaction between the effector and its target. This interaction leads to a sequence of modifications in the target cell's membrane, ultimately causing it to rupture. The cytotoxic T-lymphocyte remains unaffected by the interaction and can freely engage with other target cells. T-lymphocytes express cluster designation molecules (CDs) on their cell surface, which aid in the execution of their specific effector functions. T-helper cells exhibit the CD_4 molecule. They are essential for stimulating B-lymphocytes to generate antibodies and activating the macrophage defense system. T-helper cells identify antigens when they are displayed on cells that also exhibit class II major histocompatibility (MHC) antigens (Lofthouse et al., 2002).

Cytotoxic T-cells express CD8 molecules and can identify and eliminate target cells. T-suppressor cells can express either CD_4 or CD8 molecules and can suppress the activity of helper T-cells and regulate the immune response. Another type of small lymphocyte, known as the null cell, has also been documented. These cells do not possess surface markers specific to B-cells or T-cells. Null cells are a heterogeneous group that may include circulating hematopoietic stem cells. Peripheral blood contains a small quantity of larger lymphocytes, measuring 10 to 14 μm in diameter. These cells are referred to as large granular lymphocytes. The cytoplasm of these cells is larger in quantity and has a higher affinity for basic dyes compared to the cytoplasm of the small lymphocyte. The electron micrographs reveal an augmented quantity of ribosomes and mitochondria, a larger volume of endoplasmic reticulum, and an enlargement in the dimensions of the Golgi apparatus. There are dispersed azurophil granules. These cells exhibit direct cytotoxicity and can also cause the lysis of target cells through physical contact. Interestingly, they seem to operate independently of antibodies and without any known previous exposure to the antigen. Consequently, they have been designated as natural killer (NK) cells. Although commonly believed to be non-functional cells, there is increasing evidence suggesting that they are a distinct group of T-cells and may have a connection to immune-dependent cytotoxic T-cells. Natural killer cells are a distinct subset of lymphocytes that possess the capacity to eliminate other cells. The main function of this type of lymphocyte is to eradicate cells that are infected by viruses and certain types of tumor cells.

3.2.4.8. Stimulation by Antigens and Mitogens

Small lymphocytes possess the characteristics of "stem" cells and can generate more small lymphocytes when activated by antigens or nonspecific agents known as mitogens. They are not solely terminal effector cells involved in T- or B-cell functions. Phytohemagglutinin (PHA), concanavalin A (con A), and pokeweed mitogen (PWM) are the most extensively researched mitogens derived from plant extracts. However, other substances like liposaccharide from Escherichia coli, antilymphocyte serum, and different types of pollens also exhibit mitogenic activity. These agents possess a shared capacity to attach to surface groups on small lymphocytes, thereby initiating blastogenic transformation. During the process of transformation, small lymphocytes undergo a gradual increase in size. The nuclei of these cells also grow larger and become euchromatic, while the nucleoli become visible. Additionally, the Golgi complex enlarges, and the cell engages in the synthesis of deoxyribonucleic acid (DNA) and ribonucleic acid (RNA). Within a time frame of 36 to 48 hours, the small lymphocyte undergoes a transformation into a lymphoblast, which then undergoes division and generates new T- or B-cells. The newly formed cells have the ability to generate lymphokines, which are T-cells, or differentiate into plasma cells and produce antibodies, known as B-cells. Mitogens elicit specific responses: PHA and con A selectively activate T-cells, while E. coli lipopolysaccharide exclusively stimulates B-cells. PWM, on the other hand, triggers the activation of both types of small lymphocytes. The reaction's mechanism remains unknown, but it is specific to lymphocytes. While these agents do bind to the surface of other cells, they do not cause their transformation. The reaction of lymphocytes to mitogens is similar to their response following exposure to antigens or lymphoblastic lymphokines (Martini et al., 2019). Lymphocytes undergo repeated recirculation between the bloodstream, lymphoid organs, and lymphatic vessels. The only lymphocytes that circulate are small in size, and the majority of these (80–85%) are long-lasting cells that originate from T-cells, with a lifespan that can be measured in years. Approximately 12–15% of the cells in circulation are short-lived B-cells, which have a lifespan of several months. Lymphocytes continue to circulate until they come into contact with an antigen. A limited quantity of durable cells, derived from T and B cells, exist as memory cells. These are antigen-stimulated small lymphocytes that have not yet produced antibody or lymphokines. These cells persist for extended periods of time as primed cells that can promptly respond to the same antigen upon subsequent encounters with it. Lymphocytes are mobile cells that exit the bloodstream to enter lymphatic organs, travel through the body's connective tissues, or infiltrate epithelial tissues. They possess limited capacity to adhere to or propagate on any type of surface.

3.2.4.9. Monocytes

Monocytes are the second type of mononuclear leukocyte that is typically present in the bloodstream. Their proportions exhibit a high degree of consistency, consistently comprising 3 to 8% of the leukocytes found in circulation. Corticosteroid administration suppresses monocyte numbers. Their diameter ranges from 12 to 20 μm, and they possess a relatively large nucleus that can have a rounded, kidney-shaped, or horseshoe-shaped appearance. The nucleus does not undergo segmentation or filament formation, but it may exhibit coarse constrictions with blunt, broad lobes. The chromatin in lymphocytes is less condensed and therefore exhibits a lower density of staining. It is possible to observe two or three nucleoli. The cytoplasm is plentiful and has a bluish-gray color. It contains many small granules that give it an opaque appearance, resembling ground glass or dust. At the ultrastructural level, the nucleus exhibits one or more nucleoli, while the cytoplasm contains a limited quantity of rough endoplasmic reticulum (GER) and polyribosomes. There are small, elongated mitochondria and a well-formed Golgi apparatus. Azurophil granules are primary lysosomes that appear as dense and homogeneous structures in electron micrographs. Monocytes are a component of the mononuclear phagocyte system and serve as the mobile cells of this system. While in the bloodstream, they have limited functionality but later migrate to different organs and tissues in the body, where they undergo differentiation into macrophages. Monocytes exhibit chemotactic response to the presence of invading microorganisms and necrotic material. They exhibit elevated levels of MHC class II molecules on their surface and serve as a crucial site for the synthesis of the cytokine IL-1, which plays a significant role in the overall response to acute inflammation. Monocytes not only function as tissue scavengers, but also play a crucial role in antigen processing in the immune response. Furthermore, they have the ability to merge with each other, forming different types of phagocytic giant cells. Certain macrophages possess antigen-presenting capabilities, and these particular macrophages belong to a group of specialized cells known as antigen presenting cells. These macrophages engulf antigens that originate from within the body and break them down into smaller fragments called antigen peptides. Subsequently, these fragments are displayed on the surface of the macrophage along with class II major histocompatibility complex (MHC). $CD4^+$ helper T lymphocytes recognize the presented antigen peptide fragment and subsequently stimulate B lymphocyte differentiation. Monocytes lack genuine storage granules for their enzymes, unlike granulocytes, and primarily function as secretory cells. Their composition includes acid hydrolases, peroxidase, acid phosphatase, and aryl sulfatase.

3.2.4.10. Abnormalities

Similar to red blood cells, the overall quantity of white blood cells in circulation typically remains within a relatively limited range in healthy individuals. In the human body, the range for this measurement is 5,000 to 12,000 per cubic millimeter. Leukocytosis refers to an elevation above the usual level and can be caused by illness or heightened emotional or physical strain (Petty et al., 2004). An increase in the number of white blood cells, known as leukocytosis, ranging from 25,000 to 35,000 per cubic millimeter, has been observed following intense physical activity. The rise in numbers corresponds to the release of white blood cells that were previously trapped in small blood vessels and accumulated at the periphery of the bloodstream. Leukopenia refers to a reduction in the number of leukocytes. Activity cycles are linked to diurnal variations of varying degrees. Leukocyte number fluctuations typically involve neutrophil granulocytes and lymphocytes. Neutrophilia refers to an excess of neutrophil granulocytes, while neutropenia indicates a decrease in these cells. Lymphocytosis refers to an elevation in lymphocyte count, while lymphopenia indicates a decrease in lymphocyte count. Elevations in eosinophils, basophils, and monocytes are known as eosinophilia, basophilia, and monocytosis, respectively. Identifying reductions in these cells from smears is challenging due to their naturally low quantities, although they do indeed exist. Multiple cytologic abnormalities can occur, particularly within the granulocytes. Döhle's bodies are minute, asymmetrical blue aggregates or areas, measuring 0.5 to 2.0 μm in diameter, that can manifest within the cytoplasm of neutrophils in certain infections, post-burn injuries, cancer, or following administration of specific oncolytic medications. They seem to be composed of modified ribonucleoprotein. Toxic granulation refers to the presence of large, dark-colored granules that are randomly distributed in the cytoplasm of neutrophils. These granules indicate a change in the azurophil granules. Toxic granulation frequently coexists with Döhle's bodies and can occur alongside cytoplasmic vacuolation in cases of severe bacterial infections. Alder's anomaly is an uncommon abnormality distinguished by the presence of sizable, rough granules in the cytoplasm of neutrophils. This anomaly appears to be inherited, but it does not have any pathological significance. Granulocyte nuclei hypersegmentation is an inherited anomaly that has no significant impact and is also observed in cases of anemia caused by vitamin B12 deficiency. In this type of anemia, the cells exhibit abnormal enlargement and are referred to as macropolycytes. In the Pelger-Huët anomaly, an inherited condition, there are poorly segmented granulocytes present. All varieties of granulocytes are implicated, and the fully developed cells seldom exhibit more than two lobes; more commonly, the cells possess round nuclei devoid of filaments. The anomaly is inconsequential. Atypical lymphocytes can exhibit vacuolated cytoplasm, folded (monocytoid) nuclei, nuclear vacuolation, or prominent nucleoli. The majority of the abnormal cells are medium-sized lymphocytes. Lymphocytes in cases of gargoylism (Hurler's syndrome) have been found to contain dark, basophilic cytoplasmic granules. Similarly, children with a familial disorder exhibit lymphocytes with inclusions resembling Alder's granules (Ravelli and Martini, 2007).

3.2.5. Blood in Children

During the early stages of life, specifically infancy and childhood, the makeup of blood varies considerably in comparison to that of adults. From a hematological perspective, it is important to recognize that children are not simply miniature versions of adults. Children and infants have distinct and unique blood profiles. Typically, younger individuals exhibit more significant deviations from typical adult values and experience greater instability in their blood composition during illness. During birth, the amount of hemoglobin in red blood cells is higher than at any other time, and compared to adult levels, there is an increase in the number of red blood cells (known as polycythemia) and the cells are larger in size (macrocytic). The normal neonate is characterized by an elevation in reticulocytes and the presence of nucleated red cells (normoblasts). Macrocytes, which are abnormally large red blood cells, disappear within a few weeks after birth, and are replaced by normal-sized red blood cells found in adults. Around the third month after birth, there is a decrease in hemoglobin levels and a slight reduction in the number of red blood cells. As a result, the red blood cells appear hypochromic when compared to adult standards. The maintenance of this picture persists until approximately the second year, following which the levels of red cells and hemoglobin gradually increase until reaching adult levels during puberty. The sex differences in red cells and hemoglobin become apparent only after puberty. Neonates have a significantly higher number of leukocytes compared to adults, with neutrophil granulocytes being the most abundant. The majority of these cells exhibit a bilobed structure, with a significant number appearing as band forms. Additionally, myelocytes and even promyelocytes, which are immature forms typically found exclusively in the bone marrow, may be observed. The leukocyte count rapidly decreases and reaches adult levels by approximately the third month. During the period from the second week to approximately the second year, lymphocytes are more prevalent in the bloodstream compared to neutrophils, which are more common in adults. During disease states, a child's blood is likely to exhibit significantly more deviations and variations compared to adult blood. In adults, an infection typically causes a slight increase in white blood cells and an increase in immature white blood cells. However, in children, the same infection can cause a significant increase in white blood cells, resembling a condition called leukemoid reaction, with the presence of immature white blood cells known as myelocytes and promyelocytes. In the same way, the presence of nucleated red cells may indicate anemia in a child, whereas in adults, only polychromatophilia would be observed. Lymphocytosis is more likely to occur in children, while platelet levels tend to fluctuate significantly.

3.3. Special Connective Tissue: Hematopoietic Tissue

The cellular components of blood do not have the ability to reproduce themselves; their quantities in the bloodstream are sustained through a constant replenishment from specific blood-forming (hematopoietic hematopoietic) tissues situated outside of the blood vascular system. These comprise the bone marrow, spleen, lymph nodes, and thymus.

3.3.1. Embryonic and Fetal Hemopoiesis

In adults, blood formation is limited to the bone marrow and lymphatic tissues. However, during embryonic and fetal development, hemopoiesis initially takes place in the yolk sac and subsequently in the liver, spleen, and bone marrow. Under certain pathological conditions, the liver and spleen can regain their function in the production of blood cells.

3.3.1.1. Yolk Sac

Hematopoiesis in the embryo commences shortly after the formation of the germ layers. The initial manifestation takes place within the yolk sac walls, characterized by the emergence of blood islands. Mesenchymal cells in the yolk sac form discrete foci, which then multiply and develop into solid cell masses. These masses subsequently differentiate into two distinct lineages. The cells at the edges become flat and transform into basic endothelial cells, while the cells in the center become rounded, develop a deeply stained cytoplasm, and separate from the edge cells to become the initial precursors for blood cell formation. The majority of the initial blood-forming cells undergo differentiation into primitive erythroblasts, which produce hemoglobin and develop into nucleated red cells that are distinctive to the embryo. The blood islands that are initially separate eventually come together to form a network of vessels that ultimately connect with the vessels inside the embryo. The vessels of the embryo proper show minimal or no development of hematopoietic foci. Hemopoiesis in the yolk sac commences 19 days post-fertilization and persists until the conclusion of the twelfth week. The migration of stem cells from the yolk sac leads to the development of subsequent hemopoiesis in the liver, spleen, and bone marrow. The cells obtain entry into the embryonic circulation through vitelline and allantoic vessels (Roubenoff, 2009).

3.3.1.2. Hepatic Hemopoiesis

The liver is the second most significant hematopoietic organ in the embryo. Hepatic hemopoiesis initiates at the onset of the sixth week of gestation. Currently, hematopoietic cells constitute approximately 10% of the total cell population in the liver. Hemopoiesis reaches its maximum level at 7 to 8 weeks and remains constant until approximately the 15th week, after which it gradually decreases. Erythropoiesis is the main process during hepatic hemopoiesis, with some production of monocytes and platelets in the first 2½ weeks, but there is only a small amount of granulocyte formation. Neutrophils and eosinophils are typically generated in the connective tissue surrounding portal spaces. During the period from the third to the sixth month of gestation, the liver is the main location where red blood cells are produced. The process of erythropoiesis, although in decreasing quantities, continues until birth. Hepatic hemopoiesis bears resemblance to that in the bone marrow, and the red cell precursors in the liver are referred to as definitive erythroblasts due to their ability to generate nonnucleated red cells. The developing cells create clusters of hematopoietic tissue within the cords of developing hepatic cells, but there is no layer of tissue separating the hepatocytes and nearby blood-forming cells.

3.2.1.3. Splenic Hemopoiesis

The spleen has a limited capacity for producing blood cells, which is similar to the liver. Its main contribution is in the production of red blood cells, although it also produces some white blood cells and platelets. Erythroblastic islands and a few megakaryocytes are observed by the twelfth week of gestation. The production of blood cells in the spleen decreases as the bone marrow becomes more active, however, the spleen continues to produce lymphocytes throughout an individual's lifetime.

3.2.1.4. Myeloid Phase

The myeloid phase of hemopoiesis commences when ossification centers form in the cartilaginous models of the long bones. Hematopoietic cells are present in the clavicle of the human fetus at 2 ½ months. Erythropoietic cell clusters can be found in numerous bones by the age of 4 months, and by 6 months, the bone marrow becomes a significant contributor to the production of blood cells in circulation. Throughout the final trimester of pregnancy, the bone marrow serves as the primary organ responsible for producing blood in the developing fetus (Samad et al., 2018).

3.3.2. Bone Marrow

The bone marrow is the primary organ responsible for the production of erythrocytes, platelets, granular leukocytes, and monocytes in adults. Lymphocytes are also generated in the bone marrow and primarily reside in the lymphatic tissues. Overall, the bone marrow is an organ that is comparable to the liver in terms of weight. In humans, it is estimated to make up approximately 4 to 5% of the total body weight.

3.3.2.1. Types

Bone marrow is a highly cellular connective tissue that occupies the medullary cavities of bone. Upon initial examination, it may exhibit a red or yellow hue. The red marrow is responsible for actively producing blood cells and is also known as the hematopoietic marrow. The red color is a result of the presence of red blood cells and their pigmented precursors. Yellow marrow, also known as fatty marrow, is not active and consists mainly of adipocytes. Adipocytes are also sparsely distributed within the red marrow. The quantity and arrangement of adipose tissue within the bone marrow differ depending on age and the demand for hematopoietic cells. Active marrow is present in all bones during the late stages of fetal development and in neonates. However, as postnatal development and aging occur, the active marrow is gradually replaced by fatty marrow. The process of fatty marrow gradually replacing red marrow starts in the shafts of long bones and continues until adulthood, resulting in the majority of marrow in the limbs being of the fatty type. The active marrow is located at the extremities of the long bones and in the ribs, sternum, clavicles, vertebrae, pelvis, and skull. Approximately half of the total marrow consists of adipose tissue. Adipose tissue in the bone marrow is highly unstable and can be readily replaced by active marrow. Yellow marrow functions as a storage area for active marrow to accommodate heightened blood requirements. The active marrow initially displaces the dispersed fat cells within the red marrow. However, if there is a continued or increased need for blood, the red marrow gradually infiltrates the regions occupied by fatty marrow. When there are long-lasting or heightened requirements, the body responds by increasing the production of blood cells in other organs or tissues like the spleen, liver, or lymph nodes. Extramedullary hemopoiesis refers to the production of blood in tissues other than the bone marrow, which occurs in certain pathological conditions.

3.3.2.2. Structure

Bone marrow is a specialized type of connective tissue that can be classified as reticular connective tissue based on its fiber content. The medullary cavities of bone are filled with a loose and spongy network of reticular fibers and cells. This network, known as stroma, serves as a supporting framework for the hematopoietic cells. The network of fibers and cells is seamlessly connected to the endosteum of the bone and is closely linked to blood vessels that extensively penetrate the marrow. All the cell types typically present in blood, along with their precursors, fat cells, plasma cells, and mast cells, are contained within the reticular fiber network. These are the constituent cells of the marrow that are not restricted or limited. Reticular cells are immobile cells that lack phagocytic abilities and do not generate precursor cells for hematopoiesis. These are altered fibroblasts that have the role of creating and sustaining reticular fibers. Reticular cells possess prominent, lightly colored nuclei and unevenly divided cytoplasm that stretch out as elongated, thin projections along the reticular fibers.

3.3.2.3. Vasculature

The nutrient artery enters the marrow cavity of long bones through the nutrient canal and emits central nutrient (longitudinal) branches that travel centrally within the marrow cavity towards the extremities of the bone. These are further supported by additional branches originating from epiphyseal and periosteal arteries. The central nutrient artery gives rise to multiple branches that traverse towards the bony wall along its path. Several of these branches penetrate the bone to provide nourishment to osteons; while others reverse direction and connect directly with the venous system by merging with sinusoids. Sinusoids, also known as venous sinuses, are slender vessels with thin walls that range in diameter from 15 to 100 µm. They create a vast and intricate network throughout the marrow (Santo et al., 2018). The walls are composed of slender, flattened endothelial cells that are closely adjacent and connected by zonula adherens and gap junctions. The basal lamina is either missing or fragmented, with only sporadic patches found on the basal surface. The endothelium is partially covered by a loosely arranged layer of adventitial reticular cells, whose wide and branching extensions blend with the reticular mesh that provides support to the hematopoietic cells. The adventitial reticular cells are composed of ribosomes, GER, and bundles of microfilaments positioned directly below the plasmalemma. The extent of endothelium covered by these cells varies depending on the functional state of the marrow and can be reduced to one-third when there is a high amount of cell movement across the sinusoidal wall. Sinusoids are the initial components of veins. The sinusoids move towards the center of the marrow cavity and connect with the central longitudinal vein, either directly or after merging with other sinusoids, to create collecting sinusoids. Therefore, within the bone marrow, blood circulates from the core to the outer edges and then returns to the core. The central longitudinal vein is characterized by its thin walls, which are composed of a low endothelium, a thin yet intact basal lamina, and a thin outer layer of supportive reticular cells. The venous blood is drained from the marrow through a primary vein that exits via the nutrient canal, where it undergoes a sudden constriction. The blood supply seems to be "closed" meaning that there is uninterrupted endothelial connection between the venous and arterial parts.

3.3.3. Distribution of Marrow Elements

The hematopoietic elements are arranged in irregular cords within the sinusoids. Together, these cords of blood-forming cells constitute the hematopoietic compartment. The blood vascular components are known as the vascular compartment. When examining smears, the distribution of marrow cells seems to be random. However, when looking at consecutive sections, a certain level of cell organization becomes apparent. Fat cells are typically dispersed throughout the marrow, but they have a tendency to gather around the larger blood vessels in the central region. The distribution of blood vessels in the bone marrow leads to a high density of small vessels, particularly sinusoids, at the outer edges. The hematopoietic cells are primarily located in the vicinity of these vessels, near the endosteum. Erythrocytes undergo development in small clusters located near the sinusoids, with the cells within each cluster arranged in a specific order based on their stage of development. The outer rim of the islet is predominantly occupied by the most mature cells. Macrophages are frequently found in the midst of an erythroblastic islet, which is surrounded by multiple layers of red cells, and are typically involved in the production of red blood cells. Megakaryocytes, which are responsible for producing platelets, are in close proximity to the walls of sinusoids and often extend small cytoplasmic processes through openings in the sinusoidal wall. Granulocytes in the process of development tend to form clusters of cells that are typically found a certain distance away from the sinusoids. Blood cell formation takes place extravascularly, meaning that the cells are produced outside of the blood vessels and then enter the circulation by passing through the sinusoids. In order to enter the lumen, the blood cells need to pass through the outer layer of reticular cells and cross the endothelial lining. In regions where cells are actively passing through, the reticular sheath is significantly diminished, resulting in the vessel appearing to be composed solely of an endothelium. Blood cells traverse the endothelium by passing through openings in the cytoplasm rather than by inserting themselves between neighboring endothelial cells. The apertures are comparatively sizable, measuring 1 to 3 μm in diameter. These structures are not permanent and only form in response to and during the movement of cells (Schenck et al., 2015).

3.3.3.1. Stem Cells

The marrow contains hematopoietic cells at different stages of development, ranging from primitive stem cells to fully developed circulating elements in the blood. A stem cell is a type of cell that has the ability to undergo self-replication and differentiate into more specialized cell types. There is ample evidence to support the presence of a pluripotent stem cell in bone marrow that has the ability to generate all the various types of blood cells. When mice are exposed to a deadly amount of radiation, they quickly perish because their blood cells are destroyed, leading to the failure of their hematopoietic organs. Transfusion of bone marrow immediately after radiation exposure prevents death, and both the marrow and lymphatic tissues are regenerated by functional cells from the transfused marrow. During the process of recovery, the spleen develops visible nodules. These nodules are clusters of rapidly multiplying blood cells and contain both immature and maturing blood cells. The cells in the marrow inoculum that generate the spleen colonies are referred to as colony-forming units (CFU). Certain colonies exclusively comprise erythrocyte cells, while others contain developing granulocytes or developing megakaryocytes. However, many colonies are mixed, consisting of developing cells from all three lines. The unicellular origin of mixed colonies has been demonstrated through the transfusion of irradiated donor cells, which have been exposed to a level of radiation that allows for the formation of distinct chromosome markers without compromising their ability to replicate. When these cells develop into spleen colonies, all the cells within them carry the same marker as the cells that were injected, indicating that they must have originated from the same colony-forming unit (CFU). The distinctive chromosome marker is also present in cells that are replenishing the thymus and lymph nodes, suggesting that the CFU has the capacity to generate cells of the lymphatic lineage. Cell cultures derived from granulocytic and mixed colonies generate monocytes and macrophages that exhibit the presence of the marker chromosome. The regenerated bone marrow from these "rescued" animals, when transferred into new recipient animals, generates spleen colonies that still possess the marker chromosomes. Injecting cells from spleen colonies into irradiated animals results in the formation of new spleen colonies. Colonies that consist solely of erythrocytes or granulocytes have the ability to generate colonies of any type. Therefore, the CFU possesses the ability to differentiate and self-renew, thus meeting the criteria to be classified as a stem cell. The bone marrow must possess pluripotent stem cells that have the ability to differentiate into erythrocytes, granular leukocytes, megakaryocytes, monocytes, and lymphocytes. Aside from pluripotent stem cells, bone marrow harbors stem cells with a limited potential for differentiation. These limited stem cells are dedicated to the formation of a single specialized cell type. Empirical data confirms the presence of limited stem cells specifically for the production of erythrocytes (CFU-E), granular leukocytes (CFU-G), and megakaryocytes (CFU-Meg). The majority of studies indicate that there is a shared precursor for granulocytes and monocytes, known as CFU-GM. Restricted stem cells are derived from pluripotent stem cells and exhibit fast proliferation, but possess a limited ability to self-renew. Pluripotent stem cells have the ability to undergo extensive replication, although they have a slow rate of proliferation and serve as a reserve cell. The restricted stem cells are responsible for the continuous replenishment of blood cells on a daily basis. Three categories of restricted erythropoietic stem cells have been defined based on their size, sedimentation velocities, and response to erythropoietin. Additionally, two CFU-GM have been identified based on their growth rates, size, and sedimentation characteristics. Within a specific cell line, the different types of committed stem cells indicate advancements in development from less advanced, yet limited, stem cells to cells that are the direct predecessors of the well-defined, visually identifiable precursor cells. Although the existence of a pluripotent stem cell is unquestionable, there is uncertainty regarding its morphology. Nevertheless, there is evidence suggesting that it may bear resemblance to a lymphocyte in terms of appearance. Through the process of sedimentation column fractionation, it has been observed that CFUs (stem cells) are present in a fraction of bone marrow that consists of cells with similar size and weight to lymphocytes. Administering antimitotic drugs can increase the quantity of marrow stem cells by eliminating hematopoietic cells that are capable of dividing. Due to their slow proliferation, pluripotent stem cells are not affected and their abundance in the bone marrow is significantly enhanced. Stem cells can be further concentrated using density gradient centrifugation. This technique has been demonstrated to increase the number of stem cells in proportion to the increase in cells that resemble lymphoid cells, as evidenced by their ability to generate spleen colonies. These cells resembling lymphocytes have been referred to as potential stem cells. Although the overall structure resembles that of a small lymphocyte, the nucleus is less uniform and has fewer deep indentations compared to typical lymphocytes, and the chromatin is more evenly distributed. Mitochondria are present in limited quantities in both types of cells, but they are smaller and more abundant in the candidate stem cell. There are ribosomes that are not attached to any structure, but there is no rough endoplasmic reticulum or lysosomes (Sherman et al., 2018).

The most primitive hematopoietic cells can be found in the blood islands of the yolk sac. It has been observed that undifferentiated cells from the yolk sac circulate within the fetus and gradually colonize the liver, spleen, and bone marrow. As hepatic hemopoiesis decreases, there is an increase in the number of stem cells in circulation, indicating a significant migration of stem cells into the bone marrow. The blood island cells contain CFUs and have the ability to regenerate all the hematopoietic organs in an animal that has been exposed to radiation.

3.3.4. Development of Erythrocytes

Erythropoiesis is the term used to describe the process of red blood cell production, in which the erythrocyte undergoes gradual changes affecting both its cytoplasm and nucleus. The cell undergoes a gradual reduction in size, while the cytoplasm becomes more acidic as it accumulates hemoglobin and loses organelles. The nucleus undergoes a process of shrinking and becomes more heterochromatic and condensed, eventually leading to its complete loss from the cell. While it is feasible to delineate different "stages" in the developmental sequence, erythropoiesis does not transpire in a sequential manner. The process is a continuous one in which, at various intervals, the cells exhibit distinct and identifiable characteristics. Regrettably, the classification of the immature red blood cell precursors is muddled due to the numerous names assigned by different researchers to the different stages of maturation. The terminology utilized in this context is frequently employed, however, alternative nomenclature is also presented. The proerythroblast, also known as pronormoblast or rubriblast, is the initial identifiable precursor of the red blood cell lineage. It originates from the pluripotent stem cell and undergoes a sequence of limited stem cell divisions. The proerythroblast is comparatively large, measuring 15 to 20 μm in diameter. The cytoplasm, which lacks granules and has a bluish color, often stains unevenly. It exhibits areas that are not adequately stained, particularly near the nucleus. The presence of cytoplasmic basophilia is a crucial characteristic for identifying this early stage of red blood cells. Hemoglobin synthesis has commenced, but its visibility is hindered by the basophilia of the cytoplasm. The nucleus occupies approximately 75% of the cell body, and its chromatin has a finely and uniformly granular or stippled appearance. There are two or more nucleoli that are present and may be noticeable. The electron micrographs reveal a limited development of the endoplasmic reticulum and Golgi apparatus, while there is a high abundance of free ribosomes and scattered polysomes in the cytoplasm. The proerythroblast undergoes multiple divisions to generate basophilic erythroblasts.

The basophilic erythroblast, also known as basophilic normoblast or prorubricyte, typically has a diameter ranging from 12 to 16 µm, which is smaller than the proerythroblast. The nucleus continues to occupy a significant portion of the cell, however, the chromatin appears to be more densely aggregated and exhibits a more intense staining pattern. Nucleoli are typically imperceptible. The cytoplasm exhibits a uniform and intense basophilic staining, occasionally surpassing that observed in the proerythroblast. Electron microscopy reveals a scarcity or absence of endoplasmic reticulum profiles, while free ribosomes and polyribosomes are plentiful. Hemoglobin can be identified as small particles with low electron density. However, it may not always be visible under light microscopy due to the strong basophilia of the cytoplasm, as observed in the proerythroblast. The basophilic erythroblast has the ability to undergo multiple mitotic divisions, resulting in the formation of polychromatophilic erythroblasts. The nucleus of the polychromatophilic erythroblast, also known as the polychromatophilic normoblast or rubricyte, is located in a smaller portion of the cell. It exhibits a compact chromatin network with dispersed large clumps of chromatin. The absence of nucleoli indicates that the cell lacks the ability to divide (Simon et al., 2002). The cytoplasmic staining exhibits a range of colors, from bluish-gray to light slate gray, which corresponds to the varying ratios of ribosomes and hemoglobin. The disappearance of nucleoli leads to the cessation of ribosome formation, resulting in a decrease in ribosome concentration (which exhibits a blue stain) and a gradual increase in hemoglobin concentration (which exhibits a red stain). The size of the cells varies significantly, but they are typically smaller than basophilic erythroblasts. The polychromatophilic erythroblasts consist of multiple generations of cells, with their size indicating the number of previous divisions in the basophilic erythroblast. These cells can be conveniently categorized into "early" and "late" stages based on their size and the intensity of the cytoplasmic basophilia. Normoblasts, also known as acidophilic erythroblasts or metarubricytes, are a type of cell. At this point, the cytoplasm becomes highly saturated with hemoglobin and acquires a clearly noticeable eosinophilic coloration. The electron micrographs reveal a cytoplasm that is uniformly dense and lacks organelles, except for an occasional mitochondrion and sparsely distributed ribosomes. The nucleus is diminutive, intensely colored, and condensed, and frequently exhibits an off-center position. In the end, the nucleus is expeled from the cell along with a thin layer of cytoplasm. Reticulocytes are recently produced red blood cells that possess a small number of ribosomes. However, only a minority of these cells (less than 2%) have enough ribosomes to give color to the cytoplasm. Following the typical presence of blood stains, these cells exhibit a grayish hue rather than the transparent pink color of the more developed forms and are therefore referred to as polychromatophilic erythrocytes. The residual ribosomal nucleoprotein, when stained with brilliant cresyl blue, exhibits a reticulum or web-like structure that diminishes as the cell undergoes maturation. This structure can range from a prominent network to a few granules or threads. Reticulocytes have a volume that is approximately 20% greater than that of fully developed red blood cells. Following the loss of the nucleus, the red blood cell remains in the marrow for a period of 2 to 3 days until it reaches full maturity. Reticulocytes are only released in very small quantities unless there is an urgent need for new erythrocytes. The immature erythrocytes generate a reserve in the bone marrow that corresponds to approximately 2% of the total circulating cell count.

3.3.4.1. Loss of Nucleus

Typically, the nucleus takes on a position that is not centrally located in the cell (late normoblast) and is discarded shortly before the cell enters a marrow sinusoid. In vitro, the normoblast has been observed to actively expel its nucleus, a process that may involve a contractile protein, such as spectrin. The process of enucleation of erythrocytes occurs as the cells traverse through the pores in the sinusoidal endothelium. The pliable cytoplasm can pass through the pore, while the inflexible pyknotic nucleus is retained and detached from the cell, along with a small portion of the cytoplasm. Macrophages quickly phagocytose and eliminate free nuclei (Stavropoulos-Kalinoglou et al., 2007).

3.3.5. Development of Granular Leukocytes

Granulocytopoiesis refers to the maturation process that results in the production of mature granular leukocytes. Throughout this process, the cells gather granules, and the nucleus becomes flattened and indented, ultimately adopting the lobulated shape observed in the fully developed cell. Throughout the process of maturation, multiple stages can be distinguished. However, like the development of red blood cells, the changes that occur during maturation form a continuous sequence, and it is common to observe cells with intermediate characteristics. The commonly recognized stages are myeloblast, promyelocyte, myelocyte, metamyelocyte, band form, and polymorphonuclear or segmented granulocyte. A different terminology replaces the term "myelo" with "granulo" and the sequence of stages is as follows: granuloblast, progranulocyte, granulocyte, metagranulocyte, band form, and polymorphonuclear granulocyte. Myeloblasts are the initial identifiable precursors of granular leukocytes and are specialized stem cells dedicated to producing granulocytes and monocytes. It is found in bone marrow in limited quantities. The myeloblast is relatively diminutive, with a diameter ranging from 10 to 13 µm. The cytoplasm is minimal and exhibits a noticeable affinity for basic dyes, although to a lesser extent than in the proerythroblast, and does not contain granules. Electron microscopy shows a high concentration of unattached ribosomes, but a relatively low amount of rough endoplasmic reticulum. There is a large quantity of small mitochondria. The nucleus, which is either round or oval, takes up a significant portion of the cell. It appears pale when stained and has a somewhat vesicular appearance. There are several nucleoli present. The size of the promyelocyte ranges from 15 to 22 µm in diameter. The nucleus can exhibit a minor degree of flattening, display a small depression, or maintain its circular or oval form. The chromatin is scattered and has a pale color, and there are still multiple nucleoli present. The cytoplasm of the basophil contains purplish red azurophil granules, which become more numerous as the promyelocyte progresses in its development. The electron micrographs reveal a high presence of GER, free ribosomes, many mitochondria, and a highly developed Golgi apparatus. Azurophil granules are exclusively generated during the promyelocyte stage and are synthesized at the inner (concave) side of the Golgi complex through the merging of dense-cored vacuoles (Tello-Winniczuk et al., 2017). The divergence of granulocytes into three distinct lines takes place during the myelocyte stage, marked by the emergence of specific granules. Therefore, it is possible to differentiate between neutrophil, eosinophil, and basophil myelocytes. Myelocytes are smaller in size compared to promyelocytes, with a diameter ranging from 12 to 18 µm. The nucleus can have a spherical or concave shape, and the chromatin is highly compacted. Some myelocytes may exhibit a nucleolus that is clearly defined by a condensation of chromatin, while in others, the nucleolus is less distinct. The myelocyte represents the final stage in which mitosis is still possible. The cytoplasm of the neutrophil myelocyte contains three distinct groups of granules: azurophil granules, which are produced during the promyelocyte stage, and smaller specific granules that are formed during the myelocyte stage. Specific granules are formed through the fusion of dense-cored vacuoles. However, they are produced on the outer (convex) side of the Golgi complex, rather than the concave side. During the process of successive divisions, the myelocyte experiences a gradual decrease in the number of azurophil granules in each cell, resulting in the specific granules outnumbering the azurophil type. The cytoplasm exhibits reduced basophilic staining, and there is a decrease in the presence of free ribosomes and GER. Neutrophil granules that are specific in nature appear faintly stained in regular blood smears, exhibiting a delicate lilac-pink hue. These granules are too minuscule to be distinguished individually using a light microscope. Azurophil granules exhibit a larger size and display a purplish red color when stained with typical blood stains, although their quantity is comparatively lower. When using the electron microscope, azurophil granules exhibit a higher density compared to neutrophil granules. The granules have varying contents: azurophil granules are lysosomes and contain a complex of enzymes, including arylsulfatase, acid phosphatase, beta-galactosidase, beta-glucuronidase, esterase, and nucleotidase. Neutrophil granules contain alkaline phosphatase and proteins that have antibacterial properties. Myelocytes ultimately reach a stage where they become incapable of dividing and subsequently develop into metamyelocytes. The cells exhibit nearly all characteristics of the myelocyte, with the exception that the nucleus is significantly indented to create a horseshoe or kidney shape, the presence of nucleoli is absent, and the chromatin forms a compact network with numerous distinct masses of chromatin. Most of the granules present consist of specific granules, which account for over 80 to 90% of the total. The remaining granules are azurophilic. The neutrophil band exhibits a similar overall structure to the fully developed polymorphonuclear cell, with the distinction that its nucleus takes on a curved or twisted band-like shape. The segmentation is irregular, but it has not reached the point where distinct nuclear lobes and filaments have formed. The maturation stages of eosinophil granulocytes are identical to those of neutrophils. Eosinophil granules become evident during the myelocyte stage and can typically be recognized shortly after their emergence. At times, the granules may exhibit a faint purple-blue hue, which gradually transitions to a more pronounced orange shade as the cell develops. An uncommon eosinophil granule can be observed as early as the promyelocyte stage. The granules are significantly larger than the neutrophil type, exhibit vibrant staining with eosin, and in electron micrographs, they appear slightly less dense and smaller than azurophil granules. During the maturation of cells, the cytoplasm gradually loses its basophilic properties, while the nucleus becomes increasingly indented, forming lobes. During the late myelocyte and metamyelocyte stages, the contents of the eosinophil granules undergo crystallization. Certain granules exhibit a variable-shaped crystal located in the center, surrounded by a matrix of lower density. In contrast, other granules are dense and uniform. Eosinophil granules consist of lysosomes that contain the typical assortment of lysosomal enzymes and myeloperoxidase. The central part of the crystalloid contains a high concentration of major basic protein. The nuclei of several eosinophilic metamyelocytes divide into two parts that remain connected by a thin nuclear filament. These cells transform into eosinophils that display bilobed nuclei. The remaining eosinophilic metamyelocytes transform into band forms, with their nuclei dividing into three or four lobes that are connected by nuclear filaments. Basophil granulocytes also undergo the same maturation process. The definitive granules typically manifest during the myelocyte stage and are seldom observed in the promyelocyte stage. At first, the granules are basophilic, but they later become metachromatic and stain violet instead of blue-black when using toluidine blue or methylene blue. Aside from chemotactic and platelet factors, the granules also contain heparin, histamine, and various enzymes such as diaphorase, dehydrogenases, peroxidases, and histidine carboxylase, which catalyzes the conversion of histidine to histamine.

3.3.6. Development of Platelets

Thrombopoiesis, also known as thrombocytopoiesis, is the process by which platelets are produced. Platelets originate from megakaryocytes, which are large cells measuring 100 μm or more in diameter. Megakaryocytes are typically exclusive to bone marrow. The megakaryocyte's nucleus is characterized by its substantial size and intricate structure, consisting of numerous irregular lobes of varying sizes that are interconnected by narrow regions. The chromatin with a rough pattern stains intensely. The cytoplasm is plentiful and has an irregular outline, often with blunt pseudopods protruding from the surface. During smears, the cytoplasm is uniform and contains many azurophilic granules. At the ultrastructural level, there is a noticeable variation in the degree of zoning. Near the nucleus, there is a narrow perinuclear zone that houses a small number of mitochondria, the Golgi complex, GER, numerous polyribosomes, and some granules. The perinuclear zone is clearly separated from a sizable intermediate zone, which consists of granules, vesicles of various sizes and shapes, mitochondria, ribosomes, and components of the Golgi apparatus. The distribution of granules in megakaryocytes can vary depending on their level of development. They may be evenly distributed or grouped together in small clusters, which are outlined to different extents by a system of membranes. The outermost marginal zone is characterized by a fine granular texture, variable width, and absence of organelles. However, it does contain clusters of microfilaments. Platelets are generated through the process of cytoplasmic segmentation of megakaryocytes, facilitated by a network of demarcation membranes. The azurophil granules aggregate into small clusters, concurrently, small vesicles emerge and arrange themselves in rows amidst the clusters of granules. The vesicles initially exhibit discontinuity, but later elongate and merge to form a three-dimensional network of paired membranes (Więch et al., 2018). The narrow gaps between the membranes create fissures that enclose each prospective platelet; as they are released, the platelets disperse along the narrow fissures. Demarcation membranes are connected to the plasmalemma, meaning that each platelet is surrounded by a standard cell membrane. Megakaryocytes transport platelets by passing them through openings in the sinusoidal walls, either as individual platelets or as ribbons of platelets that later separate into individual elements within the sinusoidal lumen. Once the platelets are shed, the megakaryocyte is left with only a nucleus surrounded by a thin layer of cytoplasm and an intact cell membrane. It is commonly believed that these megakaryocytes are incapable of regenerating their cytoplasm and instead deteriorate, necessitating the formation of new generations of megakaryocytes to take their place. Abnormal megakaryocytes can be observed in the bloodstream, particularly in the small blood vessels of the lungs, where they may persist for a period of time. Megakaryocytes originate from stem cells, with the initial identifiable precursor being a sizable cell, measuring 25 to 45 μm in diameter, containing a solitary circular or oval nucleus. The chromatin exhibits a finely granular pattern, while the basophilic cytoplasm lacks granules. The cells, which are infrequent, have been termed megakaryoblasts. During endomitosis, the cell undergoes a sequence of divisions where the nucleus is replicated, but the cytoplasm does not divide. During metaphase, the chromosomes arrange themselves in multiple planes on a spindle that is becoming more intricate and multipolar. After being reconstituted, groups of chromosomes are integrated into a large lobulated nucleus. Consequently, a sequence of cells with multiple sets of chromosomes is formed, which can potentially reach a chromosome count of 64 times the haploid number in certain megakaryocytes. However, nuclei with a chromosome count of 16 times the haploid number are more frequently observed. Typically, the size of cells and nuclei is directly related to the level of ploidy. There is an interesting proposal that the division of the cytoplasm using demarcation membranes is a delayed and altered form of cytokinesis. Promegakaryocytes are often referred to as cells with 4n and 8n ploidy, measuring between 30 and 40 μm in diameter. The mature megakaryocyte exhibits a distinct marginal zone, which is absent in megakaryocytes involved in platelet formation.

3.3.7. Development of Monocytes

Monocytes are derived from a group of precursor cells in the bone marrow, which are probably the same limited stem cells that produce granular leukocytes. Within various cultures, the cells derived from granulocytic spleen colonies produce both monocytes and granulocytes. Promonocytes, which are immature monocytes found in the bone marrow, are infrequent and challenging to differentiate. Their diameter varies from 8 to 15 μm, and they have large nuclei that are round to oval. The chromatin is evenly distributed, and multiple nucleoli are present. The cytoplasm is relatively abundant and contains many free ribosomes but has a limited amount of endoplasmic reticulum. The Golgi complex, which is highly visible, is connected to multiple small granules that indicate the initial phases of azurophil granules. The fully developed monocytes found in the bone marrow closely resemble those found in the blood. They are slightly smaller than promonocytes, measuring 9 to 11 μm in diameter (Więch et al., 2018). Additionally, they have fewer ribosomes and larger, more abundant azurophil granules. Azurophil granules consist of a diverse range of hydrolytic enzymes and serve as primary lysosomes. After being released into the bloodstream, the monocyte undergoes further maturation while circulating, resulting in the formation of additional azurophil granules. Monocytes undergo maturation by differentiating into macrophages, which can be found in various tissues such as the peritoneum, alveoli of the lungs, or Kupffer cells of the liver. At these sites, they undergo additional molecular programming from the surrounding environment to perform specialized functions.

3.3.8. Marrow Lymphocytes

Lymphocytes originate from pluripotent stem cells in the bone marrow and subsequently migrate to colonize the lymphatic organs and tissues. Constrained stem cells that migrate to the thymus undergo rapid cell division and are subsequently discharged as T-lymphocytes (T-cells). Following their release from the thymus, T-cells relocate to the spleen, where they undergo the final stages of maturation and are subsequently released as durable lymphocytes. B-lymphocytes, also known as B-cells, are derived from the bone marrow. During avian migration, B-cells undergo differentiation in the bursa of Fabricius. The mammalian counterpart of the bursa has not been determined; however, it is possible that the bone marrow serves as the organ responsible for the differentiation of B-cells. Furthermore, these cells seem to undergo their maturation process within the spleen. B- and T-cells continuously move through the bloodstream and lymphatic organs. B-cells in humans have a minimum lifespan of several months, while T-cells can persist for several years.

3.3.8.1. Control of Blood Formation

Erythropoiesis is governed by humoral

control and primarily regulated by a specific erythropoiesis-stimulating factor known as erythropoietin. Nevertheless, the primary trigger to produce red blood cells is hypoxia, as the rate of erythropoietin production is inversely proportional to the amount of oxygen available to the tissues. Erythropoietin is a glycoprotein hormone primarily synthesized by the kidney. However, it is not exclusively produced by the kidney, as it can also be generated in animals that have had their kidneys removed. The specific locations where erythropoietin is produced outside of the kidneys are currently unknown. However, small quantities of a substance that stimulates red blood cell production have been found in liver perfusates. In the fetus, the liver serves as the main producer of erythropoietin. Erythropoietin stimulates the production of RNA and protein, which then leads to the start of hemoglobin synthesis and the differentiation of the limited stem cell. Erythropoietin also seems to enhance the production of hemoglobin in cells that are more specialized and still capable of RNA synthesis, and it stimulates the release of reticulocytes from the bone marrow. Additional hormones, aside from erythropoietin, have been linked to the process of blood formation. Testosterone promotes erythropoiesis and plays a crucial role in the regular maintenance of erythrocyte production, while estrogen has an inhibitory effect on this process. The existence of specific hematopoietic hormones for each cell line in the bone marrow remains uncertain. There is evidence supporting the existence of proteins that circulate in the body and regulate the process of differentiating granulocytes and megakaryocytes. The factors known as granulopoietin and thrombopoietin have not been fully characterized, and their tissue of origin is also unknown. Agents with the ability to regulate the growth and development of specific CFUs have been observed in T-lymphocytes (Sherman et al., 2018).

3.3.9. Interrelationships of Hematopoietic Cells

A pluripotent stem cell, found in the bone marrow and capable of indefinite self-renewal, generates various types of unipotent (restricted) stem cells. The latter possess a restricted ability to regenerate themselves and are dedicated to a specific pathway of growth. Therefore, there exists a dedicated stem cell for each of the cell types observed in blood, and these stem cells generate distinct stages of development that can be identified in any of the different lineages. Multiple categories of limited stem cells have been identified, indicating progressive levels of development. The morphological characteristics of the restricted and pluripotent stem cells have not been determined.

A Closer Look

Cartilage

Cartilage is a strong, flexible connective tissue that protects your joints and bones. It acts as a shock absorber throughout your body. Cartilage at the end of your bones reduces friction and prevents them from rubbing together when you use your joints. It's also the main tissue in some parts of your body and gives them their structure and shape. Damage to your cartilage can happen suddenly — like a sports injury or other trauma — but it can also build up over the course of your life and lead to osteoarthritis. Anything that injures or damages your cartilage can make it hard or impossible to use your joints the way you're used to.

Cartilage protects your bones and joints. It surrounds the ends of your bones and cushions the spaces in your joints where bones meet. Cartilage has three jobs:

- Absorbing shock: Cartilage cushions your bones and joints when you move and use them. It absorbs force and reduces how much stress an impact puts on your bones. Think about the difference between jumping up and down in bare feet and wearing running shoes. Cartilage acts like the cushion in your sneakers on the inside of your joints and around your bones.
- Reducing friction: Cartilage lubricates your joints. It helps your bones slide past each other without rubbing together. This lets your joints work as smoothly as they should and reduces wear and tear on them.

Supporting structures in your body: Cartilage helps your joints keep their shape while moving. It also connects other tissue together and to your bones. Muscles, tendons and ligaments are connected to cartilage throughout your body.

Cartilage is also the main tissue in some parts of your body including your:

- Nose.
- Ears.
- Windpipe (your trachea).

Types of cartilage

There are three types of cartilage in your body:

- Hyaline cartilage.
- Elastic cartilage.
- Fibrocartilage.

Hyaline cartilage

Hyaline cartilage is the most common type of cartilage in your body. It lines your joints and caps the ends of your bones. Hyaline cartilage at the ends of your bones is sometimes referred to as articular cartilage.

Hyaline cartilage is slippery and smooth which helps your bones move smoothly past each other in your joints. It's flexible but strong enough to help your joints hold their shape.

Hyaline cartilage locations in your body include:

- At the ends of bones that form joints.
- Between your ribs.
- In your nasal passages.

Fibrocartilage

Fibrocartilage is what its name sounds like: tough cartilage made of thick fibers. It's the strongest and least flexible of the three types. It's tough enough to hold parts of your body in place and absorb impacts.

Fibrocartilage locations in your body include:

- The meniscus in your knee.
- In disks between the vertebrae in your spine.
- Supporting muscles, tendons and ligaments throughout your body.

Elastic cartilage

Elastic cartilage is your most flexible cartilage. It supports parts of your body that need to bend and move to function. Elastic cartilage can bounce back to its original shape, even after a strong force. Your ear is made of elastic cartilage. It can bend and move without hurting you before returning to its usual shape.

Elastic cartilage locations in your body include:

- Your external ears (the parts of your ear that are outside your body).
- Your eustachian tubes (the tube that carries sounds from your external ear into your head).
- Your larynx (your voice box).

Summary

This chapter focuses on the unique category of connective tissues that have specialized functions and distinct histological features, including cartilage, bone, blood, and lymphatic tissue. These tissues are adapted to specific roles in the body, such as providing structural support, enabling movement, and facilitating transport of nutrients and waste. The chapter highlights the specialized cells, such as chondrocytes in cartilage and osteocytes in bone, as well as the organized extracellular matrix components like collagen and elastin fibers. This organization gives special connective tissues their unique properties, allowing them to withstand mechanical stress, provide elasticity, or circulate vital substances. Understanding these tissues is key for medical fields, particularly in diagnosing and treating conditions related to structural and blood-related disorders.

References

1. Dijk FS, Cobben JM, Kariminejad A, Maugeri A, Nikkels PG, van Rijn RR, Pals G. Osteogenesis Imperfecta: A Review with Clinical Examples. Mol Syndromol. 2011 Dec;2(1):1-20.
2. Ehrlich HP, Krummel TM. Regulation of wound healing from a connective tissue perspective. Wound Repair Regen. 1996 Apr-Jun;4(2):203-10.
3. Grosso G, Bei R, Mistretta A, Marventano S, Calabrese G, Masuelli L, Giganti MG, Modesti A, Galvano F, Gazzolo D. Effects of vitamin C on health: a review of evidence. Front Biosci (Landmark Ed). 2013 Jun 01;18(3):1017-29.
4. Halper J, Kjaer M. Basic components of connective tissues and extracellular matrix: elastin, fibrillin, fibulins, fibrinogen, fibronectin, laminin, tenascins and thrombospondins. Adv Exp Med Biol. 2014;802:31-47.
5. Hayakawa M, Kobayashi M, Hoshino T. Microfibrils: a constitutive component of reticular fibers in the mouse lymph node. Cell Tissue Res. 1990 Oct;262(1):199-201.
6. Heidari B. Rheumatoid Arthritis: Early diagnosis and treatment outcomes. Caspian J Intern Med. 2011 Winter;2(1):161-70.
7. Kannus P. Structure of the tendon connective tissue. Scand J Med Sci Sports. 2000 Dec;10(6):312-20.
8. Kashtan CE. Alport Syndrome. In: Adam MP, Feldman J, Mirzaa GM, Pagon RA, Wallace SE, Bean LJH, Gripp KW, Amemiya A, editors. GeneReviews® [Internet]. University of Washington, Seattle; Seattle (WA): Aug 28, 2001.
9. Last JA, Reiser KM. Collagen biosynthesis. Environ Health Perspect. 1984 Apr;55:169-77.
10. Loebel C, Burdick JA. Engineering Stem and Stromal Cell Therapies for Musculoskeletal Tissue Repair. Cell Stem Cell. 2018 Mar 01;22(3):325-339.
11. Lykkesfeldt J, Michels AJ, Frei B. Vitamin C. Adv Nutr. 2014 Jan 01;5(1):16-8.
12. Marini JC, Forlino A, Bächinger HP, Bishop NJ, Byers PH, Paepe A, Fassier F, Fratzl-Zelman N, Kozloff KM, Krakow D, Montpetit K, Semler O. Osteogenesis imperfecta. Nat Rev Dis Primers. 2017 Aug 18;3:17052.
13. Mescher AL. Macrophages and fibroblasts during inflammation and tissue repair in models of organ regeneration. Regeneration (Oxf). 2017 Apr;4(2):39-53.

14. Ogawa M, Larue AC, Watson PM, Watson DK. Hematopoietic stem cell origin of connective tissues. Exp Hematol. 2010 Jul;38(7):540-7.

15. Pinnell SR. Regulation of collagen synthesis. J Invest Dermatol. 1982 Jul;79 Suppl 1:73s-76s.

16. Ricard-Blum S. The collagen family. Cold Spring Harb Perspect Biol. 2011 Jan 01;3(1):a004978.

17. Shekhter AB. Connective tissue as an integral system: role of cell-cell and cell-matrix interactions. Connect Tissue Res. 1986;15(1-2):23-31.

18. Uitto J. Biochemistry of the elastic fibers in normal connective tissues and its alterations in diseases. J Invest Dermatol. 1979 Jan;72(1):1-10.

19. Young RA. The Ground Substance of Connective Tissue. J Physiol. 1894 May 29;16(5-6):325-50.

Chapter

NERVE AND MUSCLE

4

Contents

Introduction

Nerve and muscle tissues are essential components of the human body, playing crucial roles in movement, sensation, and communication. Nerve tissue, consisting of neurons and supporting cells called neuroglia, forms the basis of the nervous system, transmitting electrical signals throughout the body. Neurons are specialized cells capable of generating and conducting electrical impulses, allowing for the rapid transmission of information. Muscle tissue, on the other hand, is responsible for movement and maintaining posture. There are three types of muscle tissue: skeletal, cardiac, and smooth. Skeletal muscle is under voluntary control and is attached to bones, enabling body movements. Cardiac muscle is present in the heart and is responsible for pumping blood. Smooth muscle is found in the walls of hollow organs such as the intestines and blood vessels, controlling involuntary movements (Aartsma-Rus and van Putten, 2014). Histologically, nerve tissue is characterized by the presence of neurons with elongated cell bodies and branching dendrites and axons. Muscle tissue characterizes long, cylindrical cells called muscle fibers, which contain contractile proteins that allow for muscle contraction. Understanding the histology of nerve and muscle tissues is crucial for comprehending their function and dysfunction in various physiological and pathological conditions.

Orientation and Directional Terms

Term	Definition	Illustration
Skeletal Muscle	A type of striated muscle tissue that is attached to bones and facilitates voluntary movement; characterized by long, cylindrical fibers and multiple nuclei per cell.	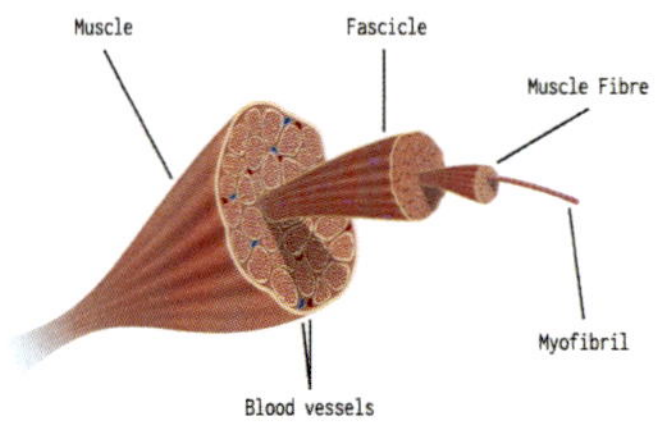
Cardiac Muscle	A specialized type of striated muscle found only in the heart; it is involuntary, has a branched structure, and contains intercalated discs that allow for synchronized contractions.	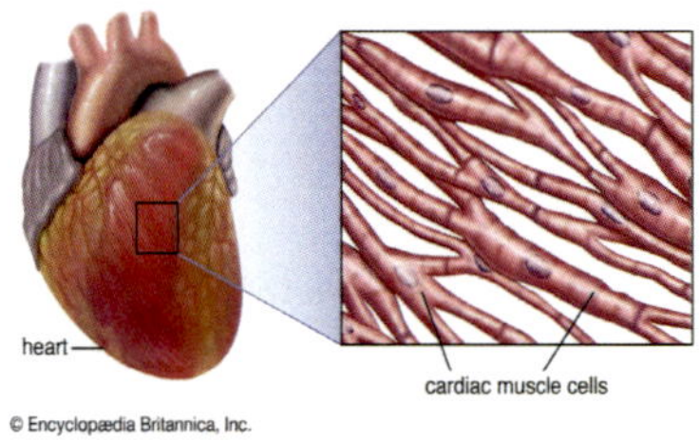
Smooth Muscle	A type of non-striated muscle tissue found in the walls of hollow organs (e.g., intestines, blood vessels); it is involuntary and responsible for peristalsis and regulating blood flow.	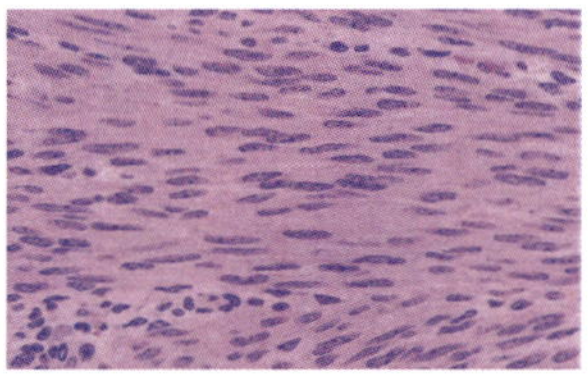
Spinal Cord	A cylindrical structure composed of nervous tissue that runs down the vertebral column, serving as a major conduit for information traveling between the brain and the peripheral nervous system.	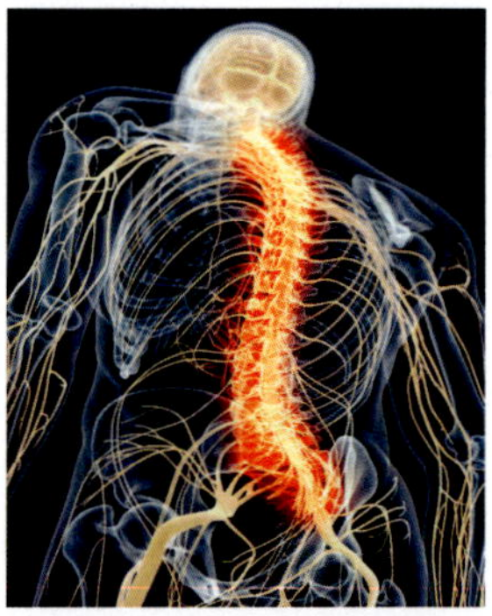
Histogenesis	The process by which cells differentiate and develop into specialized tissue types during embryonic development, involving cell proliferation, migration, and interaction.	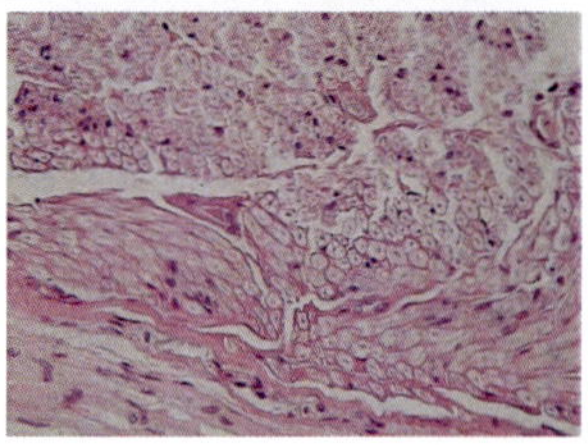

4.1. Muscle Tissue

Muscle is the fundamental tissue that exhibits the prominent characteristic of contractility. The intentional motions of the body and the upkeep of body position are achieved through the contractions of muscles that are connected to the skeleton. Muscular contraction is responsible for the rhythmic pulsation of the heart, respiration, blood vessel constriction, intestinal peristalsis, bladder voiding, and other essential physiological processes. Muscle contraction is crucial for producing heat and helps to regulate the body's temperature, which typically remains around 37°C.

The fundamental structural component of muscle tissue is the muscle cell, also known as a fiber due to its elongated shape. The shape of the cell is functionally significant as an elongated cell can achieve a greater unidimensional contraction compared to a globular cell of the same volume. The muscle fibers within a muscle mass are aligned in the direction of movement.

4.1.1. Classification

Three distinct types of muscle can be differentiated based on their physical structure and purpose. Striated muscles are characterized by a consistent arrangement of light and dark bands that span the entire width of the muscle fiber. Skeletal and cardiac muscle are the types of muscle associated with the skeleton and heart, respectively. Smooth muscle cells do not have cross-striations and are found in the walls of internal organs. They are commonly known as visceral muscles. Muscle can be classified as either voluntary, meaning it is controlled by the will, or involuntary, meaning it is not controlled by the will. Striated skeletal muscle is typically under conscious control, while smooth muscle operates without conscious control. Cardiac muscle is an involuntary striated muscle. Approximately 50% of the entire body mass is composed of muscle tissue.

4.1.2. Skeletal Muscle

Skeletal muscle is the predominant tissue in the body and comprises the structures commonly known as "the muscles." Skeletal muscle constitutes approximately 40% of the overall body mass. It allows for a broad spectrum of voluntary actions, encompassing both delicate and precise movements required for writing, as well as the swift and forceful actions involved in jumping or throwing a ball. The potential of skeletal muscle in generating power is demonstrated by the velocity achieved by a thrown ball, which can exceed 90 mph at the instant it is released from the fingertips. Skeletal muscle glycogen plays a crucial role in ATP synthesis, which provides energy for muscle activity via the process of glycolysis. Glycogen is produced from glucose through the action of glycogen synthase during a state of high blood sugar (hyperglycemia) that occurs after consuming a meal rich in carbohydrates. This process is facilitated by an increase in the ratio of insulin to glucagon hormones. Muscle glycogen phosphorylase breaks down glycogen in response to exercise because of a reduction in ATP, the release of calcium during muscle contraction, and the secretion of epinephrine, which binds to α- and β-adrenergic receptors on skeletal muscle cells. Glycogen is hydrolyzed into glucose-6-phosphate, which then undergoes glycolysis to generate ATP. Glycogen cannot be broken down into free glucose in skeletal muscle due to the absence of the enzyme glucose-6-phosphatase. As a result, glucose remains in its phosphorylated state and is unable to exit the muscle cell. Skeletal muscle cells benefit from a metabolic advantage because they can rapidly use glucose-6-phosphate, without needing to first phosphorylate free glucose. Instead, glucose is readily available to provide energy through the process of glycolysis.

4.1.2.1. Organization

The fiber, a long multinucleated cell, is the smallest visible independent unit of skeletal muscle when observed under a light microscope. Fascicles, which are composed of parallel fibers, are visible to the naked eye. Conversely, bundles of fascicles constitute a complete muscle. Fascicles exhibit size variations across different muscles, generally appearing small in muscles involved in precise movements and large in muscles engaged in activities requiring significant force. Connective tissue is present in association with muscle at all levels of organization. The complete muscle is enveloped by a connective tissue sheath, the epimysium. Septa extend from the inner layer of the epimysium to surround each bundle of muscle fibers known as the fascicle, forming the perimysium. Thin extensions of the perimysium then wrap around each individual muscle fiber, creating the endomysium (Allen et al., 2016). The connective tissue, although referred to by different names depending on its association with various structural units of muscle, remains continuous throughout the body. The composition of this structure includes collagenous, reticular, and elastic fibers, as well as various cell types such as fibroblasts, macrophages, and adipocytes. The endomysium is a fragile tissue composed primarily of reticular fibers and thin collagen fibers. It serves as a conduit for blood capillaries and small nerve branches. The major blood vessels and nerves are located within the perimysium. Connective tissue serves the dual purpose of binding muscle units together and facilitating the integration and transmission of their contraction force. The quantity of connective tissue differs among muscles, with a relatively higher amount in muscles capable of finely controlled movements. The muscles that connect to soft tissues, such as the muscles in the tongue and face, contain a high concentration of elastic tissue.

4.1.2.2. The Skeletal Muscle Fiber (Cell)

Typically, skeletal muscle fibers do not divide, but the muscles in the face and tongue may branch out when their fibers attach to mucous membranes or skin. The fibers of skeletal muscle are elongated cylindrical structures that exhibit variations in both shape and length. Some fibers have a cylindrical shape with rounded ends and span the entire length of a muscle, while others are spindle-shaped with narrow tapering ends and may not run the entire length of the muscle. One extremity of the fiber may be connected to a tendon, while the other joins with connective tissue located in the central part of the muscle, or both extremities may be situated within the muscle mass. Transverse sections of fresh muscle exhibit a circular or oval shape, whereas, in fixed material, they take on an irregular polyhedral form. The fibers have a diameter in the range of 10 to 100 μm and can reach a length of 10 cm. The size of muscles can vary both between different muscles and within the same muscle. Fibers that are longer have larger diameters and are correlated with stronger muscles. An observation has been made regarding the spatial organization of muscle fibers, where larger diameter fibers tend to be positioned more centrally. Fiber size is subject to change based on usage, with the possibility of hypertrophy (increase in size) due to continued use or atrophy (decrease in size) due to disuse. The prominent structural characteristic of skeletal muscle fibers is the presence of alternating light and dark segments, which give rise to the banding or cross-striations observed when the fiber is examined in the longitudinal section (Angebault et al., 2021). When observed under polarized light, the dark bands exhibit anisotropic properties and are referred to as A bands. Conversely, the light bands display isotropic properties and are therefore known as I bands. The Z line or Z disc is a narrow, dense line that runs transversely through the center of the I band. Electron micrographs show the presence of a pale and narrow region known as the H band, which intersects the A band. Within the H band, there is a dark M line. These features can be observed in Figures 4.1 and 4.2. The relative length of each band depends on the degree of fiber contraction. The A band maintains a consistent length, while the I band is more noticeable in a stretched muscle and shorter in a contracted muscle.

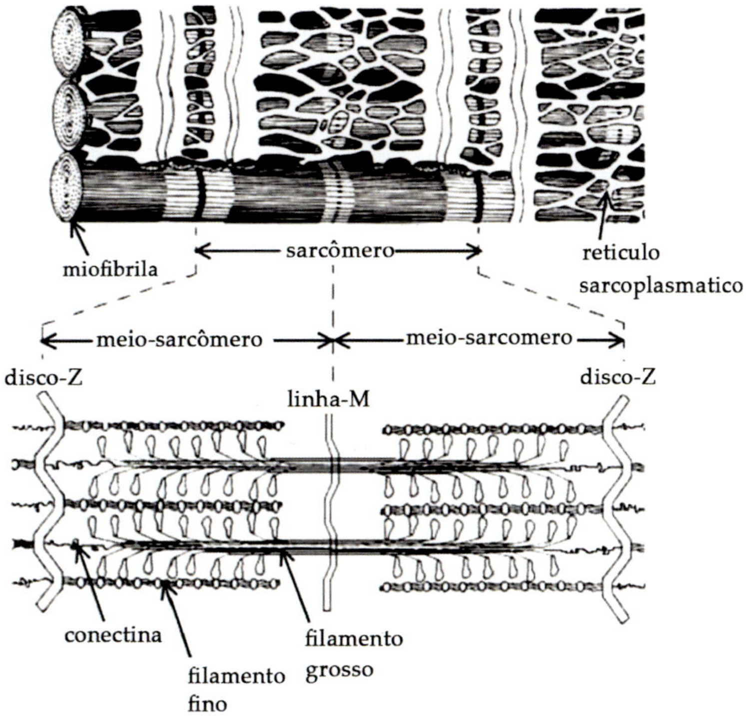

Figure 4.1. *Schematic drawing of a small section from a muscle cell showing some myofibrils and parts of the intracellular Ca^{2+} stores.*

Source: *https://www.researchgate.net/profile/Robert-Stehle/publication/23934608/figure/fig1/AS:277414346280960@1443152142537/Schematic-drawing-of-a-small-section-from-a-muscle-cell-showing-some-myofibrils-and-parts.png.*

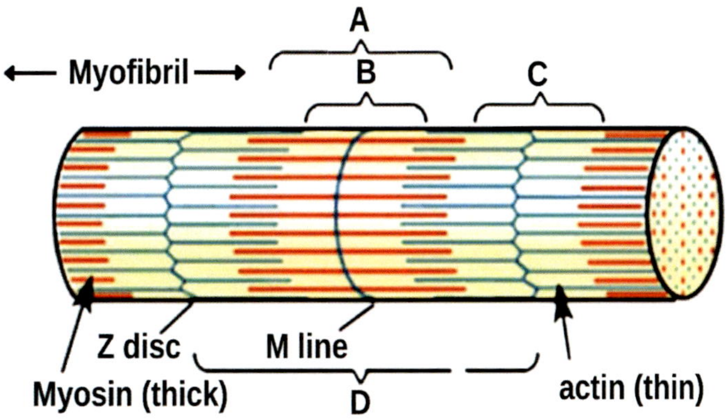

Figure 4.2. *A schematic diagram depicting the striped pattern that emerges on a solitary myofibril extracted from a skeletal muscle cell.*

Source: https://dsbihjlymzdyy.cloudfront.net/bio_images/all/Diagrams%20in%20Svg%20form%2FStructural%20Organization%20in%20Animals%2F122249.svg.svg.

4.1.2.3. Structure of Skeletal Muscle Fibers

Each skeletal muscle fiber is a long cell surrounded by a thin membrane that, when viewed under an electron microscope, can be seen as consisting of the plasmalemma and an attached outer layer made up of glycoproteins and glycosaminoglycans. The sarcolemma, which is the plasmalemma of a muscle cell, is essentially the same as the plasmalemma found in any other cell. The outer layer of glycoprotein/glycosaminoglycan corresponds to the basal lamina of epithelia and is referred to as the external lamina. It is connected to fine reticular fibers that mix with the reticular fibers of the endomysium. The striated muscle fiber is a cell with multiple nuclei. Skeletal muscle cells can possess numerous nuclei, often reaching several hundred in number. The nuclei in adult muscle are elongated in the direction of the long axis of the fiber and are positioned peripherally, directly beneath the sarcolemma. Chromatin is typically found distributed along the inner surface of the nuclear envelope, with the presence of one or two nucleoli. The nuclei are evenly distributed along the fiber; however, they become more abundant and randomly distributed in the region where the muscle attaches to a tendon. The sarcoplasm, which is the cytoplasm of a muscle cell, is equivalent to the cytoplasm of any other cell. Multiple diminutive Golgi complexes are located in close proximity to one end of a nucleus; lysosomes typically occupy a position adjacent to the nucleus. Satellite cells, which are closely connected to the muscle fiber, are positioned flat against the fiber, and are covered by the same external lamina that surrounds the muscle cell. While it is challenging to differentiate their nuclei from muscle cell nuclei using light microscopy, they have a more elongated shape, are more tightly packed, exhibit less dispersed chromatin, and lack nucleoli. The cytoplasm is limited in quantity but forms a distinct boundary between the nucleus of the satellite cell and the muscle fiber. Satellite cells in electron micrographs exhibit centrioles (which are absent in muscle cells), a limited endoplasmic reticulum, a compact Golgi complex, and a sparse distribution of mitochondria located close to the nuclei's extremities. Satellite cells potentially comprise the remaining population of primitive myoblasts and make up less than 4% of the nuclei associated with muscle tissue. Myofibrils are elongated, threadlike structures located in the sarcoplasm that extend along the entire length of the muscle fiber. Myofibrils, which have a diameter of 1 to 2 μm, are the smallest identifiable units of contractile material using a light microscope. When viewed in cross sections, myofibrils are observed as tiny dots, whereas in longitudinal sections they create a longitudinal striation along the fiber. Every myofibril exhibits a banding pattern that is the same as that of the entire fiber. The fiber banding occurs because the bands on consecutive myofibrils are aligned. The presence of cross-striations is limited to the myofibrils and does not span across the sarcoplasm between fibrils. The alignment of the striations on neighboring myofibrils is maintained by desmin, a network of intermediate filaments. These filaments connect adjacent myofibrils to each other and connect the myofibrils to the cell membrane (Ascah et al., 2011). The sarcoplasmic reticulum, which is a modified form of the smooth endoplasmic reticulum found in other cells, is connected to each myofibril. The sarcoplasmic reticulum functions as a reservoir for calcium ions in muscle tissue. The sarcoplasmic reticulum's membrane is composed of multiple transmembrane proteins, such as calcium-ATPase, which actively move calcium from the cytosol into its lumen. In this context, calsequestrin and other proteins have the ability to attach to and retain the calcium ions that have been taken into the cell. This organelle is composed of a complex and uninterrupted network of membrane-bound tubules known as sarcotubules, which encircle each myofibril in a mesh-like structure. At every intersection of the

A and I bands, there are enlarged sarcotubules called terminal cisternae. These terminal cisternae encircle each myofibril and are connected to the terminal cisternae of neighboring myofibrils. Each of the terminal cisternae is responsible for serving either an A band or an I band. Narrow, longitudinal sarcotubules extend over the A and I bands from each of the cisternae. In the A band, the tubules create a disorganized network in the H band area, while in the I band, a similar merging happens at the Z line region (Bostick et al., 2009). Therefore, each A and I band is encompassed by a "unit" or segment of the sarcoplasmic reticulum. These units are composed of the terminal cisternae located at the A-I junctions, connected by longitudinal sarcotubules that interconnect in the region of the H and Z lines of their corresponding A and I bands. The sarcoplasmic reticulum exhibits a consistent structure irrespective of the type of muscle fiber (Figure 4.3).

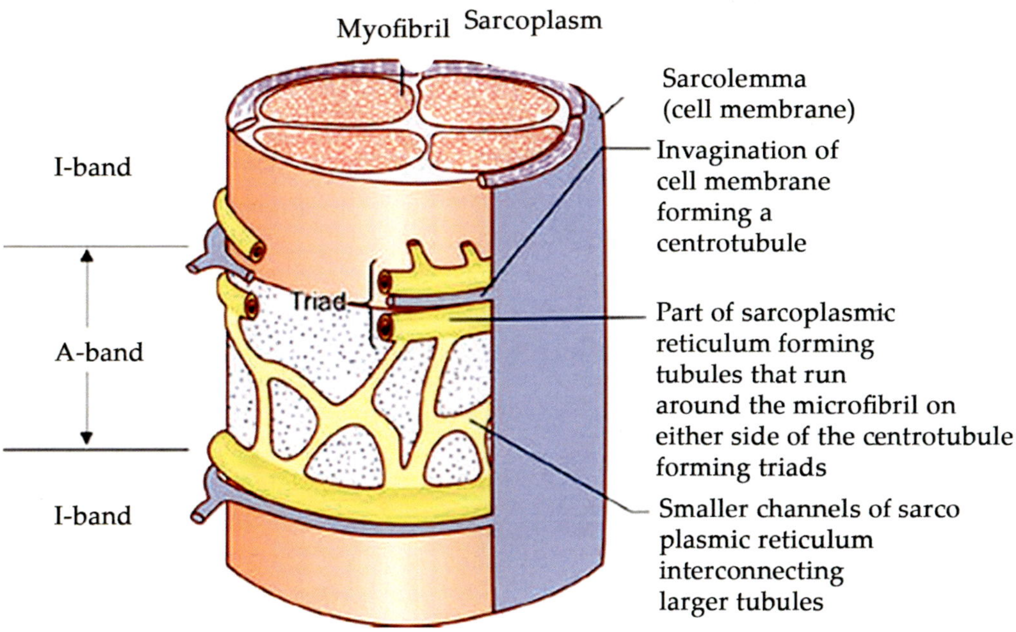

Figure 4.3. *Diagrammatic representation of the sarcoplasmic reticulum and system of T-tubules associated with skeletal muscle.*

Source: https://d45jl3w9libvn.cloudfront.net/jaypee/static/books/9789386056979/Chapters/images/255–2.jpg.

The cisternae pairs located at the A-I junctions are divided by a thin T-tubule, and these three structures – the T-tubule and two terminal cisternae – together make up the triad of skeletal muscle. T-tubules are invaginations of the sarcolemma that extend into the muscle fiber to encircle each myofibril. The T-tubules of a single myofibril establish communication with the T-tubules of neighboring myofibrils, resulting in the formation of a comprehensive network throughout the fiber. The lumen of the T-tubule does not connect to the cisternae, but it does connect to the extracellular space at the surface of the sarcolemma. T-tubules are anatomically separate from the sarcoplasmic reticulum, and together, they form the T-system (Briguet et al., 2004). The T-system efficiently propagates signals to all myofibrils within the cell, ensuring synchronized contraction. Electrical impulses passing through the sarcoplasmic reticulum cause the release of calcium ions from the sarcoplasmic reticulum into the adjacent contractile elements, which leads to their contraction. T-tubules and terminal cisternae are in proximity. Junctional feet bridge the narrow space between T-tubules and terminal cisternae, creating regions of minimal resistance that allow impulses to transmit to the sarcoplasmic reticulum. The electron micrographs reveal the presence of regularly spaced densities known as junctional feet, which extend from the T-tubules to the terminal cisternae. The cisternal membranes have evenly spaced dimples that match the locations of the feet. The junctional feet are hypothesized to be calcium ion channel proteins that span from the terminal cisternae to voltage-sensing calcium ion channel proteins of the T-tubules. During depolarization, the T-tubule channel proteins undergo a change in shape and, due to their close connection with calcium ion channel proteins of the sarcoplasmic reticulum, the latter proteins open up. This leads to the release of calcium ions into the cytosol, which then triggers muscle contraction (Bulfield et al., 1984).

4.1.2.4. Structure of Myofibrils

When observed under the electron microscope, the myofibril is observed to be composed of long, thin myofilaments. Two distinct types of myofilaments have been identified, which differ in size and chemical composition. The diameter of the thick filaments is 10 nm, while the thin filaments have a diameter of 5 nm. The thick filaments primarily comprise myosin and have a length of 1.5 μm. They possess a slightly enlarged middle section and gradually narrow towards the ends. The central section is sleek, while the extremities are adorned with numerous small protrusions. The myosin filaments can be separated into their individual molecules, with approximately 180 molecules per filament. Each molecule is composed of a head and a tail. The molecules' tails are aligned in a parallel manner, with the smooth central part of the filament composed solely of these tails. The heads protrude laterally from the filament along its tapered ends and arrange themselves in a helical pattern along the filament. The majority of the tail is composed of light meromyosin, while the heads, along with certain portions of the tails, are composed of heavy meromyosin. The length of thin filaments is approximately 1 μm (Burkin et al., 2001). These filaments consist of actin subunits that are globular in shape and are attached to each other end to end. The subunits are arranged in two longitudinal strands that are twisted around each other in a loose helix. Tropomyosin, a second protein, is located in the groove between the two actin strands and provides stability to the actin filament. A trimeric protein complex composed of troponin-T, troponin-I, and troponin-C is attached to tropomyosin at regular intervals of 40 nm. The troponin complex governs the interaction between actin and myosin. Troponin-T attaches the troponin complex to tropomyosin and places the complex at a specific location on the actin filament, allowing actin to interact with myosin. Troponin-I inhibits the binding of actin to myosin. Troponin-C forms a complex with calcium ions. Upon this event, a conformational alteration takes place in the troponin complex, enabling the binding and interaction of myosin with the actin filament. The energy required for the interaction between myosin and actin is derived from the hydrolysis of adenosine triphosphate (ATP) by ATPase activity, which is mainly found in the globular heads of the myosin molecules. Through the formation and dissolution of bonds between the myosin and actin filaments, the actin filaments move in relation to the myosin filaments, causing a decrease in the length of each sarcomere. This leads to a contraction of each myofibril. The organization of the thick and thin filaments is accountable for the striped pattern observed on the myofibrils. The I band is composed solely of thin filaments that extend in both directions from the Z line. On one side, the filaments are positioned in a way that is not aligned with the filaments on the other side. Additionally, there are connecting elements that seem to run diagonally across the Z line, forming a zigzag pattern. As the actin filament approaches the Z line, it merges with four thin threads that seem to form loops within the Z line and connect with a thread from a neighboring actin filament. Multiple accessory proteins, including α-actinin, Z protein, filamin, and amorphin, have been discovered within the Z line. α-actinin attaches the actin filaments to the Z line (Carlson, 2022). Nebulin, an extra accessory protein, is linked to the thin filaments that contain actin. The A band primarily comprises thick filaments composed of myosin, with slender cross-connections located at their midpoints. These cross-connections are responsible for the formation of the M line (Fig. 4.4). Myomesin, a protein located in the M line region, is responsible for aligning and preserving the spatial arrangement of myosin filaments. Another myosin-binding protein, known as C protein, aligns with the M-line in the outer section of the A band and assists in maintaining the proper alignment of the myosin myofilaments. Titin, also known as connectin, is a remarkably large accessory protein that possesses elastic characteristics.

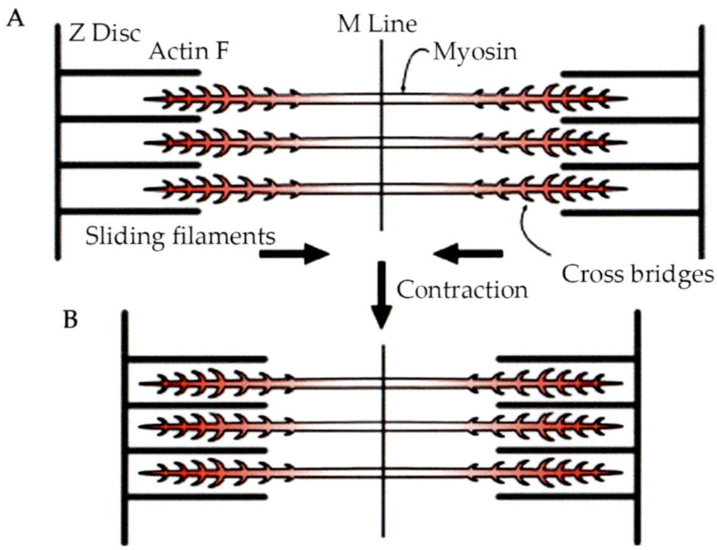

Figure 4.4. *The relationship of the cross-banding observed on a myofibril compared to the arrangement of actin and myosin myofilaments.*

Source: https://ars.els-cdn.com/content/image/3-s2.0-B9780323908016001270-f00127–04–9780323908016.jpg.

The molecule is the largest one discovered in cells of mammals. The titin molecule extends from the Z line to the M line and is believed to act as a molecular spring, generating a reactive force when a non-activated muscle is stretched. Titin, along with the connective harness surrounding the skeletal muscle cell, provides resistance against forces that attempt to dislodge actin filaments from between the myosin filaments in the A band. Recent evidence further indicates that titin may play a role in intracellular signal transduction pathways. The actin filaments protrude into the A bands, which are located between the thick filaments. The penetration of the actin filaments determines the width of the H band, which is composed solely of thick filaments. The extent of penetration is influenced by the level of muscle contraction. Each myosin filament is connected to six actin filaments. The narrow space between the thick and thin filaments at the ends of the A bands is spanned by cross-bridges comprising the heads of the myosin molecules. The function of muscles relies on the precise arrangement of actin and myosin proteins within each myofibril. This is accomplished through the utilization of accessory proteins that bind to various components of the contractile mechanism, ensuring their proper alignment with one another. The organization of the filaments also determines the structural foundation of the contractile mechanism. During muscle contraction, the A band maintains a constant length, while the I and H bands decrease in length, and the Z lines move closer to the ends of the A bands. The changes occur due to modifications in the relative positions of the thick and thin filaments (Chey et al., 2022). There is no alteration in the lengths of the filaments; instead, the actin filaments move alongside the myosin filaments to enter further into the A band. Consequently, the I and H bands experience a reduction in length. The Z lines are repositioned towards the edges of the A bands, resulting in a reduction in the length of each sarcomere (the space between consecutive Z lines), which leads to a general contraction of the myofibrils (**Figure 4.5**).

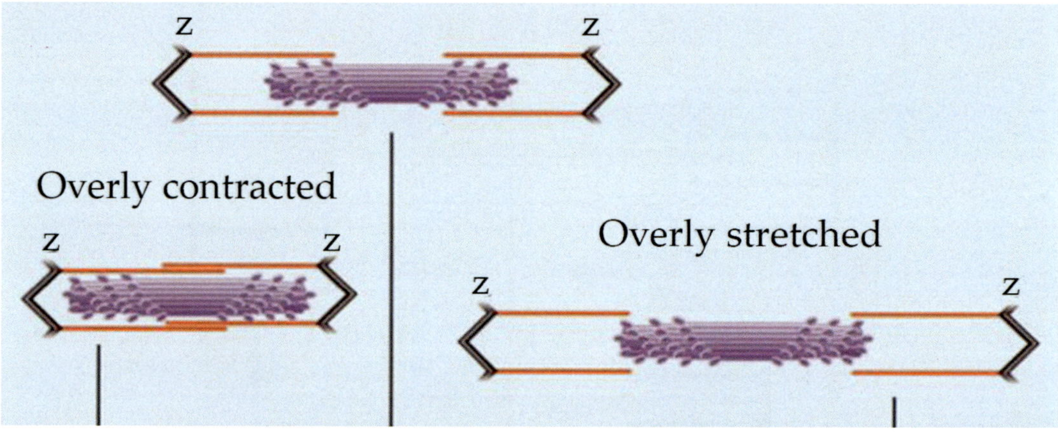

Figure 4.5. *The relationship of the cross-banding observed on a myofibril compared to the arrangement of actin and myosin myofilaments in stretched, relaxed, and contracted skeletal muscle.*

Source: https://qph.cf2.quoracdn.net/main-qimg-1550dcd18e08c1a05acc8044062f9a88-pjlq.

The movement of the filaments occurs due to the repetitive formation and separation of connections between the heads of the myosin molecules and the adjacent actin filaments. Attachments are formed at locations that are successively more distant along the actin filaments, resulting in the filaments moving in relation to each other. The movement of the filaments seems to be caused by the alteration of the angle at which the myosin heads attach to the actin filaments. To translate the contraction of a sarcomere to the contraction of an entire fiber, it is necessary for each sarcomere within the fiber to contract simultaneously rather than sequentially. The T-system induces simultaneous contraction within a single fiber and throughout the entire muscle. Link proteins facilitate the transmission of muscle contraction force to the extracellular matrix. Dystrophin serves as an anchor for actin filaments. Dystrophin is associated with multiple glycoproteins that combine to form a complex that traverses the plasmalemma (de Paepe and de Bleecker, 2013). The glycoprotein complex's outer surface is connected to a protein component called laminin 2 (merosin) in the external laminae of skeletal muscle cells. The contractile forces generated within the skeletal muscle cell are transferred to the external lamina through this linkage. The external lamina is then connected to the connective tissue harness, which is formed by the interconnections of endomysium, perimysium, and epimysium, through molecular bonding. Dystrophin is localized in high concentrations beneath the plasma membrane at the extremities of the skeletal muscle cells, specifically at or in close proximity to the junctions between muscle and tendon. Duchenne's muscular dystrophy is an inherited muscle disease that specifically affects male children. It is caused by a genetic defect in the dystrophin gene, which is responsible for producing the linking protein.

4.1.2.5. Fiber Types in Skeletal Muscle

Certain skeletal muscles exhibit a more pronounced red coloration compared to others, which is indicative of the specific type of fibers (cells) that are present. Muscle fibers are categorized as red, white, and intermediate based on their overall appearance, or as type 1, IIA, IIB, and IIC based on their reactions to histochemical staining. Type I fibers are characterized by their red coloration. These structures are rich in myoglobin (a pigment similar to hemoglobin) and fat, and they are surrounded by a large number of capillaries. Their cells possess many small mitochondria, exhibit high levels of oxidative enzymes, have low amounts of myophosphorylase and glycogen, and primarily rely on aerobic metabolism. Aerobic glycolysis is the process by which glucose is transformed into carbon dioxide and water. The mitochondria are clustered beneath the sarcolemma and are arranged in rows between myofibrils. They have numerous densely packed cristae. The Z line has a significant width. The fibers exhibit no staining when subjected to adenosine triphosphatase (ATPase) reaction at pH 9.4. However, they demonstrate a "reversal" effect and exhibit strong staining (dark) when reacted at pH 4.6 or 4.3. Type I fibers are physiological muscle fibers that are classified as slow twitch fibers. These fibers are specifically adapted to perform slow and repetitive contractions. They are also capable of sustaining long periods of continued activity (Deconinck et al., 1997). Type I fibers are typically situated in the innermost layers of a muscle, in close proximity to the bone. They are frequently found in muscles that counteract the force of gravity, such as the longitudinal muscles in the back. Type IIA fibers are red because they have a high concentration of myoglobin, but they have less fat compared to type I fibers. They possess a significant amount of glycogen and exhibit both aerobic and anaerobic metabolism. Type I fibers exhibit slightly higher activity of oxidative enzymes compared to type II fibers. The level of myophosphatase activity is elevated, the number of mitochondria is limited but their size is increased, and the Z lines appear wider than usual. The ATPase activity exhibits a high level of enzymatic activity (as indicated by the dark staining of the fibers) at pH 9.4 but demonstrates low activity at pH 4.6 or 4.3. Type IIA fibers are classified as fast-twitch muscle cells that have a high resistance to fatigue. Type IIB fibers exhibit a white coloration and possess moderate quantities of glycogen while having minimal amounts of myoglobin or fat. They can be identified by their significant diameters, reduced blood supply, decreased quantity of large mitochondria, and narrow Z lines. The fibers possess a high concentration of myophosphorylase but have a low abundance of oxidative enzymes. From a metabolic standpoint, they function anaerobically. Anaerobic glycolysis is the process by which glucose is converted into lactate. Type IIB fibers exhibit high ATPase activity at pH 9.4. However, they do not exhibit any staining at a pH of 4.3 and only display moderate reactivity at a pH of 4.6. Type IIB fibers are specialized fast twitch fibers that are well-suited for quick and brief bursts of activity, such as those found in the extraocular muscles of the eye. Type IIB fibers exhibit rapid fatigue compared to type I and IIA fibers. Additionally, Type IIC fibers have been documented. These fibers resemble type IIB fibers, but their ATPase activity is only suppressed when the pH is below 4.0. The Z lines are narrow and correspond to the intermediate fiber type. Type IIC fibers are a type of fast-twitch muscle fiber that exhibits greater resistance to fatigue compared to type IIB fibers. IID fibers have also been characterized.

4.1.2.6. Motor Nerve Endings

Each skeletal muscle receives innervation from one or more nerves that contain both efferent (motor) and afferent (sensory) fibers. A motor unit consists of a motor neuron and the muscle fibers it innervates. The motor unit size is determined by the number of muscle fibers innervated by a single nerve fiber and can vary across different muscles. Small motor units are present in situations that demand precise regulation of muscle function, while large units are found in muscles used for more coarse activities. In the extraocular muscles of the eye, each muscle fiber receives innervation from a nerve, resulting in the formation of small motor units. Conversely, in the major muscles of the limb, a single nerve fiber can innervate 1,500 to 2,000 muscle fibers, forming a large motor unit. Each motor unit consists of muscle fibers that share the same histochemical type, resulting in the presence of type I and type II motor units. The motor nerve branches terminate on the muscle fiber at a specialized area known as the motor end-plate or myoneural junction. The junction is visible as a slightly raised area on the muscle fiber where nuclei have gathered. As the nerve nears the end-plate, it sheds its myelin sheath and terminates in several swollen enlargements. The outer surfaces of these enlargements are coated by a continuation of Schwann's cells. The nerve endings are located in shallow depressions called synaptic troughs, which are found on the surface of the muscle fiber. The sarcolemma, which covers these gaps, folds inward to create multiple secondary synaptic clefts or junctional folds (Deconinck and Dan, 2007) (Figure 4.6).

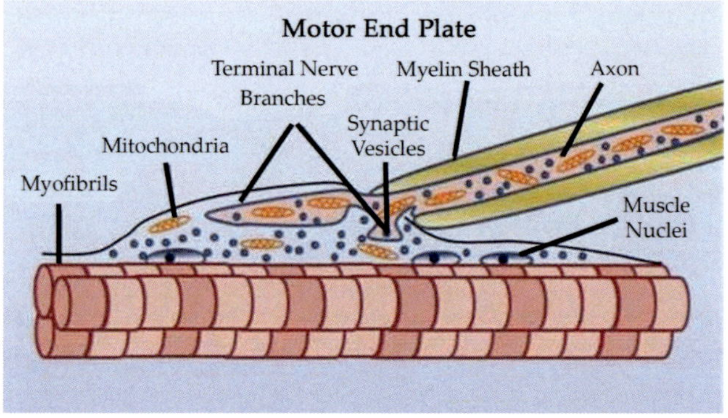

Figure 4.6. *A diagrammatic sketch of a motor end-plate.*

Source: *https://www.researchgate.net/profile/Ziad-Abu-Faraj/publication/348154430/figure/fig3/AS:975601947123716@1609613038563/The-motor-end-plate-in-a-longitudinal-section-Adapted-from-Guyton-AC-Hall-JE.jpg.*

Although nerve and muscle fibers are closely connected at the junctions, their cell membranes are separated by a glycoprotein layer that is created by the merging of the outer layers of the muscle fiber, nerve fiber, and Schwann's cells. This layer covers the primary synaptic cleft and also reaches into each secondary cleft. The sarcoplasm beneath the nerve terminal contains numerous large, vesicular nuclei, along with a substantial quantity of mitochondria, ribosomes, and GER. The nerve terminals contain a high concentration of mitochondria and a large number of synaptic vesicles that store acetylcholine, which is a neurotransmitter. An electrical signal in a nerve causes the axon terminal to become less negatively charged, which enables calcium ions to enter. This event triggers the release of acetylcholine into the narrow space between nerve cells called the synaptic cleft. Acetylcholine is discharged by synaptic vesicles via exocytosis at specific sites on the presynaptic membrane referred to as active zones. Nicotinic acetylcholine receptors are located in the sarcolemma, specifically at the outer edges of the secondary clefts.

However, acetylcholinesterase is located on the inner surface of the secondary clefts and the external lamina of this area. The acetylcholine receptors are comprised of ion channels that are formed by a complex of five homologous subunits. Upon binding of acetylcholine to these receptors, a conformational alteration takes place, resulting in the opening of the channel and the subsequent entry of sodium ions. The influx of ions depolarizes the sarcolemma, triggering an action potential. The depolarization of the sarcolemma initiates an action potential that subsequently spreads through the T-tubule network, leading to the activation of muscle contraction. Various factors can obstruct or disrupt the postsynaptic receptor site. Curare, a botanical poison, can selectively bind to the nicotinic acetylcholine receptor proteins found in the muscle cell membrane after the synapse, effectively blocking and preventing muscle contraction. Myasthenia gravis is an autoimmune disease where antibodies in the bloodstream attack and interfere with nicotinic acetylcholine receptor proteins, leading to abnormal muscle activity (Duan et al., 2021).

4.1.2.7. Sensory Nerve Endings

Skeletal muscle is equipped with numerous sensory endings, including both simple spiral terminations of nonmyelinated nerves that wrap around the muscle fibers, and more complex structures known as muscle spindles or neuromuscular spindles. The muscle spindle is composed of a stretched, oval-shaped capsule made of connective tissue. Inside the capsule, there are a small number of slender, altered skeletal muscle fibers that are connected to sensory and motor nerves. The altered muscle fibers extend through the capsule from one end to the other and create the intrafusal fibers, which differentiate them from the regular muscle fibers (extrafusal fibers) located outside the capsule. There are two different types of intrafusal fibers. Both structures exhibit striations along most of their lengths, but in the middle of the fibers, the striations are substituted by clusters of nuclei. The nuclear bag fibers are a type of intrafusal fiber that is characterized by its larger size and the presence of a cluster of nuclei in its nonstriated region. This cluster of nuclei leads to a slight expansion of the fibers in this region. The second type of fiber is characterized by its narrower diameter, and the nuclei in the central region are arranged in a single row, giving them the name "nuclear chain fiber." The nuclear bag fibers extend beyond the capsule and attach to the endomysium of nearby extrafusal fibers. The nuclear chain fibers are more abundant and have a shorter length. They connect to the capsule at the extremities of the spindle or to the coverings of nuclear bag fibers. Due to the absence of myofibrils, the central regions of the intrafusal fibers are incapable of contracting, making them noncontractile. Each spindle is innervated by a solitary, thick sensory nerve fiber that branches into multiple nonmyelinated branches. These branches terminate in an intricate network of rings and spirals located at the central regions of the intrafusal fibers. The annulospiral endings are located below the external lamina within grooves in the sarcolemma. Flower spray endings refer to the cluster- or spray-like terminations of smaller sensory nerves, primarily found on nuclear chain fibers. Intrafusal fibers also receive small motor nerve fibers that terminate either as motor end-plates or as long, diffuse trail endings that branch out over the intrafusal fibers, establishing multiple connections with them. Muscle spindles function as stretch receptors and are primarily located in slow-contracting extensor muscles that are responsible for maintaining posture. They are also found in muscles that are used for precise movements. The motor nerves provide stimulation to maintain tension on the intrafusal fibers, causing their nonstriated segments to stretch. The level of elongation is adequate to sustain the sensory nerve endings in this area in a state of excitation that is near their thresholds. When a complete muscle is elongated, it increases the tension on the intrafusal fibers and stretching of their nonstriated regions, which in turn causes the sensory nerve to release impulses. Contraction of the muscle leads to a decrease in tension on the spindle, causing the sensory nerve endings to stop firing. The rate at which the nerve endings release signals is directly related to the amount of tension on the intrafusal fibers. This, combined with the number of active spindles, guarantees an appropriate level of muscle contraction in response to the stimulus (Dubinin et al., 2021) (**Figure 4.7**).

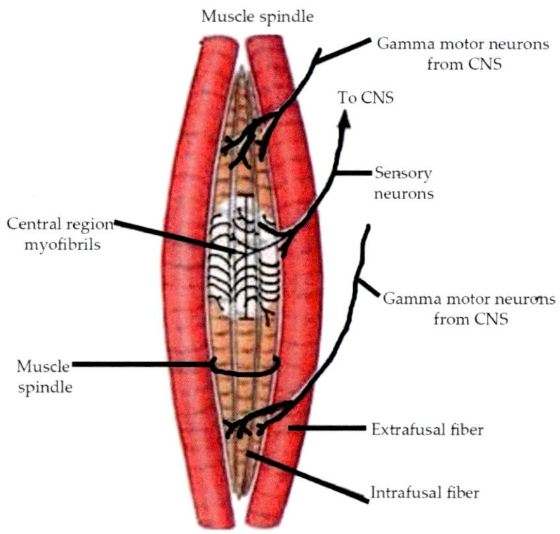

Figure 4.7. *An illustrative depiction of a muscle spindle.*

Source: https://www.researchgate.net/profile/Karin-Lienhard-2/publication/279263976/figure/fig3/AS:614272900022274@1523465480117/Schematic-illustration-of-a-muscle-spindle.png.

4.1.2.8. Tendon and Tendon-Muscle Junctions

Tendons are composed of dense collagen fibers that are tightly packed together. The endotendineum is a small amount of loose, fibroelastic connective tissue that surrounds each bundle. The peritendineum is a coarser connective tissue that wraps around poorly defined fascicles, which are made up of variable numbers of collagen bundles. The tendon is composed of clusters of fascicles, which are surrounded by a robust layer of dense irregular connective tissue known as the epitendineum. Tendons are composed primarily of collagen fibers, with fibroblasts (or tenocytes) interspersed between these fibers. Tendons exemplify dense regular connective tissue. The connective tissue of the endomysium, perimysium, and epimysium becomes highly fibrous and merges with the connective tissue of the tendon at the point where muscle and tendon meet. On the muscle side of the junction, the connective tissue fibers extend into the indentations of the sarcolemma and are firmly attached to the external lamina, to which the sarcolemma also attaches. The actin filaments of the final sarcomere within the muscle fiber are firmly attached to the sarcolemma at the fiber's end. Contraction of the muscle fiber is transmitted to the sarcolemma, the outer layer, and then to the tendon through the connective tissue sheaths. Tendon organs are sensory receptors that are enclosed in capsules and located at the junctions between tendons and muscles. The organ consists of a capsule of dense irregular connective tissue traversed by specialized collagen bundles that are continuous with collagen fibers outside the capsule. One large sensory nerve penetrates the capsule and generates multiple nonmyelinated branches that wrap around the collagen bundles. The tendon organ senses stress produced by muscle contractions, preventing them from becoming excessive.

4.1.3. Cardiac Muscle

Cardiac muscle is exclusively found in the heart, where it comprises the myocardium, the muscular wall of the heart. Cardiac muscle exhibits characteristics of both smooth and skeletal muscle. Similar to skeletal muscle, it is striated. However, like smooth muscle, cardiac muscle is involuntary. Cardiac muscle differs significantly from both types in terms of its structural characteristics and stands out by virtue of its inherent ability to contract automatically and spontaneously, without the need for any external stimulus.

4.1.3.1. Organization

In cardiac muscle, the histologic unit of structure is the cell, also known as a fiber. However, unlike skeletal muscle, the cells in cardiac muscle are connected end to end to create long tracts. The cells have the potential to undergo division at their ends prior to connecting with neighboring fibers, resulting in the formation of a complex network of branching fibers (Dubinin et al., 2020). Cardiac muscle cells are relatively small compared to skeletal muscle cells, with a length of approximately 120 μm and a width of 20 μm. The presence of a network of collagenous and reticular fibers between the muscle fibers, known as endomysium, is observed. However, due to the branching nature of the fibers, this network is more irregular compared to skeletal muscle. The perimysium, like skeletal muscle, consists of collagen and reticular fibers that envelop large clusters of cardiac muscle fibers.

4.1.3.2. The Cardiac Muscle Fiber (Cell)

Every individual cell, also known as a fiber, is surrounded by a sarcolemma. Outside the sarcolemma, there is an external lamina that is connected to delicate reticular fibers. Each fiber typically contains one or occasionally two central nuclei. Cardiac fibers exhibit a similar banding pattern to skeletal muscle, with identifiable A, I, M, H, and Z bands, although they are less prominent than in skeletal muscle.

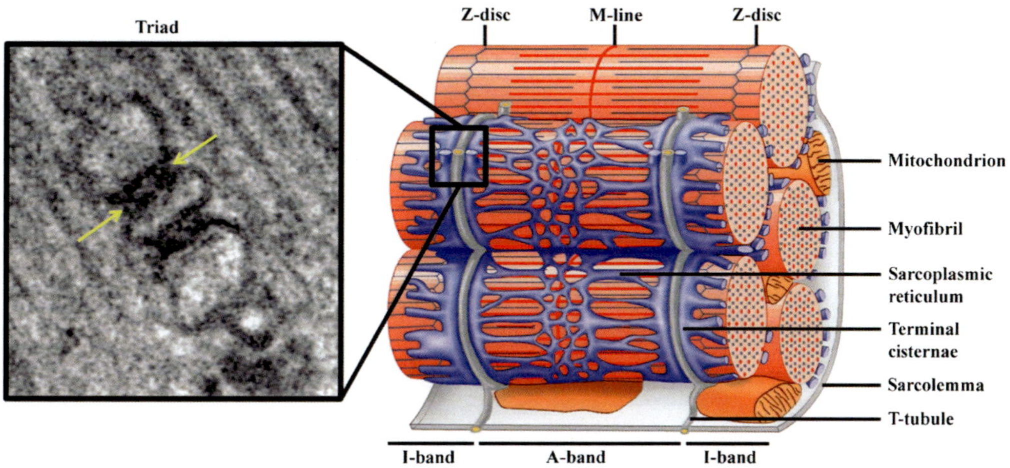

Figure 4.8. *Illustration depicting the structure of the sarcoplasmic reticulum and the network of T-tubules in cardiac muscle.*

Source: https://media.springernature.com/lw685/springer-static/image/art%3A10.1186%2F2044-5040-1-26/MediaObjects/13395_2011_Article_25_Fig1_HTML.jpg.

The banding pattern is caused by the organization of actin and myosin filaments. However, the arrangement of filaments into myofibrils is not clearly defined, and groups of myofibrils often merge with neighboring bundles or are separated by rows of mitochondria. Mitochondria constitute up to 30% of the cytoplasmic volume of cardiac myocytes, thereby endowing them with resistance to fatigue. The clusters of muscle fibers separate around the cell nuclei, creating an elongated region of cytoplasm at each end of the nucleus. These regions are inhabited by small Golgi complexes and abundant large mitochondria that possess densely arranged cristae. Cardiac muscle contains a significant amount of glycogen. The sarcoplasmic reticulum in cardiac muscle is less extensive and less developed compared to that in skeletal muscle. The sarcotubules form a continuous network throughout the entire length of the sarcomere and interconnect freely to create a plexiform pattern without any specific interconnections at the H band. The absence of terminal cisternae results in direct contact between the sarcoplasmic reticulum and the T-tubules through irregular expansions of the sarcotubules. Since the majority of T-tubules are only connected to one cisterna at a given location, the connections between T-tubules and sarcoplasmic reticulum are referred to as Dyads (**Figure 4.8**).

In cardiac muscle, the T-tubules are positioned at the Z lines instead of the A-I junctions, and they have significantly larger lumens compared to the T-tubules in skeletal muscle. The luminal surfaces of the cardiac T-tubules are covered by an extension of the outer layer of the sarcolemma. The sarcotubules located at the outer edge of the cell can be closely attached to the sarcolemma. These attachments are referred to as peripheral couplings or subsarcolemmal cisternae. In cardiac muscle, the sarcomere, which is the functional unit, is defined by two consecutive Z lines, similar to skeletal muscle.

4.1.3.3. Intercalated Discs

Cardiac muscle cells are connected to each other through specialized junctions, which can be observed as dark lines under a light microscope. The intercalated discs are structures that intersect the fibers in a sequential manner at the Z lines, resulting in both transverse and horizontal components. Across the transverse regions, the cells that face each other are intricately intertwined and occasionally connected by desmosomes. Desmosomal junctions serve to attach intermediate (desmin) filaments of the cytoskeleton to the plasmalemma. The junction between cells is generally larger than that of a desmosome and is therefore referred to as a fascia adherens. The sarcoplasm in close proximity to the cytoplasmic surface of the cell membrane contains a concentrated network of filaments, where the actin filaments are inserted (Dubowitz et al., 2020). The fascia adherens is composed of α-actinin and vinculin, which are actin-binding proteins that serve to attach actin to the plasmalemma. Transmembrane glycoproteins cadherin and plakoglobin serve as cell-adhesion molecules, effectively connecting cardiac muscle cells together at the intercalated disc. The cardiac myocytes contain large titin molecules which, similar to skeletal muscle, play a crucial role in passive force. They work in conjunction with the connective tissue surrounding the myocytes to counteract forces that attempt to separate the actin myofilaments from the myosin filaments of the A band. The membranes of adjacent cells are connected by gap junctions at various locations along the junctions. The longitudinal section of the intercalated disc is connected to the transverse part and contains a larger number of gap junctions. Gap junctions are regions of low electrical resistance that facilitate the rapid transmission of excitation impulses between cells, leading to the synchronization of muscle contraction.

4.1.4. Smooth Muscle

Smooth muscle cells are ubiquitously present in the body and have a crucial role in the functioning of organs. They constitute the contractile component of the walls of blood vessels and hollow organs, such as the digestive, respiratory, and reproductive tracts. Smooth muscle cells are found in various locations throughout the body. They can be found in the skin, where they create small muscles that are connected to hair follicles. They are also present in the iris and ciliary body of the eye, as well as in the erectile tissue of the penis and clitoris. Additionally, smooth muscle cells can be found in the stroma of the ovary and prostate.

4.1.4.1. The Smooth Muscle Fiber (Cell)

Every smooth muscle fiber is an elongated cell with a widened central region and narrowing ends. The length of cells differs across various organs, ranging from 20 μm in small blood vessels to 500 to 600 μm in the pregnant uterus. The cell contains a solitary nucleus located in the middle of its wide section, elongated along the cell's long axis. Within a contracted cell, the nucleus exhibits a crinkled or folded contour. The cells do not have cross-striations and appear uniform in typical histologic preparations. Nevertheless, longitudinal striations become visible following the process of macerating the cells in acid. These striations potentially correspond to the myofibrils. The electron micrographs reveal the presence of elongated and thin mitochondria, a limited number of GER tubules, groups of unattached ribosomes, and a small Golgi complex located at one end of the nucleus in the sarcoplasmic region.

Unlike the cells found in the heart and skeletal muscles, the presence of a basic sarcoplasmic reticulum is limited and there is no system of T-tubules. Most of the cytoplasm consists of densely packed, delicate filaments organized into bundles that align with the cell's long axis. The myofilaments are interspersed with mitochondria and glycogen granules. Oval, dense bodies are present in various locations within the sarcoplasm, serving as insertion points for the myofilaments, specifically actin. α-actinin, an actin-binding protein, is present in the cytoplasmic dense bodies (Duddy et al., 2015). Desmin, the intermediate filament that is present in the highest quantity, as well as vimentin, also attaches to these anchoring points. The sarcolemma is enveloped by a robust external lamina composed of proteoglycans and an abundance of delicate collagenous and reticular fibers that merge with the adjacent connective tissue. In certain areas, the outer layer is absent, and the cell membranes of neighboring smooth muscle cells are closely joined together through gap junctions (also known as nexuses). These junctions allow for the transmission of excitation impulses from one cell to another. Regions of heightened concentration, resembling the compact structures known as dense bodies, are present intermittently along the inner surface of the sarcolemma, becoming more abundant towards the ends of the cells. These compact areas are observed as locations where myofilaments and intermediate filaments connect to the cell membrane. They are commonly referred to as attachment plaques. Studies have demonstrated that the subplasmalemmal attachment plaques contain the actin-binding proteins, vinculin and Talin. The sarcolemma in these regions may exhibit numerous caveolae, which are formed by invaginations of the cell membrane. The caveolae are believed to serve as the functional counterpart to the T-tubule system found in striated muscle. The smooth muscle cell's caveolae contain calcium ions and are closely associated with the endoplasmic reticulum's terminal sacs, which are located beneath the plasmalemma and also contain calcium ions.

4.1.4.2. Myofilaments

Electron microscopy has revealed the presence of both thick and thin filaments in smooth muscle cells, while biochemical analysis has confirmed the presence of actin and myosin. Smooth muscle cells contain actin filaments that are linked to tropomyosin but do not possess troponin. Nevertheless, the identification of myosin filaments in typical electron microscopic preparations has proven to be challenging. It has been proposed that in smooth muscle, myosin is unstable and only forms filaments when contraction is initiated. Unfixed, rapidly frozen smooth muscle cells have revealed the presence of filamentous myosin. These cells exhibit organized arrays of thick myosin filaments, which are surrounded by rosettes of actin. The myosin found in smooth muscle differs from that in skeletal muscle in that it will only attach to actin when its light chain is phosphorylated. In smooth muscle, contraction is initiated by the release of calcium ions from the sarcoplasmic reticulum, similar to what happens in striated muscle. Calcium ions in smooth muscle form a complex with calmodulin, a protein that binds to calcium. This complex then activates myosin light-chain kinase, an enzyme required for the phosphorylation of myosin. This phosphorylation allows myosin to bind to actin. Subsequent contraction takes place. The myosin and actin myofilaments of smooth muscle interact in a similar manner as in striated muscle, suggesting that a sliding filament mechanism is responsible for the contraction of smooth muscle cells as well. The contraction of smooth muscle cells is linked to the creation of bulges in the plasma membrane, known as blebs. These blebs disappear when the cells relax (Egorova et al., 2022). The protrusions grow larger and more numerous as the cell progressively shrinks, and once the cell has contracted to 55% of its original length, it becomes entirely enveloped by blebs. Electron micrographs reveal that the blebs lack myofilaments, while filaments are clearly visible in the non-evaginated regions located between attachment plaques. In the contracted cell, the thick and thin filaments and the cytoplasmic dense bodies are arranged diagonally to the long axis, intersecting each other within the cell. On the other hand, in the relaxed cell, these components are typically aligned parallel to the cell axis. The contractile elements connect the attachment plaques to the dense bodies. During contraction, the contractile elements undergo a change in orientation, becoming oblique. As the cell undergoes contraction, it needs to widen to make room for the displaced volume. However, this is counteracted by the inward pulling force exerted by the contraction at the attachment plaques. Regions that are not directly affected by the inward force expand outward, forming bulges known as blebs. The filaments connecting the dense bodies form a contractile unit, with multiple units linked together and anchored at both ends to an attachment plaque. Besides the actin myofilaments, the dense bodies and subplasmalemmal attachment plaques also function as attachment sites for the intermediate filaments (desmin, vimentin). These intermediate filaments are crucial in providing robust cytoskeletal support for the smooth muscle cell. Smooth muscle receives abundant innervation from the autonomic nervous system, which primarily regulates the frequency and intensity of spontaneous contractions. The two distinct types of smooth muscle are recognized based on physiological differences. Tonic smooth muscle is distinguished by its absence of action potentials and its gradual contraction. Tonic smooth muscle can autonomously generate rhythmic contractions, which can be triggered by either stretching or hormonal signals. The autonomic nervous system modulates the levels of contraction rather than directly initiating contraction. Only a limited number of smooth muscle cells within the muscle sheet receive nerve supply, and the electrical impulse is transmitted through gap junctions, a phenomenon known as single unit innervation. Instances of this smooth muscle include the muscularis externa, which forms the boundary of the gastrointestinal tract, as well as the urinary bladder and uterus. Phasic smooth muscle, another type of smooth muscle, is distinguished by its specific action potentials and rapid contraction, which are precisely regulated by the autonomic nervous system. In phasic smooth muscle, each smooth muscle cell receives innervation from multiple sources (multiunit innervation). This form of smooth muscle is located in the muscular layer of the vas deferens, the iris of the eye, the erector pili muscles, and certain arteries.

4.1.4.3. Organization

Smooth muscle cells can exist either as individual entities or in small clusters within regular connective tissue, such as in the intestinal villi, the tunica dartos of the scrotum, and the capsule and trabeculae of the spleen. Additionally, they create prominent layers in the walls of the intestines and arteries. Within a single muscle sheet, the muscle fibers are generally aligned in a consistent direction but are positioned in a way that the wider parts of the cells are next to the narrowing ends of the neighboring cells. Therefore, when examining cross-sections, the size of cell outlines differs depending on the location along the lengths where the cells were sliced. The nuclei are sparse and can only be found in the largest profiles, which correspond to sections taken from the enlarged, central regions of the cells. A delicate connective tissue composed of fine collagenous, reticular, and elastic fibers stretches between the smooth muscle cells and seamlessly transitions into a denser connective tissue that binds the muscle cells together in bundles or sheets. The latter connective tissue comprises a greater number of fibroblasts, collagenous and elastic fibers, as well as a network of blood vessels and nerves. The force generated by the contraction of smooth muscle cells is transferred to the reticuloelastic sheath surrounding the cells and then to the denser connective tissue, allowing for a consistent contraction across the entire muscle layer (Grounds et al., 2020). The reticuloelastic sheath's reticular and elastic fibers are derived from smooth muscle cells.

4.1.5. Histogenesis

Skeletal muscle originates from mesenchyme in different regions of the embryo. The muscles of the limbs and trunk originate from myotomal mesenchyme, while those of the head and neck develop from the mesenchyme of the branchial arches. At first, the precursor muscle cells are spherical, noncontractile cells with a single nucleus located in the center. During the process of cell development, the cells undergo elongation and start producing myofilaments, creatine kinase, and acetylcholine receptors. This allows them to be recognized as myoblasts. The myoblasts have a spindle shape and contain a large number of ribosomes, well-developed Golgi complexes, and relatively small mitochondria. Additionally, they have a small number of myofilaments. The cells are undergoing active mitosis. At seven weeks of gestation, the myoblasts start to merge with each other, connecting end-to-end, to create primary myotubes. Primary myotubules are elongated cells, measuring 8 to 15 μm in width, that contain multiple large nuclei located centrally. Each nucleus is characterized by a prominent nucleolus. The myoblasts that undergo fusion are no longer actively producing deoxyribonucleic acid (DNA) and are in a state of cell cycle arrest. The myotubule is responsible for the synthesis of contractile proteins, which are then organized into sarcomeres that have distinct A and I bands and Z lines. Actin filaments are observed in proximity to myosin filaments. Myofibrils form clusters, come together, grow longer and thicker, and quickly develop distinct bands. Following the emergence of myofibrils, transverse tubules become visible at regular intervals of 1 to 5 μm. The fusion of Z bodies, to which actin filaments are attached, leads to the formation of Z lines that are aligned with the

T-tubule system and units of the sarcoplasmic reticulum. Subsequent cohorts of myoblasts undergo further maturation, resulting in the formation of either fresh myotubules or their fusion with existing myotubules, thereby giving rise to fibers that encompass 50 to 100 nuclei. New myotubules are likely to continue forming until their quantity matches the number of cells in a fully developed muscle. During the thirteenth week, the nuclei of the cell start shifting from the center of the tube to the outer edge, resulting in the cell being referred to as a myofiber. Nevertheless, the growth of the cell is not uniform throughout its entire length, and a single structure may exhibit characteristics of both a myotubule and a myofiber.

The central regions of the cell, where the fusion of myoblasts initially took place, are considered the most developed. The most underdeveloped regions are those located at the extremities. During a certain period, the middle of the cell may exhibit nuclei located at the outer edges, while the ends contain nuclei located towards the center due to the ongoing fusion of myoblasts. During the development of the myotubule, the quantity of mitochondria grows, and the cristae multiply and become more densely packed. In the 16th week of gestation until birth, muscle cells undergo an increase in both their length and width. Postnatal muscle mass undergoes continuous growth until the onset of puberty. There is no empirical evidence to support the notion that the quantity of cells increases after birth. However, it is observed that the cells do experience growth in length through the addition of new sarcomeres at their extremities. The enlargement in size is a result of an augmentation in the quantity of myofibrils and the volume of sarcoplasm. Cell types with histochemical characteristics can be identified during the eighteenth or seventeenth week of gestation. Before this time, all myotubules exhibit uniform reactivity as type IIC cells. Several sizable type I cells emerge around the twentieth week, but it is only after the thirtieth week that type IIB cells, followed by IIA cells, differentiate from the type IIC cells. Approximately 10% of the type IIC cells remain present at birth. Among adults, the proportion of type IIC cells is less than 3%. Damaged skeletal muscle has a restricted ability to regenerate or undergo repair. Post-injury, mature skeletal muscle cells do not undergo the process of mitosis. Instead, the satellite cells that are connected to the fully developed fibers undergo rapid reproduction and merge together to create fresh skeletal muscle cells. The forming fibers undergo differentiation in a manner that is comparable to what is observed during typical development (Hindi et al., 2013). The development of cardiac muscle occurs through the transformation of mesenchyme, specifically the myoepithelial mantle, which surrounds the endocardial tube in the embryonic heart. Initially, the cells exhibit a stellate shape and are connected by desmosomes. Primitive cardiac muscle cells undergo repeated division, unlike skeletal muscle cells.

The cells undergo myofilament synthesis, resulting in elongation and transformation into myoblasts, which promptly initiate rhythmic contractions. Cell division persists during postnatal development but is eventually replaced by hypertrophy as the primary mechanism for further growth. The locations where desmosomal connections occur between cells undergo a transformation and become intercalated discs. The final stage of mammalian cardiac muscle development is characterized by the formation of T-tubules. The tubules originate from the inward folding of the sarcolemma during the later stages of prenatal development. Cardiac muscle exhibits a significantly restricted ability to regenerate or undergo repair following injury. Instead, damaged cardiac cells are substituted with connective tissue. Smooth muscle originates from the mesenchyme at different locations in the embryo where it typically develops in the adult. The undifferentiated cells in these regions undergo continuous division until they reach a state of confluence, at which point they transform into individual cells known as myoblasts. The myoblasts undergo elongation and acquire the fusiform morphology that is typical of mature smooth muscle cells. During the early stages of development, the myoblasts exhibit a resemblance to fibroblasts. The cytoplasm is rich in free ribosomes, granular endoplasmic reticulum, mitochondria, and prominent Golgi complexes. Initially, there are only a small number of filaments, but as the smooth muscle cell matures, clusters of slender filaments emerge in connection with dense bodies. Myosin is detectable within the clusters of filaments. As filaments appear, the number of cytoplasmic organelles decreases. Attachment plaques, plasmalemmal vesicles, and an external lamina emerge simultaneously or slightly after the thick filaments. Myofilaments in newborns are diminutive and typically confined to the cytoplasmic periphery of the cell. The presence of granular endoplasmic reticulum and Golgi elements is highly noticeable and they are distributed extensively within the cell. There is evidence that new smooth muscle cells can be produced through mitotic division, even in adult organisms such as in the uterus. Typically, the enlargement of smooth muscle in adults is caused by hypertrophy. Smooth muscle exhibits a remarkable ability to regenerate and undergo self-healing after sustaining an injury. The iris's smooth muscle is typically believed to originate from cells located near the edge of the optic cup, indicating an ectodermal **source**.

4.2. Nervous Tissue

Nervous tissue, one of the fundamental tissues, comprises neurons (nerve cells) and neuroglia (supporting cells). Neurons are highly specialized to respond to stimuli and transmit the excitation from one part of the body to another. The nervous system is distinguished by its ability to respond to stimuli and transmit signals, which are crucial for the functioning of nervous tissue. Its primary functions are to facilitate communication and coordinate bodily activities.

The central nervous system (CNS) is composed of the nervous tissue found in the brain and spinal cord, while the peripheral nervous system encompasses all other nervous tissue. A receptor is a specialized type of nervous tissue that detects external stimuli. The peripheral nervous system then transmits these sensory stimuli to the CNS, which serves as a center for integration and communication. Effector neurons transmit nerve impulses from the CNS to other tissues, resulting in a specific response.

Synapses refer to the specific connections formed between neurons, through which impulses are transmitted between nerve cells via either electrical couplings or chemical transmitters. Neurons have the ability to either excite or inhibit other neurons that they come into contact with.

4.2.1. Neurons

The neuron, also known as the nerve cell, is the fundamental component of nervous tissue, responsible for both its structure and function. Typically characterized by a considerable size and intricate structure, it comprises of a central cell body called the perikaryon, along with multiple cytoplasmic processes. Dendrites are branched structures that transmit electrical signals towards the cell body and typically exist in multiple numbers. The axon is the sole conduit for transmitting the impulse from the perikaryon (Hodges et al., 1997).

The cell bodies of various neuronal types exhibit significant variations in both size (ranging from 4 to 140 μm) and shape. Typically, these cell bodies contain a sizable, centrally located, spherical nucleus with a noticeable nucleolus. The cytoplasm is abundant in organelles and can contain various inclusions. Neurofibrils gather to create a complex network that surrounds the nucleus and extends into the dendrites and axon. Neurofibrils can only be visualized using a light microscope if they are stained in a specific and targeted manner. Neurofibrils are composed of clusters of thin neurofilaments, which have a diameter of 10 nm. Additionally, they contain microtubules that are similar to those found in other cells, despite being referred to as neurotubules. Neurofilaments serve as an intrinsic framework for the perikaryon and its processes, ensuring the structural integrity of neurons. Specific membrane proteins tether the neurofilaments to the plasmalemma. The cell bodies of most neurons contain distinctive chromophilic (Nissl) substances. This substance can be visualized as basophilic masses within the cytoplasm of the cell body and dendrites when stained with dyes like cresyl violet or toluidine blue. It is not present in the axon and axon hillock, which is the area of the cell body where the axon starts.

Electron micrographs reveal that the Nissl substance is composed of multiple parallel cisternae of granular endoplasmic reticulum. Neurons have small, slender, or oval mitochondria that are distributed throughout their cytoplasm. These mitochondria contain lamellar and tubular cristae. Golgi complexes that are well developed are located near the nucleus within the cell. While centrioles may be observed on rare occasions, adult neurons typically do not undergo division. Inclusions can also be present in the perikarya. Neurons in certain areas of the brain, such as the substantia nigra, locus ceruleus, and dorsal motor nucleus of the vagus nerve, as well as in spinal and sympathetic ganglia, contain dark brown granules of melanin pigment. Lipofuscin granules are a common inclusion that tends to accumulate with age. These granules are the result of normal lysosomal activity. Neurons typically have a large number of lysosomes because the plasmalemma and other cellular components are constantly being replaced. The lipid droplets observed in numerous neurons serve as storage material or may arise due to pathological metabolism.

4.2.1.1. Nerve Processes

Nerve processes are elongated projections of the cell body that extend into the cytoplasm. These projections can take the form of dendrites or axons. Typically, each neuron possesses multiple dendrites that originate from the perikaryon and undergo repeated divisions to create branch-like extensions. Despite the significant variation in the quantity, dimensions, and configuration of dendrites, every type of neuron exhibits a comparable pattern of branching. The cytoplasm of dendrites contains elongated mitochondria, Nissl substance, dispersed neurofilaments, and microtubules that run parallel to each other. Dendrites typically possess a multitude of small protrusions known as dendritic spines or gemmules, which facilitate synaptic connections between neurons. An essential role of dendrites is to receive neural impulses from neighboring neurons. Dendrites are primarily responsible for facilitating synaptic connections between neurons, although, in certain neurons, the perikaryon and initial segment of the axon may also serve as receptor regions. The number of synaptic connections on the dendritic tree varies depending on the type of neuron, but it can reach hundreds of thousands (Johnson et al., 2022). Dendrites have a crucial function in the process of integrating numerous incoming impulses. A neuron possesses a solitary axon that transmits impulses away from the parent neuron to other neurons or effector organs that are functionally connected. The axon originates from the axon hillock, a raised area on the surface of the cell body that does not contain Nissl substance. At times, axons can originate from the base of a primary dendrite. Axons typically exhibit greater length and slenderness compared to dendrites. They may or may not generate side branches known as collaterals, which, unlike dendritic branches, generally emerge from the parent axon at right angles. Axons also exhibit a constant diameter along the majority of their length and typically have a smooth external surface. Axons terminate in multiple telodendria, which exhibit variations in both quantity and morphology and have the potential to create a network or basket-like structure surrounding postsynaptic neurons. The axoplasm, which is the cytoplasm of the axon, contains a large number of neurofilaments, neurotubules, elongated profiles of smooth endoplasmic reticulum, and long, slender mitochondria. Due to the absence of the Nissl substance in the axoplasm, protein synthesis does not take place in the axon. The protein that is broken down by the axon during nerve transmission is replenished by the protein that is produced in the cisternae of the granular endoplasmic reticulum in the Nissl substance of the perikaryon.

Neurotubules serve the purpose of conveying newly synthesized proteins and various other substances within the axon. Antegrade transport refers to the transfer of substances from the cell body to the ends of the axon and can occur at varying speeds. Rapid transportation (410 mm/day) entails the movement of membranous organelles, neurosecretory vesicles, calcium, sugars, amino acids, and nucleotides. Transport at a slow rate of 1–6 mm per day involves the movement of proteins, metabolic enzymes, and components of the cytoskeleton. Kinesin, a microtubule-associated protein (MAP), facilitates rapid antegrade transport through its ATPase activity. One extremity of the kinesin molecule binds to a transport vesicle or organelle. The remaining end engages in cyclic interaction with the microtubule wall, leading to movement towards the axon terminal. Retrograde transport refers to the movement of depleted organelles, proteins, small molecules, and recycled membranes from the axonal endings to the perikaryon. This process also serves as a pathway for certain toxins (such as tetanus) and viruses (including herpes, polio, and rabies) to invade the CNS. Retrograde rapid transport proceeds at a velocity of 200–300 mm per day and relies on another microtubule-associated protein known as dynein, which also possesses ATPase activity. Transport through dendrites also takes place, although it is not as comprehensively understood. Axons propagate signals as electrical impulses known as action potentials, originating from the axon hillock and the initial segment of the axon. An impulse exhibits a binary response, either occurring fully or not at all. The action potential is only transmitted along the axon to its terminations when the activity threshold is reached (Kornegay, 2017). These terminations either synapse with adjacent neurons or end on effector cells. An axon always induces a positive activity – for example, causing muscle cells to contract or stimulating epithelial cells to secrete. Impulses transmitted to another neuron can either stimulate or inhibit its activity.

4.2.1.2. Distribution of Neurons

The CNS is anatomically divided into two main components: gray matter and white matter. This division is based on the distribution of perikarya, or cell bodies, within these regions. Gray matter consists of the cell bodies of neurons and their closely associated processes. In contrast, white matter is primarily made up of bundles or clusters of axons and their surrounding coverings. Gray matter is centrally located within the spinal cord and is surrounded by white matter. In contrast, gray matter is found at the outer edges and covers the white matter in the cerebral and cerebellar cortices. Clusters of cell bodies are present in the gray matter of the CNS and function as separate and specialized units known as nuclei. Ganglia refer to either similar aggregates or individual neurons that are situated outside the CNS.

4.2.1.3. Types of Neurons

Neurons can be categorized based on their location, dendrite count, and the length and position of their axons. The majority of neurons in humans are located in the gray matter of the CNS. Certain neurons possess abundant, fully developed dendrites and exceptionally long axons that extend from the gray matter into the white matter of the CNS. These axons either travel upwards or downwards along the main fiber pathways of the brain or spinal cord, or they exit the CNS to help form peripheral nerves. These neurons, known as Golgi type I neurons, transmit electrical signals over long distances. Golgi type II neurons are other neurons with short axons that do not extend beyond the perikaryon region. These are particularly abundant in the cerebellar and cerebral cortices, as well as in the retina of the eye. They exhibit significant variations in both size and shape and possess multiple dendrites that branch out. Golgi type II neurons function primarily as interneurons, responsible for receiving and transmitting nerve impulses to neighboring neurons. Neurons can also be categorized based on the number of dendrites they possess. Unipolar neurons are characterized by the absence of dendrites and the presence of a single process known as the axon. While they are frequently found in the developing nervous system, they are infrequently observed in adults. Bipolar neurons possess a solitary dendrite and an axon, typically situated at opposite ends of the perikaryon. These structures can be located in the retina, olfactory epithelium, the cochlear, and vestibular ganglia. The neurons in all craniospinal ganglia initially develop as bipolar neurons in the embryo. However, as they mature, the dendrite and axon move towards the cell body and merge together to form a single process. This type of neuron is referred to as pseudounipolar in adults. The integrated process, commonly referred to as a dendraxon, can extend for a brief distance before splitting into two processes. One of these processes functions as a dendrite, receiving stimuli from the peripheral regions of the body. The other process acts as an axon, entering the gray matter of the CNS to establish synapses with other neurons. The process directed towards the periphery functions as a dendrite, but it is atypical in its morphology as it bears resemblance to an axon. This dendrite is functional, having a smooth and unbranched structure. Its primary function is to receive nervous input from a receptor organ. The most prevalent type of neuron is multipolar neurons. They exhibit significant variations in both size and shape and are distinguished by the presence of multiple dendrites. Both internuncial and motor neurons belong to this category. Among these, the internuncial neuron is the most abundant (Kumar et al., 2015).

4.2.1.4. Ganglia

Ganglia are categorized into cranial, spinal, and autonomic groups. Cranial and spinal ganglia can be observed as spherical enlargements on the sensory roots of their corresponding nerves when viewed at a macroscopic level. Every ganglion is surrounded by a connective tissue capsule and can house a varying number of neurons, ranging from just a few to as many as 55,000. A complex network of collagenous and reticular fibers, along with small blood vessels, connects individual neurons and often divides the perikarya into distinct groups, along with bundles of nerve processes. The perikarya are enveloped by two distinct capsules. The inner capsule consists of a monolayer of low cuboidal satellite cells, also known as amphicytes, which provide support. The outer capsule is located directly outside the basal lamina of the satellite cells and is composed of fragile vascular connective tissue. The cranial and spinal ganglia are sensory ganglia that consist of pseudounipolar neurons. The perikarya exhibit a spherical or pear-shaped morphology and have a diameter ranging from 15 to 100 μm. They frequently exhibit a prominent, centrally located nucleus and a clearly identifiable nucleolus. The dendritic arborization of the pseudounipolar neuron can become intricately folded to create a glomerulus. Subsequently, this neural process undergoes division: One branch, known as a functional dendrite, extends towards a receptor organ, while the other branch, known as a functional axon, extends into the CNS. The cell bodies of these pseudounipolar neurons do not receive synaptic connections from other neurons. Autonomic ganglia are clusters of cell bodies of visceral efferent motor neurons. They can be found in enlargements along the sympathetic chain or within the walls of organs that are innervated by the autonomic nervous system. Typically, they possess a connective tissue capsule. The neurons typically exhibit a multipolar morphology, displaying a diverse range of sizes and shapes. The perikarya have a diameter ranging from 15 to 60 μm. The nucleus is large, round, and frequently positioned off-center within the cell. Binucleate cells are also occasionally observed. Neurons in autonomic ganglia have a higher occurrence of lipofuscin granules compared to craniospinal ganglia. Satellite cells encapsulate the ganglia of larger sympathetic chains, although a capsule may be lacking around ganglia located in the walls of the viscera. In contrast to the craniospinal ganglia, neurons in the autonomic ganglia receive a multitude of synapses and are subject to the influence of other neurons.

4.2.1.5. Nerve Fibers

A nerve fiber comprises an axon, also known as an axis cylinder, and an encompassing sheath of cells. Myelin is a lipoprotein material that surrounds large nerve fibers, while smaller nerve fibers may or may not have this protective covering. Therefore, nerve fibers can be categorized as either myelinated or unmyelinated.

The axons of peripheral nerves are enveloped by a layer of flattened cells known as Schwann cells. These cells characteristically possess thinness, attenuated shape, and flattened, elongated nuclei positioned close to the center of the cells. Their cytoplasm is comprised of a diminutive Golgi complex, a handful of dispersed granular endoplasmic reticulum profiles, scattered mitochondria, microtubules, microfilaments, and occasionally, a multitude of lysosomes. Successive Schwann cells and the axonal surfaces of the nodes are covered by a continuous external (basal) lamina. The preservation of the external lamina is crucial for the regeneration of axons and Schwann cells following an injury. Schwann cells envelop nerve fibers from their proximal origins to their distal terminations. The neurilemma, also known as the sheath of Schwann, is connected to the satellite cell capsule that encloses the perikarya of neurons in the craniospinal ganglia. Schwann cells are responsible for the production and maintenance of myelin on nerve fibers in the peripheral nervous system. Small gaps regularly interrupt the neurilemmal and myelin sheaths along the entire length of the nerve fiber. The interruptions observed between individual Schwann cells, known as nodes of Ranvier, indicate areas of discontinuity. The neurilemmal and myelin sheaths are composed of a sequence of small individual segments. Each segment is defined as the area between two adjacent nodes of Ranvier and forms one internode or internodal segment. An internode is a segment that encompasses a solitary Schwann cell along with its myelin and typically measures approximately 1 to 2 mm in length. Myelin is not a substance that is secreted by Schwann cells, but rather a dense accumulation of lipoprotein and glycolipid. It contains a high galactocerebroside concentration, which is a distinct form of glycolipid, is being referred to. Myelin is formed by the wrapping of the Schwann cell membrane around the axon in multiple layers. Specific proteins strongly adhere to the layers of the cell membrane that constitute myelin. Myelin can exhibit a consistent appearance. However, specific techniques of preparation can expose a network of a residual protein referred to as neurokeratin. The ultrastructural level reveals myelin as a distinct pattern of evenly spaced light and dark lines. The major dense lines, also referred to as dark lines, are created when the inner surfaces of the Schwann cell plasmalemma come into contact with each other. Myelin basic protein (MBP) binds the cytoplasmic surfaces together. The Po protein forms a complex with myelin basic protein, resulting in the formation of the primary dense line. Approximately half of the protein content in the myelin of the peripheral nervous system is composed of the Po protein. The primary role of this is to aid in preserving the structural integrity of the myelin (Latroche et al., 2015). The intraperiod lines with reduced density indicate the fusion of the outer surfaces of the Schwann cell plasmalemma. These lines are situated amidst the recurring prominent dense lines. Proteolipid protein is a molecule that adheres to the outer surfaces of the Schwann cell plasmalemma. Oblique discontinuities commonly arise in the myelin of peripheral nerves, leading to the creation of Schmidt-Lantermann incisures or clefts.

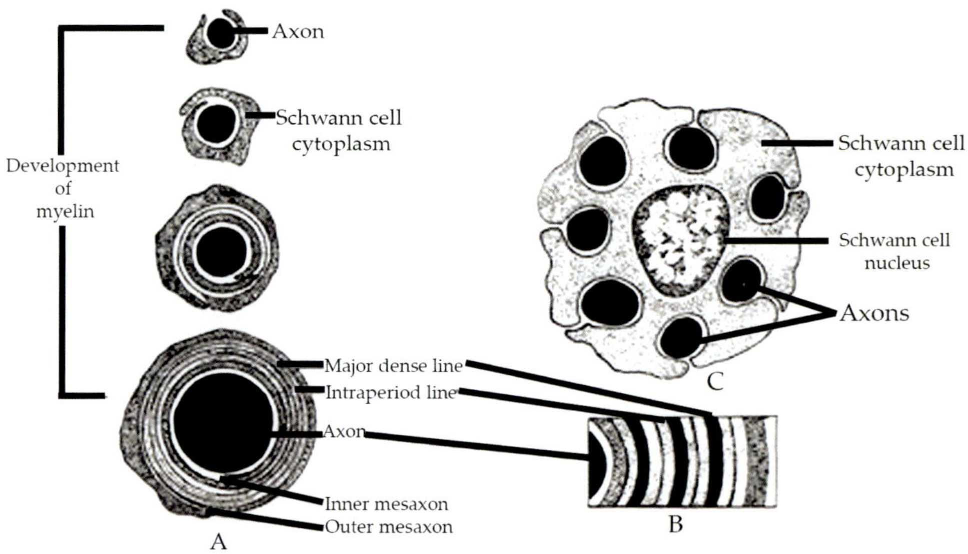

Figure 4.9. *Diagrammatic representations of a myelinated nerve fiber (A, B) and a nonmyelinated nerve fiber (C).*

The clefts represent specific divisions within the myelin lamellae. Schwann cells also surround non-myelinated axons. Electron micrographs often reveal the existence of 15 or more unmyelinated axons within the folds of a single plasmalemma of Schwann cells. The cell membrane of the Schwann cell forms a tight envelopment around each axon and is closely associated with it. The Schwann cell's cell membrane envelops the axon and creates a loop by establishing contact with itself. The precise site of contact is known as the mesaxon. The Schwann cell membrane forms primary invaginations at the junction between the axon and myelin in myelinated nerves, which are known as the internal mesaxon. The junction between the outer layers of the myelin sheath and the outer membrane of the Schwann cell is called the external mesaxon (**Figure 4.9**). The velocity at which a nerve impulse travels along a nerve fiber is directly proportional to the diameter of the fiber. While myelinated fibers typically have faster conduction due to the myelin sheath, not all myelinated fibers are necessarily larger in diameter than unmyelinated fibers. Peripheral nerves contain nerve fibers that can be categorized based on their diameter and conduction speed. Type A nerve fibers are motor and sensory fibers characterized by their large size, myelination, and diameter ranging from 3 to 20 μm.

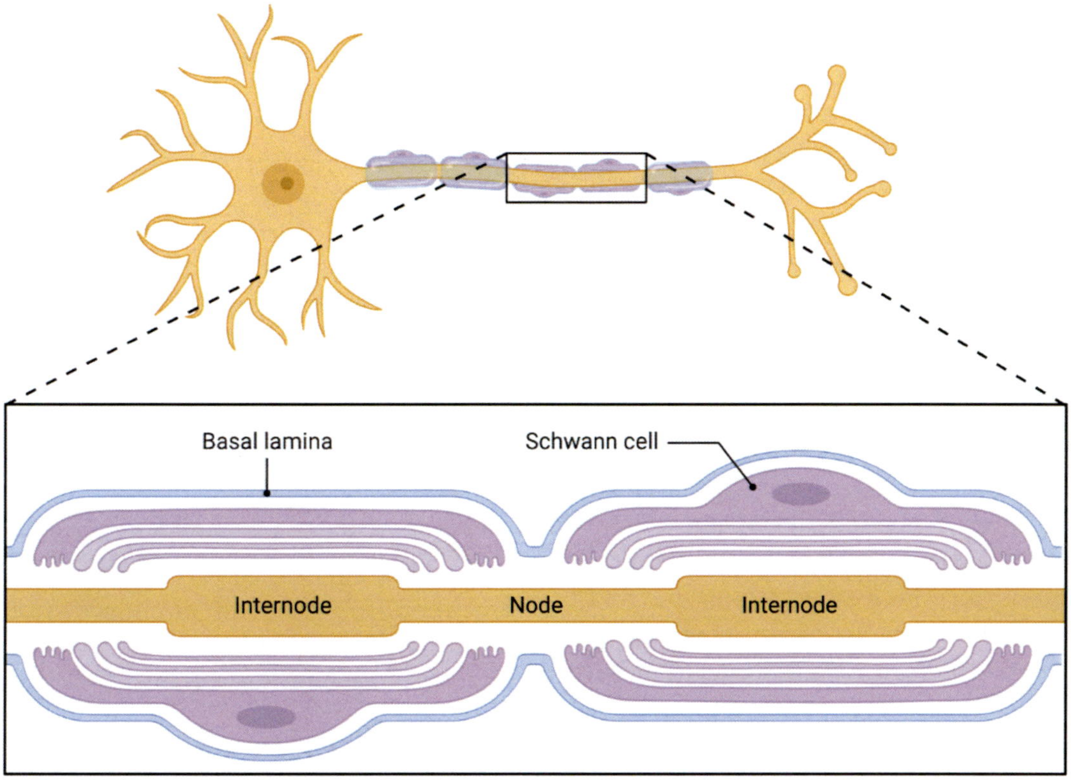

Figure 4.10. *A schematic diagram of myelinated axon in the nerve fiber.*

Source: https://www.researchgate.net/profile/Amir-Maghoul/publication/358974854/figure/fig1/AS:1136747874390017@1648033221436/A-schematic-diagram-of-myelinated-axon-in-the-nerve-fiber.png0.

These fibers can conduct impulses at speeds ranging from 15 to 120 m/second. Type B fibers are characterized by their smaller diameter of up to 3 μm and their ability to conduct impulses at speeds ranging from 3 to 15 m/second. They encompass a significant portion of the sensory fibers that pertain to internal organs. C fibers are nerve fibers that are small and lack myelin. They transmit impulses at a speed of 0.5 to 2.0 meters per second. The initial step in the formation of an action potential along a nerve fiber is a rapid rise in sodium ion permeability, leading to the depolarization of the axon and the establishment of a negative charge on the surface of the axon. The local electrical current generated between the depolarized and resting surface membranes results in an elevated permeability of the membrane to sodium ions. An iterative process of membrane activation is established, leading to the propagation of depolarization (a nerve impulse) along the nerve fiber (Meng et al., 2014). After depolarization, the electrical signal will propagate throughout the entire cell membrane of the axon. The duration of the nerve impulse is brief, and repolarization is achieved through the action of a sodium pump mechanism located in the cell membrane of the axon. The generation of a nerve impulse is a phenomenon that either occurs completely or not at all. In myelinated nerves that conduct signals at a faster rate, impulses travel from one node to another. This mode of impulse conduction is referred to as saltatory conduction. The node of Ranvier is the sole section of the axon that is not covered by the myelin sheath and is directly in contact with the extracellular fluid. Action potentials are regenerated at this specific location due to a significant concentration of ion channels. Depolarization exclusively takes place at the nodes of Ranvier, causing nerve impulses to propagate by leaping from one node to another across the internodal segment in between (Morgan et al., 2018). The axon at each node is slightly wider than the axon associated with internodal segments. The plasmalemma of the node region contains the majority of sodium voltage-gated channel proteins. These proteins are anchored to the cytoskeleton by the link protein ankyrin. This partially elucidates the greater nerve conduction speed in myelinated nerve fibers (Nonaka, 1998) (**Figure 4.10**).

4.2.1.6. Peripheral Nerves

Peripheral nerves are composed of multiple nerve fibers joined by surrounding connective tissue. These nerves are a combination of sensory (incoming) and motor (outgoing) nerve fibers, which can be either myelinated or unmyelinated. The epineurium is the connective tissue sheath that surrounds a peripheral nerve, and it serves to combine multiple bundles of nerve fibers into a single entity known as a peripheral nerve. The epineurium comprises fibroblasts, collagen fibers arranged longitudinally, and dispersed fat cells. The perineurium is a dense sheath made up of concentric layers of flattened, fibroblast-like cells enclose each bundle or fascicle of nerve fibers The perineurium is bounded externally and internally by a basal lamina. Tight junctions are present between cells; these closely adherent cells create a perineurial compartment for individual fascicles. The endoneurium is composed of delicate collagenous fibers, reticular fibers, fibroblasts, and macrophages, which are situated between individual nerve fibers within each fascicle. The epineurium contains the majority of small blood vessels, while in thicker areas of the endoneurium, they may be present as fragile capillary networks. The perineurium and epineurium of peripheral nerves merge seamlessly with the meninges of the CNS (Petrof et al., 1993).

4.2.1.7. Peripheral Nerve Endings

Nerve endings serve to augment the interface between nervous and nonnervous structures, thereby facilitating the transmission of stimuli from nerve endings to muscles, resulting in muscle contraction, or to epithelial cells, leading to secretion. Upon receiving stimulation, dendrites located at the outer edges generate electrical impulses that are transmitted along the nerve fiber to sensory ganglia and eventually reach the CNS.

Efferent nerve fibers that are located outside of the CNS can be categorized into two groups: somatic and visceral efferent fibers. Motor end-plates are the small, oval expansions where somatic efferent fibers terminate in skeletal muscle. A motor unit is formed by the skeletal muscle cells that are innervated by a single motor neuron (Roelofs et al., 2019). Muscles that possess a greater quantity of motor units can execute more accurate movements compared to muscles with a smaller number of units, even if the number of muscle cells remains constant. Visceral efferent nerve fibers activate smooth muscle, cardiac muscle, and glandular epithelium. The visceral motor endings of smooth muscle consist of multiple swellings that pass through the spaces between individual muscle cells. In cardiac muscle, many thin nerve fibers terminate near the surface of individual muscle cells, but they do not establish any specialized connections with them. The endings in glands are derived from unmyelinated nerves and create intricate and fragile networks on the outer surface of the basal lamina of the gland cells.

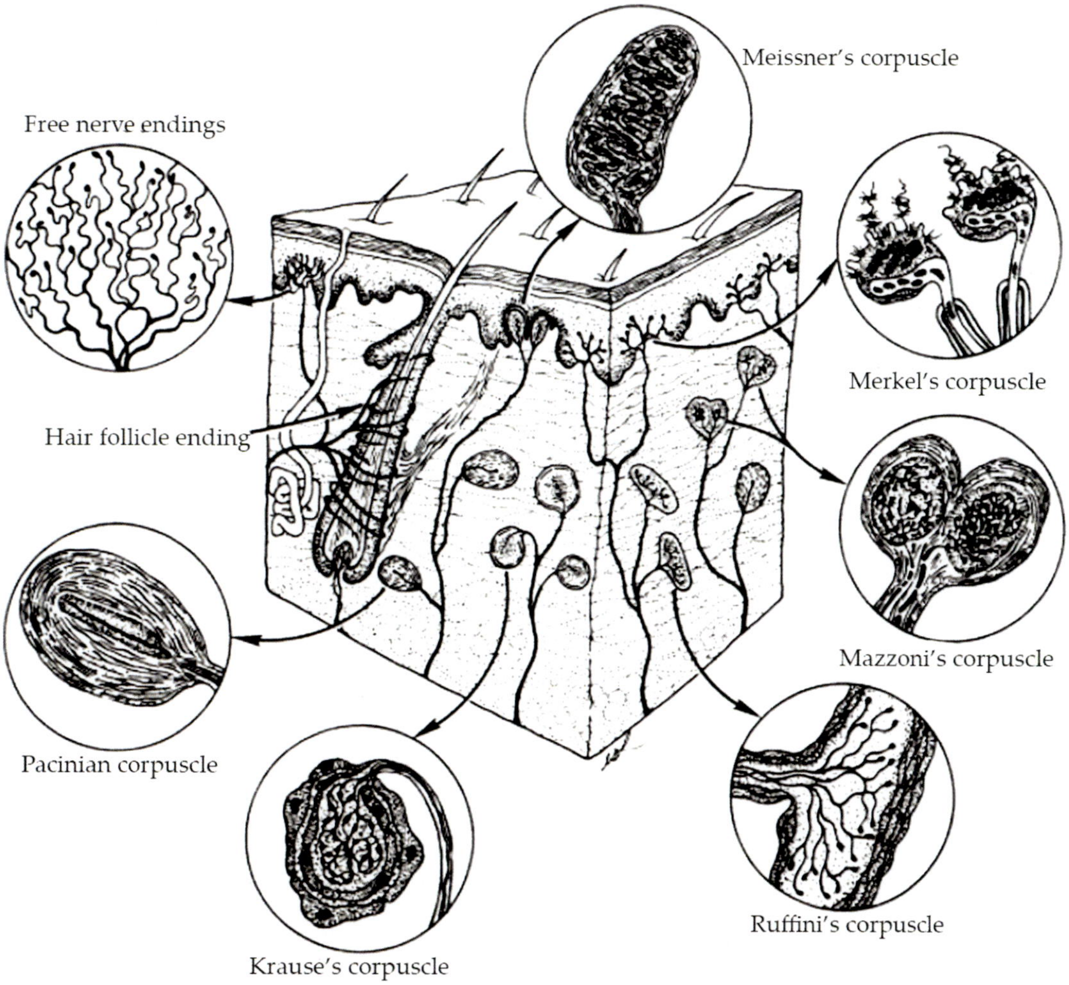

Figure 4.11. *Diagrammatic sketches of types of sensory nerve endings.*

Source: https://ars.els-cdn.com/content/image/3-s2.0-B0122272102002764-gr9.gif.

These networks consist of fine branches that penetrate the basal lamina and pass through the gaps between individual epithelial cells. Receptors are terminal peripheral nerve fibers that can be stimulated by various chemical and physical stimuli, and they have the ability to convert these stimuli into nerve impulses. Receptors exhibit diverse forms, which can be intricate, and are frequently categorized as free (uncovered), diffuse, and encapsulated nerve endings. Naked nerve endings, both myelinated and unmyelinated, originate from fibers of relatively small diameter. They are widely distributed and can be found in various locations such as the skin, connective tissue of visceral organs, deep fascia, muscles, and mucous membranes. As myelinated fibers approach their endpoints, they shed their myelin and develop unmyelinated terminal arborizations. Unmyelinated nerve fibers have multiple fibrils that end as small, knob-like thickenings. Multiple exposed nerve endings function as pain receptors. Peritrichal nerve endings, sensitive to hair movement, are formed by a diffuse type of naked receptor that encircles the base of hair follicles. Aside from the exposed interepithelial nerve endings that terminate within the layers of epithelial cells, specialized nerve endings that create concave neurofibrillar discs that attach to a single modified epithelial cell in stratified squamous epithelium. The tactile discs of Merkel refer to these more specialized nerve endings. Encapsulated nerve endings consist of terminals that are surrounded by a protective layer of connective tissue known as a capsule. They vary significantly in size, shape, location, and the types of stimuli they perceive. As the nerve fibers approach their respective capsules, they typically shed their myelin and neurolemmal sheaths and enter the capsule as exposed nerve endings (Figure 4.11).

A number of encapsulated nerve endings, their locations, and proposed functions are summarized in Table 4.1.

Table 4.1. Nerve Endings, their Locations, and Proposed Functions

Name of Receptor	**Locations**	**Functions**
Corpuscles of Vater-Pacini	The dermis of skin, mesenteries, pleura, nipples, pancreas, tendons, joint capsules, ligaments, walls of viscera, penis, clitoris	Proprioception, deep pressure, vibration
Corpuscles of Meissner	Dermal papillae of digits, lips, genitalia, and nipples	Light touch
End-bulbs of Krause	Dermis, conjunctiva, oral cavity	Proprioception, pressure
Genital corpuscles	Penis, clitoris, nipples	Touch, pressure
Corpuscles of Ruffini	Dermis, joint capsules	Proprioception, pressure
Neurotendinous endings (of Golgi)	Tendons	Proprioception
Neuromuscular spindles	Skeletal muscle	Proprioception

Source: Adapted from Guyton and Hall Textbook of Medical Physiology, 13th Edition.

4.2.1.8. Synapse

A synapse is the site where signals are transmitted from one neuron to another. This can happen between different parts of neurons, such as the axon and dendrite (axodendritic), axon and cell body (axosomatic), axon and axon (axoaxonic), dendrite and dendrite (dendrodendritic), dendrite and perikaryon (somatodendritic), or cell bodies of neighboring neurons (somatosomatic). The quantity of synapses connected to an individual neuron fluctuates depending on the specific type of neuron. Small Golgi type II neurons, specifically the granule cells of the cerebellum, possess a limited number of synaptic points. In contrast, other neurons like Golgi type I, which are the Purkinje cells of the cerebellum, can have a significantly larger amount, reaching several hundred thousand. Physiologically, both excitatory and inhibitory synapses occur. The synaptic terminations of axons typically manifest as small enlargements located at the ends of axon branches and are referred to as terminal boutons (Terry and Wells, 2016). The axon may terminate in slender branches that encircle the perikaryon or dendrites of another neuron; these terminations are referred to as calyces (basket endings). Synaptic contacts can also occur intermittently along the terminal segment of an axon, creating boutons en passage. Synaptic terminals vary significantly in morphology across neuron types, yet they typically share certain traits. Every neuron is an individual cellular entity, and there is no connection of cytoplasm between cells. Synaptic junctions bear similarities to desmosomes and potentially contribute to the preservation of communication between neurons. The presynaptic area, known as the terminal bouton, is characterized by the presence of clusters of mitochondria and several membrane-bound vesicles with diameters ranging from 40 to 60 nm. The synaptic vesicles store various neurotransmitter substances, including dopamine, norepinephrine, acetylcholine, serotonin, amino acids, and peptides. Acetylcholine is the predominant neurotransmitter found in the electron-lucent synaptic vesicles of the CNS and motor end plates. The synaptic vesicles found in most sympathetic postganglionic axons are distinguished by their electron-dense cores and contain catecholamines. The vesicles gather in close proximity to the presynaptic membrane, which is a slightly enlarged region of the axon plasmalemma at the site of synaptic connection. The pre- and post-synaptic membranes are divided by a narrow gap, measuring 20 to 30 nm in width, known as the synaptic cleft. This cleft may contain delicate filaments and glycosaminoglycans. The postsynaptic membrane exhibits heightened electron density and a slight thickening, while its internal surface is connected to a network of dense filamentous material known as the subsynaptic web. The postsynaptic cytoplasm does not contain synaptic vesicles and has a lower number of mitochondria compared to the presynaptic region. The plasmalemma of the postsynaptic cell contains multiple specialized transmembrane proteins and receptors that play a role in the transmission of neurotransmitters (Tinsley et al., 1992) (**Figure 4.12**).

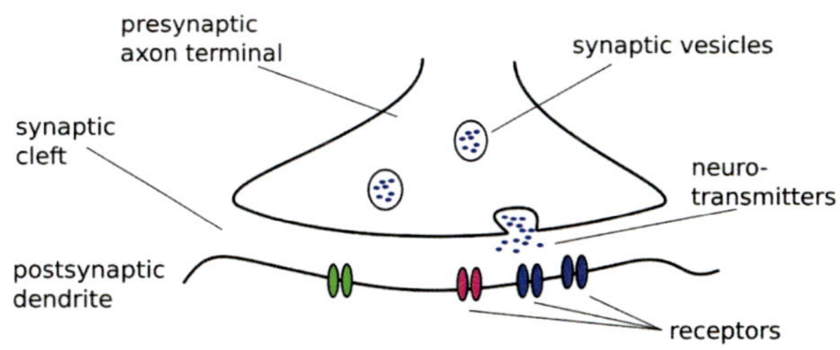

Figure 4.12. *A diagrammatic sketch of a synapse.*

Source: https://www.researchgate.net/profile/Andrea-Soltoggio/publication/37470477/figure/fig1/AS:669424038199314@1536614536557/Simplified-drawing-of-a-synapse.png.

When an action potential reaches the presynaptic region of an axon, the synaptic vesicles merge with specific locations on the presynaptic membrane and release transmitter substance into the space between neurons called the synaptic cleft. The released transmitter substance binds to specific receptors on the postsynaptic membrane, leading to a rapid increase in the permeability of the postsynaptic cell membrane to sodium ions. This results in a change in the resting membrane potential.

An action potential is transmitted by the postsynaptic neuron when the potential of the postsynaptic membrane exceeds the threshold of excitation. The axon hillock and initial segment of the axon are the first components of the postsynaptic neuron to initiate an action potential. The proximal portion of an axon is a few micrometers in length and does not possess a myelin sheath. The cell membrane in most neurons has a lower threshold of excitation in this region compared to the perikaryon or dendrites (Tulangekar and Sztal, 2021). When transmitter substances reduce the permeability of the postsynaptic membrane, it causes an increase in the threshold of excitation, resulting in an inhibitory effect. When a wave of depolarization reaches the presynaptic membrane, it causes an increase in calcium ion levels. This increase then triggers the release of transmitter substance into the synaptic cleft through exocytosis. The transmitter released interacts with receptors on the postsynaptic membrane to induce one of three potential outcomes (depolarization, hyperpolarization, neuromodulation) in the target neuron. When the transmitter substances, such as acetylcholine and glutamate, attach to particular receptor proteins on ion channels, these receptor proteins on the postsynaptic membrane open up. This opening allows positively charged ions, such as sodium, potassium, and calcium, to enter the neuron. As a result, the neuron becomes depolarized and stimulated. Alternatively, if the transmitter releases gamma-amino butyric acid (GABA) or glycine, it will bind to receptor proteins on ion channels. These proteins permit the entry of negatively charged ions, primarily chloride ions, into the cell. As a result, hyperpolarization takes place, leading to inhibition. Transmitters such as opioid proteins, dopamine, small neuropeptides, epinephrine, and norepinephrine can bind to G-protein-linked receptors instead of intrinsic ion channels in certain cases. These receptors activate second-messenger molecule systems that, through a series of intracellular events, alter the sensitivity or regulate the target neuron's response to depolarization. There are two distinct sets of synaptic vesicles in the axon terminal: a smaller set that is released when an action potential occurs, and a larger reserve set that is connected to the cytoskeleton through actin filaments. When necessary, synaptic vesicles from the reserve group transition to the releasable group. Synapsin I, a phosphorylated protein that is connected to the inner side of synaptic vesicles, serves as a bridge between actin and the vesicle surface, leading to the buildup of reserve vesicles. The phosphorylation of synapsin I, caused by the entry of calcium ions stimulated by the action potential, breaks this connection, enabling these vesicles to become part of the releasable group. Synapsin II, an extra phosphoprotein, is believed to facilitate the interaction between synaptic vesicles and the cytoskeleton. During the resting state, a protein called synaptotagmin, which is sensitive to calcium, prevents the fusion of membranes and the release of substances through exocytosis. Upon the arrival of an action potential at the terminal bouton, voltage-gated calcium ion channels undergo activation and allow the influx of calcium ions. The subsequent elevation in calcium ion concentration induces the activation of a trigger protein, facilitating the fusion of membranes and the process of exocytosis. Synaptobrevin, an anchoring protein, is present in the membrane of the synaptic vesicle. It connects the vesicle to docking proteins in the presynaptic membrane. The presynaptic membrane harbors supplementary proteins that facilitate the fusion of the membrane with the synaptic vesicle, enabling exocytosis. After the fusion of vesicles with the presynaptic membrane and the release of the transmitter, an equal amount of cell membrane is absorbed through the formation of clathrin-coated vesicles by endocytosis. These vesicles have the potential to merge with cisternae of the endoplasmic reticulum that contain transmitter substances. Additional vesicles are generated through the process of budding from these cisternae, to replenish the pool of reserve synaptic vesicles. Acetylcholine, which is released from the axon terminal, undergoes rapid hydrolysis by acetylcholine esterase in the synaptic cleft, resulting in the formation of acetate and choline. Choline is subsequently conveyed across the presynaptic membrane by a choline transporter, transformed into acetylcholine by the enzyme choline acetyltransferase, and then enclosed within newly generated synaptic vesicles. Conversely, inhibitory neurotransmitters like GABA are absorbed by specialized GABA transporters found in the plasma membrane of nearby astrocyte processes. GABA is metabolized into glutamine within the cytoplasm of astrocytes, and subsequently transported back into the nerve terminal. In this process, glutamine undergoes enzymatic conversion to form GABA, which is then stored in synaptic vesicles. Neuropeptides, in contrast to other transmitters, are produced in the perikaryon and then carried to the axon terminal. Electrical coupling is an alternative method of transmitting impulses in certain types of synapses, which takes place at gap junctions. Gap junctions function as conduits for the passage of ions (Vallejo-Illarramendi et al., 2014).

4.2.2. Neuroglia

Neurons constitute a relatively minor fraction of the cells present in the CNS. The majority of the cells are neuroglia, which are nonneuronal supporting cells. Neuroglia outnumber neurons by about 10 to 1 depending on their location in the CNS. Collectively, neuroglia comprise approximately 50% of the brain's weight and surpass neurons in number by a ratio of 10 to 1. The estimated number of glia in the CNS is approximately 1,000 billion, whereas the number of neurons is around 100 billion. Neuroglia are typically smaller than neurons and can be distinguished from them in light microscopic preparations by their small, circular nuclei that are dispersed among neurons and their processes. Neuroglia comprises ependymal cells, astrocytes, oligodendrocytes, and microglia. Astrocytes and oligodendrocytes are commonly grouped together and referred to as macroglia. Astrocytes can be classified into two types based on their morphology: protoplasmic and fibrous. Protoplasmic astrocytes are primarily located in the gray matter and are distinguished by their abundant, heavily branched processes. Fibrous astrocytes are primarily found in white matter and are characterized by elongated, slender, typically unbranched extensions. The two variations of astrocyte may be considered as a singular type that exhibits different physical characteristics depending on its location and metabolic condition. Astrocytes typically have electron-lucent cytoplasm devoid of organelles, and nuclei containing euchromatin. The cell body and its processes in the cytoplasm contain bundles of intermediate filaments known as glial filaments. These filaments are composed of glial fibrillary acid protein (GFAP). Protoplasmic astrocytes contain a high number of these filaments. Astrocytes play a crucial role in providing structural support to neurons and also contribute to their nourishment metabolic functions, maintaining the blood-brain barrier and regulating blood flow. The morphology of astrocyte processes exhibits significant variation. Some objects have a substantial and elongated shape, while others have a slender and flat structure. The processes frequently elongate to create end feet (foot processes) that are arranged in a linear fashion along the inner surface of the pia mater and surrounding the walls of blood vessels. The glia limitans is a membrane-like structure formed by the largest concentration of end feet, which are located beneath the pial surface and surround the brain and spinal cord. Oligodendrocytes are smaller neuroglial cells with fewer processes and more deeply stained nuclei. There are two types of oligodendrocytes. Interfascicular oligodendrocytes are primarily found in the fiber tracts that make up the white matter of the brain and spinal cord. Perineuronal satellite oligodendrocytes are specifically found in the gray matter and are closely linked to the cell bodies of neurons (Vulin et al., 2015). Both types of oligodendrocytes have cytoplasm that contains ribosomes, cisternae of endoplasmic reticulum, a Golgi complex, and mitochondria. The cytoplasm of the cell body and its processes contain extensive networks of microtubules that are arranged in parallel arrays. Schwann cells are absent in the CNS; oligodendrocytes function as the cells responsible for forming myelin in this area. Nodes of Ranvier are present in myelinated nerve fibers of the CNS, but unlike peripheral myelinated fibers, they do not exhibit incisures. Nodes in the CNS lack covering, whereas nodes in the peripheral nervous system are partially covered by extensions of cytoplasm from neighboring Schwann cells in the paranodal area. The myelin sheath originates shortly after the initial segment of the axon, a few micrometers away from the axon hillock, and covers the remaining length of the axon until it reaches close to its termination. A single cytoplasmic process from an adjacent oligodendrocyte wraps around the axon to form each internodal segment of a nerve fiber in the CNS. Contrary to Schwann cells in the peripheral nervous system, a solitary oligodendrocyte is responsible for producing the internodal sections of the myelin sheath for multiple distinct yet neighboring axons (**Figure 4.13**).

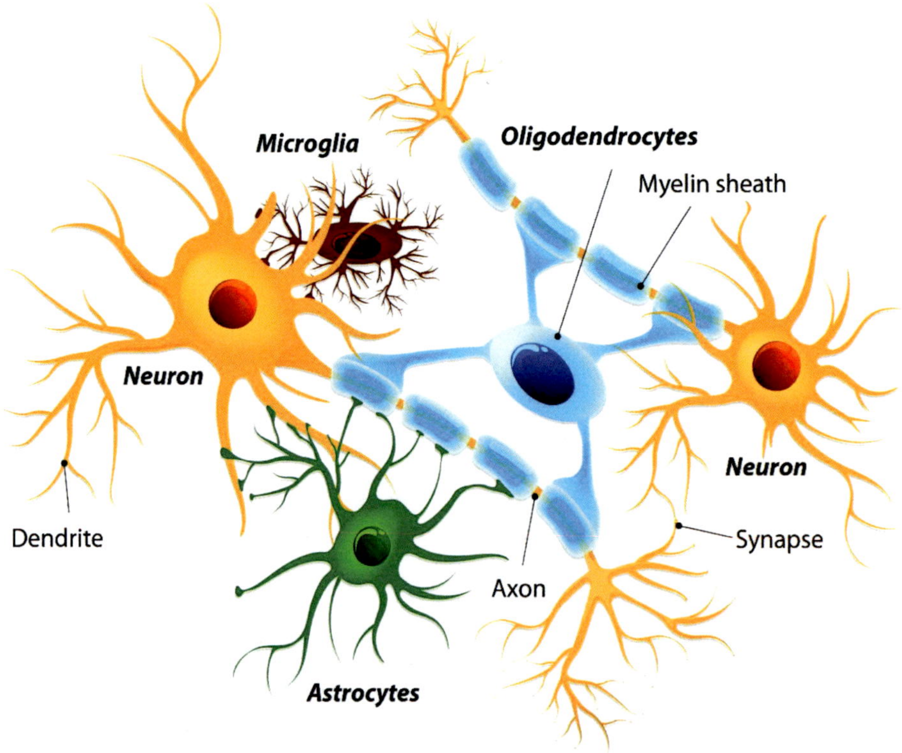

Figure 4.13. *A diagrammatic representation of myelination in the central nervous system.*

Source: https://qph.cf2.quoracdn.net/main-qimg-4f0f27f64d046ce7a5cc3cb209af3923-lq.

Within certain areas, such as the optic nerve, a solitary oligodendrocyte can be accountable for the internodal sections of approximately 40 to 50 axons. In the CNS (CNS), similar to the peripheral nervous system (PNS), specific adhesion molecules (proteolipid protein) connect the outer surfaces of oligodendrocyte plasma membare with each other. Myelin basic protein connects the cytoplasmic surfaces of the plasmalemma. Perineuronal satellite oligodendrocytes, which are located near the cell bodies of neurons, are believed to have an impact on the metabolism and nutrition of neurons. Furthermore, glia are implicated in the regulation of calcium balance and the reutilization of specific neurotransmitters. Within the CNS, perineuronal satellite and interfascicular oligodendrocytes exhibit a similar association with perikarya and their axons as the one observed between satellite cells and Schwann cells in peripheral nerve fibers. Schwann cells and satellite cells are both types of neuroglial elements found in the peripheral nervous system. Microglia, which are small cells, are also found in the CNS. Microglia possess highly branched processes, which indicates that they may function as dendritic antigen-presenting cells. Additionally, they demonstrate the presence of class II MCH molecules. In regions affected by damage or disease, it is believed that macrophages undergo proliferation and acquire phagocytic properties. Additionally, monocytes from the bloodstream are recruited and differentiate into more macrophages to supplement their numbers (Yucel et al., 2018). As the material is engulfed by phagocytosis, the cells increase in size and are subsequently referred to as Gitterzellen, or compound granular corpuscles. Monocytes are believed to be the predecessors of microglial cells, which are a component of the mononuclear system of phagocytes that ultimately originate from the bone marrow. The ependyma is a layer of cells that covers the central canal of the spinal cord and the ventricles of the brain. The ependyma is composed of a simple epithelium, with cells densely arranged in shapes ranging from cuboidal to columnar. The apical surfaces of the cells exhibit abundant microvilli and, depending on the specific site, may also display cilia. Desmosomes and zonula adherens connect neighboring cells, while zonula occludens are typically absent. Therefore, cerebrospinal fluid within the central canal and ventricles can traverse through ependymal cells to access the parenchyma of the CNS. Ependymal cells possess elongated, filamentous extensions at their base that divide, penetrate into the brain and spinal cord, and potentially reach the outer surface, where they provide end-feet to the glia limitans. The ependyma is a type of epithelium that secretes substances in the brain's ventricles. It directly contacts a highly vascular area of the pia mater called the tela choroidea. The ependyma, when modified, is referred to as choroid epithelial cells. Together with the tela choroidea, they constitute the choroid plexus, which is responsible for the production of cerebrospinal fluid. The choroid epithelial cells of the choroid plexus are tall and densely arranged, and they possess a large number of microvilli. In contrast to ependymal cells in other regions, the cell apices in this area are connected by zonula occludens, which act as barriers to prevent the movement of substances between cells. The choroid epithelial cells are positioned on a continuous basal lamina, which acts as a barrier between them and a connective tissue. This connective tissue contains small bundles of collagenous fibers, pia-arachnoid cells, and a large number of blood vessels. The capillary endothelial cells in this specific area possess a significant number of fenestrations, unlike the ones found in other parts of the brain. The movement of fluid through the capillary wall is unimpeded, but it is effectively blocked from entering the ventricles by the zonula occludens. Choroid epithelial cells actively release sodium ions into the ventricles, causing chloride ions, water, and other substances to passively follow. The concentrations of protein and glucose are relatively low. The production of cerebrospinal fluid is ongoing, and it flows at a slow pace through the brain's ventricles before entering the subarachnoid space. The meninges envelop and safeguard the CNS from physical harm and play a crucial role in the metabolic functions of the CNS (Yucel et al., 2018).

Specific compounds in the bloodstream are effectively blocked from entering the central nervous system, despite their ability to easily penetrate other bodily tissues. Astrocytes encase the capillaries located deep within the spinal cord and brain, while the nonfenestrated endothelial cells are connected by tight junctions that prevent the passage of substances. The endothelial cells in this specific location lack the characteristic transendothelial transport vesicles commonly observed in endothelial cells found in other capillaries. Moreover, the internal plasmalemma of the endothelial cells possesses unique characteristics that hinder the passage of certain substances. The blood-brain barrier is formed by the tight junctions and internal plasmalemma of the endothelial cells working together. The walls of the ventricles contain specific regions called circumventricular organs, which are highly vascularized areas. The organs mentioned are the organum vasculosum, lamina terminalis, subfornical organ, subcommissural organ, and area postrema. With the exception of the subcommissural organ, the ependymal cells in these regions undergo modifications and take on the form of star-shaped cells known as tanycytes. These cells are responsible for transporting cerebrospinal fluid to neurons in the hypothalamus. These regions lack an internal layer of glial processes called subependymal layer and an external layer called subpial layer. The capillaries beneath have an endothelium that is fenestrated. These regions do not possess the structural components of a genuine blood-brain barrier, with the exception of the subcommissural organ. However, they are capable of accumulating essential dyes. It is believed that large molecules can move through these regions, which act as areas of communication between the CNS and blood.

4.2.3. Spinal Cord

The spinal cord is divided into a central region of gray matter shaped like the letter H, and a layer of white matter that surrounds it. The gray matter primarily comprises the cell bodies of neurons, their dendrites, and the neuroglial cells that surround them. It is organized into two dorsal and two ventral horns. The dorsal horns house the cell bodies of multipolar neurons that receive sensory impulses originating from the peripheral nervous system and entering the spinal cord. The neurons located in the dorsal horns are responsible for transmitting impulses to other neurons. These neurons, found in various regions of gray matter, are commonly known as internuncial neurons. The ventral horns of the spinal cord contain multipolar neurons, which are the largest in size and responsible for transmitting motor impulses from the spinal cord to the periphery. In the thoracic and upper lumbar regions of the spinal cord, there is a cluster of small multipolar neurons known as the intermediolateral horn. These neurons are responsible for supplying preganglionic sympathetic fibers to the autonomic nervous system. The central canal of the spinal cord is located in the middle of the crossbar of the H-shaped gray matter and is surrounded by ependyma. The white matter primarily comprises axons that are coated with myelin and does not contain the cell bodies or dendrites of neurons. The structure is divided into anterior, lateral, and posterior funiculi by the dorsal and ventral horns of the gray matter. A funiculus is composed of multiple tracts, each of which contains several bundles of nerve fibers. Each tract of nerve fibers carries similar motor or sensory impulses that either travel up or down the length of the spinal cord (Zabłocka et al., 2021).

4.2.4. Cerebellar and Cerebral Hemispheres

The cerebellar and cerebral hemispheres differ from the spinal cord in terms of the arrangement of gray and white matter. In these hemispheres, the gray matter is found at the outer edges, while the white matter is situated in the central region. Both brain regions are composed of a gray matter cortex on the outside and a white matter subcortical region.

4.2.4.1. Cerebral Cortex

The cerebral cortex has a thickness ranging from 1.5 to 4.0 mm and consists of approximately 50 billion neurons, as well as nerve processes and supporting glial cells. With the exception of a small number of areas, it is distinguished by its laminated appearance. The perikarya are typically arranged into five layers. The neurons in the cerebral cortex are organized in layers, starting from the outermost layer called the molecular layer (I), followed by the external granular layer (II), external pyramidal layer (III), internal granular layer (IV), internal pyramidal layer (V), and finally the innermost layer called the multiform layer (VI). The molecular layer (I) is a region beneath the cortex surface that is mostly devoid of perikaryons. Neurons of comparable kind have a tendency to reside in the same layer within the cerebral cortex, although each cellular layer consists of multiple distinct cell types. To facilitate description, these neurons are commonly categorized into two main groups: pyramidal cells and stellate or nonpyramidal cells. The cell bodies of pyramidal cells exhibit a pyramidal shape and possess prominent apical dendrites that typically extend towards the outer surface of the cerebral cortex and penetrate the upper layers. Meanwhile, the individual axons of these cells enter the underlying subcortical white matter. They can be located in layers II, III, V, and, to a lesser degree, layer VI. The frontal lobe contains a layer called the internal pyramidal layer (V) which contains very large pyramid-shaped neurons known as Betz cells. Stellate cells, also known as nonpyramidal cells, do not have the characteristic pyramid-shaped cell bodies and the prominent apical dendrite. They are present in every layer of the cerebral cortex, but they are particularly abundant in the internal granular layer (IV). The impulses that enter the cortex are primarily transmitted to stellate cells and then passed on to pyramidal cells in different layers through the vertical axons of the stellate cells. The axons of pyramidal cells typically exit the cortex and project to various regions of the brain and spinal cord. The cerebral cortex is responsible for processing visual, auditory, and speech information, as well as controlling voluntary movements and facilitating learning.

4.2.4.2. Cerebellar Cortex

The cerebellar cortex is distinguished by its three layers: an outer molecular layer, a middle layer consisting of Purkinje cells, and an inner layer composed of granule cells. The molecular layer primarily functions as a synaptic region with a relatively low density of neuronal cell bodies. It primarily comprises unmyelinated axons originating from granule cells, with the axons aligned parallel to the cortical surface. The structure also includes prominent dendrites of the underlying Purkinje cells, as well as small scattered neurons known as stellate cells in its outer layer. Basket cells are small neurons found deep within this layer and positioned next to Purkinje cells. The Purkinje cell layer consists of the cell bodies of Purkinje cells, which are large, pear-shaped neurons arranged in a single row. These neurons are distinguished by their extensive branching dendrites that are located in the molecular layer. These neurons are Golgi type I and their total count is approximately 15 million. In three dimensions, the large dendritic trees are positioned in a narrow plane, resembling fan coral, and are arranged in such a way that each dendritic tree is parallel to the one next to it. A solitary, diminutive axon originating from the Purkinje cell traverses the granule cell layer and establishes synaptic connections with neurons in the central cerebellar region. The granule cell layer is composed of a multitude of densely clustered, diminutive neurons whose axons penetrate the molecular layer to form synapses with the dendrites of Purkinje cells. The granule cells are a type of Golgi II neurons. The nuclei are small and round, with coarse chromatin patterns and minimal cytoplasm. The dendrites are short and clawlike. The axons penetrate the molecular layer, divide into two branches, and align themselves parallel to the surface but at a right angle to the broad plane of the Purkinje dendritic tree. The axons of granule cells form synapses with approximately 450 Purkinje cells, resembling the arrangement of wires running along telephone poles. The axons of granule cells form synapses with stellate and basket neurons in the molecular layer. The Golgi cell, a distinct type of small neuron, is located in the outer region of the granule cell layer (Zabłocka et al., 2021). The cerebellar cortex receives input from two distinct types of afferent nerve fibers originating from peripheral regions of the CNS. The mossy fibers establish synaptic connections with granule cells, while the climbing fibers penetrate the molecular layer and coil around the dendrites of Purkinje cells. The primary role of the cerebellum is to modulate skeletal muscle activity, specifically in coordinating limb movement and maintaining balance. Nevertheless, there is compelling evidence indicating that the cerebellar cortex also plays a role in cognitive processes. The gray matter of the spinal cord, cerebrum, and cerebellum consists of a complex, highly ordered meshwork of dendritic, axonal, and glial processes that envelop the perikarya of associated neurons. The neuropil is a complex network that facilitates extensive synaptic connections and interactions among nerve processes, serving as a structural framework for organization. Coordinating activities in the CNS is crucial.

4.2.4.3. Meninges

The CNS is enclosed within three connective tissue membranes known as meninges, in addition to the bony covering provided by the skull and vertebral column. The outermost layer, known as the dura mater, is mainly composed of dense collagenous connective tissue. It envelops the brain in two layers and functions as a periosteum for the cranium while also acting as a protective covering for the brain. The periosteal layer contains a high concentration of blood vessels, nerves, and cells. The inner layer has a lower amount of blood vessels, and its inner surface is covered by a single layer of flat cells called simple squamous epithelium. The dura, which envelops the spinal cord, is composed of a solitary layer of dense irregular connective tissue that contains dispersed elastic fibers. The external layer is coated with a single layer of flat cells, known as simple squamous epithelium. This layer is separated from the periosteum of the vertebrae by an epidural space, which is filled with loose connective tissue containing an abundance of fat cells and veins. The inner surface of the dura of the spinal cord is covered by a single layer of flat epithelial cells. The narrow subdural space, filled with fluid, lies between the meninx, known as the arachnoid, and the adjacent meninx. The arachnoid is a delicate, net-like membrane composed of thin collagenous fibers and dispersed elastic fibers, lacking blood vessels. The outer region of the structure appears as a flat and even surface, while the inner surface produces multiple thin strands (trabeculae) that stretch into and merge with the underlying pia mater. A single layer of flat cells, known as simple squamous epithelium, covers the inner surface of the arachnoid, the trabeculae, and the outer surface of the pia. This same type of epithelium also lines a spacious area called the subarachnoid space, which holds cerebrospinal fluid. The pia mater is a delicate, blood vessel-rich membrane that tightly covers the brain and spinal cord. Due to their close relationship, the pia and arachnoid membranes are commonly referred to as the pia arachnoid. The pia mater is composed of fragile collagenous and elastic fibers, fibroblasts, macrophages, and dispersed mesenchymal cells. The blood vessels that enter and exit the brain tissue are surrounded by a layer of pia mater. The perivascular space envelops the blood vessels as they penetrate the CNS and is connected to the subarachnoid space (Zweyer et al., 2022).

4.2.5. Autonomic Nervous System

From a functional perspective, the nervous system can be further divided into autonomic and somatic subdivisions. The somatic component enables conscious regulation of skeletal muscle, while the autonomic component governs various organ functions that are not directly influenced by conscious control. Both reflex arcs are structured with afferent and efferent neurons, along with additional neurons in the CNS positioned between these two groups of neurons. The internuncial neurons serve to regulate the activity of the reflex arc. The autonomic efferent pathway comprises both preganglionic and postganglionic neurons. Preganglionic neurons extend nerve processes from the CNS to establish connections with postganglionic neurons situated outside the CNS. The autonomic outflow is divided into two subdivisions: sympathetic and parasympathetic. Sympathetic preganglionic neurons are distributed in the thoracolumbar region and their axons exit the spinal cord through nerve fibers that make up the ventral roots of the first thoracic to fourth lumbar spinal nerves. The preganglionic nerve fibers establish synaptic connections with neurons located either within the paravertebral sympathetic chain ganglia or in the collateral ganglia in close proximity to the target organ. On the other hand, parasympathetic preganglionic neurons are distributed in the craniosacral region. Their axons exit the body through cranial nerves (III, VII, IX, X) or through spinal nerves in the sacral region of the spinal cord. The parasympathetic ganglia neurons are typically situated either within the target organ or in close proximity to it. Acetylcholine is the neurotransmitter that is released by all parasympathetic postganglionic nerve endings. This neurotransmitter is also secreted at neuromuscular junctions by the somatic nervous system, as well as by nerve terminals of the sympathetic nervous system that are connected to sweat glands. The neurotransmitters released by most postganglionic sympathetic nerve endings are either norepinephrine or dopamine. In general, the sympathetic system is linked to fight or flight reactions, while the parasympathetic system is primarily associated with resting or digestive processes.

4.2.6. Histogenesis

The majority of the nervous system originates from neuroectoderm located on the dorsal aspect of the embryonic disk, specifically in the area referred to as the neural plate. The neural plate undergoes mitotic activity and cell growth, causing the lateral edges to fold upwards and create a neural groove. The boundaries of the fold come together, merge, and form a hollow neural tube that detaches from the outer layer of cells. The differential proliferation of ectodermal cells along the inner surface of the neural tube eventually leads to the development of the brain and spinal cord. Certain cells undergo proliferation and subsequently differentiate into neurons, while others develop into glial elements.

The wall of the neural tube reveals three distinct concentric zones: an internal ependymal layer, a wide intermediate mantle layer, and an outer marginal layer. The cells of the ependymal layer undergo division, migrate to the mantle layer, and then specialize into either neuroblasts or glioblasts. Neurons undergo differentiation initially, followed by astrocytes, and subsequently by oligodendrocytes. The ependymal zone in the spinal cord gives rise to the ependyma, the mantle zone transforms into the gray matter, and the white matter develops from the marginal zone. Neurons in the mantle layer initially lack polarity and are referred to as apolar neuroblasts. However, as cytoplasmic processes form at opposite ends of the cell body, these neurons transition into bipolar neurons. During the process of differentiation, a primitive axon undergoes elongation while another process is substituted by multiple small processes called primordial dendrites. This leads to the development of multipolar neurons. The axons penetrate and establish the marginal layer. Myelinization typically happens following the differentiation of oligodendrocytes, with the timing varying depending on the specific region. The areas of the neural tube that will develop into the cerebral and cerebellar cortices exhibit three zones that resemble those found in the spinal cord. Neurons in the mantle zone of the cerebral cortex undergo differentiation and then move into the marginal zone to form the outer cortical layers. The adult cerebral cortex exhibits a stratified structure due to the sequential migration of neuroblasts into the marginal zone and the subsequent differentiation of various neuronal types within the cortex. The cerebral cortex's sensory areas are distinguished by a high concentration of granular neurons, while its motor areas are characterized by a significant abundance of pyramidal neurons (Zweyer et al., 2022). At first, the developing cerebellar cortex is organized into ependymal, mantle, and marginal zones. During the process of development, certain neuroblasts originating from the mantle zone move towards the marginal zone of the cerebellar cortex and differentiate into Golgi and granular cells. Meanwhile, other neuroblasts stay in the mantle zone and give rise to cerebellar nuclei. Simultaneously, a subsequent migration transpires, during which these Purkinje cells, in conjunction with cells from the initial migration, establish the definitive structure of the cerebellar cortex. During the process of neural tube closure, a separate group of neurons called the neural crest emerges and generates both neurons and glial cells. On the top of each neural fold, cells in the outer layer of the embryo lose their characteristics as a protective layer, separate from each other, and move into the middle layer of the embryo that is located on both sides of the neural tube; they then take on the characteristics of cells that form connective tissue. The neural crest plays a significant role in the development of the peripheral nervous system. It gives rise to various types of cells, including neurons, glia, satellite cells, and Schwann cells. Specifically, it contributes to the formation of neurons and supporting cells in the spinal root ganglia, autonomic ganglia, and sensory ganglia of cranial nerves V, VII, IX, and X. However, it does not give rise to the neurons in the geniculate, acoustic, petrosal, and nodose ganglia. Additional cells from the neural crest surround the neural tube and participate in the development of the meninges.

A Closer Look

Cardiac Muscle

Cardiac muscle, also known as myocardium, is a specialized type of muscle tissue found exclusively in the heart. It is unique in its structure and function, playing a crucial role in maintaining the heart's ability to pump blood throughout the body. Cardiac muscle fibers are striated, similar to skeletal muscle, but they possess distinct characteristics that set them apart. These fibers are shorter, branched, and interconnected, forming a complex network that allows for synchronized contractions. The intercalated discs, which are unique to cardiac muscle, facilitate communication between cells, enabling them to work together efficiently. This coordinated contraction is vital for effective blood circulation, as it ensures that the heart beats rhythmically and with the necessary force to propel blood into the arteries.

Structural Characteristics

The structure of cardiac muscle is optimized for its continuous and involuntary nature. Each cardiac muscle cell, or cardiomyocyte, contains a single, centrally located nucleus, which is surrounded by a rich supply of mitochondria. This abundance of mitochondria is essential, as cardiac muscle requires a significant amount of energy to sustain its activity, relying predominantly on aerobic respiration for ATP production. The presence of myofibrils—composed of actin and myosin filaments—allows for the contraction of the muscle fibers. These myofibrils are organized into sarcomeres, the functional units of muscle contraction, which contribute to the striated appearance of the tissue. The intricate arrangement of these structures enables the heart to contract forcefully and efficiently, adapting to the varying demands placed on it during different physical activities.

Function and Regulation

The primary function of cardiac muscle is to contract rhythmically and pump blood throughout the circulatory system. This process is regulated by the heart's intrinsic conduction system, which includes specialized cells known as pacemaker cells located in the sinoatrial (SA) node. These cells generate electrical impulses that trigger cardiac muscle contractions. The autonomic nervous system also plays a crucial role in regulating heart rate and strength of contractions. Sympathetic stimulation increases heart rate and contractility, while parasympathetic stimulation decreases heart rate. Importantly, cardiac muscle exhibits a property known as automaticity, allowing it to initiate contractions without external stimuli. This inherent ability is vital for maintaining a consistent heart rhythm, ensuring that the body receives an adequate supply of oxygenated blood at all times.

Adaptations and Pathological Conditions

Cardiac muscle is remarkably adaptable, capable of responding to various physiological demands. For instance, during exercise, the heart can increase its output by enhancing the strength and frequency of contractions. Additionally, conditions such as hypertrophy may occur in response to increased workload, leading to an enlargement of cardiac muscle fibers. However, this adaptation can become pathological if it results from chronic conditions such as hypertension or valvular heart disease, potentially leading to heart failure. Other pathological conditions affecting cardiac muscle include myocardial infarction (heart attack), which results from the death of cardiac tissue due to insufficient blood supply, and cardiomyopathies, which encompass a range of diseases that affect the heart muscle's structure and function. These conditions highlight the importance of maintaining cardiovascular health through lifestyle choices and medical interventions to ensure the heart can continue to perform its vital role effectively.

Summary

This chapter explores the structure, function, and interactions between the nervous and muscular systems, emphasizing their roles in facilitating movement and communication within the body. It details the anatomy of nerve cells (neurons) and muscle fibers, highlighting how electrical impulses generated by neurons trigger muscle contraction. The chapter also explains the mechanisms of neuromuscular transmission, the role of neurotransmitters, and the process of excitation-contraction coupling in muscles. By examining different types of muscles—skeletal, smooth, and cardiac—the chapter illustrates how nerves and muscles work together to perform essential bodily functions, from voluntary movements to involuntary actions like heartbeats and digestion.

References

1. Aartsma-Rus, A., & van Putten, M. (2014). Assessing functional performance in the mdx mouse model. *Journal of Visualized Experiments, 85*, e51303. https://doi.org/10.3791/51303.
2. Allen, D. G., Whitehead, N. P., & Froehner, S. C. (2016). Absence of dystrophin disrupts skeletal muscle signaling: Roles of Ca^{2+}, reactive oxygen species, and nitric oxide in the development of muscular dystrophy. *Physiological Reviews, 96*(1), 253–305. https://doi.org/10.1152/physrev.00007.2015.
3. Angebault, C., Panel, M., Lacôte, M., Rieusset, J., Lacampagne, A., & Fauconnier, J. (2021). Metformin reverses the enhanced myocardial SR/ER–Mitochondria interaction and impaired complex I-driven respiration in dystrophin-deficient mice. *Frontiers in Cell and Developmental Biology, 8*, 609493. https://doi.org/10.3389/fcell.2020.609493.
4. Ascah, A., Khairallah, M., Daussin, F., Bourcier-Lucas, C., Godin, R., Allen, B. G., Petrof, B. J., des Rosiers, C., & Burelle, Y. (2011). Stress-induced opening of the permeability transition pore in the dystrophin-deficient heart is attenuated by acute treatment with sildenafil. *American Journal of Physiology-Heart and Circulatory Physiology, 300*(1), H144–H153. https://doi.org/10.1152/ajpheart.00455.2010.
5. Bostick, B., Yue, Y., Long, C., Marschalk, N., Fine, D. M., Chen, J., & Duan, D. (2009). Cardiac expression of a mini-dystrophin that normalizes skeletal muscle force only partially restores heart function in aged mdx mice. *Molecular Therapy, 17*(2), 253–261. https://doi.org/10.1038/mt.2008.264.
6. Briguet, A., Courdier-Fruh, I., Foster, M., Meier, T., & Magyar, J. P. (2004). Histological parameters for the quantitative assessment of muscular dystrophy in the mdx-mouse. *Neuromuscular Disorders, 14*(10), 675–682. https://doi.org/10.1016/j.nmd.2004.06.008.
7. Bulfield, G., Siller, W. G., Wight, P. A. L., & Moore, K. J. (1984). X chromosome-linked muscular dystrophy (mdx) in the mouse. *Proceedings of the National Academy of Sciences, 81*(4), 1189–1192. https://doi.org/10.1073/pnas.81.4.1189.
8. Burkin, D. J., Wallace, G. Q., Nicol, K. J., Kaufman, D. J., & Kaufman, S. J. (2001). Enhanced expression of the α7β1 integrin reduces muscular dystrophy and restores viability in dystrophic mice. *The Journal of Cell Biology, 152*(6), 1207–1218. https://doi.org/10.1083/jcb.152.6.1207.
9. Carlson, C. G. (2022). Does the pathogenic sequence of skeletal muscle degeneration in Duchenne muscular dystrophy begin and end with unrestrained satellite cell activation? *Muscles, 1*(2), 75–81. https://doi.org/10.3390/muscles1020006.

10. Chey, Y. C. J., Arudkumar, J., Aartsma-Rus, A., Adikusuma, F., & Thomas, P. Q. (2022). CRISPR applications for Duchenne muscular dystrophy: From animal models to potential therapies. *WIREs Mechanisms of Disease*, e1580. https://doi.org/10.1002/wsbm.1580.

11. de Paepe, B., & de Bleecker, J. L. (2013). Cytokines and chemokines as regulators of skeletal muscle inflammation: Presenting the case of Duchenne muscular dystrophy. *Mediators of Inflammation, 2013*, 1–10. https://doi.org/10.1155/2013/540370.

12. Deconinck, A. E., Rafael, J. A., Skinner, J. A., Brown, S. C., Potter, A. C., Metzinger, L., Watt, D. J., Dickson, J. G., Tinsley, J. M., & Davies, K. E. (1997). Utrophin-dystrophin-deficient mice as a model for Duchenne muscular dystrophy. *Cell, 90*(4), 717–727. https://doi.org/10.1016/s0092-8674(00)80532-2.

13. Deconinck, N., & Dan, B. (2007). Pathophysiology of Duchenne muscular dystrophy: Current hypotheses. *Pediatric Neurology, 36*(1), 1–7. https://doi.org/10.1016/j.pediatrneurol.2006.09.016.

14. Duan, D., Goemans, N., Takeda, S., Mercuri, E., & Aartsma-Rus, A. (2021). Duchenne muscular dystrophy. *Nature Reviews Disease Primers, 7*, 13. https://doi.org/10.1038/s41572-021-00248-3.

15. Dubinin, M. V., Starinets, V. S., Talanov, E. Y., Mikheeva, I. B., Belosludtseva, N. V., Serov, D. A., Tenkov, K. S., Belosludtseva, E. V., & Belosludtsev, K. N. (2021). Effect of the non-immunosuppressive MPT pore inhibitor alisporivir on the functioning of heart mitochondria in dystrophin-deficient mdx mice. *Biomedicines, 9*(9), 1232. https://doi.org/10.3390/biomedicines9091232.

16. Dubinin, M. V., Talanov, E. Y., Tenkov, K. S., Starinets, V. S., Mikheeva, I. B., & Belosludtsev, K. N. (2020). Transport of Ca^{2+} and Ca^{2+}-dependent permeability transition in heart mitochondria in the early stages of Duchenne muscular dystrophy. *Biochimica et Biophysica Acta (BBA)–Bioenergetics, 1861*(12), 148250. https://doi.org/10.1016/j.bbabio.2020.148250.

17. Dubowitz, V., Sewry, C., & Oldfors, A. (2020). *Muscle Biopsy: A Practical Approach* (5th ed.). Elsevier.

18. Duddy, W., Duguez, S., Johnston, H., Cohen, T. V., Phadke, A., Gordish-Dressman, H., Nagaraju, K., Gnocchi, V., Low, S. H., & Partridge, T. (2015). Muscular dystrophy in the mdx mouse is a severe myopathy compounded by hypotrophy, hypertrophy and hyperplasia. *Skeletal Muscle, 5*, 1–18. https://doi.org/10.1186/s13395-014-0026-9.

19. Egorova, T. V., Galkin, I. I., Ivanova, Y. V., & Polikarpova, A. V. (2022). Duchenne muscular dystrophy animal models. In E. Purevjav, J. Pierre, & L. Lu (Eds.), *Preclinical Animal Modeling in Medicine*. IntechOpen. https://doi.org/10.5772/intechopen.103095.

20. Grounds, M. D., Terrill, J. R., Al-Mshhdani, B. A., Duong, M. N., Radley-Crabb, H. G., & Arthur, P. G. (2020). Biomarkers for Duchenne muscular dystrophy: Myonecrosis, inflammation and oxidative stress. *Disease Models & Mechanisms, 13*(2), dmm043638. https://doi.org/10.1242/dmm.043638.

21. Hindi, S., Tajrishi, M., & Kumar, A. (2013). Signaling mechanisms in mammalian myoblast fusion. *Science Signaling, 6*(re2). https://doi.org/10.1126/scisignal.2003929.

22. Hodges, B. L., Hayashi, Y. K., Nonaka, I., Wang, W., Arahata, K., & Kaufman, S. J. (1997). Altered expression of the α7β1 integrin in human and murine muscular dystrophies. *Journal of Cell Science, 110*(Pt 23), 2873–2881.

23. Johnson, C. D., Zhou, L. Y., & Kopinke, D. (2022). A guide to examining intramuscular fat formation and its cellular origin in skeletal muscle. *Journal of Visualized Experiments, 2022*(63996). https://doi.org/10.3791/63996.

24. Kornegay, J. N. (2017). The golden retriever model of Duchenne muscular dystrophy. *Skeletal Muscle, 7*, 9. https://doi.org/10.1186/s13395-017-0124-2.

25. Kumar, A., Accorsi, A., Rhee, Y., & Girgenrath, M. (2015). Dos and don'ts in the preparation of muscle cryosections for histological analysis. *Journal of Visualized Experiments, 2015*(52793). https://doi.org/10.3791/52793.

26. Latroche, C., Matot, B., Martins-Bach, A., Briand, D., Chazaud, B., Wary, C., Carlier, P. G., Chrétien, F., & Jouvion, G. (2015). Structural and functional alterations of skeletal muscle microvasculature in dystrophin-deficient mdx mice. *The American Journal of Pathology, 185*(9), 2482–2494. https://doi.org/10.1016/j.ajpath.2015.05.015.

27. Meng, H., Janssen, P. M. L., Grange, R. W., Yang, L., Beggs, A. H., Swanson, L. C., Cossette, S. A., Frase, A., Childers, M. K., Granzier, H., et al. (2014). Tissue triage and freezing for models of skeletal muscle disease. *Journal of Visualized Experiments, 2014*(51586). https://doi.org/10.3791/51586.

28. Morgan, J. E., Prola, A., Mariot, V., Pini, V., Meng, J., Hourde, C., Dumonceaux, J., Conti, F., Relaix, F., Authier, F. J., et al. (2018). Necroptosis mediates myofibre death in dystrophin-deficient mice. *Nature Communications, 9*, 3655. https://doi.org/10.1038/s41467-018-05894-0.

29. Nonaka, I. (1998). Animal models of muscular dystrophies. *Laboratory Animal Science, 48*(1), 8–17.

30. Petrof, B. J., Stedman, H. H., Shrager, J. B., Eby, J., Sweeney, H. L., & Kelly, A. M. (1993). Adaptations in myosin heavy chain expression and contractile function in dystrophic mouse diaphragm. *American Journal of Physiology-Cell Physiology, 265*(4), C834–C841. https://doi.org/10.1152/ajpcell.1993.265.4.C834.

31. Roelofs, A. J., & de Bari, C. (2019). Immunostaining of skeletal tissues. In A. I. Idris (Ed.), *Bone Research Protocols* (3rd ed., Vol. 1914, pp. 437–450). Humana Press Inc. https://doi.org/10.1007/978-1-4939-8982-9_27.

32. Scalia, C. R., Boi, G., Bolognesi, M. M., Riva, L., Manzoni, M., DeSmedt, L., Bosisio, F. M., Ronchi, S., Leone, B. E., & Cattoretti, G. (2017). Antigen masking during fixation and embedding, dissected. *The Journal of Histochemistry & Cytochemistry, 65*(1), 5–20. https://doi.org/10.1369/0022155416676362.

33. Siemionow, M., Langa, P., Brodowska, S., Kozlowska, K., Zalants, K., Budzynska, K., & Heydemann, A. (2022). Long-term protective effect of human dystrophin expressing chimeric (DEC) cell therapy on amelioration of function of cardiac, respiratory, and skeletal muscles in Duchenne muscular dystrophy. *Stem Cell Reviews and Reports, 18*(9), 2872–2892. https://doi.org/10.1007/s12015-022-10398-8.

34. Terry, R. L., & Wells, D. J. (2016). Histopathological evaluation of skeletal muscle with specific reference to mouse models of muscular dystrophy. *Current Protocols in Mouse Biology, 6*(4), 343–363. https://doi.org/10.1002/cpmo.18.

35. Tinsley, J. M., Blake, D. J., Roche, A., Fairbrother, U., Riss, J., Byth, B. C., Knight, A. E., Kendrick-Jones, J., Suthers, G. K., Love, D. R., et al. (1992). Primary structure of dystrophin-related protein. *Nature, 360*(6404), 591–593. https://doi.org/10.1038/360591a0.

36. Tulangekar, A., & Sztal, T. E. (2021). Inflammation in Duchenne muscular dystrophy—Exploring the role of neutrophils in muscle damage and regeneration. *Biomedicines, 9*(10), 1366. https://doi.org/10.3390/biomedicines9101366.

37. Vallejo-Illarramendi, A., Toral-Ojeda, I., Aldanondo, G., & López de Munain, A. (2014). Dysregulation of calcium homeostasis in muscular dystrophies. *Expert Review of Molecular Medicine, 16*, e16. https://doi.org/10.1017/erm.2014.17.

38. Vulin, A., Wein, N., Simmons, T. R., Rutherford, A. M., Findlay, A. R., Yurkoski, J. A., Kaminoh, Y., & Flanigan, K. M. (2015). The first exon duplication mouse model of Duchenne muscular dystrophy: A tool for therapeutic development. *Neuromuscular Disorders, 25*(10), 827–834. https://doi.org/10.1016/j.nmd.2015.07.003.

39. Yucel, N., Chang, A. C., Day, J. W., Rosenthal, N., & Blau, H. M. (2018). Humanizing the mdx mouse model of DMD: The long and the short of it. *NPJ Regenerative Medicine, 3*, 4. https://doi.org/10.1038/s41536-018-0040-2.

40. Zabłocka, B., Górecki, D. C., & Zabłocki, K. (2021). Disrupted calcium homeostasis in Duchenne muscular dystrophy: A common mechanism behind diverse consequences. *International Journal of Molecular Sciences, 22*(20), 11040. https://doi.org/10.3390/ijms222011040.

41. Zweyer, M., Sabir, H., Dowling, P., Gargan, S., Murphy, S., Swandulla, D., & Ohlendieck, K. (2022). Histopathology of Duchenne muscular dystrophy in correlation with changes in proteomic biomarkers. *Histology and Histopathology, 37*(1), 101–116. https://doi.org/10.14670/HH-18-403.

Chapter 5

CARDIOVASCULAR AND LYMPH VASCULAR SYSTEMS

Contents

Introduction

Unicellular organisms obtain oxygen and nutrients through direct diffusion and other cellular membrane processes from their surrounding environment. However, in multicellular animals, the majority of cells are located internally, lacking direct exposure to the external environment. Instead, materials are transported to these cells through a closed network of branching tubes. The cardiovascular system consists of the tubular system and a muscular pump. The system comprises a cardiac organ functioning as a pump, arterial vessels transporting blood to organs and tissues, capillaries facilitating material exchange, and venous vessels returning the blood to the heart. The lymphatic system collects interstitial fluid from organs and tissues and returns it to the bloodstream. The system does not have a pumping mechanism and operates in a single direction, transporting lymph exclusively towards the heart. There is no lymphatic counterpart to blood arteries.

Orientation and Directional Terms

Term	Definition	Illustration
Endocardium	The innermost layer of the heart, consisting of endothelial tissue that lines the heart chambers and valves, providing a smooth surface for blood flow.	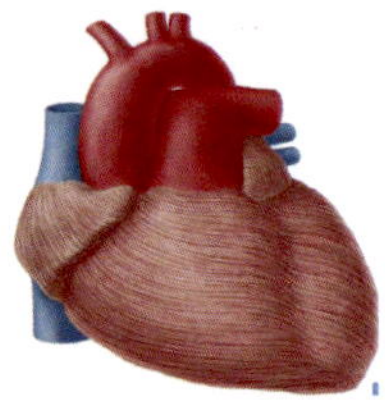
Epicardium	The outer layer of the heart wall, also known as the visceral pericardium; it is a protective layer that contains blood vessels and nerves and is involved in the heart's function.	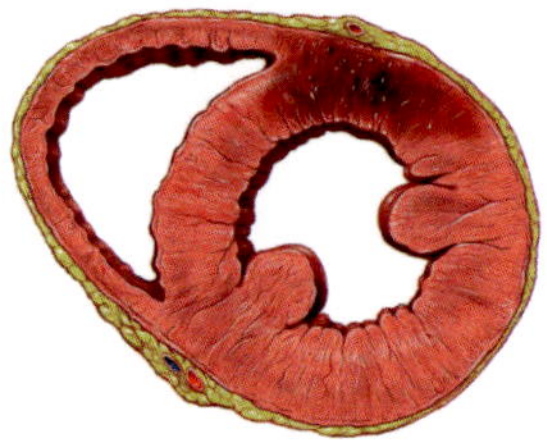
Cardiac Skeleton	A dense connective tissue structure that provides support and stability to the heart; it serves as an attachment point for cardiac muscle and helps maintain the shape of the heart.	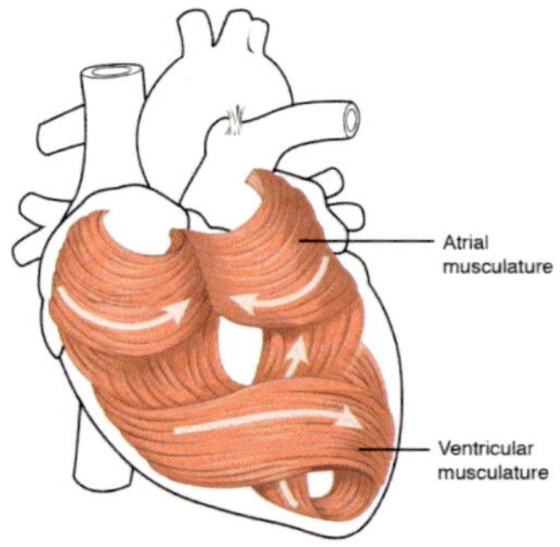
Valves	Structures in the heart and blood vessels that ensure one-way blood flow; in the heart, there are four main valves: the tricuspid, pulmonary, mitral, and aortic valves.	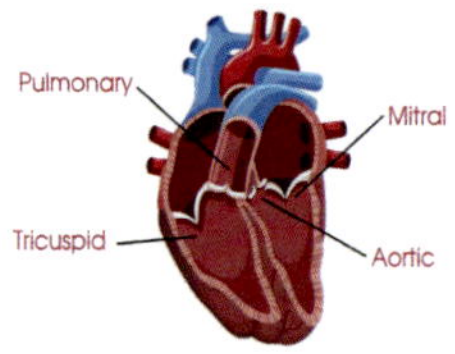
Metarterioles	Small blood vessels that connect arterioles to capillaries; they play a role in regulating blood flow and are involved in the exchange of nutrients and waste between blood and tissues.	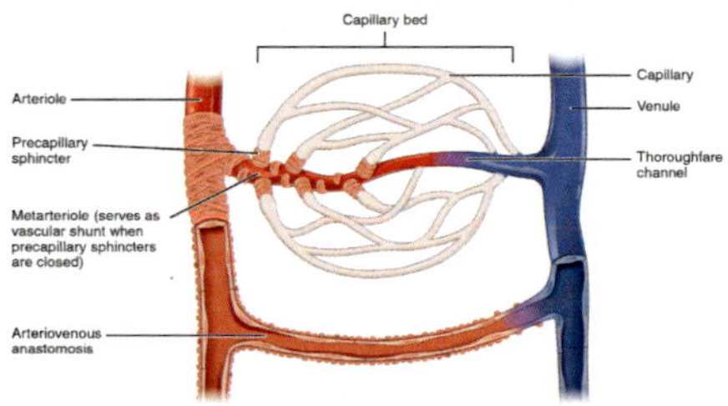

5.1. Heart

The heart is an altered blood vessel that functions as a dual pump and is composed of four chambers. Located on the right side, the atrium receives deoxygenated blood from the body, while the ventricle forcefully pumps it to the lungs. The left atrium receives oxygenated blood from the pulmonary circulation and transfers it to the left ventricle, which pumps it to all body parts. The cardiac wall is composed of an endocardium, a myocardium, and an epicardium (Ross & Pawlina, 2015).

5.1.1. Endocardium

The endocardium is the inner lining of the atria and ventricles, and it is similar to the inner lining of blood vessels. The structure is composed of a solitary layer of polygonal squamous (endothelial) cells with nuclei that are oval or rounded in shape. Tight junctions bring together adjacent cells tightly, while gap junctions allow for intercellular communication. The electron micrographs display a limited number of brief microvilli, a slender proteoglycan layer covering the inner surface, and the typical organelles within the cytoplasm. The endothelial cells are situated on a continuous layer of delicate collagen fibers, which are separated from the cells by a basement membrane. The layer composed of fibers is referred to as the subendothelial layer. Beneath it lies a substantial layer of more compact connective tissue that comprises the majority of the endocardium. This layer is rich in elastic fibers and also contains a few smooth muscle cells. The subendocardial layer is composed of loose connective tissue that attaches the endocardium to the underlying heart muscle. This tissue contains collagen fibers, elastic fibers, and blood vessels. The ventricles also house the specialized cardiac muscle fibers of the conducting system (Ames et al., 2020).

5.1.2. Myocardium

The myocardium, located in the middle layer of the heart, is primarily composed of cardiac muscle. The myocardium is a highly vascularized tissue, with an estimated capillary density of approximately 2,800 capillaries per mm^2. In comparison, skeletal muscle has a capillary density of about 350 per mm^2. The capillaries fully encircle individual cardiac myocytes and are closely attached to them by the surrounding delicate connective tissue that exists between individual muscle cells. In contrast to other tissues, the myocardial capillaries are typically fully open for perfusion, without any closed or obstructed vessels. As activity levels rise in these tissues, the number of capillaries available for perfusion also increases. The atria have the thinnest myocardium, while the left ventricle has the thickest myocardium. The myocardium is organized into concentric layers that create intricate helical patterns around the atria and ventricles. Within the atria, cardiac muscle groups create a network that is easily visible as the pectinate muscles. In the ventricles, separate groups of cardiac muscle form the trabeculae carnea. The cardiac muscle cells in the atria are comparatively smaller and possess distinct dense granules that are not found in other parts of the heart. These myocytes possess characteristics typically found in endocrine cells. The secretory granules are primarily found in the right atrium and are released upon stretching.

The granules contain atrial natriuretic factor (ANF), which is released when there is an increase in blood volume or venous pressure in the atria. Atrial natriuretic factor stimulates vasoconstriction of the afferent arteriole in the kidneys, increasing both glomerular filtration pressure and filtration rate. Atrial natriuretic peptide (ANF) also affects the distal and collecting tubules of the kidneys by reducing the reabsorption of sodium and chloride. Additionally, it hinders the release of antidiuretic hormone (ADH), aldosterone, and renin. These actions lead to the increased excretion of sodium chloride (natriuresis) in a large amount of diluted urine. The presence of elastic fibers in the ventricular myocardium is limited, while they are abundant in the atria, where they create a complex network that intertwines with the muscle fibers. The elastic fibers of the myocardium merge with those of the endocardium and the outer layer of the heart (epicardium). Cardiac muscle cells exhibit spontaneous contractions due to the generation of action potentials within themselves, which are then transmitted to adjacent cardiac myocytes through gap junctions. The generation of action potentials in cardiac muscle cells is facilitated by ion fluxes that are mediated by ion channels located in the plasmalemma and T-tubule system. The action potential plateau duration during the contraction of cardiac myocytes is significantly longer, up to 15 times, compared to that observed in skeletal muscle cells. The action potential in cardiac myocytes is generated, in part, by the abrupt activation of numerous fast sodium ion channels, which permit the influx of sodium ions. These ion channels have a brief duration of only a few 10,000th of a second before they close. Repolarization promptly follows in skeletal muscle, concluding the action potential within a mere 10,000th of a second. The action potential in cardiac muscle is generated by the activation of two distinct types of ion channels: (1) fast sodium ion channels, similar to those found in skeletal muscle, and (2) slow calcium channels, also known as calcium-sodium channels. The latter have a slower opening speed and a significantly longer duration of being open. Upon opening, both calcium and sodium ions permeate into the cardiac myocyte, leading to the sustained depolarization phase and the consequent prolonged plateau of the action potential. During this period, the plasmalemma's permeability to potassium ions also decreases due to the calcium influx. This prevents the action potential from returning to a resting level early, similar to what happens in skeletal muscle (Ames et al., 2020). A significant amount of calcium ions enter the sarcoplasm of the myocyte from the extracellular fluid by traversing the plasmalemma and T-tubules when the action potential is produced. The wide diameter of the T-tubules facilitates the entry of extracellular fluid, which contains calcium ions, into the T-tubule system. This fluid is then made accessible within the interior of the cardiac myocytes. The calcium ion influx that occurs during the action potential development is inadequate to induce contraction of the cardiac myocyte. The calcium ion that enters binds to the channel proteins of the sarcoplasmic reticulum, which then leads to the release of stored calcium. This release of calcium is what starts the contraction of the cardiac myocyte. The calcium ion that enters during the generation of the action potential is commonly known as trigger calcium due to this specific reason. The contraction mechanism of the cardiac myocyte closely resembles that of skeletal muscle.

5.1.3. Epicardium

The epicardium is the innermost layer of the pericardium, a tough fibrous sac that surrounds and protects the heart. The outer layer of the epicardium is coated with a solitary layer of mesothelial cells that range from flat to cuboidal in shape. Below this layer is a connective tissue layer that houses a large number of elastic fibers. The epicardium, located on the cardiac muscle consists of blood vessels, nerves, and varying amounts of fat. The specific term for this section is the subepicardial layer.

The parietal layer of the epicardium is composed of connective tissue that is covered by mesothelial cells, which are in direct contact with the cells covering the visceral epicardium. The two layers, lined with epithelial cells, are only separated by a thin film of fluid, secreted by the mesothelial cells. This fluid enables the layers to glide smoothly over each other when the heart contracts and relaxes (Athani et al., 2022).

5.1.4. Conducting System

The cardiac conducting system comprises specialized cardiac muscle fibers that are responsible for initiating and sustaining the heart's rhythm and ensuring the coordination of contractions between the atria and ventricles. The system comprises a sinoatrial node, an atrioventricular node, an atrioventricular bundle, and Purkinje fibers. Cardiac myocytes, including those of the conducting system, start with a resting membrane potential of approximately -90 millivolts. This potential is created by the movement of potassium ions from inside the sarcoplasm of the myocyte to the surrounding interstitial fluid. The initiation of each cardiac cycle is triggered by the autonomous generation of an action potential by cardiac muscle cells that comprise the sinoatrial node. The sinoatrial node is situated in the epicardium where the superior vena cava and right atrium meet. It takes the form of an elongated strip, measuring approximately 13 mm in length and 3 mm in width. Nodal cells are characterized by their smaller size than regular cardiac muscle cells and their reduced number of myofibrils, which are also less organized. Intercalated discs are absent between cells of the sinoatrial nodes. Due to the elevated concentration of sodium ions in the extracellular fluid surrounding them, these ions typically have a tendency to seep into the sinus muscle fibers. The self-excitation phenomenon is caused by the natural permeability of the plasmalemma of sinus nodal fibers to sodium ions through specific sodium ion channels known as If channels. Due to this leakage, the resting membrane potential of the sinus nodal fibers is reduced to a range of -55 to -60 millivolts, which is lower than the normal cardiac myocytes of the ventricles that have a resting membrane potential of -85 to -90 millivolts. Due to the reduced negativity of the resting potential, the fast sodium channels are typically inactive. In contrast, only the slow calcium-sodium channels open, leading to the generation of an action potential. The cardiac muscle fibers that comprise the sinoatrial node are directly connected to the neighboring atrial cardiac muscle cells. The action potential, which arises spontaneously, begins in the node cells and then propagates throughout the entire mass of atrial muscle. It reaches the atrioventricular node, which is situated in the posterior wall of the right atrium, behind the tricuspid valve and next to the opening of the coronary sinus. In this case, the action potential is intentionally delayed to provide sufficient time for the atria to fully empty their blood into the ventricles before the start of ventricular contraction. Compared to other areas of the heart, the sinoatrial node regulates the heartbeat due to its higher rate of rhythmic discharge. Due to its accelerated discharge rate, nodal cell activity supersedes any potential pacemaker activity from other cells (such as cells of the atrioventricular node and Purkinje cells) in the heart. Therefore, the sinoatrial node serves as the primary regulator of the heart's rhythm. The cardiac muscle tissue of the atrioventricular node serves to delay the transmission of the cardiac impulse and acts as a "gatekeeper" to ensure the continued conduction of the impulse into the ventricles. The atrioventricular node consists of cardiac myocytes with the lowest conduction velocity among all the fibers in the heart. Impulses swiftly propagate through the atrioventricular bundle located in the membranous section of the interventricular septum. The bundle bifurcates into two main branches that enter the ventricles, where they subsequently branch out into multiple smaller branches that connect with the regular cardiac muscle fibers. Therefore, the impulse is transmitted to every region of the ventricular myocardium. The specialized fibers found in these trunks and branches are called Purkinje fibers (cells) and possess distinct characteristics that set them apart from regular cardiac muscle. Purkinje fibers exhibit greater size and possess a higher amount of sarcoplasm, while myofibrils are less abundant and typically situated at the periphery (Athani et al., 2022). The fibers contain abundant glycogen and mitochondria and frequently possess two or more nuclei. Intercalated discs are infrequent, yet there are many desmosomes dispersed along the cell boundaries. Purkinje fibers are the most rapid conducting fibers in the heart. The electrocardiogram (ECG) traces the action potential of the cardiac myocytes throughout the heart. In a typical electrocardiogram (ECG), the P wave signifies the depolarization of the atria, the QRS wave complex signifies the depolarization of the ventricles, and the T wave signifies the repolarization of the ventricles. The autonomic nervous system regulates the heartbeat. The axons of parasympathetic postganglionic neurons end in the tissue of the sinoatrial and atrioventricular nodes. The nerve terminals release acetylcholine, which then binds to muscarinic acetylcholine receptors. These receptors are G-protein-linked receptors that inhibit adenylate cyclase and reduce levels of cyclic adenosine monophosphate (c-AMP), resulting in a decrease in heart rate. On the other hand, the axons of postganglionic sympathetic neurons that are spread throughout the myocardium release norepinephrine. This norepinephrine then binds to β-adrenergic receptors, which are G-protein-linked receptors. These receptors stimulate adenylate cyclase and cause an increase in c-AMP levels. As a result, the heart rate is increased.

5.1.5. Cardiac Skeleton

The ventricles of the heart do not undergo complete emptying like other hollow organs. Instead, blood is expelled from their cavities in a manner similar to wringing water out of a soaked towel. The heart possesses a complex three-dimensional network of dense connective tissue known as the fibrous skeleton, which is an anchor for its musculature. The primary component of the cardiac skeleton consists of the annuli fibrosi, which are dense connective tissue rings that encircle the openings of the aorta, pulmonary artery, and atrioventricular orifices. Among these options, the aortic ring exhibits the highest level of strength. The cardiac skeleton is further supported by triangular thickenings of fibrous connective tissue called trigona fibrosi. These thickenings connect the aortic root to the atrioventricular annuli. Additionally, the upper fibrous part of the interventricular septum, known as the septum membranaceum, also contributes to the cardiac skeleton. In certain cases, the trigona fibrosa may contain material resembling cartilage, and as it ages, it may experience calcification. The annuli fibrosi not only attach to the cardiac musculature and valve components, but also provide support and preserve the integrity of all four orifices. In the absence of these support rings, the openings would expand and the valves would lose their ability to function effectively. The annuli fibrosi, located around the atrioventricular orifices, act as a barrier that separates the atrial and ventricular myocardium. The only electrophysiological connection between them is the specialized conducting tissue of the atrioventricular bundles, which guarantees the organized sequence of events related to the cardiac cycle.

5.1.6. Valves

Valves are located between the atria and ventricles and at the entrances to the aorta and pulmonary vessels. The valves exhibit a comparable histologic structure, irrespective of their geographical location. The atrioventricular valves are connected to the annuli fibrosi, a type of connective tissue that extends into each valve and forms its central structure. Both sides of the valves are enveloped by endocardium, which is thicker on the ventricular side. Smooth muscle cells are scattered on the atrial side of the valves, whereas elastic fibers are more noticeable on the ventricular side. The ventricular sides of the valves are connected to papillary muscles, which are projections of cardiac muscle, by thin tendinous cords known as chordae tendineae. The semilunar valves of the pulmonary arteries and aorta have a thinner structure, but they exhibit the same overall histologic composition as the atrioventricular valves.

5.2. Blood Vessels

Blood vessels are a network of tubes of different sizes that form a closed circuit, allowing blood to be transported from the heart to the tissues and then returned to the heart from all areas of the body (Alberts et al., 2002). The circulatory system is responsible for distributing oxygen from the lungs, nutrients from the intestines and liver, and regulatory substances like hormones to all the organs and tissues. Excretory substances are also discharged into the bloodstream and transported to organs like the lungs and kidneys for excretion.

5.2.1. Structural Organization

While blood vessels may vary in terms of size, distribution, and function, they possess numerous shared structural characteristics. The walls of blood vessels, similar to the heart, are composed of three main coats or tunics. The variations in the appearance and functions of different components of the circulatory system are evident through structural modifications in these tunics, as well as through the reduction or even absence of certain layers. The wall of a blood vessel is composed of three layers: the tunica intima, tunica media, and tunica adventitia, starting from the innermost layer called the lumen. The tunica intima is anatomically equivalent to and forms a continuous connection with the endocardium of the heart. The structure comprises a layer of flattened squamous cells called endothelium, which is situated on a basal lamina and is upheld by a subendothelial connective tissue. The tunica media corresponds to the myocardium of the heart and is the layer that exhibits the greatest variability in terms of size and structure. The amount of smooth muscle and elastic tissue in this layer varies depending on the function of the vessel. The thickness of the tunica adventitia varies in different sections of the vascular circuit. The structure primarily comprises collagenous connective tissue and corresponds to the epicardium of the heart, although it does not contain mesothelial cells (Bäumler et al., 2020).

5.3. Arteries

As the arteries move away from the heart, they undergo a series of divisions to form multiple branches with decreasing sizes. The alterations in dimensions and the corresponding alterations in the composition of the vascular wall are continuous; however, three categories of arteries can be discerned: major elastic or conducting arteries, intermediate muscular or distributing arteries, and minor arteries and arterioles. The arterial side of the blood vasculature system is distinguished by the significant presence of smooth muscle in the tunica media.

5.3.1. Elastic or Conducting Arteries

The aorta serves as the primary conduit artery, while other arteries in this category include the common iliacs, pulmonary, brachiocephalic, subclavian, and common carotid arteries. An important characteristic of this particular artery is the significant diameter of its lumen, which, makes the vessel wall appear thin by comparison. The tunica intima has a relatively substantial thickness and is covered by a single layer of flattened, polygonal endothelial cells supported by a complete basal lamina. Endothelial cells that are next to each other can either interdigitate or overlap, and they are strongly connected through occluding and communicating (gap) junctions.

The cells possess the typical organelles, albeit in limited quantity. Distinctive membrane-bound, rod-shaped granules, composed of multiple tubules embedded in a shapeless matrix, are found and have been demonstrated to contain a factor (VIII) linked to blood clotting. This factor is produced by these cells and released into the bloodstream. The luminal surface of the cell membrane is covered by a layer called the endothelial coat, composed of proteoglycans. The endothelial cells on the basal surface are positioned apart from the basal lamina by an unstructured matrix. The plasmalemma has multiple invaginations or caveolae at both the luminal and basal surfaces. Additionally, the cytoplasm contains numerous small vesicles with a diameter of 50 to 70 nm. The transcytotic vesicles are believed to originate at one surface, detach, and traverse to the opposite side, where they merge with the plasmalemma to release their contents. In humans, approximately 25% of the overall thickness of the intima is comprised of the subendothelial layer. This layer consists of loose connective tissue containing elastic fibers and a small number of smooth muscle cells. The tunica media is the thickest layer of the structure and is primarily composed of elastic tissue. It comprises 50 to 70 concentric sheets, known as elastic laminae, which are fenestrated and measure approximately 2 to 3 μm in thickness. These sheets are spaced apart at a distance of 5 to 20 μm. Elastic fibers connect each consecutive lamina. The spaces between the laminae are filled with thin layers of connective tissue that consist of collagen fibers and smooth muscle cells arranged in a circular pattern. The smooth muscle cells exhibit a flattened, irregular, and branched morphology and are connected to neighboring elastic laminae through elastic microfibrils and reticular fibers. A significant quantity of amorphous ground substance is also present. The media of elastic arteries exclusively contains smooth muscle cells responsible for synthesizing and preserving the elastic fibers and collagen. Elastic arteries, located closest to the heart, possess a significant amount of elastic tissue, which allows them to expand. During the heart's contraction, blood is pumped and the walls of elastic arteries expand. When the heart relaxes, the elastic recoil of these vessels acts as an additional pumping mechanism, propelling blood forward between beats (Bazilevs et al., 2013). The tunica adventitia is a thin layer comprising bundles of collagen fibers (specifically type 1) and a small number of elastic fibers. These fibers are arranged in a loose, helical pattern around the blood vessel. Fibroblasts, mast cells, and infrequent longitudinally oriented smooth muscle cells are also found. The tunica adventitia gradually merges with the surrounding loose connective tissue and serves to secure the vessel to nearby structures. The walls of major arteries are too substantial to rely solely on diffusion from the inner cavity for nourishment. As a result, these vessels have their own small arteries called vasa vasorum, which may originate from the main vessel or nearby vessels. The nerves create a network in the outer layer of the blood vessel wall and typically do not extend deeply into the middle layer.

5.3.2. Muscular or Distributing Arteries

The muscular or distributing arteries are the largest group, and except for the elastic arteries, the named arteries of gross anatomy belong to this category. The small branches that arise from flexible trunks are known as muscular arteries, and the change is quite sudden, happening at the points where the arteries divide. The walls of these arteries are relatively thick and account for more than 25% of the cross-sectional diameter, when compared to the luminal diameter. The wall's thickness primarily results from the abundant smooth muscle in the media. Through contraction and relaxation, this smooth muscle plays a crucial role in regulating the blood supply to organs and tissues. The overall structure of these vessels is comparable to that of elastic arteries, although there are variations in the relative abundance of cells and fibers. The tunica intima comprises an endothelium, a subendothelial layer, and an internal elastic lamina. The endothelium and subendothelial layers exhibit similarities to those found in elastic arteries. However, as the vessel size decreases, the subendothelial layer becomes progressively thinner. The composition of this structure consists of delicate collagen fibers, a limited number of elastic fibers, and dispersed smooth muscle cells that are aligned longitudinally. The internal elastic lamina is a perforated layer made of elastin that serves as a distinct and wavy boundary separating the tunica media and the tunica intima. The endothelial cells' basal surface extends slender processes through gaps in the elastic lamina to establish contact with cells in the tunica media. The tunica media is the thickest layer and is primarily composed of smooth muscle cells organized in concentric, helical arrangements. The number of layers ranges from 3 to 4 in smaller arteries to 10 to 40 in the larger muscular arteries. The muscle cells are enveloped by basal laminae and establish communication with one another through gap junctions. Between the layers of smooth muscle, there are reticular fibers, small bundles of collagen fibers, and elastic fibers. The quantity and arrangement of elastic fibers are directly related to the diameter of the artery. Elastic fibers are distributed sporadically among the muscle cells in smaller vessels, while in larger arteries, the elastic tissue forms circular, lax networks. The elastic tissue at the point where the tunica media and the tunica adventitia meet creates a second distinct fenestrated membrane known as the external elastic lamina. In muscular arteries, the tunica adventitia is highly noticeable, and in certain vessels, it can have a thickness comparable to that of the media. The structure is composed of collagen and elastic fibers that are aligned in a longitudinal orientation. The coat seamlessly extends into the adjacent loose connective tissue without any distinct boundary. Muscular arteries exhibit a high level of contractility, primarily regulated by the autonomic nervous system and factors secreted by endothelial cells. For instance, the adrenergic sympathetic innervation of smooth muscle cells in the media of these vessels causes the muscles to contract and leads to the narrowing of the vessel, known as vasoconstriction (Cetin and Sahin, 2018).

5.3.3. Small Arteries and Arterioles

Small arteries and arterioles can be distinguished from large muscular arteries solely by their dimensions and the thickness of their walls. The differentiation between small arteries and arterioles primarily lies in their respective definitions: Arterioles are small arteries with a diameter smaller than 250 to 300 μm. They have a media layer that consists of only one or two layers of smooth muscle cells. During the transition from distributing artery to arteriole, the amount of subendothelial connective tissue gradually decreases. In arterioles, there is no subendothelial layer, and the tunica intima is composed solely of endothelium and a fenestrated internal elastic lamina. The endothelial cells are connected by tight junctions. Basal processes establish contact with smooth muscle cells via the openings in the elastic lamina. The thin basal lamina loses clarity in the tiniest arterioles. The smooth muscle cells in the media layer decrease in number as the diameter of the arterioles reaches approximately 30 μm. At this point, the muscle coat of the arterioles is composed of a single layer of cells that are oriented in a circular manner. The internal elastic membrane is characterized by its thinness and absence in terminal arterioles, while there is no distinct external elastic lamina present. The tunica adventitia also undergoes a reduction in thickness, becoming exceptionally thin in the smallest arterioles. The walls of arterioles are thicker in comparison to the luminal size. Arterioles, thanks to the presence of smooth muscle in their media layer, have the ability to regulate the blood flow to the capillary beds they supply. As a result, they play a crucial role in controlling blood pressure. Due to the high oxygen content in these vessels, they redirect the blood flow towards the capillary beds where the tissues have low oxygen levels. Arterioles exhibit a high degree of sensitivity to vascular stimuli, making them significant contributors to vascular resistance.

5.3.4. Metarterioles

Metarterioles serve as a connection between capillaries and arterioles, and they play a crucial role in controlling the blood flow within capillary beds. These areas are also referred to as capillary sphincters or precapillary arterioles. Despite lacking clear morphological definition, the lumina of these blood vessels are typically wider than the capillaries they supply. Additionally, circularly arranged smooth muscle cells are found throughout their walls. In this case, each individual smooth muscle cell is evenly spaced at a close distance around the endothelial tube, creating a surrounding configuration that resembles a cork-screw (Cetin and Sahin, 2018).

5.4. Capillaries

Capillaries are the tiniest operational components of the blood vascular system and are located between the arterial and venous sections of the circulation. They extensively divide into complex networks, the size and nature of which depend on the particular organ or tissue they are connected to (Mescher, 2015). The capillaries that are connected to certain organs are regarded as impermeable and serve as a protective barrier separating the blood from the respective organ. Some individuals demonstrate varying levels of permeability, which enables substances to move from the bloodstream into the surrounding interstitial tissues.

Capillaries are categorized as continuous, fenestrated, or discontinuous based on the visual characteristics of the endothelium and basal lamina observed in electron micrographs. Irrespective of the variety, capillaries share a fundamental structure that is comparable and represents a highly simplified version of the vessel wall. The tunica intima is composed of endothelium and a basal lamina, while the tunica media is not present and the tunica adventitia is significantly reduced.

5.4.1. Continuous Capillaries

Continuous capillaries are the predominant type of capillary that can be found in various parts of the body, including connective tissues, muscles, skin, and the CNS. Their lumina vary in diameter from 4 to 10 μm and, in the smaller vessels, may be surrounded by a single endothelial cell. In wider capillaries, the lumen may be surrounded by three or four cells. The wall is composed of an uninterrupted layer of endothelium and a slender layer called tunica adventitia. The endothelial cells are supported by a continuous basal lamina and exhibit similar characteristics to endothelial cells found in other parts of the vascular system. The cells possess typical organelles, such as caveolae and transcytotic vesicles. They also have a proteoglycan layer that covers a small number of short microvilli on the inner surfaces, as well as a varying quantity of granules enclosed by membranes. Additionally, multivesicular bodies are present. Adjacent cells can either touch each other directly, overlap at an angle, or have curving interlocking patterns. Periodically, neighboring cell membranes join in occluding junctions, although it is uncertain whether these junctions form complete belts like in other types of epithelial tissue. The tunica adventitia is a thin layer comprising a small amount of ground substance, with collagen and elastic fibers embedded within it. In addition, fibroblasts, macrophages, and mast cells are also present. Pericytes are irregular, branched, and solitary cells that are found at regular intervals along capillaries. They are surrounded by the basal lamina of the endothelium. The cells have a similar appearance to fibroblasts and typically contain a small number of dense bodies and many cytoplasmic filaments. Immunohistochemistry has shown the presence of actin and myosin in the cytoplasm, suggesting their involvement in contraction. Nevertheless, the precise purpose of these remains uncertain.

5.4.2. Fenestrated Capillaries

Fenestrated capillaries possess a similar structure to the continuous type, but they differ in that the endothelial cells contain numerous fenestrae, which are circular openings measuring 70 to 100 nm in diameter. Fenestrae can be randomly or group-wise distributed and typically have thin diaphragms that are closed by central, knoblike thickenings. The diaphragm is a thin structure consisting of a single layer, which makes it unlikely that the joining of two cell membranes forms it. The basal lamina spans uninterrupted across the fenestrae located on the basal side of the endothelium. The fenestrated capillaries of the renal glomerulus are distinct because their pores do not have diaphragms and the basal lamina is significantly thicker compared to other capillaries. Fenestrated capillaries are commonly found in the kidney, endocrine glands, and the gastrointestinal tract.

5.4.3. Discontinuous Capillaries (Sinusoids)

Sinusoids are vessels with thin walls significantly wider than capillaries and have lumina that have a more irregular outline than capillaries. Bone marrow, the liver, and the spleen all contain many sinusoids. They have attenuated endothelia, which may be continuous like those found in bone marrow, or the cells may be separated by gaps and rest on a discontinuous basal lamina. Both of these possibilities are possible. As a component of the lining, as in the liver, or closely applied to the exterior of the wall, as in the spleen, sinusoids are frequently associated with phagocytes. This is the case in both locations. Furthermore, the endothelial cells themselves do not exhibit a higher capacity for phagocytosis than those found in other vessels. In comparison to other endothelia, they exhibit a higher level of active endocytosis and a greater number of lysosomes.

5.4.4. Diffusion

The thin endothelium that lines capillaries is responsible for the exchange of nutrients and waste products between the blood and the tissues. The estimation suggests that no active cell that is located more than thirty or forty micrometers away from a capillary. The process of diffusion is the most significant method by which substances traverse the endothelium, and it has been determined that the total capillary surface area that is available for exchange is greater than one hundred square meters. Endothelial cells are responsible for the direct diffusion of lipid-soluble substances. At the same time, aquiporins, transcytotic vesicles, and the fenestrae of fenestrated capillaries are responsible for the transmission of water and water-soluble substances that are water-soluble.

In the continuous capillaries, caveolae and transcytotic vesicles have been shown to play a role in the transepithelial transport of water-soluble materials. Pinocytosis may also play a role in the transfer of substances with a high molecular weight. The term "tight capillaries" refers to a subcategory of continuous capillaries that are located in particular locations. Caveolae and transcytotic vesicles are not present in the cytoplasm of these capillaries, and the endothelial cells that make up these capillaries are tightly connected to one another through occludens type junctions (Djukic et al., 2023). The endothelium that lines these capillaries contributes to the blood brain barrier, the blood testis barrier, and the blood thymic barrier when it comes to blood circulation. Both the pressures within the blood itself and the pressures in the interstitial (connective tissue) compartment that surrounds the capillaries are responsible for controlling the movement of fluid out of or into the capillaries. Among these forces are the following: the interstitial hydrostatic pressure, the interstitial solute osmotic pressure, the capillary hydrostatic pressure, and the plasma solute osmotic pressure. If, for example, feeding arterioles dilate the hydrostatic pressure of the capillary blood increases and surpasses the plasma solute osmotic pressure as well as both surrounding interstitial pressures the movement of fluid will be out of the capillary and into the interstitial tissue. If, on the other hand, arterioles contract, thereby lowering the hydrostatic pressure, the overall effect is to draw fluid into the capillary lumen, which is driven primarily by the osmotic pressure of the plasma solute. While capillaries combine to form venules, a situation that is very similar to this one takes place in the distal (venous) portion of the capillary bed. At this location, the plasma solute osmotic pressure is high enough to draw the majority of the tissue fluid back into the bloodstream, except approximately 10% of the fluid, which is eventually absorbed by the lymphatic system and returned to the bloodstream. The liver is responsible for producing albumin, which is a highly negatively charged protein. Albumin plays a crucial role in maintaining the oncotic pressure, which is responsible for holding fluid within the vascular system. It is also possible for fluid exchange to take place through the intercellular clefts that exist between endothelial cells. Histamine, for instance, causes endothelial cells to pull away from one another and retract from further contact. Because of this, fluid and protein are able to diffuse out of capillaries and into the tissues that surround them, which results in edema. There is a possibility that this process can take place in a matter of minutes (Einstein et al., 2010).

5.4.5. Endothelial Cell Secretion

It is now known that endothelial cells secrete a number of substances that are part of the extracellular matrix that lies beneath them. These substances include collagens of types III, IV, and V, fibronectin, and laminin. Additionally, endothelial cells secrete a number of factors that are involved in the maintenance of vascular tone, blood clotting, and the emigration of leukocytes. Endothelial cells are responsible for the production and release of nitric oxide, which results in the relaxation of smooth muscle that is adjacent to them. This, in turn, leads to a reduction in the vascular tone of blood vessels. Nitric oxide is produced from arginine through a reaction that is catalyzed by nitric oxide synthase. This reaction results in the production of citrulline and not nitric oxide. The activation of guanylate cyclase in smooth muscle cells by nitric oxide results in an increase in the levels of cyclic guanosine monophosphate (cGMP) and has the effect of dilation of blood vessels. The conversion of nitroglycerin and amyl nitrates into nitric oxide is the mechanism by which these compounds exert their therapeutic effects. On the other hand, compounds like Viagra inhibit cGMP phosphodiesterase, which results in the maintenance of elevated levels of cGMP. Additionally, endothelial cells can react to anoxia by secreting a peptide known as endothelin I. This peptide is a powerful vasoconstrictor that has a long duration and binds to smooth muscle cells in the arteries, which causes an increase in blood pressure during the process. During the process of inflammation, endothelial cells can produce and insert intercellular adhesion molecules into their luminal plasmalemma. This occurs in response to cytokines that are present at the site of inflammation. Because these factors bind to leukocytes that are circulating in the bloodstream, they can move through the endothelium and arrive at the site of inflammation. In addition, endothelial cells contain thrombomodulin and tissue plasminogen activator, both of which have anticoagulant properties. Prostacyclin, which prevents platelet adhesion and causes vasodilation, is also present in endothelial cells. Endothelial cells have the ability to secrete thromboplastin, which is a thromboplastic substance that helps the blood to coagulate, as well as other thromboplastic substances, such as von Willebrand factor and antihemophilic factor VIII, which are components of the blood coagulation system within the body. Platelet adhesion to subendothelial collagen at the site of injuries is also promoted by Von Willebrand factor, which is stored in Weibel-Palade granules of endothelial cells. Consequently, endothelial cells are also capable of initiating the process of clotting and repairing minor defects in the lining of vessels, which helps to prevent the loss of blood throughout the body.

5.5. Veins

The venous side of the circulatory system is responsible for transporting blood from the capillary beds to the heart. As the veins progress through the circulatory system, they gradually expand in size and their walls become thicker. It is possible to differentiate between the three coats, which are the tunica intima, media, and adventitia, but they are not as clearly defined as the arteries. Their structure is essentially identical to that of arteries. Veins, in general, are more numerous and larger than the arteries that they accompany; however, the walls of veins are thinner due to a reduction in the amount of muscular and elastic elements. Due to the fact that their walls are less robust, veins have a tendency to collapse when they are empty, and sections of veins may appear flattened, with lumina that are irregular and slit-like. Veins are significantly more variable in their structure than arteries (Einstein et al., 2010). There is not always a correlation between the thickness of the wall and the size of the vein, and the structure of the vein can varies from one region to another within the same vein. Although the histologic classification of veins is not as satisfactory as the classification of arteries, several subdivisions are typically made up of veins. These subdivisions include venules as well as small, medium, and large veins.

5.5.1. Venules

From the union of multiple capillaries, venules emerge, resulting in vessels that range in diameter from 10 to 50 μm. Particularly significant locations for the exchange of fluids between tissues and blood are the junctions that exist between capillaries and venules. There is a thin, continuous endothelium that makes up the tunica intima. The cells that make up this endothelium are only loosely connected to one another by poorly developed intercellular junctions. Pericytes that appear to make contact with the endothelial cells are able to find their way through the thin basal lamina. In the venules that are the smallest, the tunica media is absent, and the adventitia, which is relatively thin, contains a few collagen fibers, scattered fibroblasts, mast cells, macrophages, and plasma cells. Circularly oriented smooth muscle cells that are scattered begin to appear as the vessels grow in size to reach diameters of 50 μm. These cells begin to form a tunica media that is somewhat discontinuous and incomplete. The adventitia is characterized by an increase in thickness and is made up of collagen fibers that are arranged longitudinally and form an open spiral while surrounding the vessel. There is a tendency for fibroblasts to have an irregular shape and to have thin processes.

5.5.2. Small Veins

The diameter of small veins can range anywhere from 0.2 to 1.0 millimeters. An endothelium that is continuous and rests on a basal lamina that is relatively thin is the only component of the tunica intima. In a tunica media, which can have anywhere from one to four layers of cells, smooth muscle cells provide the structure. It is possible to observe a thin network of elastic and collagen fibers that connects the smooth muscle cells. A relatively thick coat is formed by the tunica adventitia, which also contains collagen fibers that are oriented longitudinally and some thin elastic fibers at the same time.

5.5.3. Medium Veins

Medium-sized veins include the majority of the named veins in gross anatomy, except for major trunks. They can range in diameter from one millimeter to 10 millimeters. Despite the presence of a narrow subendothelial layer that may contain fine collagen fibers and scattered thin elastic fibers, the thin tunica intima is made up of endothelial cells that are resting on a basal lamina. It is possible for elastic fibers to form a network at the junction of tunica intima and media; however, only in larger vessels does a poorly defined internal elastic lamina make its appearance. Even though it is well developed, the tunica media in the majority of medium veins is thinner than the tunica media in the corresponding arteries. In comparison to the tunica media, the thick tunica adventitia constitutes the majority of the wall and is significantly larger. It is made up of collagen and elastic fibers, and it frequently contains smooth muscle cells that are oriented in a longitudinal direction. Larger vessels of this class contain vasa vasorum, which are present in these vessels. The majority of medium veins are fitted with valves, which are two flaps of tunica intima that resemble pockets and project into the lumen. The free edges of these flaps are oriented in the direction in which blood is flowing. A core of connective tissue is present, and endothelium is present on both sides of the object. The connective tissue lying beneath the endothelium on the downstream side of the valves contains a dense network of elastic fibers within its structure. When the blood flows toward the heart, the valves are pressed against the wall of the vessel. However, when the blood flows backward, the valves are pressed against each other in an outward direction to occlude the vessel and prevent the flow of blood from being reversed.

5.5.4. Large Veins

The thick tunica adventitia makes up the majority of the wall in large venous trunks, such as the venae cavae, renal veins, external iliac veins, splenic veins, portal veins, and mesenteric veins. It comprises connective tissue that is loosely knit and contains thick bundles of collagen and elastic fibers that come in longitudinal orientations. The inferior vena cava is characterized by the presence of smooth muscle bundles, which are also parallel to the longitudinal direction of the blood vessel. Vasa vasorum are present and may extend into the media. Compared to medium veins, the tunica media in large veins is poorly developed and may even be absent. In other words, it has the same organization as medium veins. Subendothelial layers, which may become more prominent in larger trunks, provide support for the tunica intima.

5.5.5. Veins with Special Features

The trabecular veins of the spleen, the veins of the retina, bone, and maternal placenta, the majority of the meningeal and cerebral veins, and the veins of the nail bed are examples of veins that do not have a tunica media. Smooth muscle is present in all three coats of the veins in the pregnant uterus. The fibers in the intima run in a longitudinal direction rather than a circular direction, just like they do in the tunica intima of the saphenous, popliteal, femoral, umbilical, and internal jugular veins. A coat of cardiac muscle covers the adventitia of the pulmonary veins and the venae cavae at their junctions with the heart. The fibers of the cardiac muscle run in a circular and longitudinal pattern around the vessels for a short distance (Haggerty et al., 2014).

5.5.6. Arteriovenous Anastomoses

It is possible for arteries and veins to join together through shunts known as arteriovenous anastomoses, in addition to the capillary connections that they share. In most cases, these originate from the side branches of arterioles that pass directly to the venules. These vessels are typically coiled and surrounded by a connective tissue sheath. They have thick walls and are muscular, and their caliber is relatively small. Both the plantar and palmar surfaces, as well as the fingertips, toes, lips, and nose, as well as the thyroid, are replete with them. The anastomoses, when open, are responsible for directing blood around the capillary bed and, as a result, regulating the blood supply to a variety of tissues. It is primarily in regulating body temperature that they perform their functions in the skin.

5.5.7. Carotid and Aortic Bodies

Numerous baroreceptors are located in the carotid sinus, which is an expanded region at the bifurcation of the carotid artery. These baroreceptors play a role in the regulation of blood pressure by mediating changes in heart rate. There are specialized regions in the carotid sinus and along the aortic arch that are home to baroreceptors, which are responsible for gathering information about blood pressure. The myelinated sensory nerve fibers that make up baroreceptors, also known as mechanoreceptors, are located close to the brain stem and project into the medulla of the brain. Baroreceptors are responsible for producing a response to stretch. When blood pressure drops, sympathetic stimulation and the release of norepinephrine are both triggered. This is because of the decrease in blood pressure. At the same time that it constricts blood vessels, norepinephrine is responsible for stimulating the activity of the heart. Increased blood pressure triggers the parasympathetic nervous system, leading to the release of acetylcholine, which slows down heart activity and causes blood vessels to dilate. In addition to contributing to the regulation of respiratory and cardiovascular reflexes, the carotid body is a limited collection of nerve endings and cells that are located in close proximity to the carotid sinus. It is responsible for detecting the partial pressure of respiratory gases and the pH of the arterial blood. These encapsulated structures are known as carotid bodies, and they are made up of masses of large polyhedral epithelioid cells, also known as glomus cells. These cells are closely related to a plentiful network of sinusoidal vessels. These cells have large and pale nuclei, and their cytoplasm is light and finely granular. Granules exhibit dense cores and contain catecholamines and 5-hydroxytryptamine, as shown in electron micrographs of the granules. A second type of glomus cell, known as type II glomus cells, is thought to be supporting glial cells. These cells have a similar appearance to type I glomus cells, but they do not contain granules. An aortic body is a similar structure that is located close to the aorta. It is located between the angle of the subclavian and carotid arteries on the right side of the body and close to the origin of the subclavian artery on the left side of the body. Glomus cells of type I and type II make up these structures, which are smaller than carotid bodies. Some people believe that they perform functions comparable to those of carotid bodies. Fibers from the vagus nerve (X) supply the aortic bodies, whereas the glossopharyngeal nerve (IX) is the primary **source** of fibers for the carotid body. The neural crest gives rise to both the carotid and aortic bodies (Jayendiran et al., 2018).

5.6. Special Circulations

The process of controlling the function of the blood vessels that are associated with a number of particular organs and/or tissues varies depending on the circumstances and requirements that are present at a particular moment in time. For instance, an increase in body temperature causes the sympathetic nerves to innervate the blood vessels of the skin, which in turn causes the blood vessels to dilate up. In order to dissipate heat, this effect pulls blood to the surface of the body. When hypoxia is present in the respiratory system, it causes vasoconstriction, which helps to move blood away from areas of the lung that have inadequate ventilation and toward areas that have adequate ventilation. Vasoconstriction is the only response that occurs in the vasculature in response to hypoxia, and it occurs only in the circulation that is associated with the lung. Vasodilation is the response that occurs in other regions of the vasculature when hypoxia is present. The blood vessels that supply skeletal muscle undergo vasodilation as a result of increased concentrations of lactate, adenosine, and potassium that occur during exercise. Via the release of norepinephrine, sympathetic innervation of smooth muscle cells in the vasculature causes vasodilatation in skeletal muscle tissue. This occurs because the release of norepinephrine stimulates both α-adrenergic and β-adrenergic receptors. Vasodilation is the response that the vasculature of the coronary circulation receives in response to hypoxia as well as adenosine, which is a byproduct of the ATP metabolism that occurs in cardiac myocytes. In response to an increase in PCO2 or a decrease in pH, the vessels that make up the cerebral circulation may dilate (Jayendiran et al., 2018).

5.7. Lymph Vascular System

Intercellular fluid, also known as tissue fluid, is recovered by the lymph vascular system, which is made up of tubes lined with endothelial cells. This fluid is then returned to the bloodstream after being collected by the blood vascular system. When fluid travels through the blood capillaries and into the tissues, a blood filtrate is produced. This blood filtrate is the fluid that is carried by the lymphatic system. The flow of lymph, in contrast to the flow of blood through the blood vessels, is only in one direction: from the tissues to the point where the lymphatic and blood vascular systems meet at the base of the neck. The lymphatic vascular system begins in the tissues as capillaries that end in a blinding manner. These capillaries then drain into larger collecting vessels, and finally, they go into two main lymphatic trunks. Filtering the lymph is the function of lymph nodes, which are located along the course of the vessels. Some tissues do not contain lymphatics, including bone marrow, the CNS, coats of the eye, the internal ear, and the placenta of the fetus. Lymphatics are present in the majority of tissues.

5.7.1. Lymph Capillaries

There is a rich network of lymph capillaries in organs and tissues. These capillaries have thin walls and are blind. They branch and anastomose freely to form this network. In comparison to blood capillaries, they are wider and more irregular in shape. There is only a thin continuous endothelium and a discontinuous basal lamina that makes up the wall of a lymph capillary. The basal lamina is only present in patches or may even be absent entirely. Endothelial cells that are adjacent to one another may overlap, but junctional complexes are uncommon, and clefts between the cells are present. There is a marginal amount of collagenous connective tissue that surrounds the endothelium on the surface of the body. Fine filaments extend in a direction that is perpendicular to the collagen bundles and attach themselves to the outer surfaces of the endothelium. These anchoring filaments are responsible for ensuring that the vessel remains open.

5.7.2. Collecting Lymph Vessels

As far as size and wall thickness are concerned, collecting lymph vessels are distinct from lymph capillaries. In spite of the fact that blood vessels are described as having three coats—the intima, the media, and the adventitia—they are not clearly differentiated from one another. A thin network of longitudinal elastic fibers provides support for the endothelium that makes up the tunica intima. The tunica media is made up of smooth muscle cells that are arranged in a predominantly circular pattern, although there are some cells that run in a longitudinal direction here and there. There are a few fine elastic fibers that are located between the muscle cells. There are bundles of collagen fibers, elastic fibers, and some smooth muscle cells that make up the tunica adventitia, which is the thickest coat. All of these fibers and cells have a longitudinal orientation. When compared to veins, lymphatic vessels have a greater number of valves and are located at more frequent intervals along their arteries. It is similar to veins in that they develop in pairs as folds of the intima.

5.7.3. Lymphatic Trunks

The thoracic and right lymphatic ducts are the two primary trunks with which the collecting lymphatic vessels ultimately come together. Compared to the other ducts, the thoracic duct is the longer one and has a larger drainage field. At the point where the left jugular vein and the subclavian vein meet, it enters the venous system. It begins in the abdomen, travels along the vertebral column, and then opens into the vein supply. The lower limbs, the abdomen, the left upper limb, the left side of the thorax, the head, and the neck all submit lymph to this organ. As it empties into the brachiocephalic vein, the right lymphatic duct is the only lymphatic vessel that receives lymph from the upper right side of the body. The structure of the trunks is generally comparable to that of a large vein, and they are identical to one another. An endothelium that is continuous and supported by a subendothelial layer of fibroelastic tissue, along with some smooth muscle, makes up the tunica intima. The elastic fibers gradually condense into a thin internal elastic lamina as they approach the junction with the tunica media. When compared to the media of large veins, the tunica media is the thickest layer because it contains a greater quantity of smooth muscle (SMT). The cells that make up smooth muscle are arranged in a predominantly circular pattern and are separated from one another by a substantial amount of collagenous tissue and a few elastic fibers (Kamada et al., 2022). Additionally, the tunica adventitia is not clearly defined and tends to blend in with the connective tissue that is all around it. Occasionally, it also has smooth muscle cells, as well as bundles of longitudinal collagen fibers and elastic fibers. Blood vessels that carry nutrients are found in the wall of the thoracic duct, which is comparable to the vasa vasorum that is found in large blood vessels. Phasic smooth muscle is the smooth muscle that is associated with the lymph vessels. In contrast to visceral smooth muscle, phasic smooth muscle of the lymphatics is responsible for the generation of action potentials and the creation of waves of contraction. These waves of contraction move lymph toward the heart and ultimately lead to its union with the blood. Lymph vessels contain valves that prevent backflow from occurring. To put it another way, the lymph vascular system can be compared to a sump pump system that is located within the interstitial compartment. This system is responsible for returning the tissue fluid that was initially absorbed by the blood vascular system to the bloodstream. It is possible for the lymph vascular system to absorb and transport up to four liters of fluid on a daily basis. Many larger molecules from a variety of organs, such as chylomicra and peptide hormones, are able to enter the bloodstream through this pathway. This is due to the fact that the majority of lymph capillaries are considered to be more leaky than the majority of capillaries.

5.8. Organogenesis

Initially, the developing embryo is nourished by simple diffusion of nutrients, at first from the uterine fluids and later, after implantation, from maternal blood lakes. With growth, these sources are unable to meet the nutritional needs of the mass of cells in the embryo, so a vascular system arises early in development.

5.8.1. Heart

An aggregation of splanchnic mesoderm that forms two longitudinal strands is the manifestation of the earliest cardiac structure. Each one develops a lumen and transforms into a straightforward tube that is lined with endothelial cells and has a fold of mesoderm. Both the mesodermal folds and the tubes come together to form a single surrounding coat, and the tubes fuse together to form a single saccular cardiac primordium. The myocardium and epicardium originate from the outer layer of mesoderm, while the endocardium is something that develops from the endothelial tube. Within the cytoplasm of differentiating cardiac muscle cells in the myocardium, myofibrils initially manifest themselves as loosely arranged groups of filaments. While the myofibrils are still in the process of developing, they will eventually acquire distinct Z bands before the appearance of A and I bands. After the two endocardial tubes have fused together, the single primitive heart tube will grow at a faster rate than the pericardial cavity. With the two ends of the cardiac tube anchored to the tissues that surround it, it is impossible for the tube to elongate, which results in the formation of a cardiac loop. The bulbus cordis, which is the caudal end of the presumptive ventricle, originates from the cephalic end. In the beginning, the endothelial tube is separated from the myocardial layer by a jelly-like fluid. This fluid is then invaded by mesenchyme, which results in the formation of the subendocardial layer. In the process of flattening into a mesothelium, the cells that are located on the exterior surface of the myocardium come together with a sublayer of connective tissue to form the epicardium at the same time. The remaining portion of the myocardial coat is composed of an outer layer of cardiac muscle that is compact and an inner layer of trabeculae that are loosely arranged upon one another (Kuchumov et al., 2021). With the exception of the trabeculae carneae of the ventricles, which continue to exist as remnants of the spongy layer, the entire muscle wall becomes compact. The atrioventricular node is the first component of the conducting system to develop. It originates from the cells of the cardiac muscle that are located around the atrioventricular canal. This is the source of the atrioventricular bundle. A different point of view proposes that the bundle originates from the muscle that is located on the dorsal wall of the atrioventricular canal. Subsequently, the bundle continues to spread out to form the atriventricular node as well as the right and left limbs of the bundle. Following the appearance of a narrow muscular band on the lateral surface of the superior vena cava, the sinoatrial node is the final node to reach its destination. After a certain point in the development of the fetus, the node becomes a part of the wall of the atrium.

5.8.2. Vessels

The extraembryonic mesenchyme is the origin of the earliest blood vessels, which initially appear as blood islands in the yolk sac and body stalk. These blood vessels later develop into blood vessels. Initially, the islands take the shape of solid cords; however, the cells that are closest to the surface eventually become the first endothelial cells, while the cells that are further inward become free and eventually become the first primitive blood cells. This changes over time. The isolated vascular spaces eventually come together to form a network of vessels that, at this stage, takes the form of simple endothelial tubes. This occurs as a result of growth and union. This canalization process takes place in a variety of different locations across the earth. The initial blood vessels of the embryo begin to form in a manner that is comparable to this description. After circulation has been established, the further extension of blood vessels is caused by the endothelial budding and growth of pre-existing blood vessels. This is the process that happens after circulation has been established. Before the development of specifically defined arteries and veins, the formation of vessels that are similar to capillaries occurs. The development of these coats will be the consequence of the differentiation of the mesenchyme that surrounds the connective tissue and the smooth muscle.

When lymphatic vessels emerge from the mesenchyme, they do so in a manner that is quite distinct and as isolated spaces. Endothelial cells can transform from cells that are located on the periphery of the spaces. The spaces are able to connect with one another through the process of progressive unions, which results in the formation of continuous channels that branch off in a variety of directions, ultimately leading to a complete set of lymphatic vessels. When it comes to the formation of the outer tunics of the larger lymphatics, the mesenchyme that surrounds the lymphatics is the one responsible for it.

5.9. Lymphatic Tissues and Organs

5.9.1. Lymphatic Tissues

Lymphatic components, which are a component of the body's defense system, can be found dispersed throughout the body in varied locations. This is because lymphatic tissues are prominent in the connective tissue coats of the gastrointestinal, respiratory, and urogenital tracts. Lymphatic tissues are generally distributed in such a way that they are quickly encountered by harmful agents that enter the body. Additionally, lymphatic structures are carried into the lymph drainage and blood circulation systems, where they perform the function of filtering both the lymph and the blood. The lymphatic system is responsible for filtering all of the body's fluids; this process takes place over time. There are two ways that lymphatic cells can be organized: either they can be grouped together within the connective tissue to form lymphatic tissues, or they can be organized into distinct structures to form lymphatic organs.

5.9.1.1. Classification

Within the connective tissue compartment, lymphatic tissue is a subtype that can be classified according to the type of fiber that is present. This is true for all connective tissues, including lymphatic tissue. It is possible to classify lymphatic tissue as reticular tissue based on this information. In addition, it is a hematopoietic tissue because it contributes cells, specifically lymphocytes, to the bloodstream. The amount of cellular material is greater than the amount of intercellular material, just like in bone marrow. It is not differences in fiber types that determine whether lymphatic tissue is diffuse or nodular; rather, it is the arrangement and concentration of the cells that determine this distinction within the tissue (Laudato et al., 2023).

5.9.1.2. Cells of Lymphatic Tissues

Both fixed and free cells are present within the lymphatic tissue. These reticular cells, known as fixed cells, are the ones that are accountable for the formation and maintenance of reticular fibers. There is a close connection between the fixed cells of lymphatic tissue and the reticular fibers, which are the two components of the reticular network. The fibers frequently reside in deep grooves within the cytoplasm of the reticular cells. Light microscopy reveals reticular cells as elongated or stellate elements with nuclei that are round or oval and palely stained. Additionally, the cytoplasm of reticular cells is scant and lightly basophilic. Due to the fact that the majority of the cytoplasm is distributed thinly along the reticular fibers, the cytoplasm is significantly more abundant than what is visible under the light microscope. A moderately well-developed Golgi apparatus and a variable amount of endoplasmic reticulum are both visible through electron microscopy. Other organelles, on the other hand, are not particularly noticeable. In the same way that bone marrow cells are unable to give rise to other cell types, lymphatic reticular cells do not exhibit any special capacity for phagocytosis. The free cells are the cells that are still present in lymphatic tissue and are found within the spaces that are contained within the reticular network. In addition to lymphocytes, macrophages, and plasma cells are also present in varying numbers. The majority of these cells are lymphocytes.

The term "lymphocyte" refers to a wide variety of cells that share certain characteristics in common with another type of cell. As a group, they have a nucleus that is rounded and positioned in the middle of the cell; their cytoplasm exhibits varying degrees of basophilia and does not contain any specific granules. The population of lymphocytes is typically classified into three categories: small, medium, and large lymphocytes. These classifications are based on the size of the lymphocytes, the nuclear morphology, and the intensity of the cytoplasmic staining. Although such a subdivision is helpful for purposes of description, it is somewhat artificial due to the fact that there is a continuum of cell sizes and morphologies that exists between the categories of small and large. The greatest number of lymphocytes are the smaller ones. Similar to the cells found in lymphatic tissues, these cells have a diameter ranging from 4 to 8 μm and are characterized by a nucleus that is deeply stained. Surrounding the nucleus is a thin rim of cytoplasm, which may be slightly expanded on one side of the cell. In the blood or lymph, the cells have a round shape; however, in tissues, the cells are closer together and take on a variety of polyhedral shapes because of compression. A nucleolus that is barely discernible unless thin sections are examined is contained within the nucleus, which is rounded or slightly indented. There are scattered masses of heterochromatin and some small patches of euchromatin that are present in the chromatin. A small Golgi complex, a few mitochondria and centrioles located in the region of the nuclear indentation, a moderate number of ribosomes, and a few lysosomes scattered throughout the cytoplasm are all visible through the use of electron microscopy. There are not many granular endoplasmic reticulum cells.

The diameter of medium lymphocytes, also known as prolymphocytes, can range from 8 to 12 micrometers. The greater dispersion of the chromatin results in their nuclei being somewhat larger and more palely stained. Additionally, their nucleoli are larger and more clearly defined than those of other cells. As a result of an increase in the number of ribosomes, the cytoplasm is more abundant and exhibits a higher level of basophilia (Lee and Griffith, 2022).

Lymphoblasts, which are large lymphocytes, can range in size from 15 to 20 μm. It is possible to find even larger forms, measuring between 25 and 30 μm, and certain authors choose to use the term lymphoblast to refer to these cells. The nucleus is rounded, shows a light stain, and has one or two nucleoli that are prominent. Additionally, the fine chromatin is more evenly distributed throughout the nucleus. Free ribosomes and polysomes are both present in the basophilic cytoplasm, which is abundant. Although mitochondria are abundant and the centrosomal region and the Golgi complex have reached a higher level of development, the granular endoplasmic reticulum has not yet reached its full potential. It is generally accepted that the direction of maturation in the development of lymphocytes is from large (lymphoblast) to small. This is the direction in which lymphocytes mature. The fact that small lymphocytes are able to respond to antigenic agents, reassume a blastlike appearance and character, and reproduce additional small lymphocytes and plasma cells is a factor that complicates the progression of this condition.

The diameter of plasma cells, also known as plasmocytes, can range anywhere from 6 to 20 μm. According to the location of the cell, light microscopy reveals that it has a polyhedral shape, a rounded shape, or a somewhat elongated shape. In most cases, the nucleus is eccentrically located and can range in shape from round to oval. When it comes to rounded cells, the nucleus may be slightly eccentric in its placement, but this is most noticeable in elongated cells. The chromatin is distributed in coarse heterochromatic blocks along the interior of the nuclear envelope, which gives the nucleus the appearance of a spoke wheel or a clock face. There is a possibility of observing binucleate cells. Except for a prominent pale area that is adjacent to the nucleus, the cytoplasm features a deep basophilic composition.

This region is a representation of the Golgi apparatus in a negative light. In some cases, the cytoplasm of plasma cells can contain globular or crystalline inclusions. Russell's bodies are the most well-known example of this phenomenon. These are acidophilic inclusions that can be round or ovoid in shape and can range in size. They are indicative of an incomplete antibody. One of the distinguishing characteristics of plasma cells, as seen in electron micrographs, is the extensive development of the granular endoplasmic reticulum, which almost entirely fills the cytoplasm. Both flat and parallel cisternae and distended cisternae with flocculent material are possible. There are a great number of free ribosomes, and the paranuclear region contains both centrioles and a Golgi apparatus that has developed to a high degree. Cisternae of the granular endoplasmic reticulum that have become distended are the locations where Russell's bodies are found when they are present. Plasma cells resemble sessile cells and eventually undergo degeneration. Forms that are intermediate between lymphocytes and plasma cells are responsible for most of the antibody production, even though endoplasmic reticulum is present in enormous quantities. B-lymphocytes are the cells that lead to the formation of plasma cells (Martinolli et al., 2021).

This system of mononuclear phagocytes is widely distributed throughout the body's tissues and organs, and the macrophages that are found in lymphatic tissue are a part of it. The diameter of the cells ranges from 10 to 20 μm, and they possess nuclei that are oval, kidney-shaped, or horseshoe-shaped.

Additionally, nucleoli are present in the nuclei of these cells. A large amount of cytoplasm that is only slightly basophilic and may be vacuolated or contain material that has been ingested is present. On the other hand, macrophages are difficult to differentiate from other large mononuclear cells, such as active fibroblasts, unless the cytoplasm does contain phagocytosed matter.

The cytoplasm exhibits a great number of folds, processes, and invaginations of the surface throughout electron micrographs. Additionally, the cytoplasm contains the typical assembly of organelles. In addition to the presence of lysosomes in large numbers, the Golgi apparatus is also noticeable, and residual bodies may be noticeable. There are macrophages in lymphatic tissue that originate from blood monocytes, just like there are macrophages in other tissues.

5.9.1.3. Diffuse Lymphatic Tissue

Diffuse lymphatic tissue is a component of lymphatic organs and is also widely distributed along mucous membranes. It is called diffuse lymphatic tissue. There is no clear demarcation between it and the surrounding tissue, which it gradually merges with. It appears to be a rather loose aggregate of cells. The fundamental component of diffuse lymphatic tissue is a three-dimensional array of reticular fibers and the reticular cells that are associated with them. Both components come together to form a framework that resembles a sponge and is filled with a large number of cells, the majority of which are lymphocytes. Regarding the connective tissue that lies beneath the epithelium of the intestine, diffuse lymphatic tissue is especially significant. On this particular occasion, the lymphatic tissue, in conjunction with the epithelium that lines the luminal surface, generates antibody. The lymphatic tissue, the cellularity of which is related to the bacterial content of the intestines, is the site where an immune response is induced by any antigen that can penetrate the epithelial lining.

5.9.1.4. Nodular Lymphatic Tissue

While nodular lymphatic tissue and diffuse lymphatic tissue both contain the same structural elements, the only difference between the two is that the components of nodular lymphatic tissue are organized into structures that are more compact and somewhat circumscribed. Despite the fact that it can manifest itself anywhere in connective tissue, it is most commonly found along the respiratory and digestive tracts. Both solitary lymphatic nodules and masses that form confluent lymphatic nodules, such as those found in the appendix and the Peyer's patches of the ileum, are examples of lymphatic nodules. Flollicles are another name for lymphatic nodules. The thymus does not contain any lymphatic nodules, in contrast to other organs, such as the tonsils, lymph nodes, and spleen, which all produce lymphatic nodules.

A primary nodule is a type of lymphatic nodule that appears as a rounded collection of densely packed small lymphocytes in ordinary histologic sections. Certain lymphatic nodules have this appearance. Other lymphatic nodules have a central region that is only slightly stained, and it is surrounded by a cuff or cap of severely stained small lymphocytes that are packed closely together. Some people have referred to the pale region as a germinal center, while others have referred to the entire structure as a secondary nodule. Only a few reticular fibers are present within the germinal center, and the free cells are supported by a cellular framework made up of stellate reticular cells. As reticular cells undergo a multitude of processes, desmosomes connect them all together. It is possible to find reticular fibers in the cuff of cells that are located on the periphery of the center, where they gather together to form concentric layers around the structure. White and dark poles are present in germinal centers. While the dark pole is densely packed with large and medium lymphocytes, cells in transition to plasma cells, macrophages, mitotic cells, and the pyknotic nuclei of degenerating lymphocytes, the light pole is sparsely populated by scattered small lymphocytes and reticular cells. On the other hand, the dark pole is densely packed with these cells. There is a zone of small lymphocytes that constitutes the cap and surrounds the center. This zone is typically thicker at the light pole, where it forms the cap. The lymphocytes that cover the dark pole are of a thinner layer. The structure exhibits a clear polarity, with the light pole always pointing in the direction of a surface. This is the case with the capsule in lymph nodes, the red pulp in the spleen, and the epithelium of a tonsil. Even though germinal centers appear to be locations where lymphocytes are formed, a significant number of newly formed cells expire in these centers. Each germinal center appears to represent a clone of cells that are derived from an antigen-stimulated lymphocyte and are active in the production of a particular antibody. In addition, they are the sites where antibodies are formed. Germinal centers are responsible for the production of B-cells, which can move out of the center through the cap and make their way to other lymphatic tissues. In regions where germinal centers are developing, follicular dendritic cells are present. These cells exhibit a wide variety of intricate cytoplasmic processes that interact with follicular lymphocytes. In contrast to the abundance of mitochondria found in the cytoplasm, ribosomes, lysosomes, and secretory granules are difficult to come by (Pons et al., 2020). Moreover, there is a distinct nucleolus and bars of heterochromatin that are located on the periphery of the nucleus, which is irregular. Antigen-presenting cells are cells that keep antigens on their surface in order to stimulate T-helper cells, also known as lymphocytes. These cells are considered to be important cellular components. Antigenic stimuli are necessary for the development of germinal centers, which do not occur until after birth. They are not present in animals that are born and raised in an environment that is free of germs. Germinal centers begin to form from scratch after the initial encounter with antigen, but they gradually diminish when antigen is not present, and they eventually vanish entirely. In response to a second stimulation by the same antigen, there is a rapid and noticeable production of germinal centers, which comes before an increase in the amount of antibody that is circulating in the bloodstream. There is a possibility that germinal centers are involved in long-term (memory) antibody responses. However, it is important to note that germinal centers are not required for the formation of antibodies. It has been hypothesized that germinal centers only emerge after repeated contact with antigen. It is possible to find aggregate or confluent lymphatic nodules in the appendix. Peyer's patches, which are located in the lower half of the small intestine, are a good example of this type of nodule. Peyer's patches are characterized by numerous solitary nodules that mass together to form grossly visible structures that lie beneath the intestinal epithelium. The epithelium is the target of the light poles that appear in their germinal centers. It is possible for individual nodules to be quite distinct and well-defined; however, in most cases, they tend to coalesce and differentiate themselves only at their apexes and by their germinal centers. It is common for children to have Peyer's patches, but as people get older, they gradually become less noticeable.

5.9.2. Lymphatic Organs

There are two categories that comprise the lymphatic system. These categories are the primary (central) organs of the lymphatic system and the secondary (peripheral) functions of the lymphatic system. Among the primary lymphatic organs, the thymus in mammals and the bursa of Fabricius in birds are the first to develop. Primary lymphatic organs are the first to develop. The bursa in mammals is comparable to the bone marrow, which is the anatomical structure that is similar to it. The lymph nodes, the tonsils, the spleen, and the lymphatic tissues associated with the gastrointestinal tract are all examples of primary lymphatic organs. The lymph nodes are considered to be secondary lymphatic organs. Collections of lymphatic tissues that are both diffuse and nodular are what make up lymphatic organs. These lymphatic tissues are arranged in distinct structures and are arranged in a specific order. The lymphatic tissues responsible for the organs' operation are separated from the surrounding tissues by a capsule that is clearly defined.

5.9.2.1. Tonsils

Tonsils are a group of lymphatic nodules that are associated with the pharynx and oropharynx. Tonsils appear in the tonsils. There is a ring of lymphatic tissue that is known as Waldeyer's ring that is located at the entrance to the esophagus and the respiratory tract. It is possible for this ring to be incomplete to varying degrees. These structures are distributed across a variety of regions, including the tongue, the oropharynx, and the nasopharynx, and they are responsible for the formation of the palatine, pharyngeal, and lingual tonsils, respectively. Figure 5.1 provides a visual representation of the general structure of a tonsil, which makes it simple to comprehend (Rousseau-Portalis et al., 2023).

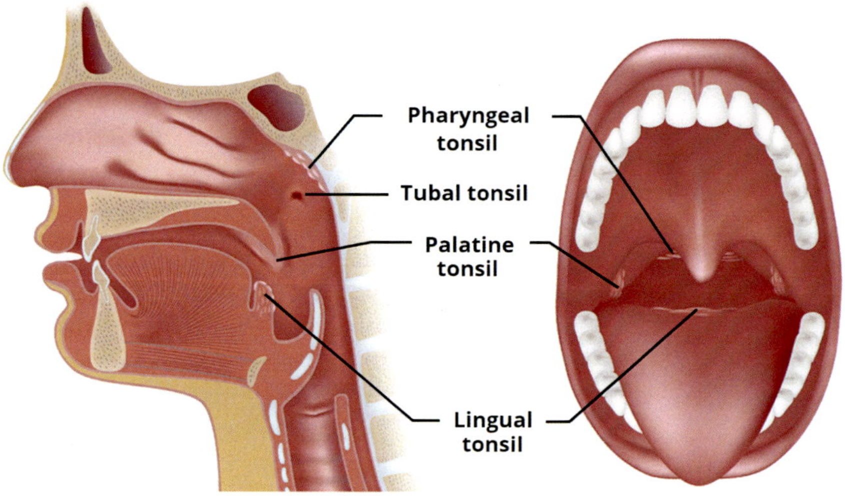

Figure 5.1. *A diagrammatic sketch illustrating the general structure of a tonsil.*

Source: https://teachmeanatomy.info/wp-content/uploads/Anatomical-Location-of-the-Tonsils-Waldeyers-Ring.png.

Tonsils are not responsible for filtering lymph because they do not have any afferent vessels that lead to them, nor do they have an internal system of sinuses that are responsible for providing lymphatic drainage. On the other hand, the beginnings of efferent lymphatic vessels are formed by plexuses of lymph capillaries that end in a blind fashion at the inner surfaces of the tonsils. Tonsils play a role in the development of lymphocytes, in which a significant number of lymphocytes migrate through the covering epithelium and manifest themselves as salivary corpuscles in the sputum. To stimulate the production of antibodies, bacteria that are able to penetrate the lymphoid tissue of the tonsils do so in the capacity of antigens (Sequí-Domínguez et al., 2020).

5.9.2.2. Palatine Tonsils

Located laterally at the junction of the oral cavity and the oropharynx, the palatine tonsils are a pair of oval lymphatic organs. For the free surface of the tonsil, there is a wet stratified squamous epithelium that is continuous with the epithelium of the oral cavity and the oropharynx. This epithelium is very closely associated with the lymphatic tissue. Deep invaginations of the epithelium are responsible for the formation of tonsillar crypts, which extend almost all the way to the base of the tonsil. Stratified squamous epithelium, which thins out in the deeper parts of the crypts, acts as a lining for secondary crypts, which can branch off from these deep pockets. Lymphatic nodules, the majority of which have prominent germinal centers, are typically arranged in a single layer beneath the epithelium and are embedded in a mass of diffuse lymphatic tissue. Lymphocytes infiltrate the epithelium in large numbers, particularly the epithelium that lines the lower ends of the crypts. This occurs frequently to such a degree that the line that separates the epithelium from the lymphatic tissue is difficult to distinguish. Within the tonsil, a partial capsule is located beneath the basal surface, and this capsule serves to separate the tonsil from the surrounding structures to which it adheres. Some septa extend from the capsule into the tonsillar tissue. These septa, composed of loosely arranged collagen fibers, partially divide the crypts. The reticular fibers of the lymphatic tissue become continuous with the fibers belonging to the septa, which spread out and become continuous with them. There is an infiltration of lymphocytes of varying sizes, plasma cells, and mast cells into the connective tissue. During inflammation of the tonsils, neutrophil granulocytes may be present in large numbers. Small compound tubuloacinar mucoserous glands are located outside the capsule, and their ducts drain to the free surface of the tonsil or, in rare cases, empty into a tonsillar crypt.

5.9.2.3. Lingual Tonsils

The lingual tonsils are nodular bulges that are located in the root of the tongue. Their general structure is comparable to that of the palatine tonsil. It is possible for crypts to be branched, and they are lined by a wet stratified squamous epithelium that invaginates from the surface. Crypts are deep as well. Two types of lymphatic tissue are associated with this condition: diffuse and nodular. The majority of the compound tubuloacinar mucous glands that are embedded in the underlying muscle of the tongue are able to drain their contents through ducts that open into the bases of the crypts.

5.9.2.4. Pharyngeal Tonsil

Placing the pharyngeal tonsil on the posterior wall of the nasopharynx is the location of this structure. The ciliated pseudostratified columnar epithelium that contains goblet cells is characteristic of its surface epithelium, which is a continuation of the epithelium that lines the respiratory passages. Patches of stratified squamous epithelium may be present, however, and tend to become more common with aging and smoking. When compared to the palatine tonsils, the crypts in the tonsils are not as deep, and the epithelium forms a large number of shallow folds. To providing fine septa that extend into the substance of the tonsil, a thin capsule serves to separate the pharyngeal tonsil from the tissues that lie beneath it (Tang et al., 2020). Underneath the capsule, there are relatively small compound tubuloacinar mucoserous glands that empty onto the surface of the folds.

5.9.2.5. Lymph Nodes

An encapsulated lymphatic organ, a lymph node is a small lymphatic organ that is located in the course of lymphatic vessels. The neck, axilla, groin, and mesenteries, as well as the course of large blood vessels in the thorax and abdomen, are also prominent locations for these structures.

5.9.2.6. Structure

When viewed from a distance, lymph nodes have the appearance of bean-shaped or flattened structures. They have a slight depression on one side, known as the hilus, the opening through which blood and lymphatic vessels enter or exit the lymph nodes. Lymph nodes are the only lymphatic structures positioned within the lymphatic circulation. As a result, they are the only lymphatic organs that possess both afferent and efferent lymphatics. On the convex surface of the node, afferent lymphatics can enter the node at a variety of locations, while efferent lymphatics exit the node at the hilus. The lymph can only flow in one direction through a node because both sets of vessels contain valves that allow for this. Regarding afferent vessels, the valves open in the direction of the node, while the valves of efferent vessels open in the opposite direction. In their most basic form, lymph nodes are made up of accumulations of lymphatic tissue that is both diffuse and nodular, and they are encased in a capsule that is significantly enhanced at the hilus. The capsule is made up of collagen fibers that are packed closely together, elastic fibers that are scattered throughout the capsule, and a few smooth muscle cells that are concentrated closer to the entrance and exit of lymphatic vessels. Branching trabeculae of dense irregular connective tissue extend into the lymph node from the inner surface of the capsule. These trabeculae serve as a kind of skeleton for the lymph node. An intricate, three-dimensional reticular network of reticular fibers and the reticular cells that are associated with them fills the spaces that are located between the capsule and the trabeculae. An outer cortex and an inner medulla are formed by the arrangement of lymphatic cells within the network's meshes, which are densely packed with lymphatic cells. In addition to extending for a variable distance toward the node's center, the cortex is a layer located beneath the capsule. Numerous lymphatic nodules, many of which contain germinal centers, are arranged in a bed of diffuse lymphatic tissue to form this structure (Tang et al., 2020). The trabeculae are arranged in a relatively regular pattern and run perpendicular to the capsule. This arrangement causes the cortex to be subdivided into a number of abnormal "compartments." Conversely, trabeculae do not form complete walls; rather, they represent bars or rods of connective tissue, and the cortex does not have a fully developed compartmentalization system. All of the cortical regions communicate with one another laterally, as well as above and below the plane of section, with the exception of the areas where trabeculae are lacking. In most cases, the cortex is divided into two distinct regions: the outer cortex, which is located directly beneath the capsule and is composed of nodular and diffuse lymphatic tissue, and the deep (inner) cortex, which is solely composed of diffuse lymphatic tissue. The two zones do not have a distinct boundary between them, and the respective proportions of each zone vary from node to node as well as depending on the functional status of the node. The nodular lymphatic tissue is where the majority of B-lymphocytes are found, whereas the diffuse lymphatic tissue is where T-cells are found (in general). Following thymectomy, the deep cortex is referred to as the thymus-dependent area because as a result of this, it loses its cell population. Additionally, this region is home to follicular dendritic cells, which are characterized by a nucleus that is pale in color, a limited number of organelles in the cytoplasm, and a multitude of lengthy processes that interdigitate with similar projections from lymphocytes in the surrounding area. In this context, they are an example of an antigen-presenting cell. Not only does the deep cortex continue into the medulla, but there is no clear demarcation or interruption along the way. In most cases, the medulla is a more pale region that generally surrounds the hilus of the node. Its width can vary. A diffuse lymphatic tissue that is arranged in the form of irregular medullary cords that are able to branch and anastomose freely makes up this structure. Plasma cells, macrophages, and lymphocytes are not in short supply in the medullary cords. Compared to the c, the trabeculae of the medulla are less regular in their arrangement ortex.

5.9.2.7. Lymph Sinuses

The lymph sinuses are a network of channel-like spaces within the lymph node. These sinuses are the conduits through which lymph percolates. Afferent lymphatic vessels are responsible for the entry of lymph into the node. These vessels can pierce the capsule at any point along the concave border. The lymph then flows into the subcapsular sinus, also known as the marginal sinus, which is located between the cortex and the capsule. The sinus does not take the form of a tubular structure; rather, it is a large space that extends beneath the capsule and is broken up at regular intervals by the trabeculae. The cortical sinuses, also known as the trabecular and intermediate sinuses, are similar to the subcapsular sinus and extend radially into the cortex, typically along the trabeculae. The subcapsular sinus contains similar structures. These, in turn, become continuous with the medullary sinuses located between the trabeculae of the medulla and the medullary cords. The medullary and subcapsular sinuses come together at the hilus, where they penetrate the capsule and become continuous with the efferent lymphatics (**Figure 5.2**).

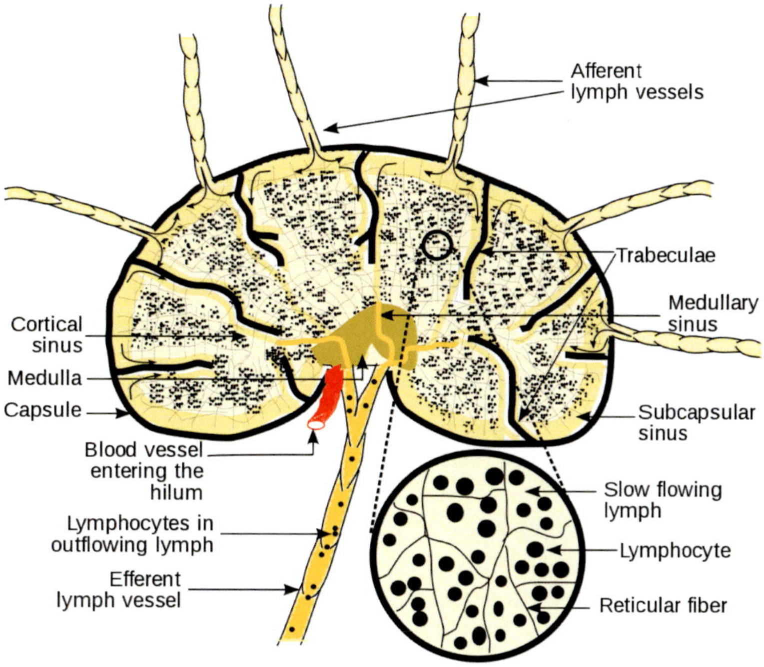

Figure 5.2. *A diagrammatic sketch illustrating the general structure of a lymph node.*

Source: https://upload.wikimedia.org/wikipedia/commons/thumb/9/92/Schematic_of_lymph_node_showing_lymph_sinuses.svg/1200px-Schematic_of_lymph_node_showing_lymph_sinuses.svg.png.

Sinuses are regions of the reticular net that are coarser and more open, and they are most noticeable when viewed in sections. Stellate cells, held together by reticular fibers, extend across the lumen in a crisscross pattern. These cells are interconnected and to the cells that border the lumen by thin processes. The luminal network contains a large number of macrophages, and these macrophages also expand outward from the sinus's boundaries. Flattened reticular cells are the cells that are considered to be the cells that form the margins of the sinuses and extend through the sinus space. On the other hand, it has also been suggested that they are endothelial cells that have been diminished, similar to the cells that line the lymphatic vessels with which they are continuous. While the medulla contains a greater number of sinuses, the cortex contains a smaller number of sinuses that are relatively narrow. In the medulla, the cells are large and irregular, and they exhibit a pattern of repeated branchings and anastomoses. They have a winding path through the medullary parenchyma, which is the reason for the irregular cord-like arrangement of the lymphatic tissue in this region (Pons et al., 2020).

5.9.2.8. Blood Vessels

It is only on rare occasions that smaller blood vessels enter the node from the convex surface. The hilus is the primary route through which the major blood supply arrives at the node. In the beginning, the arteries (arterioles) travel through the trabeculae in the medulla. However, they leave these and enter the medullary cords sooner or later to travel to the cortex. At this point, they disintegrate into a dense capillary plexus that not only forms a network around the nodules but also distributes to the lymphatic tissue that is diffuse. When the capillaries come together, they form venules, which are small veins that originate in the cortex and travel to the medullary cords. On the other hand, these are tributaries of larger veins that emerge from the node at the hilus. Postcapillary venules are the name given to the different types of venules that are found in the deep cortex because of their distinctive appearance. The high endothelium that is present in these vessels can take on a variety of shapes, ranging from cuboidal to columnar, and it can sometimes give the appearance of obstructing the lumen. It is common for the walls of these vessels to be infiltrated with small lymphocytes, which are generally thought to be traveling into the lymph node. During their passage through the endothelium, the cells indent the endothelial cells' lateral walls adjacent to them. It is not known what the significance of the tall endothelium is; however, it has been hypothesized that as the lymphocytes sink deeper between them, the adjacent endothelial cells resume their original relationship to each other above the lymphocytes. This causes the interendothelial cleft to close off, which in turn reduces the amount of plasma that is lost from the venule.

5.9.3. Spleen

It is possible to think of the spleen as a modified and enlarged lymph node that has been inserted into the blood flow. The spleen is the organ that embodies the basic structure of a lymph node. In contrast to lymph nodes, the spleen does not possess afferent lymphatics or a lymphatic sinus system. Furthermore, the lymphatic tissue of the spleen does not have a cortex and a medulla of lymphatic tissue. It indeed possesses a unique pattern of blood circulation as well as specialized vascular channels that provide assistance in the process of blood filtering.

5.9.3.1. Structure

A well-developed capsule of dense irregular connective tissue surrounds the spleen and protects it from external invasion. The deeper layers of the capsule contain the greatest number of elastic fibers, which are found in the spaces between bundles of collagen fibers to which they are attached. It is also possible for smooth muscle fibers to be present in cords or small groups, but the amount of these fibers varies. On the medial surface of the spleen, the capsule is indented to form a hilus that resembles a cleft. This hilus is the passageway through which blood vessels, nerves, and lymphatics enter or exit the lymphatic system. With the formation of a rich, branching, and anastomosing framework, the trabeculae, which are broad bands of connective tissue, extend from the inner surface of the capsule and pass deeply into the substance of the spleen. As is the case with lymph nodes, the trabeculae divide the organ into compartments that are capable of communication (Lee and Griffith, 2022). The reticular network of fibers and associated reticular cells are responsible for filling the spaces that are existing between the trabeculae. There is a wide range of sizes for the meshes, with the majority of them being smaller in areas surrounding lymphatic tissue and blood vessels. The substance that makes up the spleen is referred to as the splenic pulp, and sections taken from a fresh spleen exhibit a distinct separation of the tissue into areas that are rounded or elongated and yellowish in color, which are surrounded by a larger mass of dark red tissue. Within the white pulp, which is composed of lymphatic tissue that is both diffuse and nodular, the scattered gray areas come together to form the white pulp. Suffused with blood, the red pulp is a dark red tissue that is composed of lymphatic tissue that is diffuse and is distributed throughout the body. It is the presence of a significant number of red cells that gives the red pulp its characteristic tint. Some spleens are considered to be sinusal because they contain large blood vessels that branch off and have thin walls. These blood vessels are known as splenic sinusoids (sinuses).

5.9.3.2. White Pulp

Beginning as soon as the vessel leaves the trabeculae to enter the splenic pulp, the white pulp is typically associated with the arterial supply of the spleen. It is also responsible for the formation of the periarterial lymphatic sheaths (PALS), which are a network of lymphatic vessels that surround the arteries. Typical cellular components of lymphatic tissue are present in the sheaths, which have the structure of diffuse lymphatic tissue to begin with. Small lymphocytes, the majority of which are T-cells, constitute the majority of the cells. Throughout the sheath, the lymphatic tissue expands in certain locations, resulting in the incorporation of lymphatic nodules that are similar to the cortical nodules that surround lymph nodes. Not only do they contain germinal centers, but they also represent sites where B- lymphocytes are located. Splenic follicles are the name given to the lymphatic nodules that are found in the spleen. The reticular net is more closely meshed at the periphery of the lymphatic sheath than it is elsewhere. Additionally, the reticular fibers and cells form concentric layers, which have the tendency to delimit the lymphatic tissue from the red pulp. This constitutes the zone of marginalization. There are cells in the white pulp of the spleen that are comparable to the follicular dendritic cells that we find in lymph nodes. These cells, which are similar to dendritic cells, are known as interdigitating cells, and they are also known as antigen-presenting antibodies (Laudato et al., 2023).

5.9.3.3. Red Pulp

Along with the venous system of the spleen, the red pulp is a type of tissue that is associated with lymphatic circulation. The red pulp is filled with a large number of free cells, including all of the cells that are typically found in the blood, and the reticular meshwork is continuous throughout the entire red pulp. Therefore, the red pulp is suffused with red cells, granular leukocytes, and platelets in addition to the cells found in lymphatic tissue. On rare occasions, macrophages can be observed that contain granulocytes or red cells that have been ingested, or are loaded with a pigment called hemosiderin, which is characteristically yellowish brown and is derived from the breakdown of hemoglobin. The red pulp is filled with large blood vessels that are irregular in shape. These blood vessels are known as the splenic sinusoids. In between these sinusoids, the red pulp assumes a branching, cord-like arrangement to form the splenic cords. The lumina of the sinusoids are quite large, ranging from 20 to 40 μm in diameter, and their walls possess a distinctive structure. Endothelial cells that are fusiform and elongated and that lie parallel to the long axis of the vessel make up almost the entire wall of the cardiovascular vessel. The cells are arranged in a row around the lumen, but they are not in contact with one another and are separated by spaces that resemble slits. A basement membrane that is not continuous but rather forms thick bars that are widely spaced and encircle the sinusoid is responsible for supporting the wall outside of the endothelium. The reticular network of the splenic cords is continuous with the basement membrane bars, which are joining to each other by thinner strands of the same material. Basement membrane bars are also continuous with the reticular network (**Figure 5.3**).

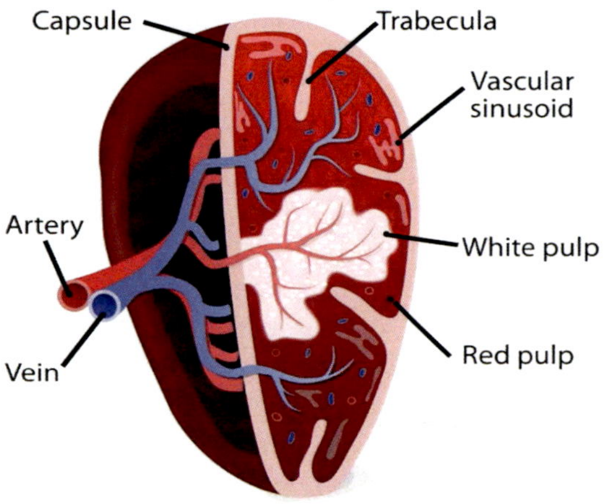

Figure 5.3. *A diagrammatic sketch illustrating the structure of a splenic sinusoid.*

5.9.3.4. Blood Supply

When viewed in relation to blood circulation, which possesses several distinctive characteristics, the architecture of the spleen is most easily comprehended. The hilus is where branches of the splenic artery enter the spleen. These branches then divide and travel through the trabeculae to reach the interior of the organ. Each main branch of these branches serves a specific region of the spleen, and the arrangement of these branches is segmental and overlaps one another above. Eventually, the trabeculae are left as central arteries, which are immediately surrounded by the lymphatic tissue of the periarterial lymphatic sheath. The trabecular arteries, as they are now called, branch multiple times from one another. When the sheath expands to form nodules, the central artery, which is more accurately referred to as the follicular arteriole, displaces itself to the side and assumes an eccentric position within the nodule. Rarely does the vessel manage to keep its central position within the nodular tissue where it is located. As it travels through the white pulp, the central artery supplies a multitude of capillaries that supply the sheath. These capillaries then travel into the marginal zone that surrounds the white pulp. No one knows for sure how these capillaries come to an end (Martinolli et al., 2021). A great number of arterial branches exhibit the appearance of opening directly into the marginal zone, and they frequently culminate in a funnel-shaped terminal part. Due to the fact that there is no direct venous return, the white pulp is only associated with the arterial supply. When a vessel reaches lymphatic tissue, it is referred to as an arteriole, even though the term "artery" is commonly used to refer to the various levels of the splenic vasculature. The central artery continues to branch, and its attenuated stem enters a splenic cord in the red pulp. There, it divides into several short penicillar arteries that are straight. Some of these penicillar arteries have a thickening of their wall, and they now form sheathed capillaries. The sheath is made up of dense masses of cells and fibers that are arranged in a concentrically arranged pattern (Kamada et al., 2022). These masses become continuous with the reticular network of the red pulp. At the periphery of the sheath, the cells exhibit a stellate appearance, in contrast to the rounded appearance of the sheath cells that are located close to the capillary. Within the sheath, the cells are phagocytic to an extreme degree. Sheathing does not cover all the capillaries, and there are times when a single sheath can cover more than one capillary. Additionally, sheathed capillaries can potentially continue functioning as simple capillaries or to divide into two to four terminal capillaries that are not sheathed. There is still some disagreement regarding the manner in which these things come to an end, which has resulted in the "open" and "closed" theories of circulation. Those who subscribe to the open circulation theory assert that the capillaries discharge their contents into the splenic cords, which contain a meshwork of red pulp. In the following step, the blood gradually penetrates the red pulp and makes its way into the venous system by way of the walls of the splenic sinusoids. Because of a decreasing pressure gradient between the two ends of the sinusoid, blood enters the sinusoid at the capillary end and exits at the venous end, according to the closed circulation theory. This is because the capillaries open directly into the lumina of the venous sinusoids of the sinusoids. Following a compromise between the two points of view, it is suggested that when the spleen is distended, a closed circulation that was present in a contracted spleen becomes open. Pulp veins are supported by a thin muscle coat and, more externally, are surrounded by reticular and elastic fibers. Splenic sinusoids drain into pulp veins, which are supported by both structures. At the junction of the pulp veins and sinusoids, smooth muscle activity resembling that of a sphincter has been described. The pulp veins come into contact with the trabeculae, where they travel alongside the artery in the capacity of trabecular veins (**Figure 5.4**). When the trabecular veins come together, they form the splenic vein, which emerges at the hilus.

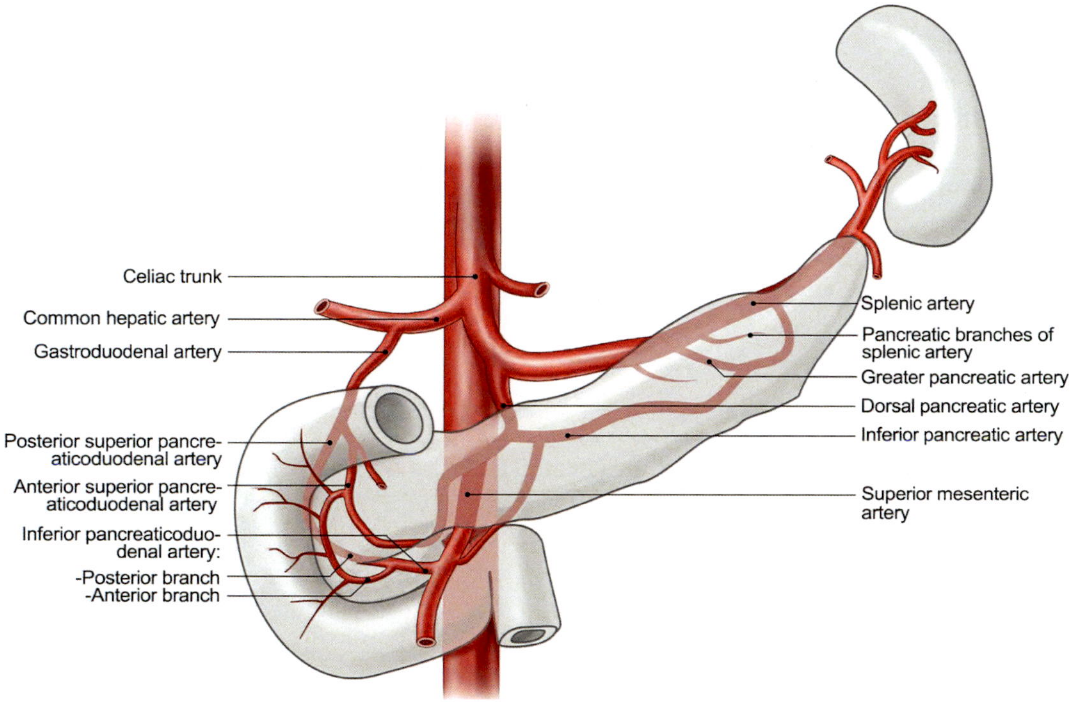

Figure 5.4. *A diagrammatic sketch illustrating the blood supply of the spleen.*

Source: https://www.researchgate.net/publication/365831185/figure/fig2/AS:11431281103566043@1669728221295/Major-blood-supply-to-spleen-and-surrounding-structures-Ref-ambosscom.png.

Efferent lymphatics originate deep within the white pulp of the spleen and converge on the central arteries. The spleen does not contain any afferent lymphatics. The lymphatics travel through the trabeculae and divide into large vessels, which then exit the body through the hilus. Lymphatics are absent in the regions of the spleen that are supplied by sinusoids, also known as the red pulp.

5.9.4. Thymus

The thymus is a lymphatic organ that is encapsulated and bilobed. It is located in the superior mediastinum, which is located dorsal to the sternum and anterior to the great vessels that emerge from the heart. In addition to being the only primary lymphatic organ, the thymus is also the first organ of the embryo to develop lymphoid potential. In contrast to the lymph nodes and the spleen, it is already significantly developed and relatively large at the time of birth. Puberty is the time when the organ reaches its maximum weight, which is between 30 and 40 grams. After this, the organ goes through a process of progressive involution, during which it is partially replaced by fat and connective tissue (Einstein et al., 2010).

5.9.4.1. Structure

The thymus is made up of two lobes that are closely connected to one another and are connected by connective tissue. In addition, there is no continuity of thymic tissue from one lobe to the other because each lobe originates from its own distinct primordium. A thin capsule of connective tissue that is loosely woven surrounds each lobe and provides septa that extend into the thymus. These septa subdivide each lobe into several irregular lobules. A cortex and a medulla are the components that make up each lobule. It is possible that the medulla will appear as isolated, pale areas that are completely surrounded by denser cortical tissue in the typical sections. Serial sections, on the other hand, demonstrate that the septa do not separate the lobules; rather, the medullary regions are continuous throughout each lobule. There is a distinction between the reticular network of the thymus and that of other lymphatic tissues in that the reticular network contains the free cells of the thymus within its meshes. When it comes to the thymus, the reticular cells are not associated with reticular fibers and instead originate from the endoderm rather than the mesenchyme. The cytoplasm of these epithelial reticular cells is highly branched and comprises a limited number of organelles. These cells have a stellate shape. Large euchromatic nuclei that are round or oval in shape display one or more nucleoli that are relatively small but prominent. Desmosomes are present at the points where the cytoplasmic processes of different reticular cells come into contact with one another, to bring them together. As a result, the stroma of the thymus is made up of a cytoreticulum that is made up of epithelial cells. It is only in relation to blood vessels that reticular fibers can typically be found.

5.9.4.2. Cortex

A thick layer that is deeply stained and extends beneath the capsule and along the septa is what makes up the cortex. Most of the cells of the cortex are lymphocytes that are closely packed with little intervening material between them. The cells have a polyhedral appearance because of the mutual compression between them. There is a presence of large, medium, and small lymphocytes, with the latter being the most prevalent; they are indistinguishable from the small lymphocytes that are available in other locations. The outer cortex, which is located beneath the capsule, is where large lymphocytes tend to congregate. These lymphocytes are representative of stem cells that have recently emigrated from the bone marrow. They constitute a relatively insignificant portion of the total cell population. Towards the deeper cortex, where degenerating cells with pyknotic nuclei are also found, the number of small lymphocytes increases and becomes more numerous. Unlike lymph nodes, there are no lymphatic nodules in the cortex of the thymus, nor is there an internal sinus system. There is a large number of lymphocytes in the cortex, which obscures the processes of the reticular cells, which are highly branched. At the periphery of the cortex, they come together to form a continuous layer that serves to separate the cortex from the capsule and the septa. These epithelial reticular cells have structures that are bound to membranes and contain tonofilaments. These structures have the appearance of being secretion granules. In the cortex, macrophages are always present, but in relatively small numbers and dispersed throughout the tissue. Except in cases where phagocytosed material is visible in their cytoplasm, it is difficult to differentiate them from reticular cells using light microscopy. Desmosomes are absent in these cells, which allows electron micrographs to differentiate them from epithelial reticular cells. The thymus contains a dispersed collection of macrophages that have consumed cells that are undergoing degeneration. These macrophages have a tendency to increase in number as they move toward the junction of the cortex and the medulla (Wang et al., 2022).

5.9.4.3. Medulla

As it forms a broad, pale band of tissue that is continuous throughout each lobule, the medulla is located in the central region of the thymus, where it occupies center stage. However, in histologic sections, it frequently appears to be isolated within a lobule, surrounded by a complete layer of cortex. This is the case. On the other hand, the number of lymphocytes is lower than it is in the cortex, and the epithelial reticular cells are not as widely distributed or as highly branched as they are in the cortex. There is a tendency for the reticular cells to be pleomorphic, and they can range from stellate cells with long processes to rounded or flattened cells with many desmosomes and an abundance of pigment fibers. The medulla and the corticomedullary region are both responsible for the presence of dendritic interdigitating cells. They serve as antigen-presenting cells for T-lymphocytes that have reached a more mature stage. A small number of macrophages are present in the medulla, but the majority of the free cells in the medulla are lymphocytes of a smaller size. One can discover eosinophil granulocytes, mast cells, and plasma cells in the body. There are not many mitotic figures. Collagen and reticular fibers wind their way between the epithelial cells between blood vessels, extending for short distances from the blood vessels. One of the most notable characteristics of the medulla is the presence of thymic corpuscles, which are epithelial structures that are either ovoid or rounded. The diameter of these bodies ranges from 10 to 100 μm or even greater, and they are made up of epithelial reticular cells that have been flattened and wrapped around one another in concentric lamellations. These lamellations are connected by a large number of desmosomes between them. Granules of keratohyalin are present in many of them. The cells that are present in the center of the structure go through a process known as hyalinization or necrosis, and they may additionally become lysed, resulting in the formation of a cystic structure. Some of the cells that are located on the periphery of the corpuscle continue to maintain their connections with the cytoreticulum that is all around them. The thymic corpuscles are considered to be nothing more than degenerated structures thus far; however, there is evidence to suggest that they may be secretory bodies. The function of these corpuscles is unknown.

5.9.4.4. Blood Supply

The arteries that supply blood to the thymus pass through the connective tissue of the septa and reach the organ. Arteriolar branches originate from these vessels and run along the corticomedullary junction. These branches supply arterioles and capillaries to the medulla, as well as capillaries to the cortex. The cortex does not contain any vessels that are larger than capillaries. Within the cortex, the capillaries run toward the capsule, forming branching arcades before passing back through the cortex to drain into venules and thence into veins accompanying the arterioles in the corticomedullary region and medulla. The veins leave via the septa and ultimately unite to form a single thymic vein. The connective tissue that makes up the collar that surrounds the cortical capillaries is a component of the barrier that separates the blood and the thymus. A continuous layer of epithelial reticular cells surrounds this envelope which, in turn, surrounds the envelope itself (Wong et al., 2013). The reticular fibers that accompany the vessel travel through the perivascular connective tissue space, which has a width that varies from position to position. Granular leukocytes, plasma cells, macrophages, and lymphocytes are all found within the perivascular space. The capillary endothelium and its basal lamina, the perivascular connective tissue sheath, and the layer of epithelial reticular cells and their associated basal lamina are the components that make up the blood-thymic barrier in the cortex. There is a limited movement of macromolecules across this barrier, and the development of cortical lymphocytes takes place in an environment relatively isolated from antigens. It is possible for circulating macromolecules to pass through the vessels that are located in the medulla and the corticomedullary junction. T-lymphocytes acquire surface marker molecules of major histocompatibility complex (MHC I and MHC II) and synthesize receptors for the recognition of foreign antigens as they differentiate in the cortex of the thymus. This process occurs during the process of peripheral blood cell differentiation. The thymus is responsible for destroying lymphocytes that can recognize self-MHC. On the other hand, T-lymphocytes that are able to react to non-self cells go on to form clones of cells that mature and are then released as immunocompetent T-lymphocytes. Within the medulla and in close proximity to the corticomedullary junction, lymphocytes exit the thymus by entering postcapillary venules.

5.9.4.5. Involution

The growth of the thymus during the life of the fetus is extremely rapid, and by the time the baby is born, the organ has reached its greatest in terms of its relative size. It persists in growing, albeit at a slower rate, until the onset of puberty, at which point it goes through progressive involution. The weight of the organ decreases, the number of cortical lymphocytes decreases, and the size and number of thymic corpuscles increase along with the organ's size. The septa also become wider as they progress. In the cortical regions, fat cells begin to infiltrate, and the replacement may become excessive in scope. By the time the process of involution begins, T-cells have already established themselves in the secondary lymphatic tissue located throughout the body. Even when an individual is very old, the thymic parenchyma does not completely disappear, and the thymus continues to be active even in adulthood (Wong et al., 2013).

5.9.4.6. Other Constituents

On a regular basis, the thymus exhibits several peculiar structural elements, the significance of which is known to be unknown. Among these structures are cyst-like spaces that are lined by cells that have brush borders, cilia, or mucus-producing cells. Additionally, reticular cells that contain microvillus-lined vacuoles are sometimes found in these structures. The cells known as "myoid" are the most peculiar because they have a semblance to striated muscle that is not entirely accurate. These cells may have characteristics similar to those of embryonal or adult muscle fibers, including typical banding patterns such as Z lines, A lines, I lines, and M lines. There is a lack of knowledge regarding whether or not these various inclusions have any functional significance or whether they represent abnormal differentiation of embryogenesis elements.

5.9.4.7. Dendritic (Antigen-Presenting) Cells

Dendritic cells, which are responsible for presenting antigens, originate in the bone marrow. However, in contrast to monocytes (macrophages), dendritic cells have low levels of lysosomal enzymes. On the other hand, they have a high concentration of class II major histocompatibility complex (MHC) molecules, which are necessary for the presentation of new antigens to T-lymphocytes. Dendritic cells can take in foreign proteins, process (partially digest) the antigens, and insert specific portions of an antigen into their cell membrane. This allows the dendritic cells to keep the product for extended periods of time. It is possible to find dendritic cells in the lymph nodes, spleen, thymus, mesenteries, and skin (Langerhans' cells), as well as beneath mucosal surfaces. Even though they share morphological characteristics, such as displaying fine ramifying cytoplasmic processes and having a relatively small number of lysosomes, it seems that every dendritic antigen-presenting cell has developed specialized surface receptors for a particular microenvironment at the location where it is located. After a certain amount of time has passed, they leave the particular environment (for example, the skin), travel to lymphoid tissue, and gradually present the antigens that were gathered in a particular environment to T-lymphocytes. Since they are responsible for monitoring a variety of different environments, dendritic antigen-presenting cells play a very significant role in the immune system.

5.9.5. Organogenesis

As a pair of endodermal outgrowths, the thymus originates from the third pharyngeal pouch, with the fourth pharyngeal pouch also contributing to its development. From the eighth week onward, each outgrowth extends caudally and medially, and by that time, it is located in the midline beneath the upper portion of the sternum. In the beginning, every outgrowth possesses a lumen that is similar to a slit and is surrounded by several layers of tall cuboidal or columnar cells. As the number of cells increases, the lumina lose their appearance. However, the cytoplasmic connections between the cells continue to exist, even though the cells become stellate and loosely arranged in the center. In the thymic cytoreticulum, these cells differentiate into epithelial reticular cells. Blood-borne stem cells that originate in the yolk sac and fetal liver are responsible for seeding the thymic rudiment at approximately 8 weeks of gestation. Additionally, lymphoid stem cells that are capable of repopulating the thymus are present in the bone marrow to a certain extent. It would appear that the chemotactic agents released by the thymic reticular cells are responsible for directing the migration of stem cells. Stem cells are responsible for the development of thymic lymphocytes, which mature into cortex and medulla by the fourteenth week of gestation. Stem cells are progenitor cells. Whether or not the lymphoid progenitor cells have already differentiated into T-cell precursors at the time of seeding or whether or not differentiation takes place in the thymus is a mystery. Condensation of the mesenchyme that surrounds the thymic primordium results in the formation of the capsule, and mesenchyme also invades the cellular mass to provide the septa.

Lymph nodes develop locally in vascular mesenchyme at sites normally occupied by lymph nodes, and their formation is related closely to development of the lymph vascular system. The formation of mesenchymal cell aggregates occurs in close proximity to lymphatic sacs and occurs around loops of lymphatic capillaries. Lymphatic vessels form isolated spaces at the periphery of the aggregates, which are separated by thin bridges of connective tissue. Condensation of the connective tissue that is located outside of the sinus and in the bridges forms the capsule and trabeculae. This occurs as the lymph spaces gradually fuse to form the marginal sinus, also known as the subcapsular sinus. Following the paths of the developing trabeculae, the sinuses subdivide and develop into the trabecular and medullary sinuses as they fuse together. Other sinuses follow the same path. The reticular cells and fibrous network of the cortex and medulla are both derived from the mesenchymal aggregates that are present in the brain. The lymphocytes that originate from the bone marrow and the thymus are responsible for seeding the entire mass, and the lymphocytes then take up their distinctive positions within the nodes. While T-lymphocytes tend to migrate into the deep cortex (paracortex) of the lymph node, B-lymphocytes have a tendency to migrate into lymphatic nodules that are located in the outer cortex when they migrate (Zhu et al., 2022).

A number of thickenings in the cranial end of the greater omentum are the initial manifestations of the spleen. The primordia eventually fuse together to form a lobulated spleen that extends into the body cavity as the developing spleen grows. During the process of expansion, the spleen loses its lobulated appearance. Mesenchymal cells in the body's cellular mass undergo differentiation into reticular cells, which are responsible for the production of the reticular stroma inside the spleen. The capsule is formed by the gradual condensation of the connective tissue that is located on the outermost layer. The trabeculae are formed by the condensation of mesenchymal projections. During this stage, which occurs between the eighth and ninth week of pregnancy, the spleen comprises a meshwork of reticular cells encased in a thin capsule. Lymphocytes derived from the bone marrow and the thymus are responsible for seeding this rudiment of the spleen. Late in the development process, the white pulp enlarges and forms nodules. Additionally, during the majority of the development process, lymphatic tissue primarily forms periarterial lymphatic sheaths. Not until after birth do germinal centers become visible. During pregnancy, the fetal spleen is responsible for producing erythrocytes and granular leukocytes; however, this function is no longer present in humans until shortly before birth.

A Closer Look

Fibrous skeleton of the Heart

The fibrous skeleton of the heart, also called the cardiac skeleton, consists of four fibrous rings (anuli fibrosi, singular: annulus fibrosis) and the membranous portions of the septa of the heart. This skeleton is located at the base of the ventricles, between the atria and the ventricles.

The rings of the fibrous skeleton are composed of dense, fibrous connective tissue that encircle the orifices of the heart valves. These fibrous rings are interconnected by connective tissue called the right and left trigones and form the structural support for the heart on which the valvular leaflets and cardiac muscle fibers are anchored.

Anatomy

The fibrous skeleton of the heart is a rigid framework of dense regular connective tissue located in a plane between the atria and the ventricles. This complex structure consist of three main components. These are the four fibrous rings, right and left fibrous trigones, and finally the membranous aspects of the interatrial, interventricular and atrioventricular septa.

The four fibrous rings surround the orifices of the pulmonary, aortic and atrioventricular valves, giving attachments to their leaflets and resisting excessive distention. The left fibrous ring encircles the left atrioventricular valve (mitral valve) and the right fibrous ring surrounds the right atrioventricular valve (tricuspid valve). The pulmonary ring corresponds to the pulmonary valve as does the aortic ring to the aortic valve.

The right and left trigones are interconnections between the fibrous rings, and the strongest parts of the skeleton. A thickened connective tissue connection between the aortic ring and right atrioventricular ring forms the right trigone, while the left trigone is formed by a similar connective tissue bridge between the aortic ring and the left atrioventricular ring.

Functions

The fibrous skeleton of the heart performs several important functions and thus plays a vital role in supporting both the structure and function of the heart.

- It helps keep the orifices of the valves it surrounds patent, and also serves as points of attachment for the leaflets and cusps of these valves.
- The fibrous skeleton separates the atrial musculature from that of the ventricles. It serves as the framework for the attachment of myocardial fibers, with atrial fibers arising from the upper border of the rings and ventricular fibers originating from the lower border of the rings.

- The fibrous skeleton serves as an electrical insulator, partitioning electrical impulses conducted through the musculature of the atria and ventricles, allowing them to contract independently. In line with this, the fibrous skeleton provides passage for the atrioventricular bundle, which serves as the only electrical connection between the atria and ventricles.

Summary

This chapter explores the structure and function of these two critical systems that circulate fluids throughout the body. The cardiovascular system consists of the heart, blood vessels, and blood, and is responsible for pumping oxygenated blood to tissues and removing carbon dioxide and waste products. It is divided into systemic and pulmonary circulation, with arteries, veins, and capillaries playing a crucial role in maintaining blood flow and ensuring oxygen and nutrient exchange. The chapter details the anatomy of the heart, including its chambers and valves, and explains how electrical impulses regulate heartbeats.

The lymph vascular system, also known as the lymphatic system, complements the cardiovascular system by draining excess fluid from tissues and returning it to the bloodstream. This system also plays a key role in immune function by filtering lymph through lymph nodes, which trap pathogens and foreign particles. The chapter explains the components of the lymphatic system, including lymph vessels, lymph nodes, and lymphatic organs like the spleen and thymus. Together, the cardiovascular and lymphatic systems maintain fluid balance, nutrient distribution, and immune protection, ensuring overall homeostasis in the body.

References

1. Ames, J., Puleri, D. F., Balogh, P., Gounley, J., Draeger, E. W., & Randles, A. (2020). Multi-GPU immersed boundary method hemodynamics simulations. *Journal of Computational Science, 44*, 101153. https://doi.org/10.1016/j.jocs.2020.101153.
2. Athani, A., Ghazali, N. N. N., Badruddin, I. A., Kamangar, S., Anqi, A. E., & Algahtani, A. (2022). Investigation of two-way fluid-structure interaction of blood flow in a patient-specific left coronary artery. *Bio-Medical Materials and Engineering, 33*, 13–30. https://doi.org/10.3233/BME-211287.
3. Bäumler, K., Vedula, V., Sailer, A. M., Seo, J., Chiu, P., Mistelbauer, G., Chan, F. P., Fischbein, M. P., Marsden, A. L., & Fleischmann, D. (2020). Fluid-structure interaction simulations of patient-specific aortic dissection. *Biomechanics and Modeling in Mechanobiology, 19*, 1607–1628. https://doi.org/10.1007/s10237-020-01288-5.
4. Bazilevs, Y., Takizawa, K., & Tezduyar, T. E. (2013). *Computational Fluid-Structure Interaction: Methods and Applications*. Hoboken, NJ: J. Wiley & Sons.
5. Cetin, A., & Sahin, M. (2018). A monolithic fluid-structure interaction framework applied to red blood cells. *International Journal for Numerical Methods in Biomedical Engineering, 35*, e3171. https://doi.org/10.1002/cnm.3171.
6. Djukic, T., Topalovic, M., & Filipovic, N. (2023). Validation of lattice Boltzmann-based software for blood flow simulations in complex patient-specific arteries against traditional CFD methods. *Mathematics and Computers in Simulation, 203*, 957–976. https://doi.org/10.1016/j.matcom.2022.09.011.
7. Einstein, D. R., Pin, F. D., Jiao, X., Kuprat, A. P., Carson, J. P., Kunzelman, K. S., Cochran, R. P., Guccione, J. M., & Ratcliffe, M. B. (2010). Fluid-structure interactions of the mitral valve and left heart: Comprehensive strategies, past, present, and future. *International Journal for Numerical Methods in Biomedical Engineering, 26*, 348–380. https://doi.org/10.1002/cnm.1318.

8. Haggerty, C. M., Restrepo, M., Tang, E., de Zélicourt, D. A., Sundareswaran, K. S., Mirabella, L., Bethel, J., Whitehead, K. K., Fogel, M. A., & Yoganathan, A. P. (2014). Fontan hemodynamics from 100 patient-specific cardiac magnetic resonance studies: A computational fluid dynamics analysis. *Journal of Thoracic and Cardiovascular Surgery, 148*, 1481–1489. https://doi.org/10.1016/j.jtcvs.2014.06.037.

9. Jayendiran, R., Nour, B., & Ruimi, A. (2018). Fluid-structure interaction (FSI) analysis of stent-graft for aortic endovascular aneurysm repair (EVAR): Material and structural considerations. *Journal of the Mechanical Behavior of Biomedical Materials, 87*, 95–110. https://doi.org/10.1016/j.jmbbm.2018.07.001.

10. Kamada, H., Nakamura, M., Ota, H., Higuchi, S., & Takase, K. (2022). Blood flow analysis with computational fluid dynamics and 4D-flow MRI for vascular diseases. *Journal of Cardiology, 80*, 386–396. https://doi.org/10.1016/j.jjcc.2022.05.014.

11. Kuchumov, A. G., Vedeneev, V., Samartsev, V., Khairulin, A., & Ivanov, O. (2021). Patient-specific fluid-structure interaction model of bile flow: Comparison between 1-way and 2-way algorithms. *Computer Methods in Biomechanics and Biomedical Engineering, 24*, 1693–1717. https://doi.org/10.1080/10255842.2021.1952063.

12. Laudato, M., Mosca, R., & Mihaescu, M. (2023). Buckling critical pressures in collapsible tubes relevant for biomedical flows. *Scientific Reports, 13*, 9298. https://doi.org/10.1038/s41598-023-36439-2.

13. Lee, J. H., & Griffith, B. E. (2022). On the Lagrangian-Eulerian coupling in the immersed finite element/difference method. *Journal of Computational Physics, 457*, 111042. https://doi.org/10.1016/j.jcp.2022.111042.

14. Martinolli, M., Biasetti, J., Zonca, S., Polverelli, L., & Vergara, C. (2021). Extended finite element method for fluid-structure interaction in wave membrane blood pump. *International Journal for Numerical Methods in Biomedical Engineering, 37*, e3467. https://doi.org/10.1002/cnm.3467.

15. Pons, R., Guala, A., Rodríguez-Palomares, J. F., Cajas, J. C., Dux-Santoy, L., Teixidó-Tura, G., Molins, J. J., Vázquez, M., Evangelista, A., & Martorell, J. (2020). Fluid-structure interaction simulations outperform computational fluid dynamics in the description of thoracic aorta haemodynamics and in the differentiation of progressive dilation in Marfan syndrome patients. *Royal Society Open Science, 7*, 191752. https://doi.org/10.1098/rsos.191752.

16. Rousseau-Portalis, M., Cymberknop, L., Farro, I., & Armentano, R. (2023). Computational clustering reveals differentiated coronary artery calcium progression at prevalent levels of pulse wave velocity by classifying high-risk patients. *Frontiers in Cardiovascular Medicine, 10*, 1161914. https://doi.org/10.3389/fcvm.2023.1161914.

17. Sequí-Domínguez, I., Cavero-Redondo, I., Álvarez-Bueno, C., Pozuelo-Carrascosa, D. P., de Arenas-Arroyo, S. N., & Martínez-Vizcaíno, V. (2020). Accuracy of pulse wave velocity predicting cardiovascular and all-cause mortality: A systematic review and meta-analysis. *Journal of Clinical Medicine, 9*, 2080. https://doi.org/10.3390/jcm9072080.

18. Tang, E., Wei, Z. A., Fogel, M. A., Veneziani, A., & Yoganathan, A. P. (2020). Fluid-structure interaction simulation of an intra-atrial Fontan connection. *Biology, 9*, 412. https://doi.org/10.3390/biology9120412.

19. Wang, C., Tang, H., & Zhang, X. (2022). Fluid-structure interaction of bio-inspired flexible slender structures: A review of selected topics. *Bioinspiration & Biomimetics, 17*, 041002. https://doi.org/10.1088/1748-3190/ac7204.

20. Wong, K. K. L., Thavornpattanapong, P., Cheung, S. C. P., & Tu, J. (2013). Numerical stability of partitioned approach in fluid-structure interaction for a deformable thin-walled vessel. *Computational and Mathematical Methods in Medicine, 2013*, 638519. https://doi.org/10.1155/2013/638519.

21. Zhu, Y., Mirsadraee, S., Rosendahl, U., Pepper, J., & Xu, X. Y. (2022). Fluid-structure interaction simulations of repaired type A aortic dissection: A comprehensive comparison with rigid wall models. Frontiers in Physiology, 13, 913457. https://doi.org/10.3389/fphys.2022.913457.

Chapter

SENSORY SYSTEM

6

Contents

Introduction

The sensory system is a marvel of biological engineering, enabling organisms to perceive and interact with their environment. Histology, the study of tissues at a microscopic level, reveals the intricate structures that underpin sensory function. The sensory system comprises specialized cells and tissues distributed throughout the body, each tailored to detect specific stimuli such as light, sound, touch, taste, and smell.

Histological examination reveals the complex layers of the retina in the eye, including photoreceptor cells like rods and cones responsible for vision. The ear's histology unveils the cochlea's spiral structure, housing hair cells crucial for hearing. Touch receptors in the skin are studied for their role in detecting pressure, temperature, and pain. Histological analysis of taste buds showcases the receptor cells responsible for detecting different taste modalities, while the olfactory epithelium in the nose contains receptors vital for the sense of smell. Understanding the histology of the sensory system provides insights into how organisms perceive and respond to their surroundings, offering a profound appreciation for the intricacies of sensory function (Birkoben et al., 2020).

Orientation and Directional Terms

Term	Definition	Illustration
Epidermis	The outermost layer of the skin, composed of stratified squamous epithelial cells that provide a protective barrier against environmental damage, pathogens, and water loss.	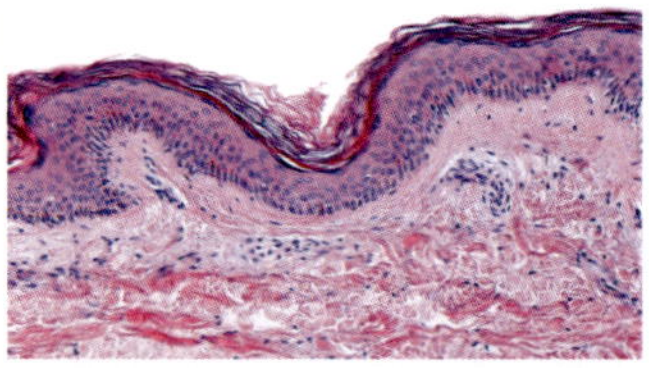
Corneoscleral Coat	The combined structure of the cornea and sclera; it provides shape and protection to the eye and is essential for light refraction and vision.	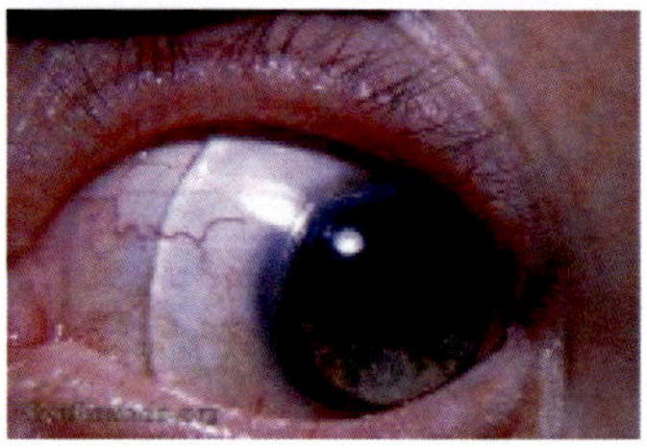
Organogenesis	The process during embryonic development where specific organs and structures form from the three germ layers (ectoderm, mesoderm, and endoderm).	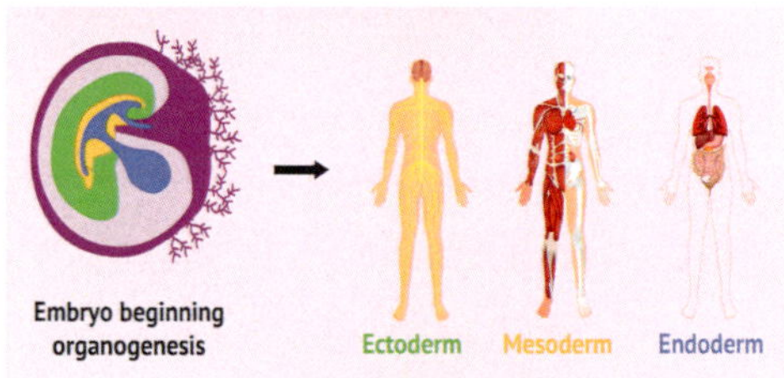
Retina	The innermost layer of the eye that contains photoreceptor cells (rods and cones) responsible for converting light into neural signals, enabling vision.	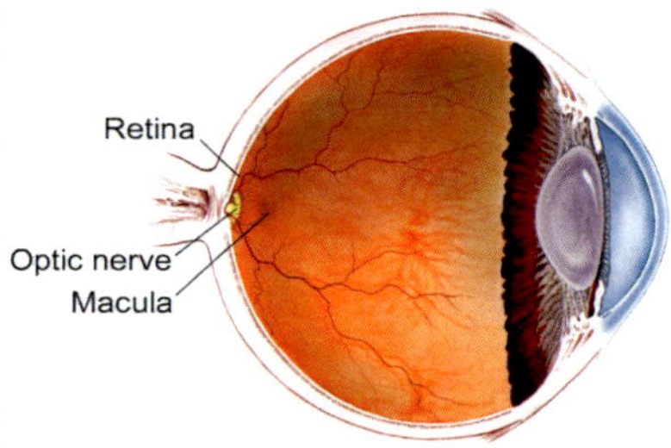
Vitreous Body	A gel-like substance that fills the space between the lens and the retina in the eye, helping to maintain its shape and providing support to the retina.	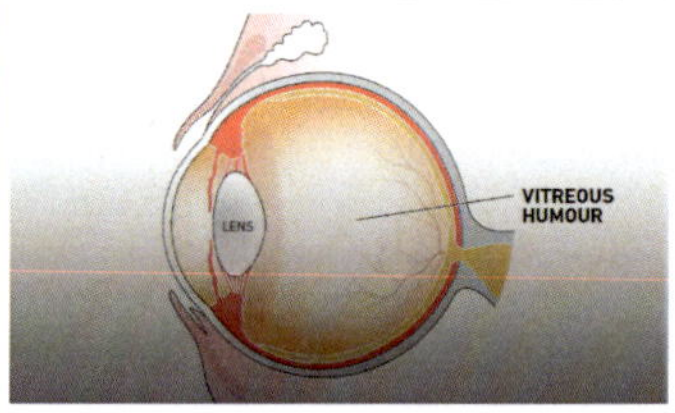

6.1. Skin

The skin envelops the outer surface of the body and serves as a substantial organ with multiple functions. The human skin comprises approximately 7% of the overall body weight and has a total surface area of approximately 1.8 m^2. The skin serves multiple functions, including safeguarding the body against physical harm and fluid loss, acting as a shield against harmful substances, assisting in maintaining optimal body temperature, eliminating waste products, and relaying information about the external environment through its receptors for heat, cold, touch, and pain sensations. Furthermore, the ultraviolet rays from sunlight stimulate the lower layer of the skin to generate vitamin D (calciferol).

6.1.1. Structure

The skin is composed of two main layers: the outermost layer, known as the epidermis, which is made up of epithelial cells, and the underlying layer, called the dermis or corium, which is made up of connective tissue. The hypodermis, a loose layer of connective tissue, connects the skin to underlying structures, although it is not classified as part of the skin. The skin appendages, including hair, nails, sweat glands, and sebaceous glands, are specialized local structures derived from the epidermis. The integument is formed by the combination of the skin and its appendages. The skin's thickness varies across different regions of the body, and the relative proportions of the dermis and epidermis also vary. The dermis is particularly thick between the scapula, while the epidermis is thickened on the palms of the hands and soles of the feet. The terms "thick skin" and "thin skin" specifically pertain to the thickness of the epidermis, rather than the overall thickness of the skin. The epidermis is highly developed in thick skin, while it is relatively thin in thin skin. The epidermis forms multiple ridge-like extensions called epidermal ridges that project into the underlying dermis at their junction. The dermal papillae are formed by complementary projections of the dermis that fit between the epidermal ridges. The surface characteristics of the skin, such as the fingerprints, mirror the arrangement of the dermal papillae (Birkoben et al., 2020).

6.1.2. Epidermis

The epidermis is the outermost layer of the skin and is composed of keratinized stratified squamous epithelium. Keratinocytes undergo a systematic process of maturation and keratinization, resulting in the formation of a superficial layer consisting of compact, flattened, lifeless cells on the surface. Melanocytes, a smaller group of cells, are responsible for the pigmentation of the skin. The epidermis is devoid of blood vessels and receives nourishment through the process of diffusion from the vessels present in the underlying dermis. The epidermis is supplied with nerves. The epidermis is composed of multiple layers (strata) that represent the successive transformation of keratinocytes as they move from the bottom of the epidermis to the surface, where they are shed. The layers of thick skin are the stratum Basale, stratum spinosum, stratum granulosum, stratum lucidum, and stratum corneum. In individuals with thin skin, the layers are narrower and less distinct, and the stratum lucidum is absent.

6.1.2.1. Stratum Basale

The stratum Basale is adjacent to the underlying dermis, with only a basement membrane separating them. The structure comprises a solitary line of columnar epithelial cells that conform to the shape of the ridges and papillae. The stratum Basale is the proliferative layer of the epidermis, where the majority, although not all, of the cell division takes place. For this reason, stratum Basale often is called the stratum germinativum. Every cell in the stratum

Basale is bounded by a characteristic trilaminar cell membrane and is connected to neighboring cells through numerous desmosomes. Hemidesmosomes play a role in anchoring the cells to the basement membrane located at the basal surface. As in other areas, the basement membrane at the dermoepidermal junction comprises three layers: a superficial lamina lucida, a lamina Densa, and a fibroreticular lamina beneath it. Type VII collagen anchoring filaments connect the undersurface of the lamina Densa to collagen fibers in the papillary dermis on the dermal side of the basement membrane. Fibrillin microfibrils connect the lamina Densa to elastic fibers. The cytoplasm of the basal keratinocytes is relatively compact and contains numerous dispersed keratin intermediate filaments. The cells exhibit prominent clusters of ribosomes, along with a moderate number of mitochondria, some profiles of granular endoplasmic reticulum, and a few Golgi saccules (Chi et al., 2018).

6.1.2.2. Stratum Spinosum

The Stratum spinosum comprises multiple layers of irregular, polyhedral cells that become partially flattened in the outermost layers. The cells are tightly adhered to each other and connected at all surfaces by numerous desmosomes. During tissue preparation, the cells undergo shrinkage and separation, except at the points where they are attached. Therefore, the cells exhibit multiple short, spiny extensions that stretch between neighboring cells and are commonly referred to as prickle cells. The projections do not represent regions of cytoplasmic connection between cells but rather serve as locations for typical desmosomes. Prickle cells in the upper layers of the stratum spinosum possess ovoid granules, measuring 0.1 to 0.5 μm in diameter, known as membrane-coating granules. These granules are not found in the basal cells. These structures are composed of parallel layers enclosed by a double membrane and contain high levels of glycols and phospholipids, contributing to the skin's ability to maintain its barrier function. Keratin intermediate filaments are abundant and can arrange into compact bundles that extend into the spinous processes, ultimately terminating in the dense plaques of desmosomes. The layers of the skin known as stratum spinosum and stratum Basale are frequently referred to collectively as stratum malpighii.

6.1.2.3. Stratum Granulosum

The stratum granulosum in thick skin comprises three to five layers of flattened cells oriented parallel to the epidermis surface. The stratum granulosum in thin skin is composed of a solitary layer of cells. The cells are characterized by the existence of amorphous, tightly packed dark granules, known as keratohyalin granules, which exhibit variation in both size and shape. The granules lack membranes and are closely associated with bundles of keratin filaments. From a chemical standpoint, these substances contain significant quantities of sulfur amino acids. In the outermost layers of the stratum granulosum, the number and size of granules increase, and the cells exhibit signs of degenerative changes. The nuclei exhibit a lighter staining, and the connections between neighboring cells become less discernible. The cells of the granular layer remain alive but experience programmed cell death as they transition into the subsequent horny layer. The number of membrane-coating granules in the cells of the stratum granulosum increases. The elongated granules merge with the plasma membrane and release their contents into the space between cells. The lipid-rich contents in this layer serve as a barrier, preventing water loss and the entry of foreign substances between cells, thus contributing to the sealing effect of the skin. Concrete evidence of this phenomenon can be witnessed when the epidermis is deeply abraded or scraped, resulting in a visible injury known as a strawberry, which occurs below the stratum granulosum. During this phenomenon, a viscous fluid of amber hue emerges and continues to exude for a considerable duration. This is the interstitial fluid that has moved through keratinocytes towards the surface to provide nutrients to the cells located deep within the stratum granulosum (Chi et al., 2018).

6.1.2.4. Stratum Lucidum

The stratum lucidum is a thin, wavy, lightly colored layer located on the stratum granulosum's surface. The structure is composed of multiple layers of densely packed cells, making it difficult to distinguish the boundaries of individual cells. Occasionally, remnants of compressed nuclei may be observed, but typically this layer is distinguished by the absence of nuclei. The cytoplasm mainly consists of aggregates of keratin intermediate filaments, which are now arranged more regularly and parallel to the skin surface. Only a small number of organelles remain. The plasmalemma exhibits increased thickness and convolutions, while the intercellular material is augmented. The stratum lucidum is highly visible in the thick dermis of the palms and soles, but it is not present in the epidermis of other body regions.

6.1.2.5. Stratum Corneum

The stratum corneum is the outermost layer of the epidermis and consists of flattened, scale-like cells known as squames. The squames are surrounded by a thickened, altered cell membrane caused by the ongoing accumulation of a protein called involucrin.

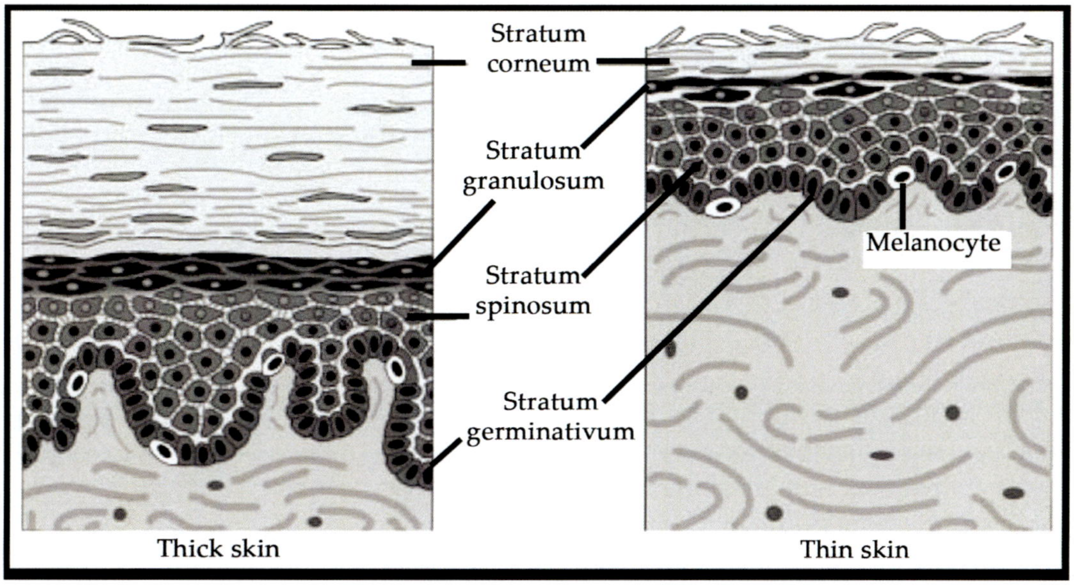

Figure 6.1. *A diagrammatic sketch illustrating the structure of thick and thin skin.*

Source: https://www.researchgate.net/profile/Noe-Ortega-Quijano/publication/252859222/figure/fig2/AS:669995033956358@1536750672111/Thick-and-thin-skin-structure-14.jpg.

This protein is first produced in cells located in the upper layers of the stratum spinosum. The squames are the remnants of cells that have lost their nuclei, all of their organelles, and their desmosomal connections to neighboring cells. The cells contain keratin, which is composed of densely packed bundles of keratin intermediate filaments embedded in an opaque, amorphous substance that is abundant in the protein filaggrin. The keratin intermediate filaments found in the stratum corneum are composed of "soft" keratin, different from the "hard" keratin found in nails and hair. Soft keratin contains less sulfur and is slightly more flexible than hard keratin. The outermost cells of the stratum corneum are regularly shed or desquamated. This area is commonly known as the stratum disjunctum (**Figure 6.1**).

Therefore, as keratinocytes migrate towards the outer layer, they are firmly connected by desmosomes. During the passage of cells through the stratum granulosum and their proximity to the surface, specific proteins, including those in the keratohyaline granules, interact with the keratin intermediate filaments and the plasmalemma. This interaction results in the formation of a dense mass of keratin. During this migration, keratinocytes also secrete a complex hydrophobic glycophospholipid, which is released upon the death of the outermost keratinocytes. This substance functions as an adhesive, binding the keratin-filled squames together and providing short-term water resistance to the surface of the epidermis. The water resistance of this product deteriorates over time when subjected to prolonged immersion in water, as demonstrated by the hands being submerged for extended periods. During this process, the keratin molecules absorb water, causing them to expand and become softer. The keratin layer serves as the primary defense against physical harm, drying out, and bacterial invasion and is chemically inert and highly resistant to water penetration. Keratinocytes undergo a life cycle that lasts approximately 40 to 55 days, from their formation in the basal layer to their shedding. As the keratinocytes move towards the surface, they transform, becoming wider and more flattened. This results in the need for only four surface squames to cover the same area requiring 100 columnar basal cells. Therefore, a minimal frequency of cell division (less than 7 out of every 1000 basal cells) is sufficient to sustain the outermost layer.

6.1.2.6. Pigmentation

Most of the keratinocytes that make up the epidermis are transparent and allow ultraviolet rays from sunlight to easily pass through the different layers of the epidermis and reach the dermis below (Chortos et al., 2016). Consequently, extended exposure can harm both the genetic composition of nuclei in the cells of the stratum Basale and the components of the underlying dermis, leading to premature aging and the formation of wrinkles on the skin. The pigments carotene and melanin, as well as the blood in the capillaries of the dermis, are responsible for determining skin color. Carotene is a yellow pigment present in the cells of the outermost layer of the skin (stratum corneum) and in the fat cells of the deeper layers of the skin (dermis and hypodermis). The brown pigment melanin is primarily found in the stratum Basale cells and the stratum spinosum's deeper layers.

Melanin is produced in specialized cells called melanocytes, which are derived from cells that migrated from the neural crest during embryonic development. Melanocytes are distributed sporadically within the basal layer and project multiple finger-like cytoplasmic extensions that stretch among the cells of the stratum spinosum. Every melanocyte forms a functional connection with approximately 36 keratinocytes in the stratum spinosum and basale layers. An epidermal-melanin unit is formed by the combination of melanocytes and keratinocytes. Epidermal melanocytes can be identified in electron micrographs based on the absence of keratin filaments and the presence of melanin granules (melanosomes) in different stages of growth. Melanocytes possess the typical assortment of cytoplasmic organelles. Although melanocytes do not have desmosomal junctions with adjacent cells, they are attached to the basement membrane through hemidesmosome-like junctions. Mature melanosomes are transported from melanocytes to keratinocytes of the basal layer and stratum spinosum through their cytoplasmic processes. In humans, melanosomes often cluster above the nuclei of basal cells, while in the outer layers of the epidermis, the granules are evenly distributed and gradually become smaller. Due to the constant shedding of epidermal cells, melanocytes are responsible for the ongoing production of melanin. While melanocytes can undergo cell death and be replenished through the division of nearby melanocytes, this process occurs randomly and does not follow a predictable cycle of melanocyte replacement. The number of melanocytes and the dimensions of the melanosomes are slightly higher in Negroid and Mongolian skin compared to Caucasian skin, although not to a significant extent that can explain the variations in skin color. Caucasoid melanosomes exhibit incomplete melanization and are organized into clusters known as melanosome complexes, which are enclosed by a membrane. The larger melanosomes found in individuals of Negroid descent are distributed more extensively within cells and do not create complexes enclosed by membranes. The distribution of pigment within the epidermis varies, with a higher concentration in the lower zones of the Malpighian layer in Caucasian skin and a more widespread distribution across most keratinocytes of this layer in Negroid skin. Lysosomes degrade the smaller melanosomes of Caucasians before they reach the upper strata. There is variation in the level of pigmentation across different regions of the body. The axilla, circumanal region, scrotum, penis, labia majora, nipples, and areola exhibit heightened pigmentation. Conversely, the palms and soles have minimal or no pigmentation. Freckles are patches of pigmentation that occur in specific areas due to abnormal groups of melanocytes. Pregnancy can lead to increased pigmentation of freckles and the areolae and nipples. Sunlight exposure leads to a general augmentation in melanization, initially through the darkening of existing melanin and subsequently through enhanced production of new melanin. The melanocytes that have been activated generate larger melanosomes. Melanin deficiency can also occur. Piebaldism in humans is characterized by the presence of white spotted patterns, which are caused by abnormalities in the morphology of melanocytes. These abnormalities result in a deficiency in the length and number of cell processes. Complete albinism is caused by the melanocytes' inability to produce melanin, rather than the absence of melanocytes (Chortos et al., 2016).

6.1.2.7. Other Cell Types

Langerhans' and Merkel's cells are two additional types of cells found in the epidermis. Langerhans' cells are distributed throughout the epidermis, with a higher concentration in the upper layers of the stratum malpighii. During regular sections, the cells exhibit prominently stained, sizable, intricately folded nuclei encased by a transparent cytoplasm. Under specific stains, these cells are observed to have a star-like shape and project elongated cytoplasmic extensions into the stratum spinosum. The nucleus exhibits a markedly irregular shape in electron micrographs, while the cytoplasm is devoid of keratin filaments, desmosomes, and melanosomes. However, it is distinguished by the presence of membrane-bound, rod-shaped granules with a consistent, granular interior. Certain granules seem to be directly connected to the cell membrane. Langerhans' cells capture antigens that enter the skin and carry them to nearby lymph nodes. These cells, known as antigen-presenting cells, are derived from a precursor cell called monocyte in the bone marrow. They play a role in a delayed immune response called type IV delayed-type reaction, mediated by T lymphocytes.

Merkel cells are typically located near exposed sensory nerve endings in the basal layer of the skin and create Merkel cell-neurite complexes. Merkel's cells, similar to melanocytes, originate in the neural crest. Morphologically, Merkel's cells exhibit similarities to cells found in the stratum Basale. However, electron micrographs reveal distinct characteristics of these cells, including indented nuclei, prominent Golgi complexes, and a high abundance of dense-cored vesicles. The vesicles exhibit a tendency to accumulate at the basal region where nerve endings converge. The precise function of Merkel's cells remains uncertain, although they are believed to potentially serve as mechanoreceptors. They potentially contribute to sensory processes and have been likened to cells containing polypeptides and hormones, although a definitive connection has not been confirmed.

6.1.3. Dermis

The dermis, also known as the corium, exhibits variations in thickness across different areas of the body. The skin is particularly thin and fragile in the eyelids, scrotum, and prepuce. It is considerably thicker in the palms and soles. It is also thicker on the back side of the body compared to the front. Furthermore, it is thicker in men than in women. The dermis is a resilient and pliable layer of skin that is composed of a network of collagen fibers interspersed with elastic fibers within a matrix containing glycosaminoglycans. The connective tissue is organized into two distinct layers: the deep reticular layer and the superficial papillary layer.

The reticular layer, which is the thicker and denser portion of the dermis, is composed of intertwined bundles of collagen fibers that predominantly align parallel to the skin's surface. The reticular layer gradually blends with the subcutaneous tissue (hypodermis), which typically consists of numerous adipose cells. The predominant type of collagen in the reticular layer is type I. The reticular layer of the dermis is a prime illustration of dense irregular connective tissue. In animals, the layer is referred to as the one used for manufacturing leather products such as shoes, belts, and coats. The reticular layer of the dermis acts as a fibroelastic covering that tightly encloses and surrounds the contents of the limbs, trunk, neck, and head (Chun et al., 2021).

The papillary layer is situated directly beneath the epidermis and protrudes into it through structures called dermal papillae. The boundary between the papillary layer and the reticular layer is not easily distinguishable, however, the collagen fibers and bundles in the papillary layer are typically thinner and less tightly organized. This layer exhibits a higher concentration of ground substance and displays a greater number of cells, resulting in a more cellular appearance. The majority of the collagen present is type III. The reticular fibers located just below the epidermis are oriented vertically. Elastic fibers are present in the deeper regions of the papillary layer.

Dermal papillae are small, cone-shaped projections with rounded or blunt tips that fit into corresponding indentations on the undersurface of the epidermis. They are most noticeable on the palm and fingers, where they are densely clustered and aligned in parallel lines that match the ridges on the skin's surface. The papillae contain capillary loops, and in certain areas, such as the palms and fingers, there are nerve endings and tactile corpuscles. The epidermis, similar to other epithelial tissues, lacks blood vessels and depends on diffusion across the basement membrane to obtain nutrients. The exchange process deep within the epidermis is facilitated by capillaries located within the dermal papillae. Smooth muscle cells are found in the deeper regions of the reticular layer in the penis, scrotum, perineum, and areola. Contraction of the smooth muscle cells causes the skin in these areas to wrinkle. The arrectores pilorum muscles are compact clusters of smooth muscle cells that are connected to hair follicles. Their contraction leads to the formation of "goose bumps."

6.1.3.1. Dermatoglyphics

The volar surface of the fingers, hands, feet, and toes all have ridges that are normal features of the skin. Additionally, it is believed that they enhance the sense of touch in addition to their function as anti-slip devices. The ridges compose three primary patterns, which are loops, whorls, and arches. In terms of patterns on the fingers, loops are the most common, while arches are the least common. Even though the ridge patterns on the toes are comparable to those on the fingers, the toes have a greater number of arches and a smaller number of whorls. The ridge pattern cn be established at an early age, and it is permanent. The pattern is different from one digit to the next in every person, and it is highly improbable that the sequence of patterns would be the same in a group of people who are entirely unrelated to one another (Chun et al., 2021).

6.1.4. Appendages of the Skin

The appendages of the skin are derived from the epidermis and include hair, nails, and sweat and sebaceous glands.

6.1.4.1. Nails

Nails are rigid, keratinized formations that encase the upper surfaces of the fingertips and toes. The nail is composed of a visible section called the nail plate and a proximal part known as the root, which is embedded into a groove in the skin. The base of the nail is covered by the proximal nail fold, a skin fold that extends along the sides of the nail and forms the lateral nail folds. The stratum corneum of the proximal nail fold covers the top surface of the nail root and extends a short distance onto the body of the nail. This creates a thin cuticular fold known as the eponychium. The skin is connected to the underside of the nail, creating the hyponychium, at the free edge of the nail. The nail is a derivative of the cornified region of the epidermis and is composed of multiple layers of flattened cells with atrophied, degenerated nuclei. The cells are firm, strongly attached, and predominantly transparent and translucent throughout the majority of the nail's structure. The pink hue of the nails is a result of the transmission of color from the underlying capillary bed. In close proximity to the base, the nail appears less transparent and takes on a curved shape, forming a crescent-shaped region known as the lunule. This lunule is most prominent on the thumb but gradually becomes smaller and less visible as it is covered by the proximal nail fold towards the little finger. The lunule is the area where nail growth starts.

The nail bed is located beneath the nail and corresponds to the stratum malpighii of the skin. The structure is composed of keratinocytes and a basal layer that is supported by a basement membrane. The dermis beneath is characterized by multiple longitudinal ridges that are highly vascularized. In close proximity to the base, the ridges exhibit reduced size and diminished vascularity. The nail matrix, located beneath the root and lunule, is a thicker and highly proliferative area responsible for the growth of the nail. The nail bed located underneath the remaining part of the nail is comparatively thinner and does not participate in the process of nail growth. The cells in the deepest layer of the matrix are cylindrical in shape and undergo frequent cell division, while above them are multiple layers of polyhedral cells and flattened squames, which are the cells that undergo differentiation to form the nail. Hard keratin, also known as nail keratin, contains a greater amount of sulfur compared to the keratin found in the epidermis (Ham et al., 2021) (**Figure 6.2**).

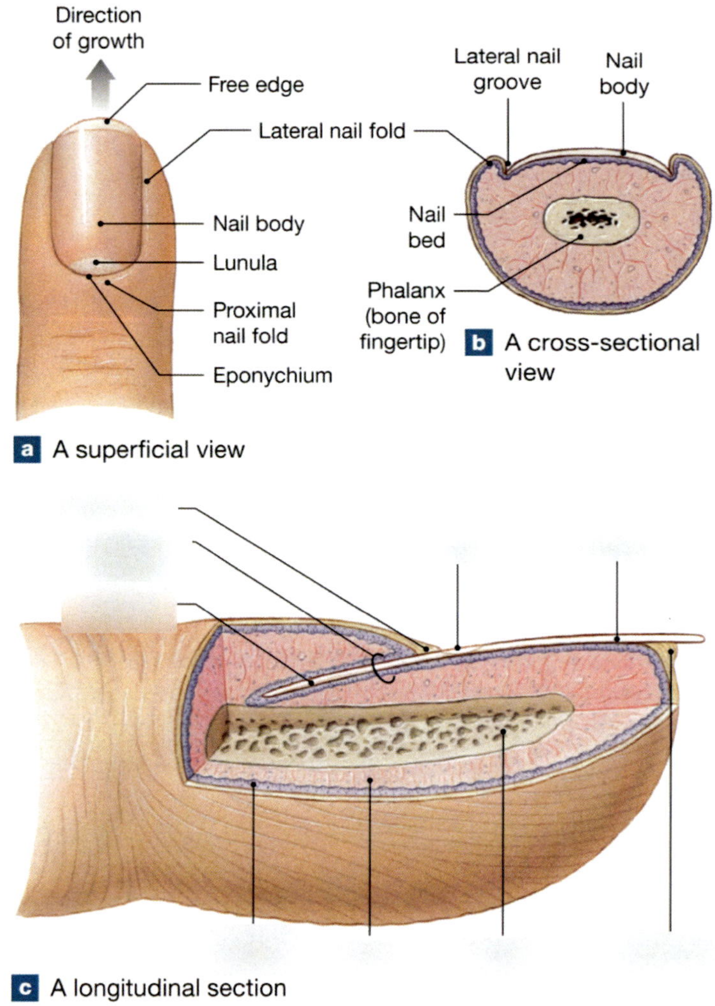

Figure 6.2. *A diagrammatic sketch illustrating a longitudinal profile through a nail.*

Source: https://o.quizlet.com/4hPZdIEvJc6s8qQXz5c2lg_b.png.

6.1.4.2. Hair

Hair is found on most areas of the skin, except for the palms of the hands, soles of the feet, edges of the lips, foreskin, penis glans, clitoris, inner labia, and inner surfaces of the outer labia. The threads are composed of flexible keratin and exhibit variations in length and thickness across different body regions and races. Starting from the midpoint of fetal development, the skin is enveloped in a delicate type of hair known as lanugo. This hair is mostly shed before birth and is subsequently replaced by soft and fine vellus hair. Vellus hair is present in most areas of the body, characterized by their short length, soft texture, and lack of color. For example, the vellus hair on the forehead is typically short, soft, and colorless. In the scalp and eyebrows, vellus hair are replaced by thicker terminal hair, which also grows as axillary and pubic hair. In men, this hair type is responsible for beard and chest hair growth.

6.1.4.3. Structure of Hair

Every hair is composed of a root that is deeply embedded in the skin and a hair shaft that extends to a varying length above the surface of the epidermis. The shaft has a circular or elliptical shape when viewed in cross-section and consists of three concentric layers. The medulla, also known as the core, consists of flattened, cornified, polyhedral cells with pyknotic or absent nuclei. Lanugo, a type of thin fine hair, lacks a medulla. Additionally, the medulla may be absent in scalp hair or only partially extend along the shaft. The cortex, which makes up most of the hair, is composed of multiple layers of highly keratinized, elongated cells densely packed together. The majority of the pigment in colored hair is located in the cortex and is distributed within the cells and the spaces between them. The cortex contains variable accumulations of air spaces located both between and within the cells. The graying of hair is caused by both the fading of pigment and an increase in the number of air spaces. The outermost layer is delicate and constitutes the cuticle (Ham et al., 2021). The structure is composed of a singular layer of transparent, flattened, squamous cells arranged in an overlapping manner, resembling shingles, from the bottom to the top. The hair root is deeply embedded within the dermis. The hair root expands at its lower end to form the hair bulb. This bulb is indented on its deep surface by a conical projection of the dermis, referred to as a papilla. Papillae house blood vessels that supply nutrients to the developing and specialized cells of the hair bulb. The root's structure varies slightly from that of the shaft. The cells in the lower root region, specifically in the medulla and cortex, are typically cuboidal in shape and have normal nuclei. As the root reaches higher levels, the nuclei become less clear and eventually disappear. The cells of the cortex gradually undergo flattening as they approach the skin's surface.

6.1.4.4. Hair Follicle

The base of every hair is contained within a cylindrical covering known as the hair follicle, comprising an inner layer of epithelial cells and an outer layer of connective tissue. The epithelial component originates from the epidermis and is composed of both inner and outer root sheaths. The connective tissue sheath originates from the dermis. The inner epithelial root sheath is formed by the outermost layers of the epidermis that have folded inward from the surface and undergone differentiation to form three distinct layers. The most internal layer is the cuticle of the root sheath, which is adjacent to the cuticle of the hair shaft. The cells are flat and plate-like, arranged in overlapping layers from top to bottom. The exposed edges of these cells interlock with the exposed edges of the cells in the hair cuticle. Huxley's layer consists of elongated cells surrounding the cuticle of the inner epithelial root sheath. The cells in question possess granules that bear resemblance to keratohyalin granules, but they differ in terms of their chemical composition. These granules are referred to as trichohyalin granules. Henle's layer, a thin layer of transparent, flattened cells containing keratin filaments, encircles Huxley's layer. The cells in these three layers contain nuclei in their distal regions, but the nuclei disappear as the inner epithelial root sheath gets closer to the surface. The outer epithelial root sheath is a direct extension of the stratum malpighii. The outermost cells are columnar and arranged in a single row. At the surface, they seamlessly connect with the stratum Basale of the epidermis (Hu et al., 2021). The inner layers of cells are indistinguishable from and seamlessly connected to the prickle cells of the stratum spinosum. The follicle's connective tissue component is composed of three layers. The glassy (vitreous) membrane, which is similar to the basement membrane, is a narrow, transparent band that tightly adheres to the columnar cells of the outer epithelial root sheath. The intermediate stratum is composed of delicate, concentrically organized collagenous fibers. The outermost layer is indistinct and consists of collagen fibers organized in lax, longitudinal bundles interspersed with a few elastic fibers. The hair root forms a swollen enlargement around the papilla. The cells within the hair bulb are not organized in layers; instead, they constitute a matrix of actively growing cells. The matrix cells located at the apex of the papilla undergo differentiation to form the medulla of a hair. The cells in the slopes differentiate into the cortex and medulla. Horizontally, the cells of the bulb create the inner epithelial root sheath. Pigmentation arises as a result of the functioning of melanocytes found in the matrix. Figure 6.3 illustrates the anatomical composition of a hair and its corresponding hair follicle.

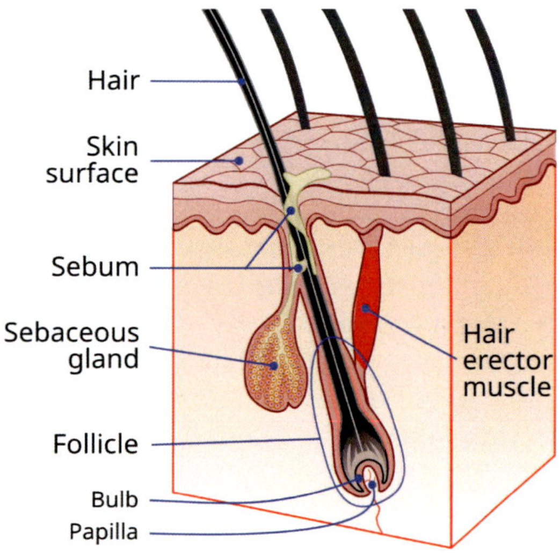

Figure 6.3. *A diagrammatic sketch illustrating the structure of a hair and a hair follicle.*

Source: https://upload.wikimedia.org/wikipedia/commons/thumb/4/4d/Hair_follicle-en.svg/800px-Hair_follicle-en.svg.png.

6.1.4.5. Hair Cycle

Hair growth occurs in cycles, including phases of active growth (anagen), diminishing growth (catagen), and rest (telogen). The cyclical activity persists throughout an individual's lifespan, although the stages of the cycle vary with age. By the fifth month of gestation, all the hairare in the anagen phase, which is characterized by a consistent and uniform growth pattern that is not observed at any other time. During the period of 8 to 10 weeks prior to birth, certain hair follicles have entered the catagen and telogen stages. Hair shedding first occurs in the frontal and parietal scalp areas, while in the occipital region, hair remains in the anagen phase until after birth. Starting approximately 6 weeks prior to birth, telogen hair reemerge on the frontal and parietal scalp, signifying the onset of a second phase of hair growth. Typically, all hair follicles transition into the telogen phase shortly after birth, resulting in a subsequent period of hair loss. Subsequently, the phases exhibit greater irregularity. Approximately 18 weeks after birth, hair growth cycles become linked to individual strands or clusters of strands. The hair cycles in adults differ depending on the region of the body. The complete hair cycle in the scalp lasts approximately 300 weeks, with telogen phase lasting for approximately 18 to 19 weeks (Hu et al., 2021).

6.1.4.6. Sebaceous Glands

Sebaceous glands are found throughout most of the skin and are particularly abundant in the scalp and face, as well as around the anus, mouth, and nose. They are not present on the palms of the hands and soles of the feet. Typically, sebaceous glands are connected to hair and empty into the upper region of the hair follicle. On the lips, glans penis, inner surface of the prepuce, and labia minora, these glands directly open onto the skin's surface, without any connection to hair. The glands exhibit size variation and are composed of a group of two to five oval alveoli drained by a solitary duct. The secretory alveoli are located in the dermis and consist of epithelial cells surrounded by a clearly defined basement membrane and supported by a thin connective tissue capsule. The cells adjacent to the basement membrane are characterized by their small size, cuboidal shape, and possession of round nuclei. The alveolus is completely filled with cells that, at the center, enlarge and become polyhedral, gradually accumulating fatty material in their cytoplasm. The nuclei undergo compression and pyknosis and ultimately vanish. The secretion is classified as holocrine, which indicates that the entire cell disintegrates and releases sebum, along with cellular debris and the secretory product consisting of triglycerides, cholesterol, and wax esters. Sebaceous glands do not have myoepithelial cells, but they are closely associated with the arrector pili muscle. Contraction of this cohesive group of smooth muscle fibers aids in the release of secretory substances from the sebaceous glands. Smooth muscle bundles are found in the connective tissue between the alveoli of the glands in the nipple. The sebaceous gland's duct is lined by stratified squamous epithelium, which is an extension of the outer epithelial root sheath of the hair follicle. The majority of secretory cells in the alveolus are replenished through the division of cells located near the walls of the ducts, particularly at their junctions with the alveoli. Cell replacement occurs at the outer edges of the alveoli. The pilosebaceous apparatus is the collective term for the hair follicle, hair shaft, sebaceous gland, and erector pili muscle. The pilosebaceous apparatus is responsible for the production of hair and sebum. Sebum serves as a protective layer for the hair and acts as a lubricant for the epidermis, safeguarding it against the dehydrating impacts of the surroundings. During puberty, the sebaceous glands become more active. This increased activity is regulated by hormones, specifically androgens, which stimulate the glands, and estrogens, which inhibit their activity (Hu et al., 2021).

6.1.4.7. Sweat Glands

There are two types of sweat glands: eccrine and apocrine. Eccrine sweat glands are the ordinary type, while apocrine glands are found in areas like the armpits and groin. Eccrine sweat glands are present in all areas of the skin except for the lip margins, glans penis, inner surface of the prepuce, clitoris, and labia minora. In other areas, the numbers differ, with a high abundance in the palms and soles and a lower quantity in the neck and back. Every gland is a basic cylindrical structure. The profound section is intricately twisted and constitutes the secretory unit within the profound dermis. The secretory unit comprises a single layer of columnar epithelial cells resting on a substantial basement membrane.

There are two types of cells: clear cells and dark cells

The basal region of the dark cells is narrow, while the luminal surface is broad. Electron micrographs reveal the presence of numerous ribosomes, secretory vacuoles, and a small number of mitochondria. The cells release glycoproteins, which have been found in secretory vacuoles. Clear cells exhibit a wide base and a narrow apex. Intercellular canaliculi connect neighboring clear cells, which are rich in glycogen, have a significant amount of smooth endoplasmic reticulum and many mitochondria, but have few ribosomes. The cell's basolateral plasmalemma exhibits extensive and intricate infoldings. Clear cells are believed to secrete sodium, chloride, potassium, urea, uric acid, ammonia, and water.

The myoepithelial cells are situated in the vicinity of the secretory part, positioned between the basal lamina and the bases of the secretory cells. These stellate cells have the ability to contract and are thought to assist in the release of secretions. Eccrine sweat glands are drained by a slender duct that initially coils and subsequently straightens as it traverses the dermis to reach the epidermis. The duct is composed of a double layer of cuboidal cells. The cells of the inner layer exhibit clusters of filaments arranged in a terminal web at their luminal surfaces. The epithelium is situated on a basal lamina and does not contain myoepithelial cells. Within the epidermis, the duct comprises a helical passageway that is essentially a gap between the epidermis cells. The cells directly surrounding the inner space of the duct are arranged in a circular manner.

Acetylcholine is released by postganglionic sympathetic neurons to regulate the function of eccrine sweat glands, which are responsible for controlling body temperature (cholinergic innervation). Conversely, in cases of emotional sweating, the eccrine sweat glands are regulated by postganglionic sympathetic neurons that secrete norepinephrine (adrenergic innervation). Apocrine sweat glands are eccrine sweat glands that have been enlarged and modified. Their secretions are more viscous than those of the typical eccrine sweat glands and consist of glycoproteins, lipids, glycolipids, and pheromones. Their histologic structure also varies from eccrine sweat glands in several aspects (Hu et al., 2019). Apocrine sweat glands are tubular glands with coiled structures. The secretory units of these glands are lined by columnar cells. The secretory tubules of these glands have a significantly larger diameter compared to the tubules of eccrine sweat glands. Their myoepithelial cells exhibit greater size and abundance, and there is a singular type of secreting cell that bears resemblance to the dark cells found in eccrine glands. The ducts of these sweat glands are analogous to those of regular sweat glands, with the distinction that they discharge into a hair follicle instead of directly onto the epidermis. Apocrine gland secretion is classified as merocrine and does not result in any loss of cellular structure. Despite being retained, the term "apocrine" is incorrectly used to describe these glands. During puberty, the apocrine sweat glands become more active due to the influence of hormones such as androgens and estrogens. Additionally, they are innervated by postganglionic sympathetic neurons that release norepinephrine (adrenergic innervation). The ceruminous glands in the external auditory canal are apocrine glands that are coiled and tubular in structure. They consist of a secretory portion and a duct, which may have branching. The glands located at the edges of the eyelids, known as Moll's glands, are simple coiled tubular apocrine glands. However, they differ from other glands in that the end portions have less coiling and wider lumina.

6.1.5. Organogenesis

The skin has a dual origin: the epidermis and its appendages originate from the ectoderm, while the dermis is formed from the mesoderm. At first, the outer layer of the embryo is coated with a solitary layer of cuboidal cells that rest on a basal lamina. Only a limited number of desmosomes connect the cells that are arranged loosely. Proliferation results in the formation of two distinct layers: an outer periderm and an inner basal layer. The periderm is the outermost layer forms in the fetus between 2 to 6 months of development. It acts as a protective covering for the "epidermis proper" before it undergoes keratinization. The structure comprises a solitary layer of flattened, polygonal cells that possess microvilli on their exposed surfaces in humans. The periderm functions to safeguard the epidermis and potentially facilitates certain exchanges between the fetus and amniotic fluid. Small protrusions resembling blebs emerge on the surfaces of the periderm cells, reaching their peak development during the early stages of the sixth week and subsequently diminishing in size. Simultaneously, blebbing occurs, and the cell membrane undergoes changes that resemble those observed during the keratinization of mature epidermal cells.

After the epidermis undergoes keratinization, the periderm sheds and its cells combine with sebaceous secretions to create the vernix caseosa, an oily layer that covers the newborn's skin. In the 1- and 2-month-old fetus, the basal layer is the sole component of the epidermis proper. The germinative layer is responsible for the generation of all epidermal cells. During the initial two months, the peridermal and epidermal cells contain glycogen and have a limited number of organelles. During the second month, clusters of filaments form within the epidermal cells, along with desmosomes and hemidesmosomes. Additional intermediate filaments, likely composed of keratin, are distributed throughout the cytoplasm. The basal cells undergo glycogen depletion and acquire adult morphology as the initial step, and as they multiply, more layers are formed between the periderm and the basal layer. The initial intermediate cells emerge between 9 and 10 weeks, and the layer reaches full development by 11 weeks. The second and third layers are added in the fourth month (Hu et al., 2023).

The cytoplasm of the intermediate cells is abundant in glycogen, while desmosomes and filaments are also highly noticeable. As the quantity of intracellular keratin filaments rises, the level of glycogen decreases. The outermost intermediate cells undergo the accumulation of laminar granules at their upper borders, followed by the differentiation into cells with cornified cell membranes, bundles of keratin filaments, and small quantities of glycogen in their cytoplasm. After the formation of the stratum granulosum, authentic cornified cells emerge, and a thin stratum corneum becomes noticeable within 6 months. Therefore, by the conclusion of the second trimester, all the strata of the epidermis have been formed. In the second month, melanocytes migrate from the neural crest into the epidermis. By the fourth month, they begin synthesizing melanin. Langerhans' cells migrate to the epidermis from the bone marrow in the third month, while Merkel's cells are initially observed in specific areas (such as the nail bed and fingertips) during the sixteenth week. Merkel's cells are derived from the neural crest. The initial surface ridges emerge on the palmar and plantar surfaces of the fingertips around the thirteenth week of development. The ridges subsequently expand to cover the complete volar surfaces of the hands and feet. The pattern that emerges during this period persists throughout an individual's lifetime. The dermis forms through the consolidation of neighboring mesenchymal cells. The fibroblasts undergo differentiation, resulting in the emergence of collagen and elastic fibers. The dermis quickly becomes clearly defined and structured into papillary and reticular layers. At first, the dermo-epidermal junction is even, but soon after, dermal ridges emerge and become distinguishable by the third to fourth month of pregnancy. The epidermal appendages, such as nails, hair, sweat glands, and sebaceous glands, develop as extensions of the original epidermis. Hairoriginate from compact strands of epidermis known as hair buds, which extend into the dermis at an inclined angle. The hair bud consists of an outer layer of columnar cells and an inner core of polygonal cells. The hair bulb, the deepest part of the hair bud, enlarges and takes the shape of a cup over a small mound of mesenchyme, known as the hair papilla. The initial dermal connective tissue that runs along the hair bud undergoes condensation to give rise to the connective tissue sheath of the hair follicle. The cells located on the outer edge of the hair bud are responsible for producing the outer layer of the root sheath, while the central mass of cells forms the main structure of the hair. Sebaceous glands originate from the thickened outer epithelial root sheath. Cell clusters develop into the adjacent mesenchyme, forming multiple flask-shaped alveoli. The cells lining the surface, originating from the stratum germinativum, rapidly multiply, causing older cells to move towards the center. In this process, they produce fats, undergo degeneration, and ultimately form sebum. The root sheath of the hair contains a cellular bulge that is located below the sebaceous glands. This bulge serves as the point of attachment for the arrectores pilorum muscles, which originate from mesenchyme separately. Eccrine sweat glands originate as solid extensions of the epidermis. As these lengthen, the inner parts become twisted to create the secretory units of the glands. A lumen is formed within each cord, which subsequently transforms into a tube that has an opening towards the surface. A bilayer of epithelial cells covers the ductal connection. Myoepithelial cells, which are connected to the secretory parts of the glands, originate from the nearby epidermal bud. Apocrine sweat glands originate from superficial epidermal swellings located on hair follicles. These glands release their secretions into the uppermost section of the follicle.

6.2. The Eye

The eyes are sensory organs with convex surfaces that capture and focus light onto a surface capable of detecting its intensity and color. The images formed in the eye are conveyed to the brain, where they are analyzed, connected, and transformed into the perception of vision (Alberts et al., 2002). The eyes have the ability to control the amount of light that enters and adjust their focal lengths. They are nearly spherical and are situated within bony sockets, which are equipped with a layer of fat for protection. Binocular vision is achieved due to the eyes' different positions, resulting in offset images. The fusion of the binocular images leads to the perception of a three-dimensional visual experience, enabling the recognition of depth and spatial orientation.

6.2.1. General Structure

The structure of the eyeball is composed of three layers: the outer corneoscleral coat, the central uvea, and the inner retina. The corneoscleral coat consists of two distinct parts: the anterior cornea, which is a smaller, transparent structure that permits the passage of light into the eye, and the sclera, a larger segment that is white in color. The sclera is a resilient fibrous membrane that safeguards the fragile internal components of the eye and aids in preserving the spherical form of the eyeball. The uveal coat comprises the choroid, ciliary body, and iris. The choroid is the highly vascularized component of the uvea, located directly beneath the retina. The iris is connected to the ciliary body, which encircles the inside of the eyeball, located just in front of the front edge of the retina. The ciliary body regulates the size and curvature of the lens, which is responsible for directing light onto the retina. The iris, the final segment of the uvea, is connected to the ciliary body and contains a central aperture called the pupil. The pupil diameter can be adjusted to control the quantity of light entering the eyeball. The retina is composed of photoreceptors that contain pigments. When these photoreceptors are exposed to light, they generate chemical energy, which is then converted into electrical energy in the form of nerve impulses. The transmission of impulses to the optic nerve occurs through a series of interconnected neurons in the retina. The optic disc is the convergence point of retinal nerve fibers, where they coalesce to form the optic nerve and exit the eyeball. The interior of the eyeball is divided into three compartments: the anterior chamber, the posterior chamber, and the vitreal cavity. Each is filled with a transparent substance that assists in preserving the form and firmness of the eye. The anterior and posterior chambers of the eye are connected by the pupil and contain a watery fluid called aqueous humor. This fluid nourishes the front structures of the eye. The vitreous cavity, which is spacious, contains a dense and clear gel known as the vitreous humor or vitreous body. Figure 6.4 illustrates the overall anatomy of the eye (Hua et al., 2021).

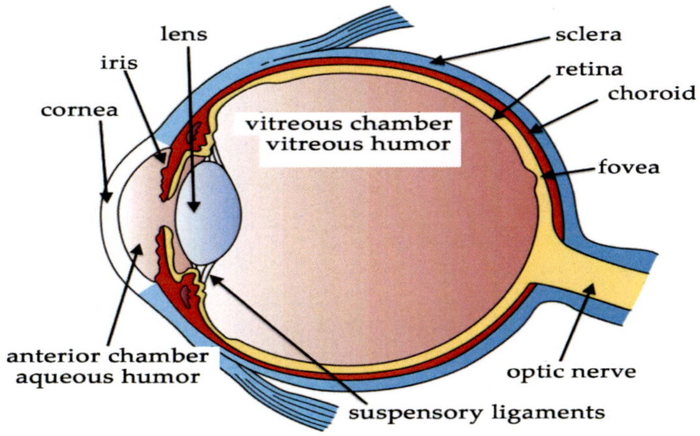

Figure 6.4. *A diagrammatic sketch of general eye structure.*

Source: https://harvardeye.com/wp-content/uploads/2018/08/Diagram-of-the-Eye.png.

6.2.2. Corneoscleral Coat

The corneoscleral coat forms the outermost layer of the eyeball and consists of the cornea and sclera.

6.2.2.1. Sclera

The sclera is the strong, non-transparent, fibrous outer layer that covers the back five-sixths of the eyeball. The thickness of the material differs across various regions but has an average measurement of approximately 0.5 mm. The structure consists of flattened bundles of collagen that are oriented in different directions, running parallel to the surface of the sclera (Hua et al., 2021). The collagen bundles are connected by intricate networks of elastic fibers and elongated, flattened fibroblasts. Melanocytes are present in the underlying scleral layers. The sclera becomes thinner and creates a fenestrated membrane called the lamina cribrosa, located where the optic nerve fibers pass through the sclera to leave the eye.

The sclera safeguards the inner part of the eye, assists in preserving its form, and acts as the point of attachment for the extrinsic ocular muscles.

6.2.2.2. Cornea

The cornea, which is transparent, is located at the frontmost part of the eye. The diameter of the object is approximately 11 mm, with a thickness of about 0.8 mm near the center and 1.00 mm at the periphery. The curvature of the anterior sclera is significantly higher than that of the posterior sclera. The cornea is structurally consistent and composed of corneal epithelium, Bowman's membrane, substantia propria, Descemet's membrane, and corneal endothelium. The corneal epithelium comprises multiple layers of flat cells and has a uniformly even outer surface. It has an average depth of approximately 50 μm. The structure typically comprises five layers of large flat cells with few cellular structures but frequently contain glycogen. The nuclei of the superficial cells remain intact, and their outer surfaces develop multiple small ridges (microplicae) that aid in retaining moisture on the surface of the cornea. The epithelium is situated on a clearly defined basal lamina. The lateral membranes of neighboring cells are intricately intertwined and connected by numerous desmosomes. The corneal epithelium is rich in numerous unencumbered nerve endings and is highly sensitive to various stimuli, particularly pain. Bowman's membrane, also known as the basal lamina of the corneal epithelium, is located on the outer layer of the substantia propria. It terminates abruptly at the peripheral edge of the cornea. Bowman's membrane exhibits a uniform appearance and comprises a mesh-like structure of small collagen fibrils (specifically type I) while lacking elastin. The substantia propria, also known as the stroma, comprises most of the cornea. The cornea is composed of multiple bundles of collagen fibers, specifically type I and type V, organized into 50–70 wide sheets known as corneal lamellae. These lamellae are aligned parallel to the surface of the cornea. The collagen bundles in each consecutive lamina exhibit distinct orientations and intersect at diverse angles. The adjacent lamellae are tightly interconnected through the interlacing of collagenous fibers. The collagen fibers, bundles, and lamellae are enclosed within a matrix that contains high levels of sulfated proteoglycans, specifically chondroitin sulfate and keratosulfate. The sclera does not contain these proteoglycans. Keratocytes, which are flattened fibroblast-like cells, can be found among the collagen fiber bundles. The substantia propria typically lacks blood vessels and lymphatics, although sporadic lymphoid wandering cells may be observed.

Descemet's membrane is a uniform membrane, with a thickness of 6 to 8 μm, located between the back surface of the substantia propria and the corneal endothelium. It is a thick basal lamina that is produced by the corneal endothelium. The material demonstrates resilience and elasticity despite the absence of elastic fibers and appears to primarily consist of collagen in the form of type VIII. The corneal endothelium is a layer of large, hexagonal squamous cells that covers the inner surface of the cornea. The uppermost points of the cells are connected by tight junctions, and the cytoplasm contains a large number of mitochondria and vesicles. The cells participate in transporting substances from the anterior chamber (Hua and Shen, 2023). The cornea's transparency results from the consistent size and organized alignment of collagen fibers, along with the specific characteristics of the ground substance. The cornea lacks blood vessels and relies on the aqueous humor and blood vessels in the surrounding limbus to provide it with nutrients. The ion pumps in the corneal endothelial cells regulate the fluid level in the substantia propria to ensure it remains crucial. When there is an excessive buildup of fluid, the cornea becomes cloudy. Corneal endothelial cells exhibit postnatal quiescence and lack regenerative capacity. Every individual is naturally endowed with a full set of corneal endothelial cells.

6.2.2.3. Limbus

The limbus is a narrow region, measuring 1.5 to 2.0 mm in width, that acts as a boundary between the clear cornea and the non-transparent sclera. The external surface features a shallow groove known as the external scleral sulcus, which is the point where the more convex cornea connects with the sclera. On the inner surface of the limbus, there is a corresponding structure called the internal scleral sulcus. The scleral spur is a ridge of tissue that extends from the back edge of the internal scleral sulcus and is connected to the tissue responsible for draining fluid from the front part of the eye. The limbus is distinguished by the terminations of Bowman's and Descemet's membranes. In this region, the collagen fibers and bundles of the cornea increase in size, and their organization becomes more disordered as they merge with those of the sclera. In this area, many small blood vessels create arcades and nourish the outer parts of the cornea, which lacks blood vessels. The spongy trabecular meshwork, which is connected to the anterior part of the scleral spur, takes the place of Descemet's membrane. The structure consists of many flattened, interconnected trabeculae of collagen fibers and ground substance. These trabeculae are covered by a thin endothelium that is connected to the endothelium of the cornea. The trabeculae create a complex network of interconnected spaces that connect with the anterior chamber. Schlemm's canal, a flattened canal lined with endothelial cells, runs around the circumference of the cornea, between the limbal stroma and the trabecular meshwork. The aqueous humor flows into the trabecular spaces from the front chamber and passes through the endothelial lining of the trabeculae, the juxtacanalicular connective tissue, and, ultimately, the endothelium of the canal to enter its inner space. Multiple channels originate from the outer wall of the canal and connect with veins in the limbus, ultimately emptying into episcleral veins. Blockage of the flow of aqueous humor leads to an increase in pressure inside the eye, which is a defining feature of the medical condition known as glaucoma (Kim et al., 2020).

6.2.3. Uveal Layer

The uvea, the middle vascular coat of the eye, is divided into the choroid, ciliary body, and iris.

3.2.3.1. Choroid

The choroid is a thin, brown, highly vascular membrane that covers the inner surface of the back part of the sclera. The suprachoroid lamina is a delicate, pigmented layer connected to the sclera by thin avascular lamellae. The lamellae primarily comprise delicate elastic fibers interspersed with numerous prominent, flat melanocytes and dispersed macrophages. The lamellae traverse the perichoroidal space, which is a potential gap located between the sclera and choroid, to reach the choroid proper. The choroid proper is composed of three distinct regions. The external layer of the vessel is composed of lax connective tissue with abundant melanocytes and houses the major branches of ciliary arteries and veins. The central choriocapillary layer comprises a network of capillaries lined by an endothelium with fenestrations. These blood vessels supply the outer layers of the retina with the necessary nutrients. The choriocapillary layer terminates in close proximity to the ora serrata. The innermost layer of the choroid is the Bruch's membrane, which is located between the rest of the choroid and the pigment epithelium of the retina. Under the light microscope, it is observed as a uniform layer, measuring 1 to 4 μm in thickness. The ultrastructure reveals five distinct layers consisting of basal laminae of capillaries in the choriocapillary layer, the pigment epithelium of the retina, and two thin layers of collagen separated by a delicate elastic network.

3.2.3.2. Ciliary Body

The ciliary body is situated between the ora serrata of the neural retina and the outer edge of the iris. It is attached to the posterior aspect of the scleral spur at the corneoscleral junction. When observed under a light microscope, it appears as a narrow triangle. It comprises an inner vascular layer and a cluster of smooth muscle located right next to the sclera. The inner surface is lined with ciliary epithelium, a continuation of the pigment epithelium of the retina and does not contain light-sensitive cells. The ciliary epithelium is composed of two layers: an inner layer of non-pigmented cells and an outer layer of pigmented cells. Each layer is supported by its basal lamina. What makes it unique is that the apices of both cell layers are closely aligned, with the apex of one layer touching that of the other.

The pigmented cell layer on the outer side is distinct from the stroma of the ciliary body by a thin basal lamina connected to the basal lamina underlying the pigment epithelium in the rest of the retina. The basal lamina of the non-pigmented layer is located next to the posterior chamber of the eye and is connected to the inner limiting membrane of the retina. The plasmalemma of the non-pigmented cells exhibits a multitude of infoldings and plays a role in the transportation of ions and fluids. The cells possess a large number of mitochondria and a highly developed Golgi complex located above the nucleus. The neighboring pigmented cells of the outer layer also exhibit prominent basal infoldings, and their cytoplasm is densely packed with melanin granules. The apices of cells in the inner, non-pigmented epithelium are connected by well-developed tight junctions. These junctions make up the anatomical part of the blood-aqueous barrier, which selectively controls the movement of substances between the blood and the interior of the eye. The ciliary epithelium produces aqueous humor, which has a different electrolyte composition and lower protein content than blood plasma. The posterior chamber is filled with aqueous humor, which serves as a **source** of nutrients for the lens. Additionally, the aqueous humor flows into the vitreous humor towards the back. It moves forward from the back chamber through the pupil into the front chamber and helps nourish the cornea. The fluid exits the front part of the eye, known as the anterior chamber, through a network of tissue called the trabecular meshwork and a canal called Schlemm's canal, and then drains into the veins surrounding the eye called episcleral veins. The inner surface of the ciliary body comprises 60 to 80 elongated ridges called ciliary processes. These processes are radially arranged and lined with ciliary epithelium. They also contain a highly vascularized stroma and scattered melanocytes. The zonule fibers, responsible for securing the lens, are primarily generated by the non-pigmented cell layer of the ciliary epithelium and are connected to its basal lamina. They span from the ciliary processes to the equator of the lens. The majority of the ciliary body is composed of smooth muscle, specifically the ciliary muscle, which regulates the shape and, consequently, the focusing ability of the lens. The muscle cells are arranged in regions characterized by circular, radial, and meridional orientations. Sparse connective tissue is formed by numerous elastic fibers and melanocytes between the muscle bundles. The ciliaris muscle plays a crucial role in adjusting the eye's focus. When it contracts, it pulls the ciliary processes forward, which in turn loosens the suspensory ligament (zonule fibers) of the lens. This allows the lens to become more curved and focus on objects that are close to the retina.

3.2.3.3. Iris

The iris is a flat, circular structure that hangs in the watery fluid between the cornea and lens. It contains a round opening in the center, known as the pupil. The iris is connected to the ciliary body at its outer edge and separates the area between the cornea and lens into two chambers: the anterior chamber and the posterior chamber. The anterior chamber is enclosed at its front by the cornea and at its back by the iris and central region of the lens. The posterior chamber is a confined area located between the outer edge of the iris and the outer part of the lens, ciliary zonule, and ciliary processes (Li et al., 2024). The two chambers are connected via the pupil. The front surface of the iris is uneven because of multiple fissures or crypts. The ciliary body is connected to the ciliary margin, while the pupil is surrounded by the pupillary margin.

The iris stroma mainly comprises lax, vascular connective tissue containing dispersed collagenous fibers, melanocytes, and fibroblasts embedded in a uniform ground substance. The front surface does not have a clear layer of endothelial or mesothelial cells, but it is partially covered by a discontinuous layer of melanocytes and fibroblasts. The tissue spaces of the stroma frequently seem to be connected to the anterior chamber. The back surface is coated with two rows of cuboidal, pigmented cells connected to the ciliary epithelium. The inner non-pigmented layer of the ciliary epithelium becomes heavily pigmented as it reaches the posterior surface of the iris. The cells in the outer layer have a reduced amount of pigment and undergo modifications to become myoepithelial cells, which then form the dilator of the iris. The pupil dilator comprises a single layer of myoepithelial cells arranged in a radial pattern. Contraction of these cells enlarges the pupil. The sphincter muscle is composed of a densely packed, circular arrangement of smooth muscle cells located near the edge of the pupil. The sphincter muscle contraction causes a decrease in the pupil's diameter. The iris functions as a diaphragm, regulating the quantity of light that enters the eye, thereby enabling a wide range of vision in different lighting conditions (Li et al., 2023).

The pigmentation of the iris dictates its coloration. In blue eyes, melanin is limited to the back surface of the iris. In contrast, in gray and brown eyes, melanin is present in higher amounts within melanocytes distributed throughout the stroma of the iris. In individuals with albinism, the absence of melanin pigment results in a pink coloration of the iris, which is caused by the presence of blood vessels in the stroma of the iris.

6.2.4. Retina

The retina, the innermost layer of the eye, is a fragile sheet of nervous tissue that serves as the photoreceptor. The outer surface of the object is in direct contact with the choroid, while the inner surface is positioned next to the vitreous body. The posterior retina comprises an outer pigment epithelium and an inner neural retina, also known as the retina proper. The retina gradually becomes thinner towards the front, and its nervous component terminates at an irregular boundary known as the ora serrata. The retina's thin extension extends forward to cover the ciliary processes as the ciliary epithelium. It also covers the back part of the iris, forming the iridia retinae. The anterior extension of the retina comprises solely the pigmented layer and an inner layer of columnar epithelial cells, without the presence of nervous tissue. The neural retina is attached solely at the optic disc, where nerve fibers gather before traversing the sclera to create the optic nerve, and at the ora serrata. While the cells of the pigment epithelium interlock with the photoreceptor cells of the neural retina, there is no physical link between the two parts of the retina. As a result of injury or illness, the neural retina can become separated from the pigment epithelium. The precise midpoint of the back part of the retina aligns with the axis of the eye, and at this specific location, vision is optimal. The macula lutea is a visible diminutive, yellow, oval region. The fovea centralis, located at the center of the retina, is a depression measuring approximately 1.5 mm in diameter. This area contains the highest concentration and most organized arrangement of sensory elements. Moving towards the outer edges of the retina, the neural elements become larger, less numerous, and more unevenly distributed. The optic disc, where the optic nerve forms and exits, is approximately 4.0 mm towards the nasal side of the macula lutea. This region of the retina, lacking photoreceptors, is unresponsive to light and constitutes the "blind spot."

6.2.4.1. Neural Retina

The neural retina, except for the outermost edge and the fovea centralis, consists of nine distinct layers, arranged in the following order under a light microscope, starting from the choroid: The retina is composed of nine distinct layers: (1) a layer of rods and cones, (2) the external limiting membrane, (3) the outer nuclear layer, (4) the outer plexiform layer, (5) the inner nuclear layer, (6) the inner plexiform layer, (7) the ganglion cell layer, (8) the layer of nerve fibers, and (9) the internal limiting membrane. The layer composed of rods and cones corresponds to these photoreceptor cells' inner and outer segments. The rod outer segments are characterized by their darker staining and higher abundance compared to the cone outer segments. The latter are bigger and have a conical form. The external (outer) limiting membrane is situated between this layer and the outer nuclear layer. The line is visible as a distinct and interrupted structure created by the junctional complexes connecting the scleral tips of Müller's cells with neighboring photoreceptor cells. The outer nuclear layer comprises the cellular bodies and nuclei of the rods and cones (Liu et al., 2020). The outer plexiform layer mainly comprises rod spherules, cone pedicles, and dendrites of bipolar neurons. The inner nuclear layer comprises the nuclei and cell bodies of bipolar neurons, horizontal cells, amacrine cells, and Müller's cells. The inner plexiform layer consists of axons from bipolar neurons, dendrites from ganglion cells, and processes from amacrine cells. The ganglion cell layer is composed of ganglion cells and dispersed neuroglial cells. The nerve fiber layer consists mainly of unmyelinated axons derived from ganglion cells and the processes of Müller's cells. The internal limiting membrane, which is extremely thin, is created by the vitreal processes of Müller's cells and their basement membrane. The neural retina, which is structurally intricate, primarily comprises a conducting chain of three neurons that ultimately give rise to the nerve fibers found in the optic nerve. The fundamental components of the conducting chain are photoreceptors (rod and cone cells), bipolar neurons, and ganglion cells (Figure 6.5).

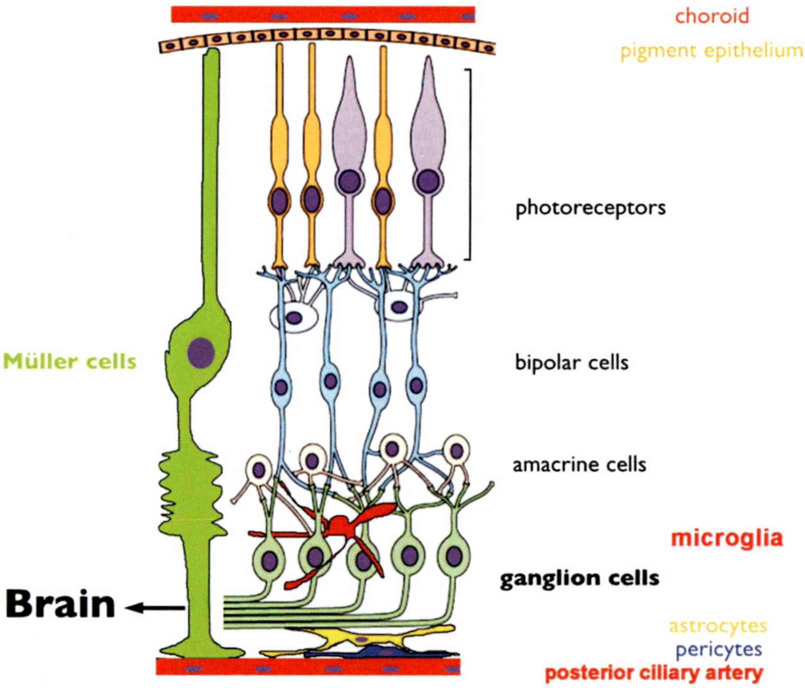

Figure 6.5. *A schematic diagram depicting the fundamental three-neuron chain system of the retina.*

Source: https://www.researchgate.net/profile/Daniel-Ryskamp/publication/265649076/figure/fig1/AS:392055131000832@1470484635131/A-schematic-of-the-retina-showing-overall-arrangement-of-retinal-layers-and-relationship.png.

When exposed to light, photoreceptor cells generate an electrical signal transmitted to bipolar neurons, which then form connections with ganglion cells. Unmyelinated axons originating from the ganglion cells penetrate the layer of retinal nerve fibers and converge at the optic disc to create the optic nerve, which conveys the electrical signal to the brain. Additional intraretinal cells consist of association neurons, such as horizontal cells and amacrine cells, as well as glial cells. The components are arranged in distinct layers within the retina (Luo et al., 2023).

6.2.4.2. Glial Cells

Müller's cells, which span from the outer to the inner limiting membranes of the neural retina, are the largest and most prominent glial elements in the retina. Their cytoplasmic processes traverse the space between the cell bodies and processes of neurons in the retina, offering physical support to the neural components. Müller's cells have a basal lamina that is located next to the vitreal body and serves as the inner limiting membrane of the retina. Müller's cells connect to neighboring photoreceptor cells through junctional complexes, creating the outer limiting membrane. The cytoplasm is abundant in the smooth endoplasmic reticulum and contains a large amount of glycogen. Müller's cells not only provide structural support but also play a role in nourishing other components of the retina. They have been compared to astrocytes in the CNS. A few spindle-shaped glial cells are found surrounding ganglion cells and interspersed among the axons that make up the nerve fiber layer of the retina.

6.2.4.3. Photoreceptor Cells

There are two distinct categories of photoreceptors, namely rod cells and cone cells. Rod cells are elongated, slender cells positioned at a right angle to the layers of the retina. The length of these structures ranges from 40 to 60 μm, while their width varies from 1.5 to 3.0 μm, depending on their position in the retina. The number of these structures in each retina falls between 75 million and 170 million. The rod proper, which constitutes the outer third of each rod, is situated between the pigment epithelium and the outer limiting membrane. The scleral end of the rods is anchored in the retinal pigment epithelium, which plays a crucial role in the phagocytosis of the rod's outer segments. The vitreal end of the rods extends into the outer plexiform layer. The rod proper comprises outer and inner segments linked by a thin stalk containing nine peripheral doublets of microtubules. The doublets arise from a basal body located at the vitreal end of the inner segment. However, the connecting stalk is distinct from a typical cilium as it does not possess a central pair of microtubules (Luo et al., 2021).

The outer segment consists of numerous flattened membranous sacs or discs that have a consistent diameter. These sacs house rhodopsin, the substance accountable for the absorption of light. Following light exposure, rhodopsin undergoes a molecular transformation from cis to trans and degrades subsequently. This process leads to the hyperpolarization of the plasmalemma of the rod cell, causing the generation of an electrical potential that is then transmitted to the dendrites of the associated bipolar cells. Rhodopsin reconstitution occurs in the dark after it is degraded following light absorption. The inner segment comprises an outer scleral region known as the ellipsoid, which contains a large number of mitochondria, and a vitreal portion that contains the Golgi complex, free ribosomes, and myoid. There is a large quantity of microtubules in both regions. The myoid region comprises components of granular and smooth endoplasmic reticulum. It is responsible for the synthesis and packaging of proteins. These proteins are then transported through the connecting stalk to the scleral end of the outer rod segment. They are utilized in the construction of new membranous discs. During the morning hours, older sacs are discarded from the tips of the rods and are subsequently substituted with new discs. The discarded discs undergo phagocytosis and are subsequently destroyed by pigment epithelium cells. The remaining components of the rod cell include an outer fiber, a cell body, and an inner fiber. The outer fiber is a slender projection that connects the inner segment of the rod to the cell body, which houses the nucleus. The intracellular fiber connects the soma to the spherule, which is a synaptic terminal shaped like a pear. The spherule houses multiple synaptic vesicles and a synaptic ribbon. The latter refers to a compact protein plaque that is positioned at a right angle to the presynaptic surface, typically surrounded by multiple vesicles. The rods' cell body and nucleus are situated in the outer nuclear layer of the retina, while the spherule is found in the outer plexiform layer. The length of cone cells at the fovea is 75 μm or greater, and it decreases to 40 μm at the periphery of the retina. The retina of the human eye typically consists of a range of 6 to 7 million cone cells. Typically, cone cells have a similar structure to rods, but they have a flask-like shape with short, conical outer segments and relatively wide inner segments. These segments are connected by a modified stalk, which is similar to the stalk found in rod cells. The membranous sacs of the outer cone segments exhibit variation in their attachment to the surrounding cell membrane and undergo a reduction in diameter as they approach the tip of the cone. The inner segment, known as the ellipsoid portion, exhibits a region abundant in mitochondria and a myoid part that houses the Golgi complex as well as components of smooth and granular endoplasmic reticulum. In rods, cones synthesize proteins that are subsequently transported to the outer segments, where they contribute to the production of new membranous sacs. It seems that older sacs are discarded in the evening and then engulfed by the pigment epithelial cells through a process called phagocytosis. Contrary to the rod cells, the sacs become smaller as they get closer to the tip of the cone. Iodopsin, the visual pigment found in cone cells, is linked to the outer segments. The process of light absorption and the generation of an electrical impulse in this context is analogous to what happens in rods. Cones play a role in color perception and visual acuity by detecting light that is of relatively high intensity. The perception of color is thought to rely on the existence of multiple pigments in the cones, while the rods are believed to possess only a single type of pigment (Mohammadi et al., 2021) (**Figure 6.6**).

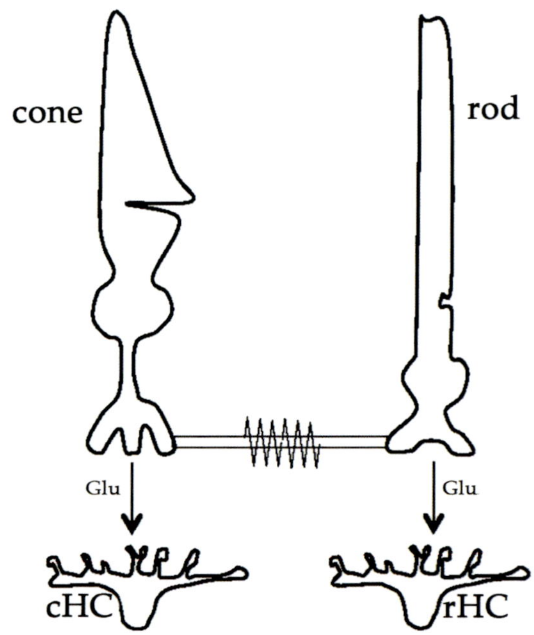

Figure 6.6. *A diagrammatic sketch illustrating rod and cone cells.*

Source: https://www.researchgate.net/publication/335461224/figure/fig1/AS:797050870431745@1567043144562/Schematic-diagram-showing-signaling-between-cone-and-rod-photoreceptor-cells-and.png.

There have been three distinct classifications of cones that have been identified. Long wavelength cones are most sensitive to the red range, middle wavelength cones are most sensitive to the green range, and short wavelength cones are most sensitive to the blue range. With the exception of cones located in the outer fovea, cones do not have an outer fiber. Instead, the inner cone segment merges with the cell body. The nuclei of cone cells are comparatively larger and lighter in color than those of the rods. They are arranged in a single row in the outer nuclear layer, which is located next to the outer limiting membrane. The cones in the retina contain a dense inner fiber that extends to the outer plexiform layer. In this layer, the fiber forms a synaptic ending called the cone pedicle, which connects with the processes of bipolar and horizontal neurons.

Photoreception occurs when light is absorbed by visual pigments in the rods and cones. The pigment that is activated by light triggers the activation of a G protein called transducin. This, in turn, stimulates a phosphodiesterase enzyme to break down cyclic GMP molecules inside the cell. This process involves the closure of sodium channels, which results in the hyperpolarization of the photoreceptor. Additionally, it leads to a decrease in the release of glutamate at the synaptic terminal. Photoreceptor cells detect light and transmit the resulting action potential to neurons in the inner retina, which then relay the signal to the brain.

6.2.4.4. Bipolar Cells

Bipolar cells, similar to photoreceptor cells, are positioned at a right angle to the layers of the retina, with their cell bodies and nuclei located in the inner nuclear layer. They generate one or more dendrites extending into the outer plexiform layer, forming synapses with terminals of photoreceptor cells. A solitary axon extends into the inner plexiform layer and forms synapses with processes originating from ganglion cells. Various classifications of bipolar neurons have been documented: Rod bipolar cells establish connections with multiple rod cells, while flat cone bipolar cells form synapses with multiple cone pedicles. Invaginating midget and flat midget bipolar cells synapse with only one cone pedicle. Bipolar cells transmit signals from the rod and cone cells to the ganglion cells in the subsequent layer.

6.2.4.5. Ganglion Cells

The dendrites of ganglion cells form synapses with the axons of bipolar neurons, serving as the final and third connection in the chain of neurons. The axons of different ganglion cells traverse the vitreal surface within the nerve fiber layer of the retina. They converge with other axons at the optic disc to create the optic nerve. While there are multiple morphologic variations of ganglion cells, their synaptic connections with bipolar neurons have led to the identification of two distinct forms. Diffuse ganglion cells form synapses with multiple types of bipolar cells, while midget ganglion cells, which are monosynaptic, form synapses with only one midget bipolar cell (Nahavandi et al., 2022).

6.2.4.6. Association Neurons

The soma and nuclei of horizontal cells are located in the inner nuclear layer. The dendrites of the neurons extend into the outer plexiform layer and form connections with a single cone pedicle. The axons also penetrate the outer plexiform layer and travel parallel to the neighboring retinal layers, ultimately terminating on terminal twigs that establish synaptic connections with multiple rod spherules. The functional role of horizontal cells remains uncertain, as they form synapses with cones in one region, rods in another region, and bipolar cells. However, it has been proposed that they may modulate the functional threshold of these cells, either increasing or decreasing it. Amacrine cells are neuronal cells with a pear-shaped morphology characterized by the absence of axons and the presence of multiple dendrites. The somata are located in the inner nuclear layer, while their dendrites project into the inner plexiform layer. The cell bodies of interplexiform cells are also located in the inner nuclear layer and extend processes to both plexiform layers. Amacrine cells provide input to them and transmit their output to both horizontal and bipolar neurons. The three types of association neurons are believed to regulate the transmission of impulses from the photoreceptors to ganglion cells. Association neurons facilitate the integration of signals among neighboring clusters of photoreceptors.

6.2.4.7. Fovea Centralis

The fovea centralis is a concave depression located on the back surface of the retina, directly aligned with the visual axis. Currently, the vitreal layers of the retina that are located beyond the outer nuclear layer are shifted to the side, allowing light to pass almost unhindered to the photoreceptors. The central region of the fovea, measuring approximately 1.5 mm in diameter, exclusively comprises elongated and slender cones that differ in shape from cones found in other parts of the retina. The objects are densely clustered, and their quantity ranges from approximately 25,000 to 35,000. The visual acuity is highest in this region of the retina.

6.2.4.8. Pigment Epithelium

The retinal pigment epithelium comprises a single layer of hexagonal cells that tend to enlarge in size towards the ora serrata. Their basal cell membranes exhibit a multitude of infoldings accompanied by mitochondria and are believed to be involved in transportation. The basal lamina is a component of the Bruch's membrane in the choroid, which can be observed using a light microscope. The lateral cell membranes of neighboring cells exhibit interdigitations and are connected by tight junctions near the apex. There are two types of cytoplasmic processes that originate from the tips of the cells: cylindrical sheaths cover the ends of the rod and cone outer segments, and elongated microvilli extend towards photoreceptor cells. The cytoplasm is distinguished by a plentiful presence of mitochondria close to the cell's base and numerous lipofuscin and melanin granules. Pigment epithelial cells may exhibit many residual bodies containing remnants of phagocytized membrane material shed by rod outer segments. Pigment epithelium absorbs light after it has passed through the neural retina, thereby preventing reflection within the eye, and the apical tight junctions prevent undesirable substances from entering the intercellular spaces of the neural retina. The pigment epithelium functions as a storage site for vitamin A, which serves as a precursor for rhodopsin and is necessary for the outer rod membranes (Peng et al., 2021).

6.2.4.9. Vascular Supply of the Retina

The outer nuclear and plexiform layers, as well as the layer of rod and cone inner segments, are devoid of blood vessels. The capillaries of the choriocapillary layer of the choroid provide nourishment to these specific areas of the retina. Nutrients traverse the pigmented epithelium to access the intercellular spaces of the outer neural retina. The inner layers of the retina receive blood supply from retinal vessels originating from the central retinal artery. This artery enters the eye through the optic nerve. The capillary networks originating from this source are located within the nerve fiber layer and the inner plexiform layer.

6.2.5. Lens

The lens is a transparent, biconvex structure located directly behind the pupil, positioned between the iris and the vitreous body. The object has a diameter of approximately 10 mm and a thickness ranging from 3.7 to 4.5 mm. The posterior surface exhibits a greater degree of convexity compared to the anterior surface. The lens comprises a capsule, anterior lens cells, and lens substance. The lens is enveloped by a uniform capsule rich in proteoglycan and has a thickness of 10 to 18 μm on both its front and back surfaces. The anterior lens cells, a layer of cuboidal cells, are located directly under the capsule and make up the epithelium of the lens. This layer is limited to the front surface of the lens. The posterior surface lacks epithelium. The anterior lens cells have apices that are oriented inward, towards the lens, while their basal surfaces are in contact with a basal lamina. The anterior lens cells possess ion pumps that regulate the optimal hydration of the lens. Near the equator of the lens, the cells experience an elevation in height and progressively undergo specialization into lens fibers, which constitute the majority of the lens and are commonly known as the lens substance. The lens undergoes growth throughout an individual's lifespan through the addition of new fibers to its outer edge. The cortex is comprised of the outer layers of the lens substance. The lens nucleus, located closer to the center, is composed of densely packed fibers arranged in concentric patterns, resulting in a uniform appearance. At the equator of the lens, the cells in the front part of the lens stretch and move inward, positioning themselves below the outer layer of cells in the front and the outer covering in the back. As the cells elongate, they undergo a loss of their nuclei and basal attachment to the capsule, transforming into lens fibers. These fibers exhibit a uniform, finely granular cytoplasm with a limited number of organelles. Their cross section is hexagonal, and their length ranges from 7 to 10 μm. The lateral membranes of the lens fibers in the cortex exhibit prominent projections that interlock with depressions in neighboring fibers, resembling a ball and socket arrangement. Nexus junctions frequently occur at these locations. The ball and socket joints ensuring the fibers' relative positions are maintained while the lens undergoes shape changes during focusing. The lens is devoid of blood vessels and obtains nutrients exclusively through diffusion from the aqueous humor and vitreous body. The lens is secured by a network of fibers known as zonule fibers, which form the suspensory ligament of the lens. Zonule fibers originate from the ciliary epithelium that covers the ciliary processes and connect to the lens capsule at the front and back of the lens's equator. Zonule fibers comprise compact clusters of slender threads, measuring around 12 nm in width, which likely correspond to the microfibril (glycoprotein) constituent of elastic fibers. The ciliary muscle regulates the thickness and convexity of the lens. When the ciliary muscle contracts, it pulls the ciliary body and choroid forward and towards the center, which reduces tension on the zonule fibers. As a result, the lens becomes thicker and more curved. This allows for the ability to concentrate on objects that are close in proximity. When the ciliary muscle is relaxed, the zonule fibers experience tension, causing the lens to become thinner and less curved to focus on distant objects (Price and Duman, 2020).

6.2.6. Vitreous Body

The vitreous body is a colorless, transparent, gelatinous substance that occupies the vitreal cavity. The composition of this substance consists of 99% water, hyaluronic acid and other hydrophilic glycosaminoglycans. It also contains thin fibrils of collagen (specifically type II and type XI) arranged in a random network. The fibrils are most noticeable or conspicuous towards the outer edge. The outermost regions of the vitreous body contain a small number of cells, specifically hyalocytes, and sporadic macrophages. Hyalocytes are potentially accountable for the creation and upkeep of the vitreous body. The hyaloid canal, a slender and tubular arrangement of fibrils, stretches from the optic disc to the back surface of the lens. It denotes the location of the developing hyaloid artery in the embryo. The vitreous body nourishes the lens and nearby structures while also preserving the proper texture and form of the eye.

6.2.7. Accessory Structures

6.2.7.1. Eyelids

The eyelids shield the front parts of the eyes. They are composed of a central connective tissue core that is externally covered by a layer of thin skin. The conjunctiva is a mucous membrane that covers the interior surface of each lid and the anterior surface of each eye, excluding the cornea. The palpebral conjunctiva is the inner lining of the eyelid, while the bulbar conjunctiva is the outer covering of the front part of the eye. Both structures are composed of a stratified columnar epithelium with goblet cells, supported by a dense connective tissue abundant in elastic fibers and may contain many lymphocytes. Goblet cells secrete mucus, which lubricates and protect the corneal epithelium from abrasion. The palpebral conjunctiva is connected to the keratinized stratified epithelium of the skin at the edge of the eyelid. The outer layer of the eyelid is composed of keratinized stratified squamous epithelium, while the inner layer is made up of loose connective tissue containing numerous elastic fibers. Delicate strands of hair are present, accompanied by numerous small sebaceous and sweat glands. The lid contains skeletal muscle derived from the orbicularis oculi and superior levator palpebrae muscles. The lid contains a significant structure called the curved tarsal plate, which comprises dense fibrous connective tissue. It adheres to the contour of the eyeball and preserves the shape of the eyelid. The tarsal (meibomian) glands, which are big sebaceous glands, are located within the tarsal plate. They are organized in a single row and their ducts open at the edge of the eyelid. Each gland comprises an elongated central duct encircled by multiple secretory alveoli. They produce a lipid secretion that lubricates the edges of the eyelids. Eyelashes are dense, truncated, and curved filaments organized in two or three asymmetrical lines along the edge of the eyelid. Their hair follicles penetrate the tarsal plate. The sebaceous glands that are connected to the eyelashes are referred to as the glands of Zeis. The modified apocrine sweat glands situated between the hair follicles are known as Moll's glands. Moll's glands secrete several types of antimicrobial proteins, including IgA, lysozyme, lactoferrin, and β-defensin-2. These proteins help protect the eye from infections.

6.2.7.2. Lacrimal Glands

The lacrimal glands are highly developed, complex tubuloalveolar glands of the serous variety. They are situated in the superior temporal region of the orbit. Each gland comprises multiple distinct glandular units that discharge into the conjunctival sac through 6 to 12 ducts. The secretory units are composed of tall columnar cells that contain prominent, light-colored secretory granules. Multiple myoepithelial cells are located between the bases of the secretory cells and their basal lamina. The ducts are initially covered by a layer of simple cuboidal epithelium, which then transitions to stratified columnar epithelium in the larger ducts. Accessory lacrimal glands may be present on the inner surface of the eyelid. Accessory lacrimals are present in two locations: the fornix of the conjunctiva, specifically in the glands of Krause, and just above the tarsal plate, specifically in the glands of Wolfring. The lacrimal gland secretes fluids that moisten, lubricate, and cleanse the front surface of the eye and the inner part of the eyelids. Tears that are in excess accumulate at a part of the conjunctival sac that expands towards the center, and are then drained by the lacrimal duct into a lacrimal sac located at the inner corner of each eye (Sangwan and Hersam, 2020). The lacrimal duct is covered by stratified squamous epithelium. The lacrimal sac and the nasolacrimal duct, responsible for draining the sac into the inferior meatus of the nasal cavity, are covered by a layer of pseudostratified columnar epithelium. The remaining portion of their walls is composed of compact connective tissue. The tear film maintains an ideal refractive surface and serves as a protective barrier against mechanical and microbial threats on the corneal surface. The lipid component is derived from the Meibomian glands and constitutes the outermost layer of the tear film. The aqueous component comprises water, electrolytes, and a diverse array of proteins, peptides, and glycoproteins (mucins) secreted by the lacrimal glands. Furthermore, the tear film is supplied with antimicrobial proteins secreted by the Moll glands.

6.2.8. Organogenesis

The formation of the eyeball is derived from the neuroectoderm of the embryonic forebrain, the surface ectoderm of the head, and the mesenchyme that surrounds or lies between these structures. Table 6.1 presents a summary of the contributions made by these embryonic tissues to the adult structures of the eye. The process of eye development initiates with the creation of shallow optic grooves on both sides of the developing forebrain. During the process of neural tube closure, the optic grooves enlarge and transform into optic vesicles, which remain connected to the brain through a hollow optic stalk. The surface ectoderm undergoes thickening over the optic vesicles, resulting in the development of lens placodes. These placodes then expand along their lateral walls, forming lens pits. Eventually, lens vesicles emerge from these pits. The lens vesicles are composed of surface ectodermal cells. The loss of the superficial (epitrichial) cells of the surface ectoderm and the connecting stalk to the surface leads to the transformation of the underlying cuboidal cells of the lens vesicles into the definitive cells of the lens. At the same time, the far end of the optic vesicle collapses inward to create a two-layered optic cup, where the top edges of the cube-shaped cells in both layers are directed towards each other. During the formation of the optic cup, the lens vesicle moves downward into the cavity of the cup, where it undergoes further development. The optic cup remains connected to the brain via the optic stalk. The optic cup develops into the retina, while the optic stalk transforms into the optic nerve. Simultaneously, the infiltration of mesenchyme from the paraxial region aids in the segregation of the lens vesicle from the surface ectoderm. A portion of the mesenchymal ingrowth undergoes differentiation to form the corneal endothelium, while the remaining part contributes to the anterior chamber. A second invasion of mesenchyme occurs, spreading between the outer layer of skin and the inner layer of cells lining the cornea, resulting in the formation of the cornea's substantia propria. The surface ectoderm, previously a single layer of cells, has now become a bilayer and gives rise to the corneal epithelium. A third invasion of mesenchyme originates from the lateral side near the lens. It penetrates into the optic cup, creating a loosely arranged, non-cellular structure between the lens and corneal endothelium. The gel-like substance located behind the central cornea becomes liquid and creates a preliminary space in front of the eye. As this space expands, it separates the corneoscleral area from the developing iris. Bowman's and Descemet's membranes become visible in the fourth month, while collagen fibrils in the substantia propria reach their maximum thickness (Schuman et al., 2022). The cornea undergoes thickening as the corneal epithelium and substantia propria develop, reaching its maximum size by the end of the first year after birth. The outer layer of the double-walled optic cup undergoes pigmentation to create the pigment epithelium of the retina. The choriocapillaris is formed by endothelial cells in the neighboring undifferentiated mesenchyme. The collagenous component of the glassy (Bruch's) membrane forms initially, with the elastic portion appearing approximately six weeks later. By the fifth month, melanocytes have migrated from the neural crest and are found in the outer layers of the choroid. Eventually, they also appear in the inner layer of the choroid. The sclera forms when mesenchyme condenses around the optic cup, located just outside the developing choroid. Condensation initiates at the equator of the sclera, and by month five, it develops into a fully formed layer.

Table 6.1. Summary of Contributions Made by Embryonic Tissues to Adult Eye Structures

Embryonic Tissue	Adult Structure Contribution
Neural ectoderm	Retina, optic nerve,
	iris, ciliary body,
	anterior chamber
Surface ectoderm	Lens, corneal epithelium
Mesoderm	Corneal stroma, sclera,
	uvea (choroid, ciliary body,
	iris stroma)

Source: Gilbert, S. F. (2000). Developmental Biology. 6th edition. Sunderland (MA): Sinauer Associates.

The neural retina is formed by the thickening of the posterior four-fifths of the inner layer of the optic cup, which occurs because of cell proliferation and migration. The inner layer of the optic cup undergoes differentiation, resulting in the formation of distinct inner and outer neuroblastic layers. The neurons and glial elements of the adult retina are derived from the cells in the inner neuroblastic layer. At the same time, the rods and cones are formed from ciliated cells in the outer neuroblastic layer. The developing retina contains a peripheral layer that receives axons that extend toward the optic stalk in a posterior direction. Retinal cell differentiation initiates in the posterior region of the optic cup and progressively extends anteriorly towards the area of the ora serrata in adult individuals. The neuroblastic layers in the macular region undergo initial development, causing the axons that develop later in the periphery to navigate around this region to reach the optic disc. Retinal differentiation, particularly in the macular region, continues after birth, and the density of the retinal pigment also increases after birth. The cells in the front 20% of the inner layer of the optic cup, located past the ora serrata region of the adult eye, continue to exist as a single layer. The cells are positioned so that their apexes are in contact with the cells of the pigment layer. These cells of the pigment layer extend to the edge of the optic cup and cover the developing ciliary region and iris. The ciliary body originates from the neuroectoderm of the anterior optic cup along with its associated mesoderm. The neuroectoderm gives rise to the pigmented and non-pigmented epithelia that cover the ciliary body and ciliary processes, while the mesenchyme forms the ciliary muscle, stroma, and blood vessels. As the ciliary muscle undergoes differentiation, folds form in the outer layer of neuroectoderm, located outside the margin of the optic cup. Every fold generates a ciliary process, consisting of a central core of mesenchyme and blood vessels, and is covered by two epithelial layers with cells arranged in an apex-to-apex manner (Shi et al., 2023). Zonule fibers originate in the vitreous and stretch from the inner surface of the ciliary process to the lens capsule. The suspensory ligament of the lens emerges in the third month of development. The iris is derived from both neuroectoderm and mesenchyme. The iris is covered by a double layer of epithelium that originates from the double cell layer of the optic cup. The smooth muscle of the sphincter and dilator muscles of the iris are unique in that they originate from the neuroectoderm. The iris is formed by the invasion of mesenchyme at the periphery of the optic cup, which gives rise to the stroma and vasculature of the iris. The optic nerve originates from the axons of retinal ganglion cells, as well as from neuroectodermal cells and mesoderm that are connected to the optic stalk. The mesoderm is responsible for the development of the blood vessels and supportive tissue of the nervous system, which includes the meninges. Initially, the optic stalk includes a ventral groove called the choroid fissure, which serves as an entry point for mesenchyme into the optic cup. The hyaloid vessels, responsible for nourishing the lens and inner surface of the retina during their growth, as well as the axons connecting the brain to the retina, both traverse through the groove. During the closure of the choroid fissure, the optic stalk undergoes a transformation and becomes the optic nerve. At the center of the optic nerve is the central retina artery, which was previously known as the hyaloid artery. The segment of the hyaloid artery responsible for nourishing the lens undergoes degeneration and is subsequently absorbed. The mesenchyme that occupies the back part of the optic cup transforms into the gelatinous and transparent vitreous. The lamina cribrosa originates from neuroectoderm through the condensation of glial cells. The mesenchymal component, which generates fibroblasts and collagenous septae, enhances its strength as it intermingles with the neuroglial cells (Skedung et al., 2013).

6.2.8.1. Accessory Structures

Folds of integument adjacent to the eyeball differentiate to form the eyelid. The Ectoderm on the exterior of the developing eyelid becomes the outer layer of stratified squamous epithelium (epidermis) that covers the cornea, and the anterior part of the sclera forms the conjunctiva. As development proceeds, the folds meet and fuse temporarily. The epidermal union breaks down prior to the opening of the eyes. Eyelashes and sebaceous, sweat, and tarsal glands develop along the edge of each eyelid while they still are fused. The follicles of the lashes and their associated glands arise as epidermal ingrowths that then develop as hair elsewhere in the body. Lacrimal glands develop as a series of solid cords of cells from the conjunctival epithelium. The cords grow, branch, and acquire lumina, thus establishing the ductal system. Secretory alveoli are the last components to form. The lacrimal sac and nasolacrimal duct first appear as a solid outgrowth of epithelium from the nasolacrimal groove; a second growth from the epithelium of each eyelid joins it. The distal end of the cord grows toward the nasal cavity and fuses with the nasal epithelium prior to acquiring a lumen.

6.3. The Ear

The ear is a complex organ responsible for auditory perception and balance, consisting of three main parts: the external ear, middle ear, and inner ear. The external ear, including the pinna and ear canal, collects sound waves and directs them toward the eardrum (tympanic membrane). The middle ear contains three small bones (ossicles) called the malleus, incus, and stapes, which transmit and amplify vibrations from the eardrum to the oval window, a membrane-covered opening leading to the inner ear. This conversion of sound waves into mechanical vibrations in the middle ear is crucial for efficient transmission of auditory information.

The inner ear, housed within the temporal bone, contains the cochlea, which is responsible for hearing, and the vestibular apparatus, which is responsible for balance. The cochlea is a spiral-shaped, fluid-filled structure containing sensory hair cells that convert mechanical vibrations into electrical signals, which are then transmitted to the brain via the auditory nerve for processing as sound. The vestibular apparatus includes the semicircular canals and otolith organs, which detect head position and movement, sending this information to the brain to maintain balance and coordinate eye movements (Figure 6.7).

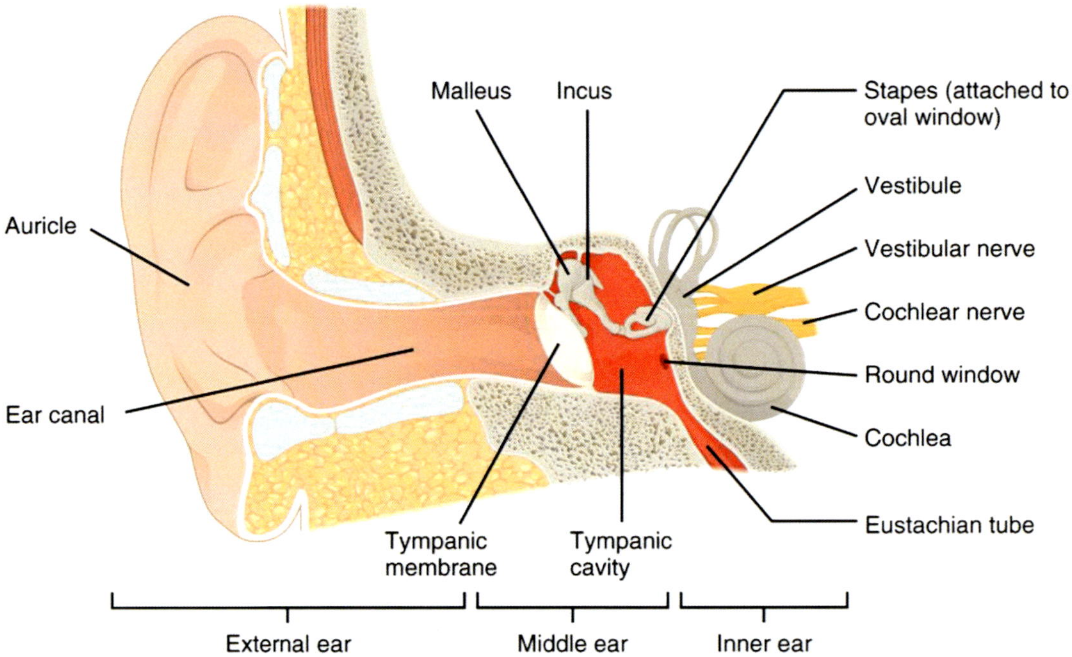

Figure 6.7. *A diagrammatic sketch illustrating the general structure of the ear.*

Source: https://s3-us-west-2.amazonaws.com/courses-images-archive-read-only/wp-content/uploads/sites/18/2014/07/19182020/1404_The_Structures_of_the_Ear.jpg.

6.3.1. External Ear

The pinna, or auricle, of the outer ear is composed of a non-uniform structure made of flexible cartilage. It is enveloped by a dense perichondrium that contains a high concentration of elastic fibers. The integumentary system comprises a limited number of fine hair, along with their corresponding sebaceous glands and sporadic eccrine sweat glands. The skin tightly adheres to the perichondrium, except for the posterior surface, which has a subcutaneous layer. The auricle is connected to layers of skeletal muscle. The external auditory meatus measures approximately 2.5 cm in length and follows a curved path resembling the letter S. The structure comprises an external section with cartilaginous walls that connect to the auricular cartilage and an internal section with walls made of the temporal bone. The external auditory meatus is covered by a layer of keratinized stratified squamous epithelium, which is connected to the outer layer of skin on the auricle. The epithelium is securely attached to the adjacent perichondrium or periosteum through a dense collagenous connective tissue. The outer part of the meatus contains a multitude of small hair that are connected to large sebaceous glands in the underlying connective tissue. The ceruminous gland, a unique type of coiled tubular apocrine sweat gland, is found in the skin lining the meatus. The shape of secretory cells can range from cuboidal to columnar, depending on their activity level. The secretory tubules are enveloped by a myoepithelial cell network between the basal lamina and the bases of the epithelial cells. The ducts can open directly on the surface or, in conjunction with neighboring sebaceous glands, into hair follicles. Their excretion is cerumen, a substance with a waxy consistency that prevents the skin lining the external auditory meatus from drying. Hair and glands are mainly found on the superior surface of the osseous portion of the external auditory meatus (Sun et al., 2021).

6.3.2. Middle Ear

The tympanic cavity is a non-uniformly shaped void located in the petrous section of the temporal bone. The structure is connected to the auditory (eustachian) tube at the front and to the mastoid air cells (cavities) of the temporal bone at the back. The lateral wall primarily comprises the tympanic membrane, also known as the eardrum. This membrane is a barrier separating the tympanic cavity from the external auditory meatus. The osseous wall of the middle ear connects with the inner ear through two small apertures, known as the oval and round windows, which are covered by membranes. The oval window membrane houses the stapes, which is an auditory ossicle. The membrane that envelops the round window is commonly known as the secondary tympanic membrane. The tympanic cavity houses the auditory ossicles, which are a sequence of three bones (malleus, incus, and stapes) that connect the tympanic membrane of the middle ear to the oval window of the inner ear. The ossicles are composed of dense bone and are connected by small synovial joints. The bones within the tympanic cavity are held in place by delicate strands of connective tissue known as ligaments. The tensor tympani and stapedius are two small skeletal muscles connected to two of the ossicles in the ear. The tendon of the tensor tympani is attached to the malleus, while the tendon of the stapedius is attached to the stapes. Most muscles are situated within narrow canals in the temporal bone. A thin mucous membrane, composed of a simple squamous epithelium resting on a thin layer of connective tissue, covers the auditory ossicles, their suspending ligaments, and the inner walls of the tympanic cavity. The mucous membrane is securely adhered to the periosteum of the temporal bone, forms the mastoid air cells lining, and covers the inner surface of the tympanic membrane. The lining epithelium at the junction of the tympanic cavity and auditory tube consists of ciliated columnar cells, which are mixed with secretory cells.

The auditory tube, also known as the eustachian tube, is approximately 4 cm in length and serves to connect the front part of the tympanic cavity to the nasopharynx. The auditory tube serves as a conduit for ventilating the tympanic cavity and facilitates the equalization of pressure between the middle ear and pharynx. The wall adjacent to the tympanic cavity is composed of dense bone, while the inner two-thirds of the auditory tube is supported by a J-shaped elastic cartilage. The osseous portion is covered by a single layer of columnar epithelial cells, which transitions into a ciliated pseudostratified columnar epithelium in the cartilaginous region. The cilia move in the direction of the pharynx. The lining epithelium near the pharynx contains goblet cells, while the underlying connective tissue often contains mixed, compound, tubuloalveolar glands. The tubal tonsil, a cluster of lymphoid tissue, occupies the connective tissue and penetrates the lining epithelium near the pharyngeal opening of the eustachian tube (Sydnor, and Satterthwaite, 2023).

The tympanic membrane comprises most of the lateral wall of the tympanic cavity and consists of three layers. The outer layer is composed of stratified squamous epithelium, which is reflected onto the tympanic membrane from the external auditory meatus. The middle layer is composed of two layers of collagenous fibers and fibroblasts. The fibers in the outer layer are arranged in a radial pattern, while those in the inner layer follow a circular pattern. The third layer consists of a simple squamous epithelium and its accompanying connective tissue, seamlessly connecting with the mucosa that lines the tympanic cavity. The fibrous layers of the tympanic membrane are connected to the surrounding bone through a ring of fibrocartilage that encircles the eardrum. The inner surface of the tympanic membrane is connected to the malleus. The tympanic membrane is set into vibration by the sound waves it receives. The vibrations are subsequently conveyed to the fluid-filled chambers of the inner ear through the ossicles. The size of the tympanic membrane is approximately 18 times greater than that of the oval window in the inner ear, which houses the foot plate of the stapes. Due to this configuration, the eardrum and auditory ossicles function as pistons, applying pressure to the enclosed fluid in the inner ear. Therefore, the tympanic membrane and auditory ossicles not only convey vibrations but also can enhance weak forces of sound waves without using energy. The tensor tympani and stapedius muscles safeguard the fragile structures in the inner ear by reducing the movement of the ossicles caused by loud or abrupt sounds. Additionally, they are believed to control the level of tension in the tympanic membrane, enabling the detection of sounds of moderate intensity in a noisy setting.

6.3.3. Inner Ear

The inner ear comprises the cochlea, which is responsible for hearing, and five vestibular sense organs that are dedicated to maintaining balance and detecting head position. The structure consists of a network of canals and hollow spaces located within the petrous part of the temporal bone. The dense bone that directly encloses the canals and cavities constitutes the bony labyrinth and contains a fluid known as perilymph. The perilymph contains a collection of fluid-filled membranous structures known as the membranous labyrinth. The membranous labyrinth contains endolymph, a fluid that has a similar ionic composition to intracellular fluid. It is high in potassium ions and low in sodium ions. Perilymph is similar to extracellular fluid in that it contains a large amount of sodium ions and a low amount of potassium ions. The stria vascularis in the cochlear duct is responsible for producing endolymph, while the specific location where perilymph is formed remains unidentified (Toricelli et al., 2021). The bony and membranous labyrinths comprise two main parts: the vestibular labyrinth, which houses sensory elements responsible for maintaining balance, and the cochlea, which houses sensory structures responsible for detecting sound.

6.3.3.1. Vestibular Labyrinth

The vestibular labyrinth comprises three semicircular canals connected to an elliptical structure known as the utricle. The utricle is connected to the saccule, a spherical part of the vestibular system, through a thin duct that joins with another duct from the saccule. The two ducts come together to create the slender endolymphatic duct, which ends in a small enlargement known as the endolymphatic sac. Most of the membranous labyrinth, which constitutes the vestibular section of the inner ear, is covered by a single layer of flat epithelial cells. The remaining portion of this wall is composed of delicate connective tissue fibers and star-shaped fibroblasts. Delicate strands of connective tissue extend from the wall of the membranous labyrinth and traverse the perilymphatic space to merge with the periosteum of the adjacent bone. The trabeculae support the membranous part of the semicircular canals, utricle, and saccule, filled with perilymph and located within the bony labyrinth. The perilymphatic connective tissue contains a high concentration of blood capillaries that provide nourishment to the different parts of the membranous labyrinth.

The epithelium in certain areas of each section of the membranous labyrinth exhibits a stratified structure and functions in sensory perception. The sensory epithelium of each semicircular canal is limited to the widened ampullary section and, along with a connective tissue core beneath it, creates a horizontal ridge that extends into the interior of the ampulla. The connective tissue is rich in nerve fibers. The cristae ampullaris are formed by the sensory neuroepithelial regions of the semicircular canals. The utricle and saccule contain neuroepithelial regions similar in structure and are known as the macula utriculi and the macula sacculi, respectively. The macula utriculi occupies an area of approximately 2 square millimeters along the superoanterior wall. The macula sacculi is located on the anterior wall of the saccule and is perpendicular to a plane. This area measures 2 × 3 mm (**Figure 6.8**). The macula of the utricle is located on a horizontal plane The macula of the saccule is positioned on a vertical plane that is perpendicular to the macula of the utricle. The sensory epithelium of the cristae and maculae comprises type I and type II sensory hair cells and supporting (sustentacular) cells.

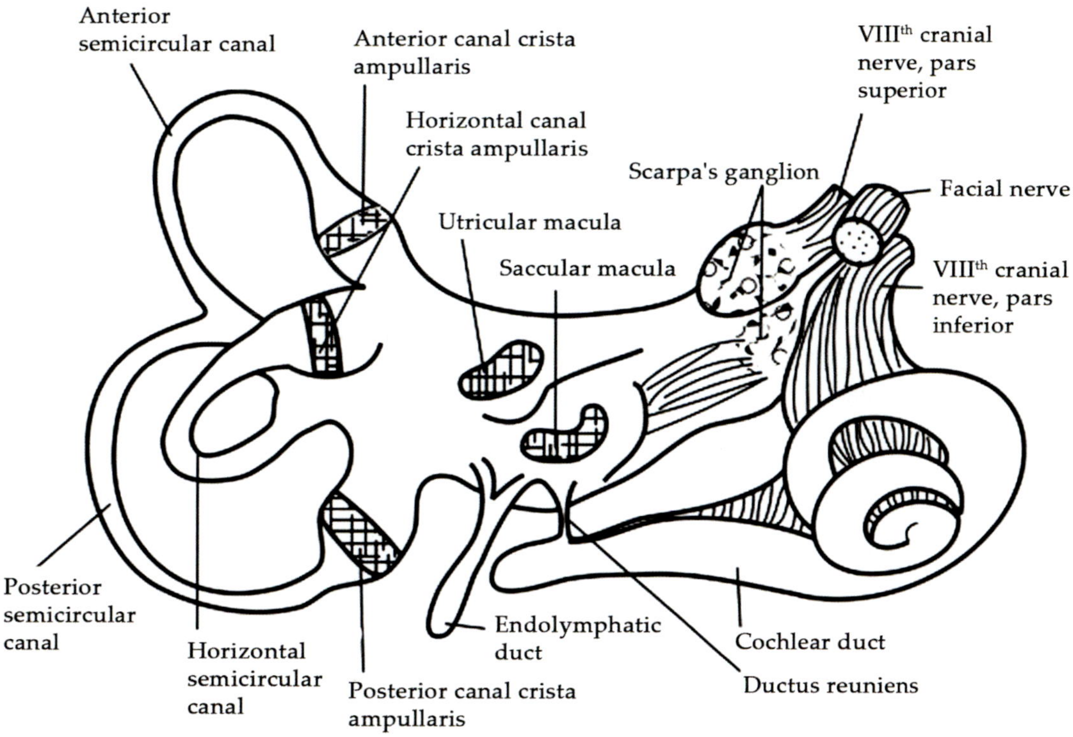

Figure 6.8. *A diagram showing the positions of the sensory regions in the membranous labyrinth.*

Source: https://ars.els-cdn.com/content/image/3-s2.0-B9780123742360100355-f35–01–9780123742360.jpg.

The type I hair cell has a flask-shaped morphology, characterized by a slender apical region and a rounded base housing the nucleus. A significant portion of the cell is surrounded by a cup-shaped afferent nerve ending known as a calyx. The nerve calyx is in close proximity to efferent nerve endings, but there is no direct contact between the type I hair cell and the nerve endings. A narrow intercellular cleft, measuring 30 nm in width, separates the hair cell from the nerve ending. The gap junctions, dispersed between the two compartments, create a space that is reduced to about 5 nm in width. Synaptic ribbons are frequently located in the cytoplasm of type I hair cells, positioned directly next to the plasmalemma. Mitochondria are primarily located near the nucleus and at the top of the cell, while a large number of microtubules are found, particularly in the top region. The nerve calyx's cytoplasm contains dispersed mitochondria and numerous vesicles with diameters ranging from 50 to 200 nm (Sun et al., 2021). The apical cell membrane of the type I hair cell possesses 50 to 100 prominent, specialized microvilli, referred to as "hair." These immobile components are restricted by a plasma membrane, have cytoplasmic centers that contain many thin filaments, and are narrowed at their base just prior to connecting with the rest of the cell. The longitudinal filaments emerge from the microvilli and penetrate a dense network of filaments, which constitutes a terminal web in the apical cytoplasm of the cell. The height of the microvilli gradually varies from approximately 1 μm on one side to around 100 μm on the opposite side of the cell. Individual microvilli in each row are connected by fine extracellular filaments. A single cilium is located in an unusual position on the top surface. It is unique because the two central microtubules stop shortly after starting from the basal body. The cilium is commonly referred to as a kinocilium and is believed to be immotile.

Type II hair cells are characterized by their simple columnar shape and are surrounded by multiple distinct afferent and efferent nerve endings. In contrast, type I hair cells are surrounded by a single afferent nerve ending (as shown in Figure 6.9). The type II hair cell possesses a solitary, off-center, immotile cilium and 50 to 100 sizable microvilli organized in the same manner as those found in type I cells. The cytoplasm contains dispersed structures of granular endoplasmic reticulum, plentiful mitochondria, smooth-surfaced tubules, and numerous vesicles measuring 20 nm in diameter. The Golgi complex is located above the nucleus and is highly developed. Synaptic ribbons are located within the cytoplasm of type II hair cells, directly across from the adjacent nerve terminals.

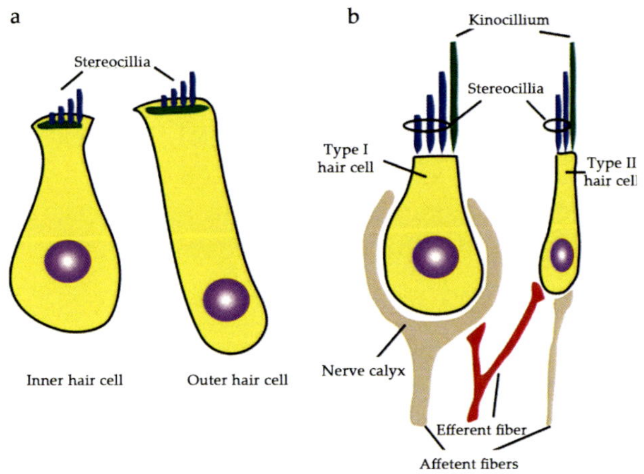

Figure 6.9. *A schematic diagram depicting the characteristics of type I and type II hair cells.*

Source: https://entokey.com/wp-content/uploads/2017/03/A322688_1_En_3_Fig3_HTML.gif.

Sustentacular cells, which are columnar-shaped supporting cells, extend from the basal lamina to the free surface of the sensory epithelium in an adjacent manner. The cells exhibit a highly irregular path within the epithelium, and electron micrographs reveal the presence of a fully developed terminal web at the top of the cell, a noticeable Golgi complex, multiple secretory granules, and bundles of microtubules that extend from the bottom of the cell to the terminal web (Shi et al., 2023). Microtubules are essential components of the cytoskeleton and contribute to the structural stability of the cells. The precise function of the supporting cells remains uncertain, but it has been proposed that they are involved in the metabolism of endolymph or in providing nutrition to the hair cells. The peripheral region of the sensory epithelium contains supporting cells that are arranged in a single layer called the planum semilunatum. This layer does not contain any hair cells. The hair cells in the cristae have microvilli that are surrounded by a gelatinous structure called the cupula cristae ampullaris. This structure is made up of viscous proteoglycans that extend from the surface of the crista into the ampullary lumen of each semicircular canal. Supporting cells within the sensory epithelium may also play a role in the formation of the cupula. The planum semilunatum is capable of secreting sulfated proteoglycans. The hair cells in the maculae of the utricle and saccule have a row of microvilli that are the tallest. These microvilli are embedded in a thick proteoglycan substance, which forms the otolithic membrane. Furthermore, a multitude of crystalline structures known as otoliths (otoconia) are held in suspension within this layer. These organisms are composed of protein and calcium carbonate. The gelatinous cupula of the cristae extends into the lumen of the ampullary region of the semicircular canal, resembling a swinging door. During angular movement of the head, the cupula is shifted by the motion of endolymph within this section of the membranous labyrinth. The movement of the cupula stimulates the sensory hair cells, which then produce an action potential detected by nearby nerve endings. Likewise, the gravitational forces acting on the otolithic membrane and the otoconia contained within it result in a sliding motion on the microvilli of the hair cells located beneath the macula. Linear acceleration additionally leads to the activation of hair cells in the macula. The precise mechanism by which the sensory epithelium in the vestibular organs converts the mechanical energy of endolymph movement into electrical energy for nerve impulses is currently unknown. The flexion or movement of microvilli is believed to activate mechanoreceptors, leading to the polarization of hair cells. This action potential is then transmitted to adjacent nerve endings, resulting in the production of a nerve impulse. Efferent nerve endings likely possess inhibitory functions to regulate the activity threshold of hair cells. The movement of microvilli towards the tallest row is believed to cause depolarization (excitation) of the hair cell, while movement towards the shortest row is believed to cause hyperpolarization (inhibition) of hair cell activity (Wang et al., 2018).

6.3.3.2. Cochlea

The cochlea, similar to the vestibular portion of the inner ear, is composed of a bony outer section and a central membranous part filled with perilymph. The bony portion of the cochlea forms a spiral shape, wrapping around a cone-shaped axis made of porous bone known as the modiolus, completing two and three-fourths rotations. The modiolus contains blood vessels, nerve fibers, and the perikarya of afferent bipolar neurons, known as the spiral ganglion. The spiral lamina, a bony projection, extends from the modiolus into the lumen of the cochlear canal throughout its entire length. The basilar membrane, a fibrous structure, stretches from the spiral lamina to the spiral ligament, which is a thickening of the periosteum located on the outer bony wall of the cochlear canal. The slender vestibular membrane stretches diagonally across the cochlear canal, connecting the spiral lamina to the outer wall of the cochlea. The cochlear canal is divided into three parts: the upper scala vestibuli, the intermediate cochlear duct, and the lower scala tympani, by the basilar and vestibular membranes. Figure 6.10 displays a cross-section of the cochlear canal.

The cochlear duct is a component of the endolymphatic system and is linked to the saccule of the membranous labyrinth through the small ductus reuniens. The cochlear duct terminates at the apex of the cochlea as the blindly ending cecum cupulare. The scala vestibuli and the scala tympani are filled with perilymph and connect at the top of the cochlea via a small opening known as the helicotrema. The scala tympani, located at the base of the cochlea, is sealed by the secondary tympanic membrane, which occupies the round window. This membrane acts as a barrier between the perilymph in the scala tympani and the middle ear. The scala vestibuli traverses the perilymphatic channels of the vestibule and terminates at the oval window, which is sealed by the foot of the stapes. The motion of the stapes bone within the oval window applies force on the perilymph fluid in the scala vestibule (Wang et al., 2018). Due to the inability of fluid to be compressed, pressure waves either propagate through the cochlear duct, causing displacement and entry into the scala tympani, or directly enter the scala tympani via the helicotrema. The elasticity of the secondary tympanic membrane causes it to bulge into the tympanic cavity of the middle ear, thereby releasing pressure from the confined perilymphatic spaces of the cochlea (**Figure 6.11**).

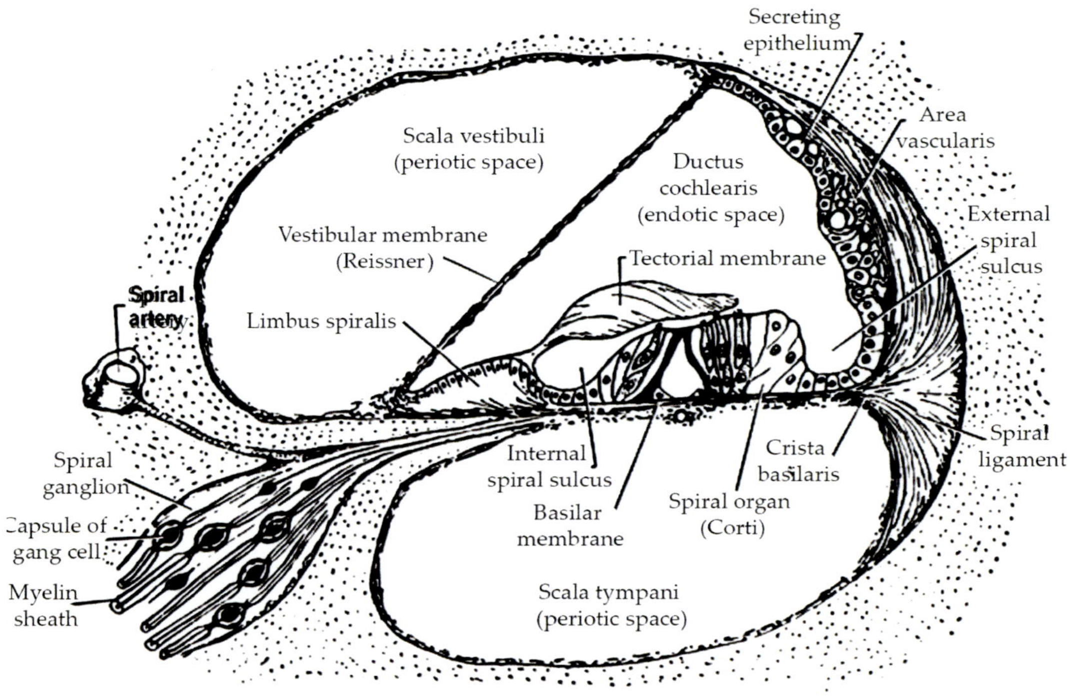

Figure 6.10. *A schematic diagram depicting a cross-sectional perspective of the cochlear canal.*

Source: https://www.researchgate.net/profile/David-Hill-53/publication/327384334/figure/fig2/AS:666213680177152@1535849127621/Cross-section-of-the-cochlear-canal-Cross-section-of-cochlea-canal-1117-From-Handbook.png.

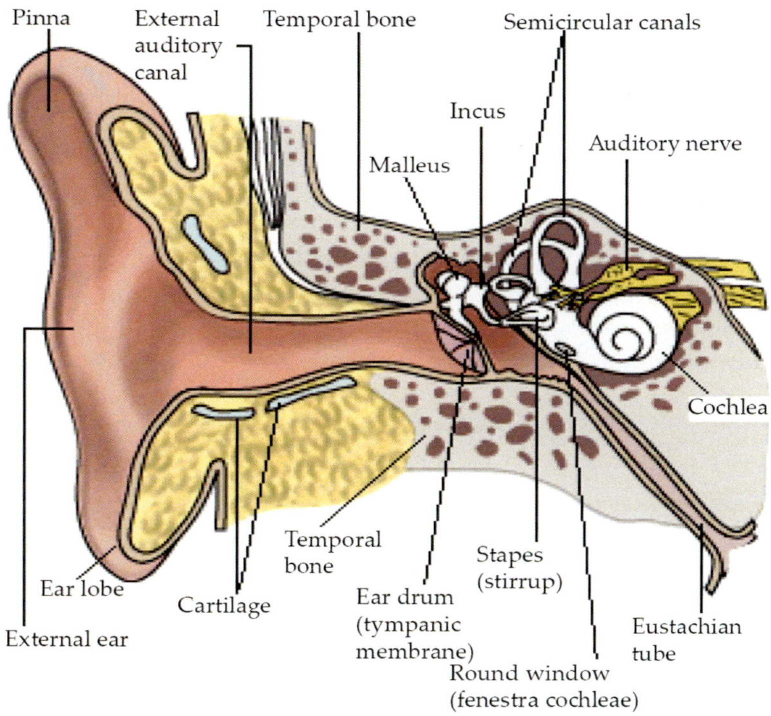

Figure 6.11. *An illustrative diagram depicting the mechanics involved in the process of hearing.*

Source: https://drfasih.com/wp-content/uploads/2014/10/hear1.jpg.

6.3.3.3. Cochlear Duct

The cochlear duct is a triangular cavity that traces the spiral path of the cochlea. The basilar membrane forms the floor of the structure, while the vestibular membrane forms the roof.

The basilar membrane is composed of collagen-like fibers embedded in a shapeless matrix. It stretches from the osseous spiral lamina of the modiolus to the spiral crest, which is a well-vascularized periosteal region located along the outer wall of the cochlea. The vestibular membrane is composed of two layers of simple squamous cells that are primarily separated by their basal laminae (Wang et al., 2023). The stria vascularis is the vascular area that forms the outer wall of the cochlear duct. The structure is present throughout the entire cochlear duct and is composed of a pseudostratified columnar epithelium that is supported by a vascular connective tissue. It contains basal and marginal cells. The epithelium is contiguous with the simple squamous epithelium that forms a lining on the inside of the vestibular membrane. The marginal cells exhibit extensive invaginations of the basal and lateral cell membranes and are accompanied by a large number of mitochondria, indicating their involvement in the transportation of fluids. They can contribute to the formation of endolymph. Basal cells exhibit a limited number of mitochondria or basal infoldings. The epithelium of the stria vascularis is distinct from epithelium found in other parts of the body due to the presence of intraepithelial capillaries. The epithelium of the stria vascularis is connected to a single layer of thin cells that covers the spiral prominence, has a thickened area of the periosteum with a lot of blood vessels. The spiral prominence is located below the stria vascularis and spans the entire length of the cochlear duct. The cells transition into a cuboidal shape as the epithelium bends towards the basilar membrane from the outer wall of the cochlear duct.

6.3.3.4. Organ of Corti

The cochlear duct houses a section of specialized cells known as the organ of Corti, which converts vibrations from the basilar membrane into nerve signals. The avascular organ of Corti spans the entire length of the cochlear duct and is situated on the basilar membrane. The composition primarily comprises supporting and hair cells.

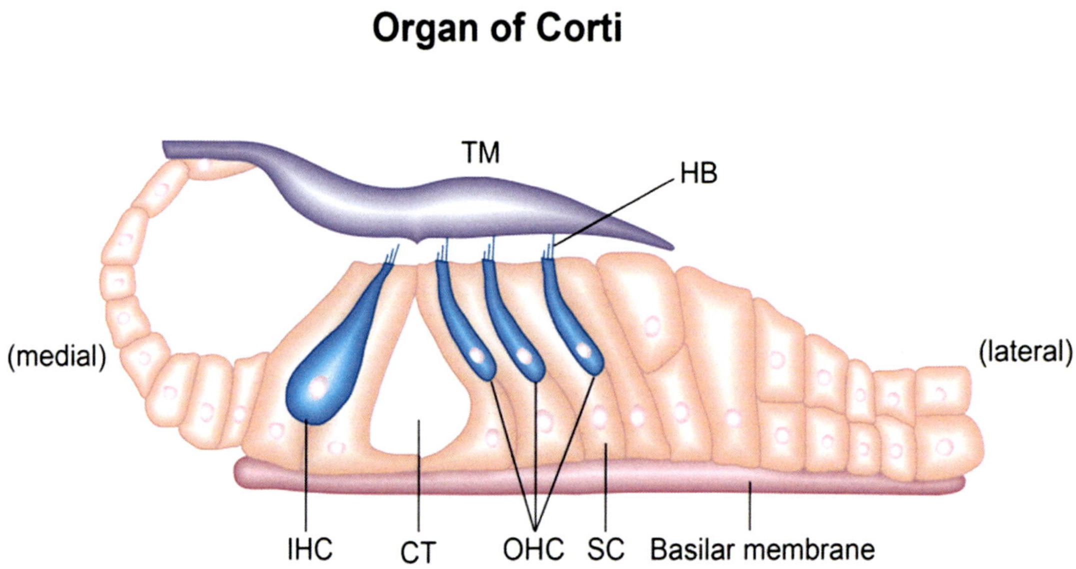

Figure 6.12. *A diagrammatic sketch of the organ of Corti.*

The supporting cells are characterized by their tall columnar shape and include the inner and outer pillar cells, inner and outer phalangeal cells, border cells, Hensen cells, and Claudius cells. The inner and outer pillar cells delineate the boundaries of the inner tunnel, a cavity that is located within and runs the entire length of the organ of Corti. The nucleus is situated in the wide base of both types of pillar cells. The elongated cell bodies possess a multitude of microtubules that constitute a cytoskeleton. The inner pillar cells are slightly enlarged at the top and cover the outer pillar cells. The uppermost points of the outer pillar cells also enlarge slightly to fit into the curved upper surface of the inner pillar cells. The pillar cells not only define the boundaries of the inner tunnel but also offer structural reinforcement to neighboring cells. The phalangeal cells function as structural components for the sensory hair cells. The inner phalangeal cells are positioned in a single row directly next to the inner pillar cells. They encircle the sensory inner hair cells, except for their uppermost regions. On the other hand, the outer phalangeal cells that are shaped like columns are organized into three or four rows. These cells provide support to the outer hair cells, which are also arranged in rows. The top part of each outer phalangeal cell forms a cup-like structure that encloses the lower one-third of an outer hair cell. The afferent and efferent nerves are situated at the base. Every outer phalangeal cell produces a thin cytoplasmic extension filled with microtubules. The process continues to the surface, forming a flat plate that connects to the apical edges of the outer hair cell. This plate is supported laterally by the outer phalangeal cells and neighboring outer hair cells" for better flow. The apical plates of the outer phalangeal cells offer supplementary support to the outer hair cells, specifically the upper two-thirds that lack support from neighboring cells and are enclosed by sizable intercellular spaces filled with fluid. The fluid in these cavities is considered similar to that in the inner tunnel (Yang et al., 2019) (**Figure 6.12**).

Border cells are a type of supportive cells that are found along the inner edge of the organ of Corti. The elongated cells transform into the flat cells that form the lining of the inner spiral tunnel. The space in question is created by the spiral limbus, which is composed of periosteal connective tissue that extends from the osseous spiral lamina and protrudes into the cochlear duct. The limbus contains vertically aligned collagen fibers, also known as auditory teeth. Interdental cells are specialized cells located on the superior surface of the spiral limbus. The cells traverse the collagen fibers to access the lumen of the cochlear duct. On the superior surface of the limbus, they create an uninterrupted layer and are connected by tight junctions. The interdental cells produce a layer of substance that creates the tectorial membrane. This membrane is composed of a gel-like structure that contains a high amount of proteoglycans and a protein that is believed to be similar to epidermal keratin. The tectorial membrane covers the interdental cells and extends beyond the spiral limbus to overlay the hair cells of the organ of Corti. The microvilli of both the outer and inner hair cells make contact with the undersurface of the tectorial membrane (Yang et al., 2019).

Located in close proximity to the outer phalangeal cells, near the outer border of the organ of Corti, there exists a distinct cluster of columnar supporting cells known as Hensen's cells. The cells decrease in height and undergo a transformation into the neighboring cells of Claudius, which make up the outer boundary of the organ of Corti (**Figure 6.13**).

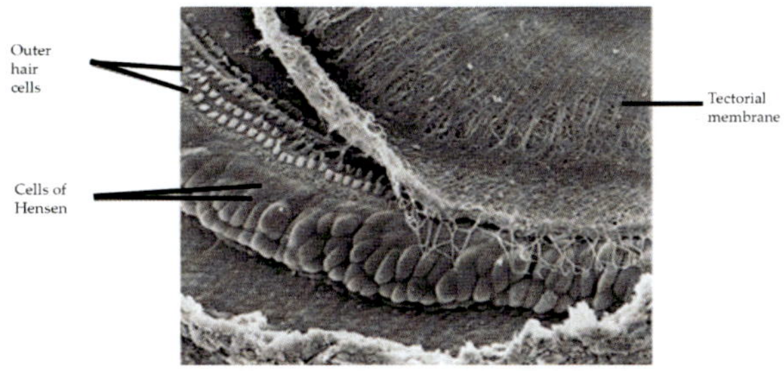

Figure 6.13. *This image is a scanning electron micrograph that displays the outer edge of the tectorial membrane and its connection to the Hensen cells. Observe the visible outer hair cells where the tectorial membrane is elevated. Micrograph courtesy of M. Lenoir, University of Montpellier, France.*

The sensory hair cells are categorized into inner and outer hair cells. The inner hair cells are arranged in a singular row along the inner part of the organ of Corti and span the entire length of the cochlea. The inner hair cells of the cochlea, similar to the type I hair cells of the vestibular labyrinth, are compact cells with a short, flask-like shape and narrow necks. The inner hair cells possess well-developed microvilli that extend from their apical surface. However, unlike type I hair cells, they do not have a kinocilium. The microvilli possess multiple filaments that protrude into a compact terminal web in the uppermost region of the cytoplasm. Mitochondria cluster directly below the terminal web and are also dispersed throughout the rest of the cytoplasm, which contains scattered ribosomes and smooth endoplasmic reticulum profiles. Multiple nerve endings form synapses with the bases of the inner hair cells at a level below the nucleus. The outer hair cells are typically arranged in three or four rows and are supported by the apices of the outer phalangeal cells. The microvilli are organized in a V-shaped pattern, as shown in **Figure 6.14**. There is an absence of cilium. Mitochondria cluster at the basal region of the outer hair cell, establishing connections with both afferent and efferent nerve fibers. With regards to all other aspects, the outer hair cells bear resemblance to the inner hair cells, and both serve as sound receptors in the organ of Corti.

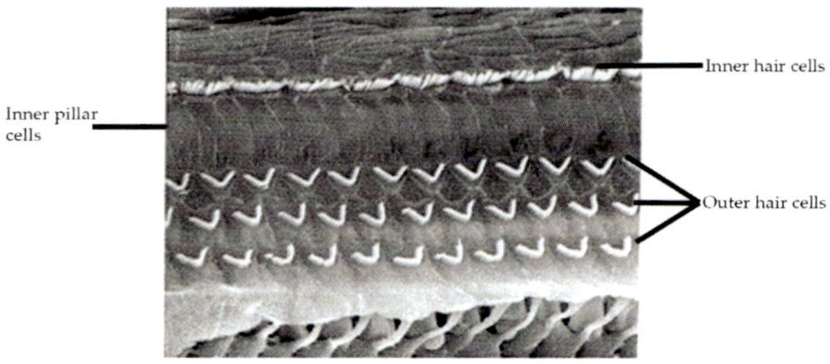

Figure 6.14. *This is a scanning electron micrograph displaying the surface of the organ of Corti. It clearly shows the arrangement of microvilli that extend from both the inner and outer hair cells. The hair cells are divided into inner pillar cells. Micrograph courtesy of M. Lenoir, University of Montpellier, France.*

6.3.4. Organogenesis

6.3.4.1. External Ear

The auricle is formed by the proliferation of mesenchymal cells around the borders of the first and second pharyngeal arches, along with the surface ectoderm. The proliferations emerge near the openings of the developing external auditory meati and progressively merge to create the final auricles. The external auditory meatus originates from the first pharyngeal groove and the surrounding arches. As the pharyngeal groove expands towards the center, it takes on the shape of a funnel with a lining of ectoderm and is surrounded by mesoderm (cartilage). An epithelial plate of significant thickness is produced in the ectoderm, originating from the bottom of the pit and extending towards the developing tympanic cavity. The connective tissue that forms between the two layers of epithelium originates from mesenchyme. At first, the eardrum is positioned horizontally, nearly parallel to the floor of the meatus. However, as the meatus continues to develop, the eardrum gradually becomes more upright (Zhang et al., 2022).

6.3.4.2. Middle Ear

The tympanic cavity originates from the first pharyngeal pouch and is lined with endodermal epithelium. The terminal section of the pouch, known as the tubotympanic recess, expands to create a temporary tympanic cavity. The slender proximal attachment to the area of the developing nasopharynx transforms into the auditory tube. The mesenchyme originating from the first and second pharyngeal arches, located above the provisional cavity, undergoes cartilaginous transformation and gives rise to the initial structures of the ossicles. The spongy mesenchyme retains these until the tympanic cavity expands and the mesenchyme deteriorates. During this process, epithelium undergoes expansion to form a lining on the recently developed cavity and the inner surface of the eardrum. It also covers the ossicles in a manner similar to a mesentery. The ossicles are suspended within the tympanic cavity, but they are located outside the epithelium of the cavity. Endochondral ossification occurs in each ossicle. The tensor tympani and stapedius muscles originate from mesenchyme of the first and second pharyngeal arches, respectively, and are located outside the lining of the tympanic cavity. The ligaments that support the ossicles originate from the mesenchyme located between the folds of the covering epithelium, resembling mesentery. The mucosa that covers the inside of the tympanic cavity gradually expands and eventually covers the mastoid air cells located in the temporal bone.

6.3.4.3. Inner Ear

The inner ear's epithelium originates from the ectoderm. The ectoderm undergoes thickenings known as auditory placodes, which develop symmetrically along the sides of the midbrain and then fold inward to create cup-shaped auditory pits. These structures enlarge, disconnect from the surface ectoderm, and transform into separate oval-shaped sacs known as auditory vesicles or otocysts. The endolymphatic duct, a slender and cylindrical cavity, arises from the area most recently in contact with the ectoderm, and gradually enlarges into a closed sac called the endolymphatic sac. The otocyst undergoes elongation, and a tubular outgrowth emerges at the ventral end, spiraling for two and three-fourths rotations into the adjacent mesenchyme. The cochlear duct is connected to the saccule through a narrow ductus reuniens. The posterior section of the otocysts undergoes expansion and maturation, resulting in the formation of the semicircular canals. The middle portion gives rise to the utricle and saccule. The epithelial lining of the different sections of the membranous labyrinth is initially composed of a simple layer of low columnar cells. As nerve fibers extend into the cells of the cristae ampullaris, maculae of the utricle and saccule, and organ of Corti, the epithelium becomes thicker and undergoes specialization into distinct sensory and supporting cells. It is believed that the supporting cells secrete and preserve the cupula cristae ampullaris and otolithic membranes in the maculae. The differentiation of the organ of Corti proceeds gradually, commencing with a thickening of the epithelium at the basal region of the cochlea and advancing towards the apex (Zhang et al., 2022). The epithelium consists of large inner and small outer ridges, both of which are connected to a tectorial membrane. The peripheral ridge generates the supporting cells and inner and outer hair cells of the organ of Corti. The prominent central ridge undergoes involution to become the lining of the spiral sulcus. Initially, the structures of the developing membranous labyrinth are surrounded by mesenchyme, which later undergoes chondrification and is subsequently replaced by bone to form the bony labyrinth. The cartilage next to the membranous labyrinth undergoes degeneration, resulting in the formation of a syncytial reticulum. This reticulum then transforms into the perilymphatic spaces filled with perilymph. Within the developing cochlear duct, the cartilage is absorbed, resulting in the formation of two perilymphatic spaces known as the scala vestibuli and scala tympani, located on either side of the cochlear duct. The modiolus of the cochlea originates directly from the mesenchyme as a membranous bone.

A Closer Look

The Sensory System

The sensory system is a vital component of the human body, responsible for processing and interpreting external stimuli, enabling individuals to interact with their environment. Comprising various sensory modalities, including vision, hearing, taste, smell, and touch, this intricate network relies on specialized receptors that convert physical stimuli into neural signals. These signals are then transmitted to the brain for interpretation, allowing for the perception of the world around us. The sensory system not only facilitates basic survival functions, such as detecting danger or finding food, but also enriches our experiences and emotional responses. Understanding the sensory system is essential for comprehending how we perceive reality and interact with our surroundings.

Mechanisms of Sensation

The process of sensation begins with sensory receptors, which are specialized cells or structures designed to respond to specific types of stimuli. For example, photoreceptors in the eyes respond to light, mechanoreceptors in the skin detect pressure and touch, and chemoreceptors in the nose and mouth respond to chemical substances, enabling the senses of smell and taste. Each receptor type is tuned to a particular stimulus, ensuring that the brain receives accurate information about the external environment. Once stimulated, these receptors generate electrical impulses that travel along sensory neurons to the central nervous system. The pathways of sensation vary depending on the type of sensory input. For instance, the visual pathway involves light entering the eye, being focused by the lens onto the retina, and then converted into neural signals that travel via the optic nerve to the visual cortex in the brain.

Processing and Interpretation

After sensory information is received by the brain, it undergoes complex processing in various cortical areas tailored to specific sensory modalities. The primary sensory cortex for each modality—such as the visual cortex for sight or the auditory cortex for hearing—initially processes the incoming signals. This processing involves distinguishing patterns, intensities, and temporal sequences, allowing the brain to create a coherent representation of the stimuli. For example, in the visual system, the brain interprets color, motion, and depth to form a complete image of the environment. Furthermore, higher-order processing areas integrate sensory information from different modalities, enabling multisensory perception. This integration is crucial for tasks such as locating a sound **source** in a crowded room or associating a smell with a specific memory, highlighting the interconnectivity of the sensory system.

The Role of Sensation in Experience and Behavior

The sensory system plays a critical role not only in perception but also in shaping behavior and emotional responses. Sensory experiences are intricately linked to memories and learning. For instance, the scent of a particular food may evoke nostalgic memories of childhood, influencing an individual's appetite and food preferences. Additionally, sensory input can trigger emotional reactions, such as fear in response to loud noises or delight from pleasant smells. The sensory system also contributes to social interactions; for example, the ability to interpret nonverbal cues, such as facial expressions and body language, relies heavily on sensory perception. Disorders of the sensory system, such as sensory processing disorder or agnosia, can significantly impact an individual's quality of life, underscoring the importance of proper sensory functioning for effective communication and interaction in daily life.

Summary

The sensory system is a complex network responsible for detecting and processing sensory stimuli from the environment, allowing organisms to perceive and respond to various external and internal cues. It comprises specialized sensory organs and receptors that detect stimuli such as light, sound, touch, taste, and smell. Each sensory modality has its own pathways and processing centers in the brain, ensuring that information is accurately interpreted and integrated to facilitate appropriate responses. The sensory system plays a vital role in survival, enabling organisms to navigate their environment, find food, and avoid danger.

Sensory processing begins with the activation of sensory receptors, which convert external stimuli into neural signals. These signals travel along specific pathways to designated areas of the brain, where they are processed and perceived as sensations. The sensory system also involves intricate mechanisms of adaptation and modulation, allowing individuals to adjust their sensitivity to persistent stimuli. Understanding the sensory system is essential for fields such as neuroscience, psychology, and medicine, as it provides insights into how perception influences behavior, decision-making, and overall quality of life.

References

1. Birkoben, T., Winterfeld, H., Fichtner, S., Petraru, A., & Kohlstedt, H. (2020). A spiking and adapting tactile sensor for neuromorphic applications. *Scientific Reports, 10*, 17260. https://doi.org/10.1038/s41598-020-74153-2.
2. Chi, C., Sun, X., Xue, N., Li, T., & Liu, C. (2018). Recent progress in technologies for tactile sensors. *Sensors, 18*(4), 948. https://doi.org/10.3390/s18040948.
3. Chortos, A., Liu, J., & Bao, Z. (2016). Pursuing prosthetic electronic skin. *Nature Materials, 15*, 937–950. https://doi.org/10.1038/nmat4671.
4. Chun, S., Kim, J. S., Yoo, Y., Choi, Y., Jung, S. J., Jang, D., Lee, G., Song, K. I., Nam, K. S., Youn, I., et al. (2021). An artificial neural tactile sensing system. *Nature Electronics, 4*, 429–438. https://doi.org/10.1038/s41928-021-00607-4.
5. Ham, D., Park, H., Hwang, S., & Kim, K. (2021). Neuromorphic electronics based on copying and pasting the brain. *Nature Electronics, 4*, 635–644. https://doi.org/10.1038/s41928-021-00642-1.
6. Hu, G., An, H., Xi, J., Lu, J., Hua, Q., & Peng, Z. (2021). A ZnO micro/nanowire-based photonic synapse with piezo-phototropic modulation. *Nano Energy, 89*, 106282. https://doi.org/10.1016/j.nanoen.2021.106282.
7. Hu, J., Wang, W., & Yu, H. (2019). Endowing soft photo-actuators with intelligence. *Advanced Intelligent Systems, 1*, 1900050. https://doi.org/10.1002/aisy.201900050.
8. Hu, Z., Lin, L., Lin, W., Xu, Y., Xia, X., Peng, Z., & Sun, Z. (2023). Machine learning for tactile perception: Advancements, challenges, and opportunities. *Advanced Intelligent Systems, 5*, 2200371. https://doi.org/10.1002/aisy.202200371.
9. Hua, Q., & Shen, G. (2023). Full-system-integrated neuro-inspired memristor chips for edge intelligence. *Science Bulletin, 68*, 3108–3110. https://doi.org/10.1016/j.scib.2023.04.014.
10. Hua, Q., Cui, X., Ji, K., Wang, B., & Hu, W. (2021). Piezotronics enabled artificial intelligence

systems. *Journal of Physics: Materials, 4*(2), 022003. https://doi.org/10.1088/2515-7639/abf3fb.

11. Kim, S., Lee, Y., Kim, H. D., & Choi, S. J. (2020). A tactile sensor system with sensory neurons and a perceptual synaptic network based on semi volatile carbon nanotube transistors. *NPG Asia Materials, 12*, 76. https://doi.org/10.1038/s41427-020-00244-5.
12. Li, L., Zhang, W., Ren, Z., Chang, L., Xu, X., & Hu, Y. (2024). Endowing actuators with sensing capability: Recent progress on perceptive soft actuators. *Chemical Engineering Journal, 479*, 147550. https://doi.org/10.1016/j.cej.2023.147550.
13. Li, T., Su, Y., Zheng, H., Chen, F., Li, X., Tan, Y., & Zhou, Z. (2023). An artificial intelligence-motivated skin-like optical fiber tactile sensor. *Advanced Intelligent Systems, 5*, 2200460. https://doi.org/10.1002/aisy.202200460.
14. Liu, Y., Bao, R., Tao, J., Li, J., Dong, M., & Pan, C. (2020). Recent progress in tactile sensors and their applications in intelligent systems. *Science Bulletin, 65*(1), 70–88. https://doi.org/10.1016/j.scib.2019.09.007.
15. Luo, Y., Abidian, M. R., Ahn, J. H., Akinwande, D., Andrews, A. M., Antonietti, M., Bao, Z., Berggren, M., Berkey, C. A., Bettinger, C. J., et al. (2023). Technology roadmap for flexible sensors. *ACS Nano, 17*(5), 5211–5295. https://doi.org/10.1021/acsnano.2c12571.
16. Luo, Y., Li, Y., Sharma, P., Shou, W., Wu, K., Foshey, M., Li, B., Palacios, T., Torralba, A., & Matusik, W. (2021). Learning human-environment interactions using conformal tactile textiles. *Nature Electronics, 4*, 193–201. https://doi.org/10.1038/s41928-021-00554-5.
17. Mohammadi, A., Tan, Y., Choong, P., & Oetomo, D. (2021). Flexible mechanical metamaterials enabling soft tactile sensors with multiple sensitivities at multiple force sensing ranges. *Scientific Reports, 11*, 24125. https://doi.org/10.1038/s41598-021-03408-7.
18. Nahavandi, D., Alizadehsani, R., Khosravi, A., & Acharya, U. R. (2022). Application of artificial intelligence in wearable devices: Opportunities and challenges. *Computer Methods and Programs in Biomedicine, 213*, 106541. https://doi.org/10.1016/j.cmpb.2021.106541.
19. Peng, Y., Yang, N., Xu, Q., Dai, Y., & Wang, Z. (2021). Recent advances in flexible tactile sensors for intelligent systems. *Sensors, 21*(16), 5392. https://doi.org/10.3390/s21165392.
20. Price, R. B., & Duman, R. (2020). Neuroplasticity in cognitive and psychological mechanisms of depression: An integrative model. *Molecular Psychiatry, 25*, 530–543. https://doi.org/10.1038/s41380-019-0551-z.
21. Sangwan, V. K., & Hersam, M. C. (2020). Neuromorphic nano electronic materials. *Nature Nanotechnology, 15*, 517–528. https://doi.org/10.1038/s41565-020-0724-5.
22. Schuman, C. D., Kulkarni, S. R., Parsa, M., Mitchell, J. P., Date, P., & Kay, B. (2022). Opportunities for neuromorphic computing algorithms and applications. *Nature Computational Science, 2*, 10–19. https://doi.org/10.1038/s43588-021-00144-2.
23. Shi, Y., Hua, Q., Dong, Z., Wang, B., Dai, X., Niu, J., Cui, Z., Huang, T., Wang, Z. L., & Hu, W. (2023). Neuro-inspired thermoresponsive nociceptor for intelligent sensory systems. *Nano Energy, 113*, 108549. https://doi.org/10.1016/j.nanoen.2023.108549.
24. Skedung, L., Arvidsson, M., Chung, J. Y., Stafford, C. M., Berglund, B., & Rutland, M. W. (2013). Feeling small: Exploring the tactile perception limits. *Scientific Reports, 3*, 2617. https://doi.org/10.1038/srep02617.

25. Sun, J., Hua, Q., Zhao, M., Dong, L., Chang, Y., Wu, W., Li, J., Chen, Q., Xi, J., Hu, W., et al. (2021). Stable ultrathin perovskite/polyvinylidene fluoride composite films for imperceptible multi-color fluorescent anti-counterfeiting labels. *Advanced Materials Technologies, 6*, 2100229. https://doi.org/10.1002/admt.202100229.

26. Sydnor, V. J., & Satterthwaite, T. D. (2023). Neuroimaging of plasticity mechanisms in the human brain: From critical periods to psychiatric conditions. *Neuropsychopharmacology, 48*, 219–220. https://doi.org/10.1038/s41386-023-01549-5.

27. Toricelli, M., Pereira, A. A. R., Souza Abrao, G., Malerba, H. N., Maia, J., Buck, H. S., & Viel, T. A. (2021). Mechanisms of neuroplasticity and brain degeneration: Strategies for protection during the aging process. *Neural Regeneration Research, 16*, 58–67. https://doi.org/10.4103/1673-5374.286954.

28. Wang, Z., Dong, C., Wang, X., Li, M., Nan, T., Liang, X., Chen, H., Wei, Y., Zhou, H., Zaeimbashi, M., et al. (2018). Highly sensitive integrated flexible tactile sensors with piezoresistive Ge2Sb2Te5 thin films. *NPJ Flexible Electronics, 2*, 17. https://doi.org/10.1038/s41528-018-0030-x.

29. Wang, Z., Xiao, C., Roy, M., Yuan, Z., Zhao, L., Liu, Y., Guo, X., & Lu, P. (2023). Bioinspired skin towards next-generation rehabilitation medicine. *Frontiers in Bioengineering and Biotechnology, 11*, 1196174. https://doi.org/10.3389/fbioe.2023.1196174.

30. Yang, J. C., Mun, J., Kwon, S. Y., Park, S., Bao, Z., & Park, S. (2019). Electronic skin: Recent progress and future prospects for skin-attachable devices for health monitoring, robotics, and prosthetics. *Advanced Materials, 31*, 1904765. https://doi.org/10.1002/adma.201904765.

31. Zhang, J., Yao, H., Mo, J., Chen, S., Xie, Y., Ma, S., Chen, R., Luo, T., Ling, W., & Qin, L. (2022). Finger-inspired rigid-soft hybrid tactile sensor with superior sensitivity at high frequency. *Nature Communications, 13*, 5076. https://doi.org/10.1038/s41467-022-32754-3.

Chapter 7

RESPIRATORY AND DIGESTIVE SYSTEM

Contents

Introduction

The respiratory and digestive systems are essential anatomical systems responsible for gas exchange and nutrient absorption, respectively, crucial for maintaining human life. Histologically, these systems exhibit specialized structures that facilitate their functions. In the respiratory system, the histology of the trachea, bronchi, and alveoli reflect their roles in conducting air and facilitating gas exchange. The trachea and bronchi are lined with pseudostratified ciliated columnar epithelium, containing goblet cells that secrete mucus to trap particles and pathogens. This epithelium helps in the movement of mucus and particles out of the respiratory tract through ciliary action. Alveoli, the site of gas exchange, are lined with simple squamous epithelium, allowing for efficient diffusion of oxygen and carbon dioxide (Alves et al., 2021). The digestive system histology is tailored for the processing and absorption of nutrients. The alimentary canal, including the esophagus, stomach, and intestines, exhibits varying histological features. For instance, the stomach has gastric pits lined with mucous-secreting cells and gastric glands that produce digestive enzymes and hydrochloric acid. In contrast, the small intestine is lined with simple columnar epithelium containing microvilli, which increase surface area for nutrient absorption. Understanding the histology of these systems is vital for comprehending their physiological functions and pathophysiology.

Orientation and Directional Terms

Term	Definition	Illustration
Respiratory System	The organ system responsible for the intake of oxygen and the expulsion of carbon dioxide, consisting of structures such as the nose, trachea, lungs, and diaphragm.	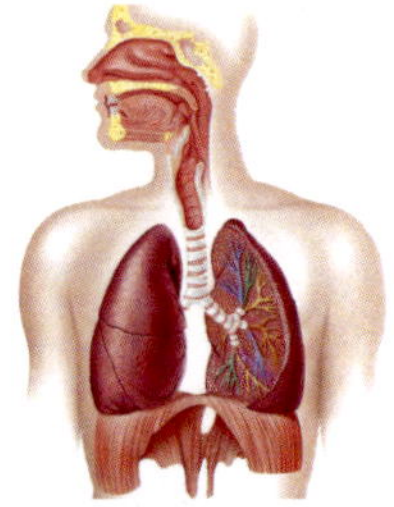
Respiratory Tissue	Specialized tissue involved in gas exchange, primarily found in the alveoli of the lungs; it includes epithelial cells and connective tissue that facilitate respiration.	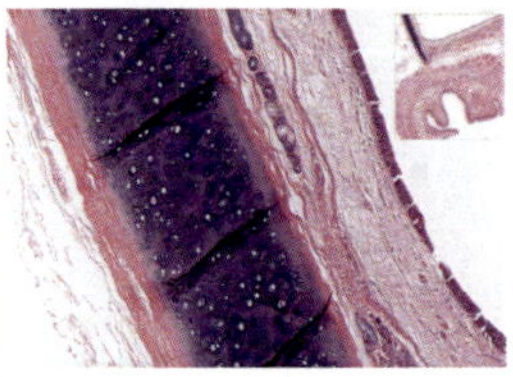
Salivary Glands	Glands located in and around the mouth that produce saliva, which contains enzymes for digestion, lubricates food, and helps maintain oral health.	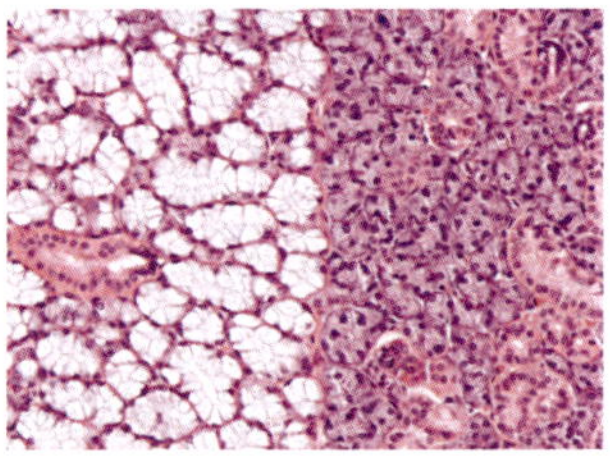
Pharynx	A muscular tube that connects the nasal and oral cavities to the esophagus and larynx; it plays a role in both the respiratory and digestive systems.	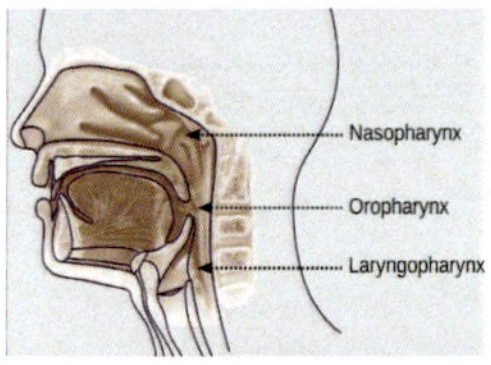
Gastrointestinal Mucus	A viscous secretion produced by the mucous membranes lining the gastrointestinal tract, serving to protect the lining, lubricate food passage, and aid in digestion.	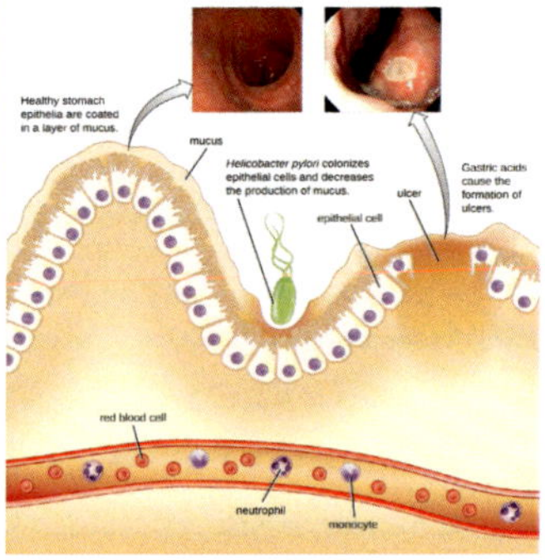

7.1. Respiratory System

The respiratory system is crucial for gas exchange, with its components divided into the conducting and respiratory portions. The conducting portion includes the nasal cavities, pharynx, larynx, trachea, and bronchial tree branches, which transport air to the respiratory tissues. These structures are characterized by rigid walls that maintain their shape and keep the airways open. The respiratory portion, located in the lungs, is where gas exchange occurs between air and blood. This region is characterized by its intimate association between capillary blood vessels and air chambers, facilitating efficient gas exchange. Both intrapulmonary (within the lungs) and extrapulmonary (outside the lungs) components make up the conducting system, further emphasizing its role in ensuring air reaches the respiratory tissues. Understanding the anatomy and function of these components is essential for comprehending respiratory physiology and diagnosing respiratory disorders.

7.1.1. Nose

The dermis that envelops the outer layer of the nose extends briefly into the vestibule of the nasal cavity, where rigid hair and their accompanying sebaceous glands assist in the filtration of the inhaled air. The vestibule is lined with nonkeratinized stratified squamous epithelium, located towards the back. Most of the remaining nasal cavity is covered by a respiratory passage lined with ciliated pseudostratified columnar epithelium, which includes goblet cells. However, the roof of the nasal cavities contains a distinct olfactory epithelium.

The epithelium is underlain by a layer of connective tissue called the lamina propria, which is separated from the epithelium by a basement membrane. The lamina propria contains mucous glands, serous glands, and thin-walled venous sinuses. The venous sinuses play a role in heating the air that enters and are particularly noticeable in the lamina propria that covers the middle and inferior conchae. Lymphatic tissue is found and becomes prominent near the nasopharynx. The innermost layers of the lamina propria combine with the periosteum or perichondrium of the nasal bones and cartilage. In these areas, the nasal mucosa creates a mucoperiosteum or mucoperichondrium, respectively. The epithelial lining is covered by a thin layer of mucus, which is continuously propelled towards the pharynx by the ciliated epithelial cells. The mucus originates from goblet cells on the surface and secretions from mucoserous glands in the lamina propria. The mucus layer serves to humidify the air and trap particulate matter. The mucous layer contains immunoglobulins, including IgA, which provide protection against localized infection. IgA is synthesized by plasma cells located in the lamina propria and is subsequently internalized by secretory cells in nearby glands. Subsequently, the IgA is bound to the secretory component of these cells, conveyed, and discharged onto the exterior of the nasal mucosa. The paranasal sinuses have a similar mucosa as other areas, but with some differences. The epithelium is thinner, there are fewer goblet cells, the lamina propria is thinner and has fewer glands, and there are no venous sinuses present. The paranasal sinuses, including the maxillary, sphenoid, frontal, and ethmoid sinuses, are located within corresponding bones that surround the nasal cavity. These sinuses are connected to the nasal cavity through small openings. The cilia in the lining epithelium of the paranasal sinuses typically move towards the nasal cavity. However, the ciliated epithelial cells are organized in a coordinated manner, following a wide, open spiral pathway. This spiral pathway becomes narrower at the opening to the nasal cavity (Alves et al., 2021).

7.1.1.1. Olfactory Epithelium

The olfactory epithelium is located in the upper part of the nasal cavities, covering the superior conchae and a small area on both sides of the nasal septum. Additionally, it exhibits a pseudostratified columnar epithelium structure, although it does not possess goblet cells and has a significantly greater thickness compared to the respiratory lining epithelium.

There are three main types of cells: supporting cells, basal cells, and sensory or olfactory cells. Sustentacular cells are characterized by their tall stature, narrow bases, and broad apical surfaces adorned with long, slender microvilli. The cell contains an oval nucleus positioned slightly above its center. At the apical region, fully developed junctional complexes connect the supporting cells with the neighboring olfactory cells.

The olfactory cells, which are bipolar nerve cells, are evenly distributed among the supporting cells and serve as the sensory component. The cells have a spindle-like shape, with nuclei that are rounded and positioned centrally within an enlarged region of cytoplasm. At the apex, the cell narrows down to a thin, elongated structure (a modified dendrite) that stretches between the surrounding cells to reach the surface. At the surface, it enlarges into a rounded olfactory vesicle (knob). Six to eight elongated olfactory cilia protrude from the olfactory vesicle and run parallel to the epithelial surface, immersed in a layer of fluid. The olfactory hair are specialized, immotile cilia that serve as the responsive part of these cells. The olfactory hair initially possess a ciliary structure, but they quickly narrow and undergo a sudden decrease in the number of microtubules, transitioning from doublets to singlets. Essentially, the olfactory cells become narrower and form a thin process called an axon, which then enters the lamina propria. In this region, the axon combines with similar fibers to create small bundles of nerves. The fila olfactory directly connects to the olfactory bulb. The nasal cavity contains approximately 50 million olfactory receptor neurons.

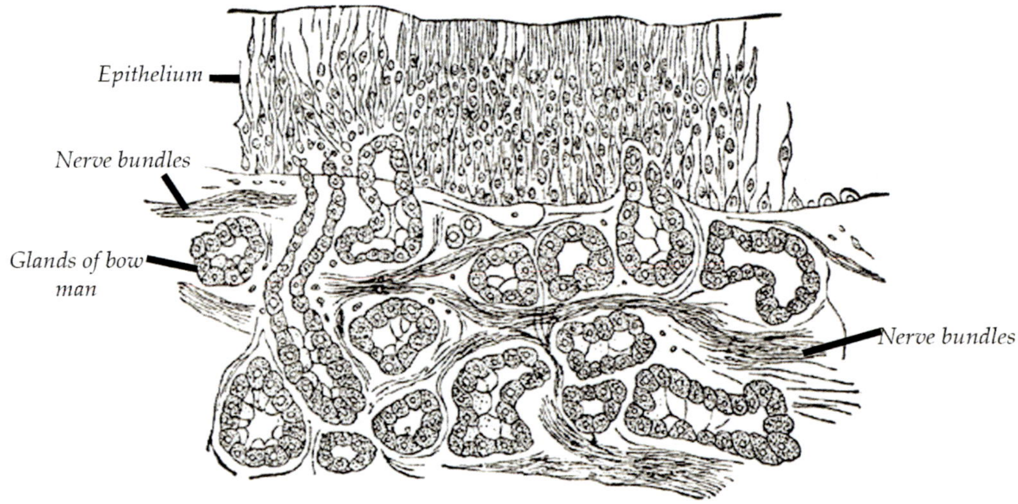

Figure 7.1. *A diagrammatic sketch of the olfactory epithelium.*

Source: https://upload.wikimedia.org/wikipedia/commons/4/4d/Gray857.png.

Odorants, which are airborne substances that stimulate olfactory sensory neurons, attach to a nasal-specific protein called olfactory binding protein. This protein helps attach the odorant molecules to receptors found in the plasmalemma of olfactory cilia. Odorant receptors are a type of G-protein coupled receptor that consist of seven transmembrane molecules. These receptors can detect and differentiate between thousands of specific molecules. Basal cells are small, triangular cells that are tightly packed between the bases of sustentacular and olfactory cells (**Figure 7.1**). These cells are pluripotent and can differentiate into either of the two other cell types. Olfactory cells possess a distinctive characteristic in that they directly interface with the external environment and, unlike other neurons, undergo continuous replacement every 30 to 60 days. Olfactory cells are generated through the process of differentiation of the basal cells. The olfactory epithelium's thickness is partially due to varying numbers of receptor neurons that become more differentiated as they progress from the luminal surface to the basal cells.

The lamina propria contains intricate networks of blood vessels and branched, tubuloacinar serous glands. The olfactory glands, known as Bowman's glands, produce watery secretions that cleanse the surface of the olfactory epithelium. This prevents constant stimulation from a single odor and acts as a solvent for odorant substances. Contrary to earlier reports, vomeronasal organs (VNO) are indeed present in the nasal cavities of most adult humans. The human VNO comprises two small sacs, each approximately 2 mm in depth, which connect to shallow indentations on both sides of the nasal septum. The sacs are lined with an epithelium that bears resemblance to olfactory epithelium. This epithelium consists of supporting cells and cells that have a similar appearance to olfactory receptor bipolar neurons. These bipolar neurons can attach to antibodies that target neuron-specific enolase and protein gene product 9.5, which is a characteristic shared by most neurons. The neural connectivity between these cells and the brain remains unidentified in humans. The precise function of the VNO in humans remains uncertain. Other extensively studied mammals have demonstrated that the VNO is connected to an accessory olfactory bulb, which is subsequently linked to the limbic system of the brain. The VNO in these mammals is responsible for detecting pheromones, which play a role in regulating sexual and territorial behaviors (Alves et al., 2021).

7.1.2. Pharynx and Larynx

The nasal cavities extend backwards into the pharynx, which consists of nasal, oral, and laryngeal sections. The highest region, known as the nasopharynx, is directly connected to the nasal cavities and is covered by the same type of respiratory passage epithelium – specifically, ciliated pseudostratified columnar epithelium with goblet cells. A nonkeratinizing stratified squamous epithelium may develop in areas that are prone to abrasion, such as the edge of the soft palate and the posterior wall of the pharynx. These surfaces come into contact with each other during the act of swallowing. The connective tissue beneath contains mucous, serous, and mixed mucoserous glands, as well as a large amount of lymphatic tissue. Lymphatic tissue is dispersed sporadically within the connective tissue and creates tonsillar structures, including the pharyngeal tonsils located on the back wall of the nasopharynx, the tubal tonsils surrounding the openings of the eustachian tubes into the nasopharynx, and the palatine and lingual tonsils at the junctions of the oral cavity and oropharynx. This lymphatic tissue is a component of the mucosa-associated lymphoid tissue (MALT) and makes up Waldeyer's ring. Lymphoid tissue is occasionally found in the connective tissue beneath the epithelium of the trachea, bronchi, and true bronchioles. The lymphoid tissue located in the bronchi is known as bronchus-associated lymphoid tissue (BALT). The larynx serves as the anatomical link between the pharynx and trachea. The framework of the structure is composed of multiple cartilages, specifically the thyroid, cricoid, and arytenoid cartilages, which are made of hyaline cartilage. On the other hand, the epiglottis, corniculate cartilages, and the tips of the arytenoid cartilages are made of elastic cartilage. The cartilages in this structure are connected and attached to the hyoid bone by layers of dense fibrous connective tissue, which create the cricothyroid and thyroid membranes. The epithelium of the lining varies depending on its location. The front side and approximately half of the back side of the epiglottis are coated with nonkeratinized stratified squamous epithelium, which may have a small number of taste buds. The vocal cords are also coated with a moist stratified squamous epithelium, while the rest of the larynx is lined with respiratory passage epithelium. The larynx's lamina propria is dense and consists of mucous and a few serous or mucoserous glands (Buddington and Krogdahl, 2004).

7.1.3. Trachea and Extrapulmonary Bronchi

The trachea and its primary bronchi have walls that contain 15 to 20 C-shaped rings made of hyaline cartilage. These rings help keep the airway open and unobstructed. The interstices between adjacent rings are occupied by compact fibroelastic connective tissue, while the spaces between the branches of the cartilages are filled with clusters of smooth muscle known as the trachealis muscle. The gaps are oriented towards the back, and when viewed in cross-section, the trachea and extrapulmonary bronchi appear compressed. The lining epithelium is composed of a ciliated pseudostratified columnar epithelium that contains many goblet cells and is supported by a thick basal lamina. The cilia move in the direction of the pharynx. Aside from the ciliated and goblet cells, various other cell types have been identified in the tracheobronchial epithelium. Brush cells are characterized by the presence of glycogen granules, long and straight microvilli on their upper surfaces, and contact with nerve processes at their base. These cells are uncommon in humans and their purpose is not yet understood. However, they could potentially be sensory cells, depleted goblet cells, or transitional cells between short cells and fully developed ciliated cells. Pulmonary neuroendocrine cells, characterized by their small size and granulated appearance, are sparsely distributed in the lungs. The pulmonary neuroendocrine system is present throughout the entire respiratory tree. These cells are components of a widespread network of cells that contain amines, such as serotonin (5-HT), and amine precursors, along with several peptides. These substances are believed to have localized effects on neighboring cells, as well as on smooth muscle cells in the trachea and bronchi. The pulmonary neuroendocrine cells located in the epithelium of the trachea and bronchi are believed to be responsive cells that can detect low oxygen levels. They can release substances that can either relax or contract nearby airway smooth muscle cells, thereby influencing their contraction. Undifferentiated cells, known as short cells, are present in the lower layers of the epithelium, specifically between the bases of other cell types. These short cells can generate goblet and ciliated cells. A network of dendritic cells is located beneath the tracheal epithelium. They act as antigen-presenting cells with the ability to bind and present antigens to T-lymphocytes. The lamina propria of the trachea consists of numerous small seromucous glands and sporadic clusters of lymphatic tissue. The compound tubuloacinar glands consist of serous units that generate a thin, aqueous secretion abundant in glycoproteins, lysozyme, and IgA obtained from neighboring lymphoid cells. Myoepithelial cells are connected to the secretory units of the tracheal glands and assist in the release f secretory products. The cartilage is surrounded by a fibroconnective tissue layer called the adventitia. This layer consists of elastic, collagenous, and reticular fibers, as well as blood vessels and nerves.

7.1.4. Intrapulmonary Air Passages

The primary bronchi branch out to form multiple levels of intrapulmonary bronchi, where the C-shaped cartilaginous rings of the primary bronchi are substituted with irregular plates of hyaline cartilage that fully enclose the structure. The intrapulmonary bronchi are cylindrical and lack the flattened shape of the main bronchi and trachea. The large intrapulmonary bronchi have a mucous membrane that is internally lined. This membrane is continuous with and identical to the mucous membrane of the trachea and primary bronchi. It consists of a ciliated pseudostratified columnar epithelium with goblet cells. The lamina propria consists of scattered lymphatic tissue and is distinctively separated from the epithelium by a prominent basal lamina. Below the lamina propria is a layer of smooth muscle cells that are arranged irregularly and form spirals around the bronchus, either in a left or right direction. The muscular layer acts as a barrier between the lamina propria and the connective tissue of the submucosa, which is located directly inside the hyaline cartilage plates. The submucosa contains both mucous and mucoserous bronchial glands, which have ducts that extend through the muscle layer and open onto the epithelial surface. The glands in question and other glands in the respiratory system produce secretions that contain IgA. This IgA, derived from nearby lymphoid tissue, provides immunological defense to the larger respiratory passages (Buddington and Krogdahl, 2004).

Through consecutive divisions, the intrapulmonary bronchi gradually diminish in size. While they maintain the fundamental structure described earlier, the layers of their walls become thinner. The bronchial tree can have up to 25 branches or as few as 10 before reaching the respiratory part of the lung. The intrapulmonary bronchi of the smallest size exhibit isolated cartilage plates and are no longer encased by cartilage. The epithelium is transformed into a layer of ciliated simple columnar cells that contain goblet cells. The bronchial glands are present in the same location as the extent of the cartilage. The medium-sized bronchi are the main sites where airway resistance occurs during breathing. The resistance can be altered by either increasing or decreasing the contraction of bronchial smooth muscle. Activation of the parasympathetic nervous system causes the contraction of the smooth muscles in the bronchi, leading to the narrowing of the airway passages and an increase in resistance to airflow. Activation of the sympathetic nervous system causes bronchial smooth muscle relaxation, leading to the widening of the airways and a reduction in airway resistance. Once the tube's diameter reaches approximately 1 mm, the cartilage vanishes from the wall, transforming the structure into a bronchiole. The glands and lymphatic tissue undergo regression, while the smooth muscle becomes notably prominent and assumes the primary role in providing support. The epithelium lining of the bronchioles exhibits variation, ranging from ciliated columnar epithelium with goblet cells in the larger bronchioles to ciliated cuboidal epithelium without goblet cells in the terminal bronchioles. Terminal bronchioles are the most diminutive divisions of the exclusively conducting system. Intermingled with the ciliated cells are a small number of nonciliated cells with protruding apical surfaces in the lumen and possess a limited number of microvilli. The Clara cells, also known as bronchiolar secretory cells, are present in the respiratory system. They release protease inhibitors, oxidases, glycosaminoglycans, and immunosuppressive proteins. Cytochrome P450 enzymes are believed to have a protective effect against inhaled toxins and carcinogens, and they may also play a role in preventing conditions like emphysema. The Clara cell may also contribute to the removal or generation of surfactant in this area.

Neuroepithelial bodies are clusters of nerve endings located in the lining of the airways within the lungs, and they can also be found in the small air sacs called alveoli. They are absent from the trachea. The corpuscles are observed as oval or triangular structures, measuring 20 to 40 μm in width. They are embedded in the respiratory epithelium, spanning from the inner space to the basement membrane. Fundamentally, the neuroepithelial body is intimately associated with a capillary. The entire structure is abundantly supplied with nerves, and a significant number of nerve endings establish contact with cells of the corpuscle. The neuroepithelial bodies consist of 4 to 10 elongated neuroendocrine cells that lack cilia and have a slightly acidophilic cytoplasm, which exhibits a positive reaction to argyrophil (silver) staining. The oval nuclei are positioned at the base and aligned with the long axis of the cells. These cells contain a large number of mitochondria, moderately well-developed granular endoplasmic reticulum, small Golgi complexes, and some glycogen and multivesicular bodies. These cells are characterized by the presence of numerous dense-cored vesicles. Neuroepithelial bodies are considered chemoreceptors that respond to the chemical makeup of inhaled air. When the level of oxygen in the air we breathe decreases, the neuroepithelial body releases dense-cored vesicles that contain serotonin, a powerful substance that constricts blood vessels, and other peptides that may affect the tone of the airways. Therefore, in the event of local hypoxia, blood is redirected from poorly oxygenated and ventilated regions of the lungs to areas with higher oxygen levels. Under conditions of decreased oxygen availability, three processes take place to enhance ventilation and redirect pulmonary blood flow towards more well-ventilated areas of the lung. The events involved in this process include: (a) an elevated rate of communication between glomus cells in the carotid body and respiratory centers in the brain, (b) the narrowing of pulmonary arterioles due to low oxygen levels, and (c) the regulation of this process by pulmonary neuroendocrine cells located in the respiratory epithelium of the major airways. Each of these tissues can detect sudden alterations in oxygen levels, generate a signal, and activate compensatory mechanisms. The highly innervated neuroepithelial bodies serve as transmitters of the hypoxia stimulus through neural input, influencing the regulation of respiration and other pulmonary functions. Neuroepithelial bodies, similar to glomus cells in the carotid body, secrete serotonin when exposed to low oxygen levels. The plasmalemma of cells comprising the neuroepithelial bodies exhibits the membrane characteristics of excitable cells (Buddington and Krogdahl, 2004). The oxygen-sensing mechanism in these cells relies on the interaction between the oxygen-sensing protein (NADPH oxidase) and an oxygen-sensitive potassium channel located in the plasmalemma. Therefore, the presence of oxygen concentration can stimulate oxygen sensors in both solitary pulmonary neuroepithelial cells and innervated clusters of pulmonary neuroepithelial cells (neuroepithelial bodies), which can then regulate various pulmonary processes such as airway tone, pulmonary circulation, and even the control of breathing. Significant evidence suggests that the solitary neuroepithelial cells have a crucial role in the development of the lungs. This is supported by the presence of bombesin and other peptides in human fetal lung tissue, which possess properties similar to growth factors.

7.1.5. Respiratory Tissue

The exchange of gases between the air and blood only occurs when they are in close proximity. This condition initially manifests in the respiratory bronchioles, which serve as a bridge between the conducting and respiratory areas of the lung. The walls of respiratory bronchioles are composed of collagenous connective tissue containing interlacing bundles of smooth muscle and elastic fibers. The respiratory bronchioles of greater size are covered by a layer of simple cuboidal epithelium, which contains only a small number of ciliated cells and does not have goblet cells. A significant proportion of the cuboidal cells are Clara cells. Within the smaller respiratory bronchioles, the epithelium undergoes a transformation into a low cuboidal shape, devoid of cilia. The alveoli emerge from the walls of the respiratory bronchioles and serve as the respiratory sections of these air passages. The number of alveoli increases as we move towards the distal end. The respiratory bronchioles terminate by dividing into alveolar ducts. Alveolar ducts are slender tubes with thin walls with multiple openings for alveoli or groups of alveoli. As a result, the duct wall is mostly composed of these alveolar openings. The presence of a tube is only observed in a limited number of locations, where clusters of cuboidal cells are found between consecutive alveoli. These cells also cover the fibroelastic tissue and smooth muscle bundles beneath them. The alveolar ducts terminate in irregular cavities encircled by clusters of alveoli known as alveolar sacs. Alveoli are polygonal structures with thin walls that come in different sizes and have an opening on one side to allow air to enter their cavities. The lungs contain a population of approximately 300 to 800 million structures and offer a surface area of 70 to 95 square meters for the exchange of gases. The alveoli that are next to each other are divided by a shared interalveolar septum, which is characterized by a prominent network of capillaries that protrude from the wall of the septum (Buddington and Krogdahl, 2004). Reticular and elastic fibers create a delicate structure for the septa. The septal wall contains small openings, known as alveolar pores of Kohn, which have a diameter ranging from 1 to 10 μm. These pores allow for the exchange and equalization of air pressure between the alveoli. Pores can have a significant impact on obstructive lung disease by acting as a bypass mechanism to provide air to the alveoli beyond the obstruction. The alveolar wall is coated with a thin epithelium on both sides, supported by a basal lamina underneath. The epithelial basal lamina and the basal lamina of the capillary are separated by a narrow space of only 15 to 20 nm in many areas. However, in some regions, the two laminae are fused. Therefore, at its narrowest point, the blood-air barrier is composed of a thin layer of liquid, the thin epithelium of the alveolar lining cell, the merged basal laminae, and the endothelium of the capillaries in the septal wall (**Figure 7.2**). The thickness of the blood-air barrier ranges from 0.2 to 0.5 μm.

The septa contain various types of cells. The pulmonary epithelial cells, also known as type I pneumonocytes, are attenuated squamous cells that create a continuous lining for the alveolar wall. Furthermore, septal cells, alveolar macrophages, and endothelial cells form a lining along the blood capillaries. Septal cells, also known as type II pneumonocytes, are cells that have a rounded or cuboidal shape. These cells can be found either deep in the surface epithelium or protruding into the alveolar lumen, which is the space between the pulmonary epithelial cells (type I). Their exposed surfaces possess small projections called microvilli, and the cells are connected to pulmonary epithelial cells through junctional complexes (Figures 7.3 and 7.4). The defining characteristic of septal cells is the existence of multilamellar bodies within their cytoplasm (Buddington and Krogdahl, 2004).

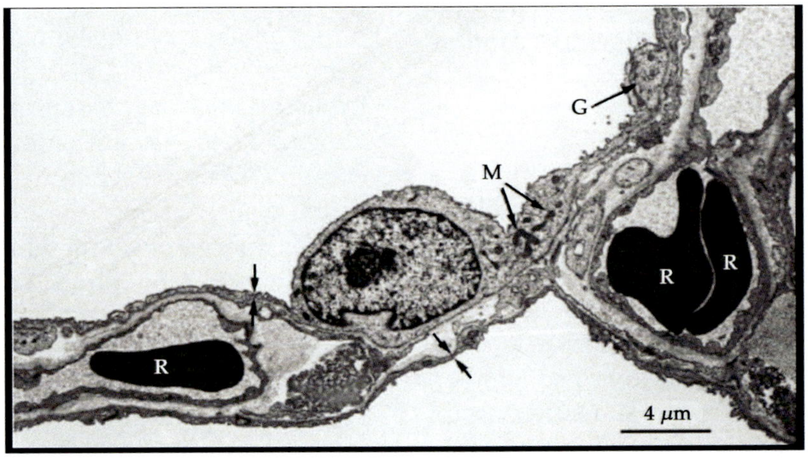

Figure 7.2. *Type I cell. Transmission electron micrograph of rat alveolar septum. The nucleus of a type I cell can be seen in the center of the image. Arrows indicate the thin cytoplasmic extensions of type I cells on both sides of the alveolar septum. M: mitochondria; G: Golgi apparatus; R: red blood cells in capillaries. (Original magnification 2500 6; image courtesy of Lennell Allen.).*

Source: https://www.researchgate.net/profile/Meshell-Johnson/publication/6496303/figure/fig1/AS:322642679746560@1453935417513/Type-I-cell-Transmission-electron-micrograph-of-rat-alveolar-septum-The-nucleus-of-a.png.

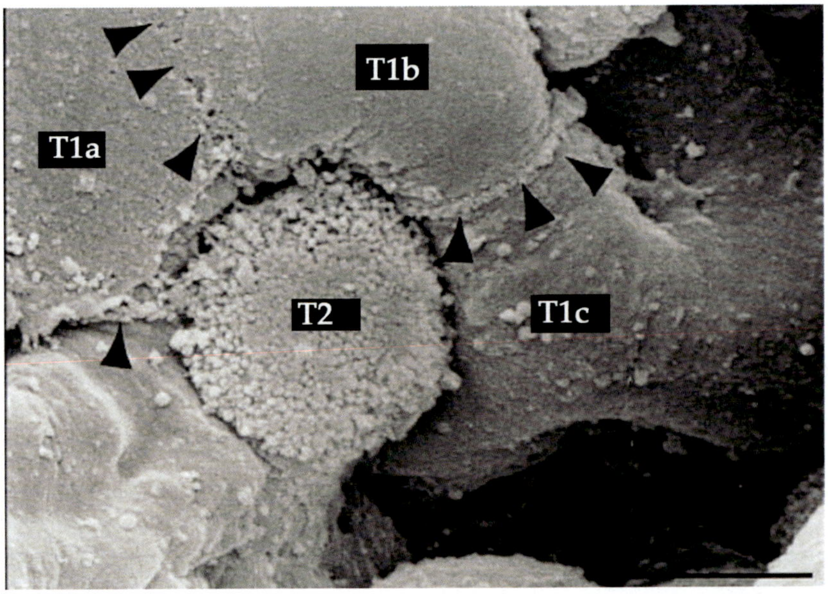

Figure 7.3. *Scanning electron micrograph of type 2 (T2) pneumocyte surrounded by protruding capillaries covered by squamous type 1 (T1) pneumocytes (T1a, T1b, T1c). T1 pneumocyte borders (arrowheads) converge at the margin of the T2 pneumocyte. This is an area much like the one that was reconstructed.*

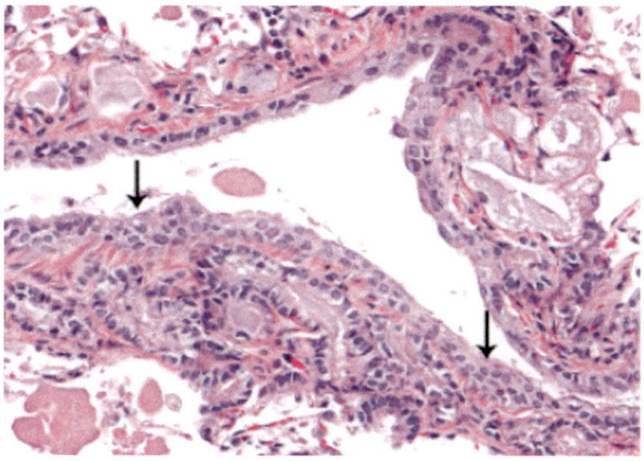

Figure 7.4. *A transmission electron micrograph showing a type II pneumocyte located in the limiting wall of an alveolus.*

Source: https://ars.els-cdn.com/content/image/3-s2.0-B978012391448400023X-f23-17-9780123914484.jpg.

These structures are composed of thin, concentric layers and serve as the locations where surfactant is stored. It is produced by septal cells and released through exocytosis. The surfactant that is released forms a single layer over the thin layer of fluid that covers the alveoli. It acts as a detergent, reducing the surface tension between the liquid and the air. Reducing surface tension helps to prevent the collapse of alveoli at the end of exhalation. Therefore, pulmonary surfactant creates the surface-active layer essential for the proper functioning of the lungs.

This substance is composed of a complex mixture of phospholipids, with dipalmitoyl phosphatidylcholine being the primary component. Additionally, it contains four proteinaceous elements referred to as surfactant-associated proteins: SP-A, SP-B, SP-C, and SP-D. SP-A is the predominant and water-soluble oligomeric glycoprotein that aids in the creation of a film with surface-active properties. Additionally, it plays a part in the body's defense against microorganisms. Type I pneumocytes constitute approximately 40% of the cell population that lines the alveoli, yet they cover more than 90% of the total surface area. On the other hand, type II pneumocytes constitute approximately 60% of the total alveolar cell population, yet they only contribute to 8 to 10% of the overall alveolar surface area. Type I pneumocytes have limited ability to undergo cell division. In contrast, type II pneumocytes have maintained their ability to divide and act as a reservoir of replacement cells for both type I and type II pneumocytes (Buddington and Krogdahl, 2004).

Alveolar macrophages can be found in the interalveolar septa and alveolar lumina. These cells often contain particles of inhaled material and are commonly referred to as "dust" cells. Alveolar macrophages, like all macrophages, are derived from blood monocytes. The majority of these cells are eventually expelled through the air passages and can be found in the sputum. A few cells may enter the lymphatic system and exit the lungs through this pathway. It is important to understand that the lungs receive blood from two separate blood supplies. Understanding that the lungs receive blood from two separate blood vessels is crucial. The bronchial vascular system supplies oxygenated blood to the main structures of the bronchial tree. The bronchial artery originates directly from the thoracic aorta, while the bronchial veins of the main parts of the bronchial region drain into the azygos and hemiazygos veins. The terminal branches of the bronchial veins empty into the pulmonary veins.

On the other hand, the capillaries of the pulmonary vascular system are specifically where gaseous exchange takes place. The pulmonary arteries deliver oxygen-depleted blood, which is high in carbon dioxide, from the body tissues to the lungs through the right side of the heart. Pulmonary vessels are typically characterized by their short and wide structure, which results in increased distensibility due to the reduced presence of smooth muscle in their walls. Pulmonary vessels exhibit low pressure and low resistance. Additionally, because all cardiac output from the right side of the heart passes through the lungs, they have a high flow rate. The pulmonary capillaries are organized in a planar manner, unlike the systemic vessels which are arranged in a branching pattern similar to the roots of a plant. The capillaries are located between and around the alveoli. The capillaries surrounding the alveoli are known as septal or alveolar capillaries. The capillaries located at the corners between alveoli are commonly referred to as extra-alveolar or corner capillaries. The lung's capillaries create one of the most extensive areas for exchange in the body, measuring approximately 90 m^2. After undergoing gaseous exchange in the pulmonary capillaries, the blood that has been re-oxygenated is gathered by pulmonary venules and veins. It is then transported back to the body tissues through the left side of the heart. The arterioles of the pulmonary vascular circuit exhibit a distinct behavior in contrast to the systemic arterioles. In ischemic areas of the lung, these arterioles tend to divert blood away from such regions, rather than directing it towards an area with low oxygen levels, as is the case with systemic vessels. The lymphatic capillaries originate around the respiratory bronchioles and progressively combine to create larger vessels that trace the bronchial tree towards the hilum and exit the lung. Another set of lymph capillaries is situated in the visceral pleura and connective tissue septa, which divide each lung into separate lobes. It is believed that these substances flow into the pleural cavity. When the pressure in the pulmonary capillaries rises, the fluid part of the blood easily moves through the very thin alveolar wall and into the alveolar lumen. This event occurs in cases of pulmonary edema caused by left heart failure. In this scenario, there is an incomplete emptying of the left ventricle of the heart, resulting in an accumulation of pressure in both the left atrium and the pulmonary veins. Elevated pressure in the pulmonary veins causes fluid to be pushed from the capillaries into the alveolar spaces within the lung. This excess fluid overwhelms the lymphatic system, which starts in the smaller airways, and results in the accumulation of fluid in the respiratory part of the lung, hindering the exchange of gases (Cao and Wang, 2009).

7.1.6. Pleura

The pleura consists of thin membranes composed of collagenous and elastic fibers, enveloped by a single layer of mesothelial cells. The parietal pleura is the layer that lines the wall of the thoracic cavity. It extends from the thoracic wall to cover the surface of the lungs, where it transforms into the visceral pleura. The pleura secrete a small amount of fluid between the two layers of mesothelium covering to facilitate smooth movement without friction.

While the two pleurae can move smoothly across each other, their separation encounters significant resistance. Consequently, the lungs firmly attach to the inner surface of the thoracic wall and expand or contract in response to changes in the volume of the thoracic cavity during breathing. The diaphragm contracts, causing the thoracic cavity to increase in its vertical dimension (superior-inferior diameter). Additionally, the intercostal and other accessory respiratory muscles contract, raising and elevating the ribs, which expands the anterior-posterior diameter of the thorax. The contraction of intercostal muscles causes the rotation of rib arches 2 to 7, at the costosternal and costovertebral joints. The bucket-handle movement refers to the upward movement of the ribs and the outward movement of their lower edges, leading to an expansion of the width of the thorax. The sternal ends of the ribs and costal cartilage are raised, pushing the sternum forward to expand the front-to-back diameter of the thorax. This motion is referred to as the pump-handle movement. Furthermore, the intercostal muscles reinforce the rigidity of the thoracic wall, thereby preventing alterations in the configuration of the thorax caused by the suction effect generated by the diaphragm's contraction. As the volume of the thoracic cavity increases, the pressure within the pleural cavity and lungs decreases. Consequently, air is drawn into the respiratory system from the surrounding atmosphere. Expiration is predominantly a passive phenomenon. As the diaphragm ascends and the intercostal muscles relax, the rib cage contracts, resulting in a reduction in the volume of the thorax and lungs. The abdominal muscles are used during forced expiration. Concurrently, the elastic tissue in the lungs contracts, resulting in an elevation of pressure within the lungs, which in turn expels air from the lungs.

7.1.7. Control of Respiratory Rate

The main respiratory center responsible for controlling respiration is situated in the reticular formation of the medulla (specifically, the rostral ventrolateral medulla) in the brain. The neurons in this region serve as a pacemaker, producing a fundamental respiratory rhythm. The fundamental rhythm can be altered by input from other brain regions, as well as input from receptors that detect variations in the chemical composition of the arterial blood. Chemoreceptors detect increases in carbon dioxide levels, decreases in oxygen levels, and alterations in pH. The chemoreceptors that detect these changes can be divided into two main categories: central chemoreceptors, primarily found in the medulla of the brain, and peripheral chemoreceptors located in the carotid and aortic bodies. The carotid bodies transmit their sensory information to the medulla primarily via the glossopharyngeal nerves, while the aortic bodies transmit their information through the vagus nerves.

7.1.8. Organogenesis

Respiratory passages emerge during the 4th week of gestation as an endodermal bud originating from the caudal end of the laryngotracheal groove. As the lung bud expands, it becomes enveloped by mesenchyme, which subsequently undergoes differentiation into blood vessels and the supportive structures such as cartilage, smooth muscle, and connective tissues that uphold the walls. The endoderm forms the epithelial lining of the entire respiratory tract. The lung bud elongates downward and goes through a series of divisions, with the initial branches forming the primary bronchi. Successive subdivisions yield increasingly intricate ramifications of an intricate respiratory tree, ultimately culminating in diminutive dilations known as infundibula. Over time, these small sacs develop into the final alveoli. Throughout their development, the lungs undergo significant morphological changes, and histologically, three distinct phases can be observed. The initial or glandular phase spans from weeks 5 to 17 and primarily involves the growth of the branching airway passages. The lung's gland-like appearance is achieved through the repeated divisions of the endodermal tubes within a mesenchyme bed. The tubes are composed of undifferentiated columnar cells that possess a limited number of organelles, but are abundant in glycogen and contain fat. The size of nuclei varies and they typically exhibit one or two nucleoli. Mitoses are frequently observed. The cells are connected at their uppermost points by tight junctions and desmosomes. From the very beginning, the epithelial cells are distinguished from the mesenchyme by a fragile basement membrane. The cells subsequently transform into cuboidal shape, and by the 13th week, cilia and goblet cells emerge, initially in the trachea and then in more distal regions of the respiratory tree. At the age of 16 weeks, Clara cells undergo differentiation and endocrine cells become detectable. The canalicular phase occurs between the seventeenth and 26th week of development.

During this phase, there is rapid growth of the tubular elements, which form the smaller branches of the respiratory tree. Additionally, the respiratory parts become more distinct and defined. The terminal buds, also known as infundibula, undergo a change in shape from spherical to a less rounded form and establish a close connection with networks of capillaries. The process of tubules transforming into canaliculi involves the epithelium becoming flattened and undergoing significant cytodifferentiation. Epithelial cells that produce surfactant contain osmiophilic lamellar bodies. These cells also have well-developed endoplasmic reticulum and abundant ribosomes. The presence of type II pneumocytes and surfactant becomes detectable during the 28th week of gestation. In this phase, the cells decrease in height and their intercellular junctions are located in the lower half of the cell instead of at the top as in the glandular phase. These cells at a low level are the early forms of type I pneumocytes found in the saccules and alveoli. The alveolar (terminal sac) phase lasts from the 26th week of pregnancy until the baby is born. At this stage, the respiratory bronchioles can be identified as tubes with flattened epithelium on one side and ciliated cuboidal epithelium on the other side. The buds on the branches have developed into clusters of saccules, which are now composed of five to six generations. These saccules are lined by flattened epithelial cells that are closely connected to capillaries (Cao and Wang, 2009). The septa separating capillaries are initially thick, but gradually become thinner. During the time of birth, the alveoli are small and not very deep. Additionally, there are only a few individual alveoli found in the respiratory bronchioles. Alveolar inflation takes place after birth when respiration begins, starting in the hilar region and then spreading to the central part of the lungs. The distal alveoli become inflated only after several hours of breathing. Alveoli, which are tiny air sacs in the lungs, continue to develop after birth. However, it takes until around the eighth year after birth for the lungs to reach their full adult capacity of alveoli.

7.2. Digestive System

The digestive system, also known as the alimentary canal or gastrointestinal tract, is a complex system responsible for the breakdown and absorption of nutrients from food. It consists of several components, including:

1. **Mouth**: The oral cavity where digestion begins. Teeth break down food mechanically, while saliva contains enzymes that start the chemical digestion of carbohydrates.
2. **Pharynx**: A muscular tube that connects the mouth to the esophagus. It plays a role in swallowing, moving food from the mouth to the esophagus.
3. **Esophagus**: A muscular tube that connects the pharynx to the stomach. It moves food from the mouth to the stomach through a series of muscular contractions called peristalsis.
4. **Stomach**: A muscular organ that stores food and secretes gastric juices, which contain acids and enzymes that further break down food. The stomach also helps regulate the release of food into the small intestine.
5. **Small Intestine**: The longest part of the digestive tract, where most digestion and absorption of nutrients occur. It is divided into three parts: the duodenum, jejunum, and ileum. Enzymes from the pancreas and bile from the liver aid in the digestion of fats, proteins, and carbohydrates.
6. **Large Intestine (Colon)**: Absorbs water and electrolytes from the indigestible food residue, forming

feces. It also houses bacteria that aid in the fermentation of undigested material.

7. **Rectum**: The final section of the large intestine, where feces are stored before being expelled from the body through the anus.

In addition to these components, there are accessory digestive organs that play a role in digestion but are not part of the alimentary canal. These include the liver, gallbladder, and pancreas. The liver produces bile, which is stored in the gallbladder and released into the small intestine to aid in the digestion of fats. The pancreas produces digestive enzymes and bicarbonate, which help neutralize stomach acid in the small intestine (Cao and Wang, 2009).

7.2.1. General Structure

The alimentary tract exhibits various characteristics that serve as shared structural elements throughout its entirety. The innermost layer of tissue in the digestive tract is referred to as the mucous membrane or mucosa. It is composed of a lining epithelium and a layer of delicate, interconnected connective tissue fibers known as the lamina propria.

The muscularis mucosae, a muscular element of the mucosa, is exclusively located in the tubular section of the tract. Directly below the mucosa lies a layer of connective tissue composed of thick, loosely arranged collagen fibers and sporadic elastic fibers. The submucosa is a layer that contains larger blood vessels and nerves, and it allows the mucosa to have a significant amount of mobility. In areas where it is not present, the mucosa is stationary and securely connected to nearby structures. The tubular section of the tract is surrounded by a muscular wall called the muscularis externa, which is made up of a thick layer of smooth muscle. This muscular wall is further enclosed by either connective tissue called adventitia or a layer of connective tissue covered by mesothelium known as serosa.

7.2.2. Oral Cavity

The oral cavity is a non-uniformly shaped structure that includes the lips, cheeks, tongue, gingiva, teeth, and palate. The mucosa is composed of a stratified squamous epithelium and a relatively compact lamina propria. In certain areas of the oral cavity, there may exist a layer called the submucosa (Cao and Wang, 2009).

7.2.2.1. Lip

The outer layer of the lip is enveloped by a delicate layer of skin and includes sweat glands, hair follicles, and sebaceous glands. The lip is covered by a nonkeratinized, translucent, stratified squamous epithelium at the vermilion border, which does not have hair follicles or glands. The lamina propria extends into the epithelium above it, creating multiple tall connective tissue papillae that are rich in capillaries. The red color of this part of the lip is due to the presence of tall vascular papillae and translucent epithelium. The red portion is anatomically contiguous with the oral mucosa internally and with thin skin externally. The absence of glands results in the red part of the lips being kept moist through the action of licking. The inner surface of the lip is covered by a layer of nonkeratinized (moist) stratified squamous epithelium, which sits on top of a dense lamina propria containing many connective tissue papillae. The orbicularis oris muscle lies between the oral mucosa and the skin. The submucosa contains fibrous connective tissue that forms strong connections between the mucosa and the surrounding muscle. The submucosa contains multiple mixed mucoserous labial glands, whose ducts release fluid and lubrication onto the internal surface of the lip. These small bumps can be detected when the tongue is firmly pressed against the inside of the lip.

7.2.2.2. Cheek, Palate, and Gingiva

The interior of the cheek, soft palate, floor of the mouth, and underside of the tongue are all lined by a comparable mucous membrane. The mucosa of the cheek and soft palate, as well as the lips, is connected to the underlying skeletal muscle fibers through thick connective tissue elements in the submucosa. This allows for significant movement of the oral mucosa in these areas. The submucosa contains mucoserous glands, adipose tissue, larger blood vessels, and nerves. The cheek and soft palate consist of skeletal muscles, specifically the buccinator and palatine muscles, respectively. Superficially, the cheek is enveloped by a layer of delicate skin. The noncornified, stratified squamous epithelium of the oral cavity transitions into a typical respiratory passage epithelium when it reaches the posterior aspect of the soft palate and enters the nasopharynx. The hard palate, gingiva, and dorsum of the tongue, which experience mechanical trauma during chewing, do not have a submucosa and are covered by a layer of cornified, stratified squamous epithelium. The lamina propria in these regions is fixed in place due to its connection to the underlying structures. A mucoperiosteum is formed when the mucosa directly attaches to the bone. The gingival mucosa is directly connected to the periosteum of the alveolar bone. A similar connection is found in the midline raphe of the hard palate and at the junction between the hard palate and the gingiva. Beneath the remaining portion of the hard palate, there is a layer called the submucosa. This layer is composed of a significant amount of fatty tissue in the front and small glands that produce mucus in the back.

By using the tip of the tongue, one can determine the presence or absence of a submucosa and the texture of the mucous membrane in different regions of the oral cavity through self-examination. The mucous membrane lining the upper and lower lips, cheeks, mouth floor, and soft palate is characterized by a slippery and moist texture. It is composed of nonkeratinized stratified squamous epithelium. Similarly, the mucosa in all of these areas can be drawn between the teeth (lips and cheek region) or exhibit flexibility when prodded by the tongue (mouth floor and soft palate), indicating the presence of a submucosa that allows for movement in these regions. In contrast, the hard palate, gingiva, and dorsum of the tongue do not have a submucosa. Instead, the mucosa is directly attached to bone or muscle in these areas. The texture of these regions also varies, suggesting a level of epithelial cornification.

7.2.2.3. Tongue

The tongue's mucous membrane is tightly connected to a skeletal muscle core, without a submucosa. The tongue musculature consists of intertwined fascicles that are oriented in three perpendicular planes. The ventral surface of the tongue is sleek, while the anterior two-thirds of the upper surface exhibits numerous small protrusions known as papillae. The posterior one-third does not have papillae, but it does have mucosal ridges and mound-like elevations. The latter arises from the lymphatic tissue that is located beneath the lingual tonsils. The anterior portion of the tongue is associated with four types of papillae. Filiform papillae measure 2 to 3 mm in length and consist of a conical core of connective tissue that is connected to the underlying lamina propria. The stratified squamous epithelium is covered with varying levels of cornification. Papillae of this type are the most abundant. The fungiform papillae, which have a mushroom-like shape, are dispersed individually among the filiform papillae. The small red dots are most abundant at the tip of the tongue. The color is a result of the abundance of capillaries in the cores of their connective tissue. This type of papilla may be linked to taste buds. The circumvallate papillae, which are the largest among the papillae, are situated along the V-shaped sulcus terminalis that separates the tongue into anterior and posterior regions. In humans, their quantity ranges from 10 to 14. The circumvallate papillae seem to have receded into the mucosa of the tongue and are encircled by a barrier of lingual tissue, with a deep groove separating them. Each entity comprises a substantial central mass of connective tissue, accompanied by a multitude of blood vessels and small nerve fibers. Small serous glands may be present at times. The lateral surfaces of these papillae are covered by an epithelium that contains a large number of taste buds, with a potential count of 250 or more per papilla. The lingual minor salivary glands, also known as Serous (von Ebner's) glands, are located in the lamina propria and have openings at the base of the furrows. Their slender serous secretions consistently cleanse the groove and create a conducive environment for sensory perception by the taste buds. In humans, foliate papillae are underdeveloped, while in species like rabbits, they are well-developed and contain numerous taste buds. The oval bulges are located on the back and sides of the tongue, and they are made up of ridges and furrows that run parallel to each other. Taste buds are located in the epithelium on the sides of the ridges, and small serous glands empty into the bottoms of the nearby furrows (Alves et al., 2021).

7.2.2.4. Taste Buds

The average human tongue typically possesses approximately nine thousand taste buds. Taste receptors are located in fungiform, circumvallate, and foliate papillae and can also be found throughout the epithelium of the soft palate, glossopharyngeal arches, pharynx, and epiglottis. They manifest as faintly discolored, elliptical formations that stretch from the basement membrane nearly to the surface of the lining epithelium. A minuscule taste receptor pore facilitates communication with the surrounding external environment. Taste buds are composed of sustentacular cells, which are surrounded by neuroepithelial cells. These cells are organized in a manner similar to the segments of a peeled orange. Both types of cells possess prominent microvilli known as taste hair, which extend into the taste pore and are immersed in an amorphous polysaccharide substance. Tastant molecules that enter the taste pore stimulate neuroepithelial cells. Tastants bind to taste receptor proteins on the microvilli of neuroepithelial cells. The taste sensation is conveyed to nerve endings shaped like clubs, which pass through both cell types of the taste bud but appear to only make synaptic connections with neuroepithelial cells. Receptor binding causes depolarization of the neuroepithelial cells, leading to the release of glutamate. This, in turn, triggers an action potential in nearby afferent nerve terminals. Peripheral and basal cells, which are also linked to taste buds, are believed to be undifferentiated progenitors of the supporting and neuroepithelial cells (Alves et al., 2021).

There are five distinct taste sensations that can be perceived by humans: bitterness, sweetness, saltiness, sourness, and umami. The sensations can be localized to specific regions of the tongue, with sweetness and saltiness detected at the tip, sourness at the sides, and bitterness in the area of the circumvallate papillae. However, no structural variations in taste buds have been observed between these regions. Activation of the umami receptor leads to the perception of pleasant taste in the foods consumed.

7.2.3. Salivary Glands

The salivary glands in the oral cavity can be classified into major and minor glands, all of which are complex tubuloacinar glands. The primary salivary glands consist of the parotid, submandibular, and sublingual glands, which are located external to the oral cavity. The oral cavity and tongue contain many smaller salivary glands that are an integral part of the surrounding tissue. These glands, known as minor salivary glands, are responsible for continuously producing saliva to keep the mucosa of the oral cavity, vestibule, and lips lubricated (**Table 7.1**).

Table 7.1. Minor Salivary Glands

Name	**Location**	**Type of Gland**
Labial glands	Upper and lower lips	Mixed
Buccal glands	Cheeks	Mixed
Anterior lingual glands	Tip of tongue	Mixed
von Ebner's gland	Near circumvallate papillae	Serous
Posterior lingual glands	Root of tongue	Mucous
Palatine glands	Palate	Mucous

Saliva is a combination of secretions from different types of salivary glands and consists of water, ions, mucins, immunoglobulins, desquamated epithelial cells, and deteriorating granulocytes and lymphocytes (salivary corpuscles). Amylase, maltase, and salivary lipase are also present to initiate the breakdown of certain carbohydrates and fats. Saliva lubricates the mouth, breaks down food, cleanses the mouth, and allows for the perception of taste. Certain toxic metals are excreted in the saliva, and reduced saliva production during dehydration triggers the feeling of thirst. The salivary mucins, specifically those produced by the submandibular gland, exist primarily as individual molecules and possess the ability to attach to and group together with the microorganisms present in the mouth. This process helps regulate the population of microorganisms. Subsequently, the glycoproteins, along with the attached microbes, are ingested and expelled from the oral cavity. This is one mechanism that helps regulate the bacterial population in the oral cavity. Additional constituents present in saliva play a crucial role in regulating the abundance of bacteria in the oral cavity. The serous cells of the salivary glands not only produce lysozyme but also contribute to the production of immunoglobulin, which helps to inhibit the growth of bacteria. Immunoglobulin A (IgA) is produced and secreted by B-lymphocytes and plasma cells. It is then absorbed by the serous cells and bound to a protein called secretory piece. Finally, it is released into the oral cavity. The secretory piece is produced by the epithelial cells and serves to inhibit the degradation of IgA. The submandibular gland releases epidermal growth factor (EGF) and nerve growth factor (NGF) into the mouth. The salivary glands secrete approximately 1,000 ml of fluid on a daily basis.

7.2.4. Major Salivary Glands

The primary salivary glands, namely the parotid, submandibular, and sublingual glands, exclusively produce saliva when they receive nervous stimulation. The response is inherently reflexive and can be triggered by olfactory, visual, or even cognitive stimuli related to food (Carrassón et al., 2006).

7.2.4.1. Parotid Gland

The parotid gland, which is the largest among the primary salivary glands, is situated beneath and anterior to the external ear. The primary excretory duct traverses the cheek and terminates in the vestibule of the mouth, directly across from the upper second molar tooth. The gland is a compound tubuloacinar structure and in humans, it consists entirely of serous cells. The parotid gland in adult humans contains a significant number of dispersed adipocytes. The parotid gland is surrounded by a fibrous capsule and divided into lobes and lobules by connective tissue septa. The secretory units and ducts are enveloped by a fragile stroma that houses a multitude of blood capillaries and sporadic nerve fibers. Myoepithelial cells are located between the basement membrane and the bases of the secretory cells. They play a role in facilitating the movement of secretions from the secretory units into the duct system. Acini consist of pyramidal-shaped cells that are serous in nature. These cells have oval nuclei located at the base, basophilic cytoplasm, and distinct secretory granules at the apex. Narrow passageways, known as intercellular secretory canaliculi, are present between serous cells and serve as an alternative pathway for secretory products to reach the lumen. The intercalated duct is the first part of the duct system and is particularly noticeable in the parotid gland. The lining of the structure consists of a thin layer of flat or slightly cubed-shaped cells, and it may be accompanied by neighboring myoepithelial cells. Intercalated ducts are connected to striated ducts, which are lined by columnar cells exhibiting multiple basal striations. The complex folding patterns of the basolateral plasmalemma enhance the surface area, while the mitochondria located within these folds generate ATP to support cellular energy needs. This interplay between the infoldings and mitochondria is crucial for facilitating fluid and ion transport during the process of secretion. The intralobular ducts of the major salivary glands are closely associated with a surrounding network of capillaries, which assist in their function. The intercalated and striated ducts make up the duct system inside the lobule and together create the intralobular duct system. The remaining ducts are located within the connective tissue between lobules and are known as interlobular ducts. The intralobular ducts are directly connected to these ducts, which initially have a simple columnar epithelium lining. As the duct diameter increases, the epithelium transitions from pseudostratified to stratified. The amount of connective tissue increases as these ducts merge to create the main excretory duct. The terminal section of the primary excretory duct is covered by nonkeratinized stratified squamous epithelium, which seamlessly connects with the inner lining epithelium of the cheek.

7.2.4.2. Submandibular Gland

The submandibular gland, similar to the parotid gland, is a complex tubuloacinar gland that possesses a fibrous capsule with septa, lobes, lobules, myoepithelial cells, and a well-developed duct system. The gland is classified as a mixed gland, with the serous secretory units being the predominant type in humans. The mucous tubules typically exhibit serous demilunes (crescents) at their terminal points. Narrow passageways, known as intercellular secretory canaliculi, connect the mucous cells and extend between the serous cells of the demilune. Therefore, the substance produced by the demilunes can directly enter the lumen of the mucous tubule. Myoepithelial cells are located between the secretory cells and the basement membrane. They surround the secretory units and the first parts of the ductal system. In general, the duct system of the submandibular gland is similar to that of the parotid gland. However, the striated ducts in the submandibular gland are longer and therefore more noticeable in sections. The primary excretory duct of each submandibular gland drains into the oral cavity floor adjacent to the lingual frenulum on both sides (Carrassón et al., 2006).

7.2.4.3. Sublingual Glands

The sublingual gland is a compound gland consisting of multiple glands of different sizes. Each gland has its own separate opening either on the floor of the mouth or into the excretory ducts of the submandibular gland. The capsule lacks clear definition, despite the presence of septa. The gland is a combination of tubuloacinar structures, with the majority of the secretory units producing mucous. The majority of serous cells are organized in a demilune arrangement. Myoepithelial cells are located in proximity to the secretory units. The segments of the intralobular duct system are relatively brief and less visible compared to those in the other two primary salivary glands.

7.2.5. Teeth

Humans have two sets of teeth: primary (deciduous) and permanent. The eruption of primary teeth occurs between 6 to 8 months after birth, and a full set of 20 teeth is formed by the age of 2. The deciduous teeth are shed between the ages of six and thirteen, and are gradually replaced by the permanent set of 32 teeth.

7.2.5.1. Structure

All teeth exhibit identical histologic structure. Each entity possesses a coronal region and a subterranean structure, and the juncture where these two parts converge is referred to as the neck. The base of the tooth is inserted into a socket, also known as an alveolus, located in either the mandible or maxilla. Each tooth has a compact pulp cavity that conforms to its external shape. The pulp cavity connects with the alveolar cavity and periodontal membrane via the apical foramen, a minute aperture located at the apex of the root. The tooth's hard tissues comprise enamel, dentin, and cementum. The soft tissues that are connected to the tooth include the pulp, periodontal membrane, and gingiva.

7.2.5.2. Dentin

The tooth is primarily composed of dentin, which encloses the pulp chamber. Cortical bone, which is denser than compact bone, is composed of 80% inorganic material and 20% organic substance. The majority of the organic substance is composed of collagen, whereas the inorganic constituent exists in the form of hydroxyapatite crystals. The dentin exhibits a radial striated pattern caused by the presence of numerous small canals known as dentinal tubules. These tubules follow an S-shaped path as they extend from the pulp chamber to the dentinoenamel junction. The dentinal tubules house delicate cytoplasmic extensions, referred to as dentinal (Tomes') fibers, which originate from a specific cell type called odontoblasts. Neumann's sheath refers to the thin layer of dentin that surrounds each dentinal tubule and exhibits higher refringence compared to the rest of the dentin. The soma of the odontoblast is located within the pulp cavity, in close proximity to the dentin. The odontoblasts secrete the organic matrix of dentin, known as predentin, and remain active throughout an individual's lifespan. As a result, the pulp cavity gradually becomes narrower as a person ages. Predentin is abundant in collagen, comprises glycosaminoglycans, and lacks mineralization. Predentin undergoes mineralization after it is formed outside of the cell. The interglobular spaces are formed by areas of dentin that are not fully calcified. Dentin exhibits sensitivity to cold, pain, tactile stimuli, and hydrogen ion concentration. The perception of sensation is believed to be mediated by the activities of odontoblasts, which subsequently transmit the sensory stimulation to neighboring nerves within the pulp chamber.

7.2.5.3. Enamel

The crown of each tooth is protected by a layer called enamel, which is the most durable substance in the human body. The substance is devoid of cells and is primarily composed of calcium salts in the shape of apatite crystals. The organic material constitutes only 1% of the enamel substance. Enamel is composed of slender structures known as enamel prisms, which are positioned at a right angle to the dentin surface and stretch from the dentinoenamel junction to the tooth's outer surface. Every prism, with a diameter ranging from 6 to 8 μm, takes a meandering and irregular path towards the tooth's surface. The prismatic rod sheath refers to the organic matrix that encloses each enamel prism. The main components of the enamel's organic matrix are proteins known as enamelins, which attach to the crystallites of the enamel prisms. The interprismatic substance, located between the enamel prisms, is composed of a small quantity of organic matrix along with apatite crystals. Every enamel prism is formed by a solitary ameloblast, which are the cells responsible for producing enamel and are shed during tooth eruption. Consequently, the tooth is incapable of producing fresh enamel once it has emerged.

7.2.5.4. Cementum

The tooth root is enveloped by cementum, which overlays the dentin. The cementum closest to the tooth's neck is thin and devoid of cells, creating the acellular cementum. The remaining portion of the tooth root, known as the apex, consists of cells called cementocytes. These cells are located within small spaces called lacunae and are surrounded by a calcified matrix that is similar to the structure of bone. The specific term used to describe this type of cementum is cellular cementum. The amount of organic material in cementum increases as an individual gets older. Sharpey's fibers, which are bundles of collagen fibers, penetrate the cementum and serve as anchors, connecting the tooth root to the alveolar bone in the socket (Carrassón et al., 2006).

7.2.5.5. Pulp

Pulp refers to the fibrous material that occupies the pulp cavity. It consists of multiple slender collagenous fibers that are embedded in a plentiful gelatinous ground substance. The pulp is primarily composed of stellate fibroblasts, with a smaller presence of mesenchymal cells, macrophages, and lymphocytes. The cell bodies of the odontoblasts are located in the pulp, specifically along the edge of the pulp cavity that is next to the dentin. The apical foramen serves as the entry and exit point for blood vessels, lymphatics, and nerves into and out of the pulp cavity.

7.2.5.6. Periodontal Membrane

The periodontal membrane is composed of dense bundles of collagen fibers that extend between the cementum, which covers the tooth root, and the alveolar bone that surrounds it. Sharpey's fibers extend into the bone and cementum. The arrangement of the fibers in the periodontal membrane differs at various levels within the alveolar socket.

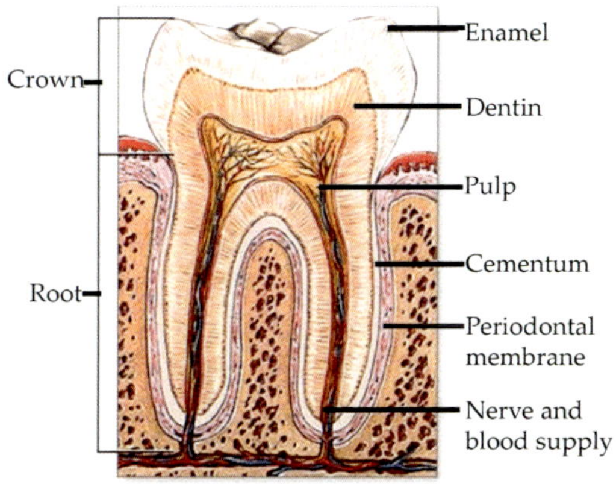

Figure 7.5. *A diagrammatic representation of the structures associated with a tooth.*

Source: https://www.researchgate.net/profile/Sergey-Dorozhkin/publication/291786544/figure/fig5/AS:989703947956224@1612975217020/A-schematic-drawing-of-a-tooth-Other-very-good-graphical-sketches-of-the-mammalian-tooth.ppm.

Despite being securely connected to the adjacent alveolar bone, the fibers are not tense, allowing the tooth to exhibit slight mobility in all directions. The periodontal membrane serves as a ligament that suspends the tooth. Osteoblasts and osteoclasts are present at the interface between the periodontal membrane and the alveolar bone, along with other connective tissue cells. The periodontal membrane possesses a plentiful vascular supply and is responsive to alterations in pressure. The sensory nerve fibers connected to the mesencephalic nucleus of the fifth cranial nerve serve to inhibit excessive pressures on the teeth during chewing, thus preventing self-inflicted tooth damage (Carrassón et al., 2006) (**Figure 7.5**).

7.2.5.7. Gingiva (Gum)

The gingiva, also known as the gum, encircles each tooth in a collar-like fashion and is firmly connected to the periosteum of the underlying alveolar bone. In close proximity to the tooth, the collagenous fibers of the gingival lamina propria merge with the outermost fibers of the periodontal membrane. The gingival ligament, comprised of collagenous fibers, extends from the lamina propria into the upper cementum of the tooth, ensuring a strong attachment. The gingiva is composed of keratinized stratified squamous epithelium. In this area, it forms the epithelial attachment cuff. The connection between the cuff and the tooth is upheld by a thickened basal lamina and hemidesmosomes, which create a seal at the dentogingival junction.

7.2.6. Pharynx

The oral cavity extends backwards into the pharynx, which stretches from the base of the skull to the level of the cricoid cartilage. At this point, it connects seamlessly with the esophagus. The digestive and respiratory systems briefly converge in the pharynx, which is divided into nasal, oral, and laryngeal sections. The pharyngeal walls are composed of three layers: a mucosa, a muscularis, and an adventitia.

7.2.7.1. Oropharynx

The oropharynx is covered by a nonkeratinized stratified squamous epithelium that is upheld by a compact, fibroelastic lamina propria. Directly below the lamina propria lies a highly developed layer of elastic fibers that seamlessly connects with the muscularis mucosae of the esophagus. The elastic layer merges with the connective tissue located between the muscle bundles of the pharyngeal wall in close proximity. The submucosa is found exclusively at the junction of the pharynx and the esophagus, as well as in the side walls of the nasopharynx. The pharyngeal wall's muscularis is composed of the skeletal muscle from the three pharyngeal constrictor muscles. These muscles are then surrounded by the connective tissue of the adventitia (Carrassón et al., 2006).

7.2.7. Tubular Digestive Tract

The digestive tract is composed of a series of tubular organs, including the esophagus, stomach, small intestine, colon, and rectum. Every segment of the digestive tract is composed of the four fundamental layers, although the composition of these layers differs depending on the specific functions of each segment.

7.2.7.1. Esophagus

The esophagus is a 25 cm long muscular tube. It maintains a continuous connection with the oropharynx at the lower edge of the cricoid cartilage, and below it forms a continuous connection with the cardia of the stomach.

7.2.7.2. Mucosa

The esophageal mucosa is composed of an epithelial lining, a lamina propria, and a muscularis mucosae. The epithelial lining is thick and composed of nonkeratinized stratified squamous epithelium, which is uninterrupted and shares similarities with the epithelium lining the oropharynx. Antigen-presenting cells, specifically Langerhans cells, have been found in the esophageal epithelium.

At the point where the stomach and junction meet, there is a sudden change in the epithelium to a simple columnar epithelium. The lamina propria is a type of connective tissue that is loose and contains scattered lymphatic tissue, both in diffuse and nodular forms. The muscularis mucosae is composed of smooth muscle cells that are arranged longitudinally in a delicate, elastic network. Smooth muscle cells may also be found arranged in a circular pattern. The muscularis mucosae and the elastic layer of the pharynx are connected at the level of the cricoid cartilage.

7.2.7.3. Submucosa

The submucosa is mainly composed of dense collagenous fibers and elastic fibers organized within a substance known as ground substance. Contained within it are sizable blood vessels, lymphatic vessels, nerve fibers, sporadic autonomic ganglia, and glands. The mucosa of the non-distended esophagus has a distinct pleated appearance due to the presence of long folds in the submucosa. During the act of swallowing, the mass of food flattens these folds and causes the inner space to temporarily expand, allowing for the passage of the swallowed material.

7.2.7.4. Muscularis Externa

The upper portion of the muscularis externa is exclusively composed of skeletal muscle. The muscle of the pharynx becomes more organized as it extends from the lower border of the inferior constrictor muscle, with inner circular and outer longitudinal layers. The second quarter of the esophagus contains a combination of skeletal and smooth muscle, whereas only smooth muscle is found in the distal half (Carrassón et al., 2006).

Based on histochemical studies, it has been determined that the skeletal muscle fibers in the esophageal wall are classified as type IIa fibers. These fibers are known for their fast contraction speed and ability to resist fatigue. The autonomic ganglia (Auerbach's plexus) contain nerve cells that are located between the inner and outer layers of smooth muscle. The upper esophageal sphincter (UES) and the lower esophageal sphincter (LES) are areas of high pressure within the esophagus. Both the lower esophageal sphincter (LES) and the upper esophageal sphincter (UES) are functional rather than structural sphincters. Normally, the pressure created by the LES inside the esophagus is strong enough to prevent the backflow of stomach contents into the esophageal passage. For certain individuals, the lower esophageal sphincter (LES) malfunctions, leading to a persistent exposure of the lower esophageal mucosa to gastric acid and pepsin. Chemical exposure causes long-term inflammation of the esophagus, leading to a transformation of the esophageal lining from a moist, layered squamous epithelium to a single-layered columnar epithelium resembling the lining of the stomach. Barrett's esophagus can lead to significant ulceration in this region. Gastroesophageal reflux disease (GERD) is the term used to describe this condition. The primary role of the upper esophageal sphincter is to prevent the entry of air into the upper part of the esophagus. Gastrin hormone stimulates the contraction of the lower esophageal sphincter.

7.2.7.4. Adventitia

The esophagus is covered by a layer of loosely arranged connective tissue called the adventitia, which serves to bind it to the surrounding structures. A serosa covers a small portion of the esophagus located below the diaphragm.

7.2.7.5. Glands

The esophagus contains two types of glands: esophageal cardiac glands and esophageal glands proper. There are two sets of esophageal cardiac glands: one set is found in the upper part of the esophagus close to the pharynx, and the other set is located in the lower part of the esophagus near the cardia of the stomach.

Both are tubuloacinar glands of the mucous type and are found exclusively in the lamina propria. The esophageal glands proper are compound tubuloacinar glands that produce mucus. They are located in the submucosa and are scattered throughout the entire length of the esophagus. Lysozyme and pepsinogen have been detected in certain secretory cells, but not in all of them. Myoepithelial cells are connected to the secretory units of the esophageal glands in humans.

7.2.7.6. Stomach

The stomach is an enlarged section of the tubular digestive tract located between the esophagus and small intestine. The human stomach is anatomically divided into four main regions: the cardia, which is a short section where the esophagus connects to the stomach; the fundus, a dome-shaped protrusion of the stomach wall located above the junction between the esophagus and stomach; the corpus, which is the large central part of the stomach; and the pylorus, a narrow region situated just above the junction where the stomach meets the small intestine. The stomach performs both mechanical and chemical processes to break down the materials that are consumed.

7.2.7.7. Mucosa

The mucosa of the stomach, when empty, contains multiple folds or ridges known as rugae, which largely diminish when the stomach is filled or stretched. The gastric lining epithelium is a single layer of columnar cells that starts abruptly at the point where the wet stratified squamous epithelium of the esophagus meets it, and ends just as abruptly at its junction with the intestinal epithelium. The lining epithelium in the stomach is structurally consistent and is composed of secretory columnar cells that together create a secretory sheet. The surface epithelium continuously secretes a neutral mucin that forms a protective mucous film. This film serves to safeguard the mucosa from the acid and pepsin in the gastric lumen, as well as to lubricate the surface (Collie and Ferraris, 1995).

The tops of the columnar cells are tightly connected by tight junctions, and the side cell membranes have many desmosomes. The apical surfaces contain scattered and short microvilli, while the apical cytoplasm is filled with numerous distinct mucin granules. The basal cytoplasm contains granular endoplasmic reticulum, while the supranuclear region is occupied by well-developed Golgi complexes. The gastric mucosa consists of approximately 3 million small tubular infoldings of the surface epithelium, known as gastric pits or foveolae. These pits are lined by the same type of simple columnar epithelium that covers the surface (Figure 7.6).

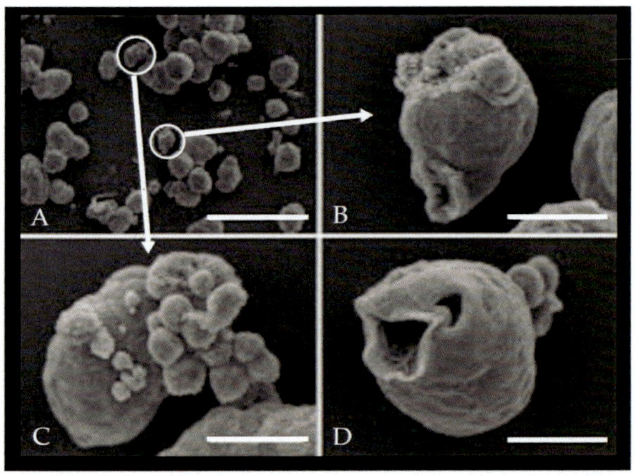

Figure 7.6. *An image captured by a scanning electron microscope shows the inner surface of a human fundic stomach, revealing many gastric pits.*

The surface epithelial cells undergo replacement every 4 to 5 days. The generation of new cells occurs through the differentiation of a limited number of undifferentiated cells situated in the lower regions of the gastric pits. Cells from this area progressively move upwards along the walls of the gastric pit to substitute the cells of the surface epithelium. There are three distinct types of glands that can be found in the gastric mucosa: cardiac glands, gastric (oxyntic) glands, and pyloric glands (Collie and Ferraris, 1995).

7.2.7.8. Cardiac Glands

The cardiac glands originate directly around the opening of the esophagus and continue for approximately 3.4 cm along the upper part of the stomach. Their maximum depth is reached in close proximity to the esophageal-gastric junction. In this case, the tubular glands exhibit extensive branching and seem to be grouped together into lobule-like structures due to the connective tissue of the lamina propria that surrounds them. Close to the point where it meets the fundus, the cardiac glands exhibit reduced branching, the clear clustering diminishes, and the thickness of the glandular region decreases. Cardiac glands are primarily composed of simple branched tubular glands that directly connect to the gastric pits above them. The depth of the gastric pit and the length of the cardiac gland are approximately the same. The secretory units primarily comprise mucous cells, with sporadic presence of parietal cells that seem indistinguishable from those found in gastric glands. There are also several undetermined endocrine cells present.

7.2.7.9. Gastric (Oxyntic) Glands

The gastric (oxyntic) glands, which number approximately 15 million, are the predominant glands in the stomach and are distributed throughout the entire corpus of the stomach. These glands are primarily characterized by their simple branching and tubular structure. The glands are oriented at a right angle to the mucosa's surface, and one or multiple glands may empty into the base of each gastric pit. The length of the gastric glands is approximately four times greater than the length of the pits in which they open. The gland consists of mucous neck cells, parietal cells, chief (zymogen) cells, and endocrine cells.

Mucous neck cells are predominantly found in the upper portions of the gastric glands, where the glands connect to the gastric pits. The cells frequently appear to be positioned between other types of cells, and their irregular shape is distinctive. Some objects exhibit wide bases and narrow apices, while others display narrow apices and broad bases. The nucleus is located at the base of the cell and is surrounded by cytoplasm that has a high affinity for basic dyes. The apical cytoplasm is filled with secretory granules. Contrary to the mucous cells that cover the gastric surface and gastric pits, mucous neck cells generate an acidic mucin. Parietal cells are primarily located in the central region of the gastric glands, but they can also be found dispersed among mucous neck cells in the upper portions of the gland. These cells are sizable and round, with their bases frequently protruding from the outer edge of the glands into the lamina propria. Parietal cells can be identified in routine sections by their acidophilic cytoplasm. Every cell possesses a prominent nucleus located in the center, along with a multitude of mitochondria, and is distinguished by the presence of intracellular canaliculi. Approximately 40% of the volume of parietal cells is composed of mitochondria, which are responsible for the presence of eosinophilia in hematoxylin and eosin stained preparations. The canaliculi are indentations of the cell membrane that create passageways close to the nucleus and open at the top of the cell into the interior space of the gland. The intracellular canaliculi contain multiple microvilli that extend into the lumina. The quantity and size of these microvilli depend on the secretory function of the cell. The tubulovesicular system, composed of smooth cytoplasmic membranes, is located directly next to each canaliculus and consists of small tubules and vesicles. The tubulovesicular membranes contain a high concentration of a distinct hydrogen, potassium ATPase enzyme, which functions as a proton pump in the stimulated parietal cell. The membranes additionally comprise proteins that function as ion channels for potassium and chloride ions. Hydrochloric acid is secreted by the cell membrane that lines the canaliculi (Gustafsson, and Johansson, 2022). When parietal cells are stimulated, the tubulovesicular membranes decrease, there is an increase in the number of canalicular microvilli, and the canaliculi become longer. On the other hand, when acid is inhibited, the opposite happens. After the parietal cells are stimulated, actin microfilaments form and interact with myosin, which causes the tubulovesicular membranes to move and merge with the canalicular membranes. This leads to an expansion of the canalicular membrane area, which now contains hydrogen, potassium-ATPase, and ion channel proteins. Parietal cells possess a significant amount of carbonic anhydrase, an enzyme that facilitates the combination of carbon dioxide and water to produce carbonic acid (H_2CO_3). The cell receives carbon dioxide and water through diffusion from nearby capillaries. Upon formation, H_2CO_3– rapidly undergoes dissociation into hydrogen ions (H^+) and bicarbonate ions (HCO_3–). The process involves the active transport of hydrogen ions into the lumen of the canaliculus, while bicarbonate ions move back into the bloodstream of the gastric mucosa. This results in an increase in pH, which is referred to as the alkaline tide. Ion channels facilitate the transport of potassium and chloride ions into the canalicular lumen. The hydrogen, potassium-ATPase transports the potassium ion back into the parietal cell in exchange for a hydrogen ion. The ultimate outcome of this process is the creation of hydrochloric acid within the canalicular lumen. The canaliculi are filled with water through osmosis, which is facilitated by the movement of ions. The augmentation of the surface area of the canalicular membrane during the activation of parietal cells enables the occurrence of these events.

Parietal cells in the human stomach secrete a glycoprotein called gastric intrinsic factor, which combines with vitamin B12 from the diet. This complex is then absorbed in the lower part of the small intestine. An insufficiency of intrinsic factors leads to reduced absorption of vitamin Bl2, a vital vitamin for the development and generation of red blood cells. Deficiency of this vitamin leads to pernicious anemia and is a condition commonly linked to atrophic gastritis. The vagus nerve initiates and regulates the stimulation of parietal cells during the cephalic phase of digestion in response to sensory stimuli such as taste, smell, sight, chewing, or even thoughts of food. This activity leads to the secretion of acetylcholine from postganglionic cholinergic muscarinic neurons, which in turn stimulates both parietal and ECL (enterochromaffin-like) cells. During the gastric phase of digestion, the stretching of the stomach, along with the presence of proteins and amino acids, triggers G-cells in the pyloric mucosa to release gastrin, which also affects parietal and ECL cells. The histamine released by stimulated ECL cells has a synergistic effect with both gastrin and acetylcholine, resulting in an increase in parietal cell secretory activity. Gastrin, histamine, and acetylcholine, which are physiological agonists, bind to specific transmembrane receptors in the parietal cell plasmalemma. The somatostatin produced by the D cells in the pyloric mucosa has a suppressive effect on the nearby G cells, preventing the release of gastrin and consequently reducing the activity of parietal cells. Chief (zymogen) cells are primarily located in the lower half of the gastric glands and can be identified by their basophilia in routine sections. The cells possess a large amount of granular endoplasmic reticulum in the lower part of the cytoplasm, well-developed Golgi complexes in the upper part of the cytoplasm, and zymogen granules at the top, which are characteristic features of cells that are involved in the secretion of proteins (enzymes). The chief cells secrete pepsinogen, which is a precursor of the enzyme pepsin (Gustafsson, and Johansson, 2022). Pepsin has its highest level of activity at a pH of 2.0. Parietal cells are responsible for creating the acidic environment in the gastric lumen. Pepsin plays a crucial role in the breakdown of proteins during gastric digestion, by catalyzing the hydrolysis of proteins into peptides. Endocrine cells, which contain specific granules enclosed by smooth membranes, are also found scattered within the bases of the gastric glands. These cells produce peptides and amines. The orientation of these cells indicates that they release substances into the bloodstream or the spaces between cells rather than into the cavities of gastric glands. The endocrine cells of the gastric glands contain gastrointestinal hormones such as somatostatin, glucagon, pancreatic peptide, histamine, and the amine 5-hydroxytryptamine (5-HT, serotonin). Gastric cells secrete glucagon, which promotes the breakdown of glycogen in the liver and raises glucose levels in the blood.

7.2.7.10. Kinetics of the Gastric (Oxyntic) Glands

The pluripotent stem cells found at the junction of a gastric gland and the bottom of a gastric pit, known as the isthmus, undergo division to both sustain themselves and generate various specialized cell types, including pre-pit, pre-mucous neck, pre-parietal, and pre-endocrine cells. Chief cells originate from mucous neck cells during a pre-zymogenic phase. All pit cells migrate towards the gastric lumen to differentiate into gastric lining epithelial cells. Eventually, these cells are shed into the lumen after approximately 5 days. Mucous neck cells migrate towards the base of the gastric glands and undergo transformation into pre-chief (zymogenic) cells within a span of approximately 2 weeks. Once fully differentiated, chief cells migrate to the basal region of the gastric glands and maintain their activity for a period of 6 months. Afterwards, they are either eliminated due to necrosis and expelled into the lumen, or if apoptosis takes place, they are engulfed by nearby chief cells or macrophages that enter the region. Endocrine cells originate from the isthmus and migrate towards the base of the glands, where they are plentiful. Their time to turnover is approximately 3 months. Conversely, parietal cells that differentiate can migrate in two directions, with approximately equal numbers migrating towards either the gastric lumen or the lower parts of the gastric glands. The turnover rate of these cells is approximately 60 days. If they become necrotic, they are expelled into the gland's lumen. When the parietal cells undergo apoptosis, they are engulfed by adjacent cells or macrophages through phagocytosis.

7.2.7.11. Pyloric Glands

The pyloric glands are limited to the last 4 or 5 centimeters of the stomach. These glands are either simple or branched tubular structures made up of mucous cells that resemble the mucous neck cells found in the fundic region. There may be a rare occurrence of a parietal cell. The pyloric glands discharge into gastric pits that are similar in length to the glands. There are many endocrine cells, primarily G cells, that are present. The unicellular endocrine glands produce gastrin, a peptide hormone that stimulates acid secretion by the parietal cells in the rest of the stomach. Pyloric glands contain a significant amount of endocrine cells that secrete somatostatin (D cells) and serotonin (5-HT). Therefore, besides producing mucus, pyloric glands also have significant endocrine functions. Serotonin enhances gut motility, while somatostatin suppresses the secretion of neighboring endocrine cells (Hernández et al., 2009).

7.2.7.12. Lamina Propria

The lamina propria of the stomach is not clearly visible due to the glands in the gastric mucosa being closely packed together. The structure comprises an intricate arrangement of collagenous and reticular fibers that encircle and stretch between the glands and gastric pits. The lamina propria is rich in a multitude of capillaries. The lamina propria contains many lymphocytes, along with plasma cells, eosinophils, and mast cells. Lymphatic nodules may also be present.

7.2.7.13. Muscularis Mucosae

The muscularis mucosae consists of an inner circular, an outer longitudinal and, in some places, an additional outer circular layer of smooth muscle. Slips of smooth muscle extending into the lamina propria form a loose network around individual glands and extend to the gastric lining epithelium. The contraction of these smooth muscle cells acts to compress the contained gastric glands. The muscularis mucosae gives additional mobility to the gastric mucosa.

7.2.7.14. Submucosa

The submucosa is composed of a dense connective tissue that contains a high concentration of mast cells, eosinophils, and lymphatic cells. This layer comprises lymphatic vessels and major blood vessels. The parent vessels arising from the celiac axis penetrate the stomach wall at lesser and greater curvatures and provide smaller branches that encircle the stomach within the submucosa. The mucosa receives its vascular supply from smaller branches of the submucosal vessels.

7.2.7.15. Muscularis Externa

The muscularis externa comprises three layers of smooth muscle: an outer longitudinal layer, a middle circular layer, and occasionally an inner oblique layer in the body and fundic regions. The forceful contractions of the stomach's muscle wall generate a vigorous churning motion that mechanically aids in the digestion of consumed substances. The middle circular layer in the pylorus undergoes thickening to create the pyloric sphincter, which is believed to assist in regulating the process of stomach emptying. Isotonic substances have a stimulating effect, while fats have an inhibitory effect on gastric emptying.

Elevated levels of hydrogen ions in the proximal duodenal lumen also impede the process of gastric emptying.

7.2.7.16. Serosa

The muscularis externa is covered by a thin layer of loose connective tissue, which is in turn covered by the mesothelial lining of the peritoneal cavity, known as the visceral peritoneum. This arrangement forms a serosa.

7.2.7.17. Small Intestine

The small intestine spans from the stomach to the colon and is partitioned into three sections: the duodenum, jejunum, and ileum. While there may be slight microscopic variations among these subdivisions, they all share the same fundamental structure as the rest of the digestive tube, which includes the mucosa, submucosa, muscularis externa, and serosa or adventitia. The shift from one segment to another is gradual. The first 12 inches of its length are typically referred to as the duodenum, the next two-fifths closest to the beginning are called the jejunum, and the last three-fifths are known as the ileum. The small intestine transports chyme from the stomach to the colon and finalizes the digestive processes by incorporating enzymes released by the intestinal mucosa and accessory glands (liver and pancreas). However, its main purpose is absorption (Hernández et al., 2009). The small intestine receives a daily influx of around 8 to 9 liters of fluid. The volume of food and liquid intake accounts for 1–2 liters, while the remaining volume is derived from endogenous sources like salivary, gastric, intestinal, pancreatic, and biliary secretions. Out of the total volume, approximately 6–7 liters are absorbed in the small intestine, while only 1–2 liters enter the colon. The majority of absorption takes place in the small intenstine. The colon primarly absorbs water and electrolytes. Only a minute quantity of fluid is expelled in the stool. Most of the water is absorbed through passive means in the gastrointestinal tract and relies heavily on an osmotic gradient.

7.2.7.18. Specializations for Absorption

Three specific adaptations – plicae circulares, intestinal villi, and microvilli – significantly augment the surface area of the intestinal mucosa to enhance the process of absorption. The morphological features are estimated to have an absorptive surface area of 200 square meters. Plicae circulares are enduring, extensive folds composed of the intestinal mucosa and a submucosal core. The intestinal lumen is encircled by shelflike folds that spiral around it, covering approximately one-half to two-thirds of its circumference. These folds may also divide into branches. Plicae originate in the upper portion of the duodenum, reach their peak development in the proximal section of the jejunum, and subsequently decrease in size and vanish in the lower half of the ileum. The small intestine is covered by numerous finger-like projections called villi, which are projections of the intestinal mucosa. Their composition includes a central lamina propria and an outer layer of intestinal epithelium. Villi are between 0.5 and 1.5 mm long and are most prominently present in the duodenum and jejunum. In these regions, they take the shape of wide, spatula-like structures. In the ileum, they undergo a reduction in length and adopt a more digit-like appearance.

The luminal surfaces of the intestinal absorptive cells are densely covered with microvilli, increasing the surface area of the intestine by approximately 30-fold. The striated border observed through light microscopy is composed of microvilli. Every microvillus is a cylindrical projection of the plasma membrane that surrounds a small cytoplasmic core. The apical cytoplasm of each microvillus contains multiple slender actin filaments that contribute to the terminal web. The terminal web is a network of delicate filaments located just beneath and parallel to the border of the microvillus. The actin filaments in the microvillus core are interconnected to create a bundle through the action of the proteins fimbrin and villin. A brush border myosin connects the actin bundle to the adjacent plasmalemma. In close proximity to the outer side of the cell, the filaments combine with those connected to junctional complexes. The filaments and terminal web play a role in the cytoskeleton and provide stability to the microvillus border. The contraction of the terminal web region can cause the tips of microvilli to spread out, thereby enhancing absorptive efficiency.

7.2.7.19. Mucosa

The intestinal mucosa is composed of a single layer of column-shaped cells called simple columnar epithelium, along with a layer of connective tissue called lamina propria, and a layer of smooth muscle called muscularis mucosae. The extensive villi in the mucosal lining contribute to the smooth and velvety texture of the interior of the small intestine. The crypts of Lieberkühn, which are simple tubular intestinal glands, empty into the spaces between the bases of the villi. The glands have a depth ranging from 0.3 to 0.5 mm and reach the level of the muscularis mucosae by passing through the mucosa. They are separated from each other by the connective tissue of the lamina propria. The intestinal glands secrete substances that assist in digestion, but their primary function is the regeneration of intestinal epithelial cells, which are shed at the ends of the villi (Ji et al., 2016) (**Figure 7.7**).

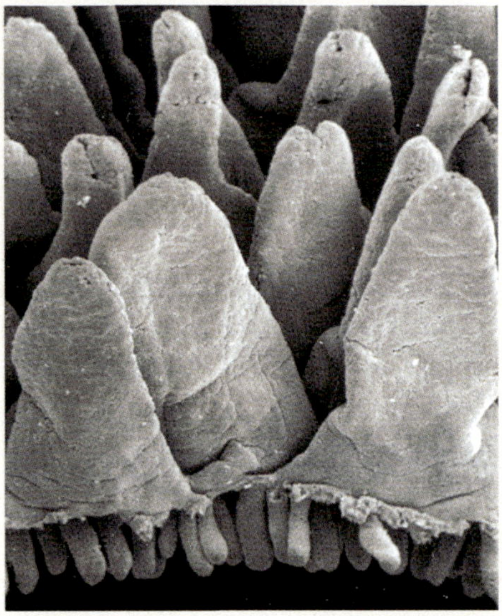

Figure 7.7. *A scanning electron micrograph showing isolated villi and intestinal glands of the duodenum.*

Source: Courtesy of J.E. Magney, University of Minnesota.

7.2.7.20. Epithelial Lining

The intestinal lumen is lined by an epithelium that consists of a diverse population of simple columnar cells. The primary cell type is the enterocyte, which is a tall and cylindrical cell located on a fragile basement membrane. It exhibits a distinct striated (microvillus) border on its exposed surface. The intestinal absorptive cells are joined together at their apices by prominent terminal bars, and desmosomes located along the lateral surfaces assist in maintaining close contact between the cells. The striated border, composed of microvilli, is coated with a glycocalyx layer produced by the intestinal epithelial cells. The glycoprotein layer is referred to as the surface coat and is impervious to substances that break down mucus and proteins. It is hypothesized that it serves a protective role and is involved in digestion.

While pancreatic enzymes and bile salts contribute to digestion in the intestinal lumen, a substantial portion of digestion also takes place near the microvillus surface before absorption. The enzymes involved in the degradation of disaccharides and polypeptides are found in the glycocalyx or on the plasma membrane of the microvilli. Several enzymes are found at this site, including enterokinase, peptidases, sucrase, maltase, and lactase. Lactose intolerance occurs when the enzyme lactase is not present. The intestinal absorptive cells play an active role in absorbing tripeptides, dipeptides, amino acids, monosugars (glucose, galactose, fructose), and lipids from the intestinal lumen, in addition to their contribution to the digestive process. Materials that have been absorbed and are moving through the epithelium need to enter the cell by passing through the apical plasmalemma. They are prevented from passing between the cells by the zonulae occludens, which create a tight seal around the upper part of the cells. The metabolic byproducts of sugars and proteins traverse the basal plasmalemma to gain access to blood capillaries located in the connective tissue cores of the villi (Ji et al., 2016). The process of lipid absorption is unique due to its pathway through the intestinal absorptive cells and the fact that lipids enter the lymphatic channels instead of the blood-vascular system. Bile salts emulsify fats, primarily triacylglycerols, and pancreatic lipase breaks them into fatty acids and monoacylglycerols. Long-chain fatty acids, cholesterol, monoacylglycerol, and fat-soluble vitamins (A, D, E, and K) are subsequently enclosed in micelles and taken up. Triacylglycerols are resynthesized in the smooth ER of the apical cytoplasm. The modified lipid migrates to Golgi complexes, where it combines with apoproteins to create lipoprotein droplets known as chylomicrons. Chylomicrons lack limiting membranes and are released through the lateral cell membranes of the intestinal absorptive cells into the intercellular space near the nucleus, thereby avoiding the basal regions. The chylomicrons traverse the intercellular spaces, cross the basal lamina, and subsequently enter lymphatic channels known as lacteals, following their passage between endothelial cells. Conversely, that are short- and medium-chained are able to penetrate the bloodstream. Most of the absorption of fat takes place in the ileum. Similar to other types of epithelia involved in transportation, the zonula occludens junction tightly connects the uppermost parts of enterocytes to form a continuous layer of epithelial cells. Additionally, it plays a crucial role in clearly dividing the enterocyte plasmalemma into distinct apical and basolateral domains. Each domain possesses distinct transmembrane proteins that are specific to it. The apical cell membrane domain contains a high concentration of transmembrane proteins involved in the transport of electrolytes and the movement of ions, allowing materials to enter the cell from the intestinal lumen. The process of enterocyte absorption is largely dependent on the sodium transport mechanism. Sodium can be transported into the cell either through a transmembrane protein ion channel or through transmembrane proteins that require binding to both sodium and chloride ions before allowing their entry into the cell. This process is known as coupled cotransport. Furthermore, sodium can be assimilated through a sodium-solute-coupled cotransport mechanism. This mechanism involves the cotransport of solutes, including galactose, glucose, dipeptides, tripeptides, amino acids, water-soluble vitamins, and certain bile acids, along with sodium, through the apical plasmalemma and into the cell. After entering the cytosol, the solute moves along a concentration gradient and exits the cell through the basolateral plasmalemma. The apical plasmalemma contains mechanisms for exchanging sodium-hydrogen ions and chloride-bicarbonate ions, which are typically linked to the absorption of sodium chloride. The sodium-potassium ATPase in the basolateral plasmalemma maintains the sodium gradient necessary for absorption. It moves excess sodium out of the cell and into the extracellular space, in exchange for potassium ions. The flow of water typically aligns with the movement of sodium, chloride, and solutes (such as glucose and amino acids) from the intestinal lumen. Typically, the sodium ion is transported initially, establishing a transepithelial gradient, followed by the chloride ion and water transport (Kirschbaum and Formicki, 2019).

Fructose is taken up through a process called facilitated diffusion. The absorption of calcium relies on the existence of the active form of vitamin D (1, 25-dihydroxycholecalciferol), which stimulates the production of a protein (calbindin) that binds to calcium ions in the cells of the intestines (enterocytes). Enterocytes in the small intestine absorb phosphate by using a sodium/phosphate transporter. The activity of this transporter is also enhanced by the active form of vitamin D. The main forms in which iron is absorbed are ferroheme (bound to myoglobin or hemoglobin) or as free Fe++ ions. It is then carried in the blood plasma by a protein called transferrin. Depending on the specific situation, ion trapping can also occur in the intestinal tract. Ammonia (NH_3) is capable of dissolving in lipids and gains access to the intestinal lumen by traversing the epithelial lining of the intestine. When hydrogen ion reacts with ammonium (NH_4^+), the hydrogen ion becomes trapped as ammonium. Ammonium is not soluble in lipids and is excreted in the feces. Goblet cells are dispersed among the intestinal absorptive cells, and their quantity increases towards the end of the intestinal tract. The unicellular exocrine glands secrete mucus to provide lubrication and protection to the mucosal surface. The apical regions of goblet cells frequently expand due to the accumulation of secretory granules. The base of the cells consists of a thin region that contains the nucleus, scattered profiles of granular endoplasmic reticulum, and occasional Golgi complexes. Goblet cells are located in the lining epithelium and are connected to intestinal absorptive cells through apical tight junctions and scattered desmosomes on the lateral surfaces. Goblet cells also migrate from the intestinal glands and eventually shed at the apex of the villus. The lifespan of goblet cells in humans is approximately 4 to 5 days. While they can secrete continuously, it is generally believed that they only go through one secretory cycle. Mucin granules are discharged through exocytosis and rapidly undergo a significant increase in volume, expanding by several hundred times, owing to their hydrophilic properties. The resulting mucus is a sticky gel-like substance composed of glycoproteins. The viscosity of mucus is lower near the intestinal glands.

Endocrine cells are also found in the epithelial lining, dispersed within the epithelium of the villi and intestinal glands, but their quantity is significantly lower compared to goblet cells. Endocrine cells release peptides and amines that impact the secretion and movement of gastric and intestinal fluids, the contraction of the gallbladder, and the functioning of the pancreas and liver (**Table 7.2**). These entities are distinguished by their high concentration of secretory granules, dispersed profiles of granular endoplasmic reticulum, and a cytoplasm that appears light under electron microscopy. Aside from the hormones produced by the enteroendocrine cells, there are also several peptide hormones (neurotensin, substance P, vasoactive intestinal polypeptide, somatostatin, galanin, calcitonin gene-related peptide, gastrin-releasing peptide, neuromedin U, enkephalins, dynorphin) present in the neurons of the enteric plexus. Peptides like VIP and galanin are present in neurons of the enteric system that span the entire gastrointestinal tract. Neuromedin U, along with other substances, is specifically found in the neurons of the duodenum and jejunum. In addition, opioids such as enkephalin are present in the intrinsic nerves of the stomach and pyloric sphincter. At the same time, dynorphin is primarily found in the submucosal plexus of the duodenum and ileum. The regulatory peptides in the gastrointestinal tract, whether in endocrine cells or enteric neurons, serve as local regulatory molecules and function as neurotransmitters and/or neuromodulators. They impact all aspects of digestive function, encompassing secretion, motility, absorption, growth regulation, and potentially even mediating inflammation in the gastrointestinal tract (Kirschbaum and Formicki, 2019).

The epithelial lining may occasionally exhibit another type of cell called the caveolated cell. The cell has a shape resembling that of a pear, with a broad base and a narrow apex that extends slightly into the lumen. Tight junctions and desmosomes maintain close proximity between these cells and adjacent epithelial cells. Caveolated cells possess prominent microvilli that usually house clusters of actin filaments, which extend extensively into the supranuclear region. Caveolae are small elongated channels that form between the bundles of filaments and extend from the apical cell membrane into the deep, apical cytoplasm, passing through the microvilli. This particular type of cell is found in other parts of the gastrointestinal tract and in other organs originating from the endoderm. Chemoreceptors may exist in certain areas, such as the respiratory system, but their purpose in the intestine remains unclear.

Table 7.2. Hormones and Related Factors Found in Endocrine Cells of the Gastrointestinal Epithelium

Hormone	Primary Location of Endocrine Cell	Primary Action
Gastrin	Mucosa of stomach (antrum) and duodenum (G cell)	Stimulates gastric acid secretion, trophic factor for the mucosa of stomach body
Secretin	Mucosa of duodenum and jejunum (S cell)	Stimulates pancreatic bicarbonate secretion in the ductal system
Cholecystokinin	Mucosa of duodenum and jejunum (I cell)	Stimulates pancreatic enzyme secretion by pancreatic acinar cells; gallbladder contraction
Enteroglucagon	Mucosa of ileum and colon (L cell)	Inhibits gastric acid secretion
Gastric inhibitory peptide	Mucosa of duodenum and jejunum (K cell)	Inhibits gastric acid secretion; stimulates insulin secretion
Motilin	Mucosa of duodenum and jejunum (Mo cell)	Acts to regulate the interdigestive myoelectric migrating complex (MMC)
Somatostatin	Mucosa of stomach, small intestine, and colon (D cell)	Paracrine inhibitor
Neurotensin	Mucosa of ileum (N cell)	Stimulates contractions of muscularis externa
Histamine	Mucosa of the body of the stomach (enterochromaffin-like (ECL) cell)	Stimulates gastric acid secretion
Peptide tyrosine tyrosine	Co-localized with enteroglucagon in the mucosae of ileum and colon (L cell)	Inhibits gastric acid secretion

7.2.7.21. Intestinal Glands

The origin of all epithelial cells that form the lining of the intestine is from cells located in the intestinal glands. The upper portions of the glands are covered by a layer of simple columnar epithelium, which is comparable to and uninterrupted with the lining of the intestinal lumen. The structure consists of cells capable of absorption, cells that produce mucus, cells that release hormones, and a small number of cells with small cavities. The basal half of the intestinal glands is lined with undifferentiated cells that undergo frequent mitoses. The mid-gland region contains intestinal absorptive cells (enterocytes) and oligomucous cells, which are intermediate stages of goblet cell differentiation. Intestinal epithelial cells are constantly generated in the lower part of the glands, move upwards by displacing other cells, and eventually spread to cover both the villi and the entire surface of the intestines. The oldest intestinal epithelial cells are discarded at the ends of the villi. The epithelial lining of the intestine undergoes a complete turnover every 4 to 5 days. During the migration of absorptive intestinal cells up the villus, their height increases and the striated border becomes more noticeable. The role of the enterocyte varies based on its position along the villus-crypt axis. The enterocytes located deep within the intestinal glands are relatively undifferentiated. In contrast, the enterocytes that line the upper one-third of the intestinal glands and cover the lower one-third of villi are mainly responsible for secretion. The enterocytes that line the upper two-thirds of the villi are mainly responsible for absorption, although they also participate in secretion to a lesser degree. Enterocyte function undergoes alterations throughout its lifespan as it moves along the villus-crypt axis, ultimately being shed at the tip of the villus. The chloride ion is actively transported into enterocytes for secretion through a sodium, potassium-2 chloride cotransport mechanism (Lipscomb et al., 2020). These proteins are located in the basolateral membrane.

Potassium protein channels and sodium-potassium pumps, found in the basolateral plasmalemma, work together to maintain high levels of intracellular chloride. This allows for the passive outflow of chloride through chloride channel proteins and CFTR (cystic fibrosis transmembrane regulator protein) chloride channels in the apical plasmalemma. The CFTR protein functions as an active transporter, necessitating energy utilization in the form of ATP to facilitate the transportation of chloride ions. Transcellular chloride secretion is believed to be the main factor responsible for the movement of water and sodium through the paracellular pathway. This ultimately leads to the secretion of a solution containing high levels of sodium chloride and water into the intestinal lumen. The process of water secretion by the small intestine begins with the transportation of chloride ions, which creates a transepithelial gradient. This is then followed by the transportation of sodium ions and finally water. The transmembrane conductance regulator protein, which controls the movement of chloride ions across the apical plasmalemma, is believed to be influenced by two intestinal peptide hormones known as guanylin and uroguanylin. Some types of harmful enteric bacteria release heat-stable enterotoxins that imitate the effects of these peptides. This leads to the occurrence of "traveler's diarrhea" and demonstrates the extent of fluid production in this system when left uncontrolled. Paneth cells, which are pyramid-shaped and have prominent granules, are located at the base of the intestinal glands. They differ from other cells in the intestinal epithelium by maintaining a relatively stable population with a low turnover rate. Paneth cells have been demonstrated to possess lysozyme and release defensins, which serve as a defense mechanism against infection. Intraepithelial lymphocytes frequently reside in the spaces between and within the intestinal epithelial cells that form the protective layer over the villi or line the intestinal glands, also known as crypts of Lieberkühn. The intraepithelial lymphocytes consist mainly of T-lymphocytes, with approximately 80% of them being T-suppressor cells and the remaining portion being T-helper lymphocytes.

7.2.7.22. Lamina Propria

The connective tissue of the lamina propria forms the central structure of the villi and fills the spaces between the intestinal glands. It contains a dense network of reticular fibers that form a delicate meshwork. This meshwork is populated by various types of cells, including reticular cells, lymphocytes, plasma cells, macrophages, and eosinophils, giving the lamina propria a highly cellular appearance. The lamina propria is a specialized form of lymphatic tissue and plays a critical role in the gut-associated lymphoid tissue (GALT), contributing to immune defense in the intestinal tract. The unfilled spaces within the lamina propria serve as a safeguarding layer that surrounds the intestinal lumen directly below the epithelium. Lymphocytes are the predominant cells and serve as a large reservoir of immune-competent cells. T-lymphocytes make up the majority of immunocompetent cells in the diffuse lymphatic tissue of the gut lamina propria. Approximately 70% of these cells are T-helper cells, while the remaining 30% are T-suppressor cells. Nevertheless, the lymphatic nodules and Peyer's patches do possess both B- and T-lymphocytes. Plasma cells in the lamina propria produce immunoglobulin A (IgA), which is absorbed by the intestinal absorptive cells and combined with a protein called secretory piece, made by the enterocyte. Subsequently, the complex is discharged from the cell, forming a safeguarding layer for the epithelial cells, acting as an immunological barrier against viruses and bacteria. The secretory piece functions as a transporter for IgA and potentially shields it from degradation by lysosomes while inside the cell and from enzymatic breakdown on the luminal surface. Lymphocytes frequently exit the lamina propria to traverse the intestinal epithelium and enter the intestinal lumen.

Lymphatic nodules of varying sizes are present in the lamina propria, distributed throughout the entire intestinal tract. However, they increase in size and number as you move towards the end of the tract. The lymphoid follicles are abundant and highly developed in the ileum, often spanning the entire thickness of the mucosa. The lymphatic nodules can exist as individual entities or be clustered together to form collections known as Peyer's patches. These elliptical formations can reach a considerable size of 20 mm in length and can be observed without the aid of magnification. Peyer's patches can extend throughout the entire thickness of the mucosa and submucosa.

The M-cell, a distinct cellular type, is located within the intestinal epithelium that lines the lymphatic nodules. The cells exhibit distinct microplicae on the inner surface, as opposed to microvilli. M-cells capture undamaged macromolecules from the inside of the intestine and carry them in vesicles surrounded by a membrane to intraepithelial lymphocytes. After becoming sensitized, the lymphocytes travel to different clusters of lymphatic tissue in the lamina propria or mesenteric lymph nodes, transmitting information to locations where antibodies are produced. M-cells enable the immune system to continuously monitor the gut lumen and respond accordingly to any alterations in the environment. Monitoring of the intestinal lumen by M-cells is not exclusive (Lipscomb et al., 2020). The Langerhans' cells in the epidermis monitor the external environment and transmit information to the immune system. Both are classified as antigen-presenting cells. Lymphatic vessels are present in the lamina propria and play a crucial role in the absorption of fat. The dilated lymphatic channels originate within the cores of villi near their tips and give rise to the central lacteals. The walls are composed of slender endothelial cells encased by basal lamina and reticular fibers. The lymphatic capillaries at the bases of the villi connect with those running between intestinal glands and create a network before traversing the muscularis mucosae. Within the submucosa, they converge with larger lymphatic vessels. Vessels that penetrate the muscularis mucosae may possess valves.

7.2.7.23. Muscularis Mucosae

The muscularis mucosae is clearly delineated and comprises an internal circular layer and an external longitudinal layer of smooth muscle. It has a close and direct connection with slender elastic fibers. The smooth muscle fibers detach from the muscularis mucosae and penetrate the central region of the villi, enabling the contraction of the villi. The continuous contraction of villi ensures that the intestinal epithelium covering the villi is constantly exposed to a fresh environment, which maximizes its ability to absorb nutrients efficiently. The contraction of the muscles also facilitates the movement of absorbed substances into the blood and lymphatic capillaries. This helps to remove these substances from the vessels in the lamina propria and transport them into the larger vessels of the submucosa, thereby enhancing the process of absorption (Miller et al., 2021).

Within the muscularis mucosae, there are small arteries that travel along its inner surface. These arteries then divide into capillary networks, creating a closely packed arrangement of fenestrated capillaries just below the intestinal epithelium. Close to the ends of the villi, the capillaries empty into small veins that descend to connect with a network of veins surrounding the intestinal glands before joining veins in the submucosa.

7.2.7.24. Submucosa

The submucosa is composed of abundant collagenous fibers and a multitude of elastic fibers. It frequently includes lobules of fat tissue along with the cells typically found in loose connective tissue. The ileum may contain substantial clusters of lymphoid cells that form lymphatic nodules known as Peyer's patches. The duodenal (Brunner's) glands are located in the submucosa of the duodenum. Their ducts penetrate the muscularis mucosae and empty into the intestinal glands above. The branched tubular glands are initially found right after the pyloric sphincter and continue all the way to the proximal jejunum.

They frequently appear in the submucosal cores of the plicae circulares. The duodenal glands are the sole submucosal glands found in the gastrointestinal tract. They are composed of secretory cells that exhibit both serous and mucous characteristics at the ultrastructural level. Brunner's glands have been demonstrated to produce various factors, along with mucin glycoproteins and possibly a small quantity of bicarbonate. Epidermal growth factor is hypothesized to have a significant role in the development of the alimentary canal and is considered crucial for wound healing (cytoprotective effects) and liver regeneration. Epidermal growth factor is a peptide that strongly suppresses the production of gastric acid and may regulate the growth and movement of cells in the inner lining of the upper part of the small intestine. Brunner's glands have been shown to contain bactericidal factors, such as lysozyme and proteinase inhibitors. These factors are believed to serve as a protective mechanism for the duodenal mucosa against the effects of microbial and pancreatic proteolytic enzymes in the surrounding environment. Apolipoprotein J, a sulfated glycoprotein, safeguards the mucosal barrier cells in the luminal environment by shielding them from surface-active substances like bile. Therefore, the mucus layer contains substances that protect against the breakdown of the mucus layer and underlying mucosa by pancreatic enzymes and other agents present in this area. It also contains substances that stimulate the growth and specialization of cells.

The submucosal plexus, known as Meissner's plexus, comprises nerve fibers and parasympathetic ganglia. It is present in the submucosa of the esophagus, stomach, small intestine, and large intestine. This plexus supplies motor innervation to the muscularis mucosae and the strands of smooth muscle that penetrate villi or other areas of the mucosa and contribute to movement. The submucosa contains significant blood and lymphatic vessels. The sizable mesenteric vessels penetrate the muscularis externa where it is connected to the mesentery and subsequently enter the submucosa. They then divide into smaller branches and encircle the entire circumference of the intestinal tube. The submucosal vessels provide blood supply to the mucosa above and also receive small branches from it.

7.2.7.25. Muscularis Externa

The muscularis externa is composed of an inner layer of smooth muscle arranged in a circular pattern and an outer layer of smooth muscle arranged in a longitudinal pattern. Both layers spiral around the intestinal tube. The fibers in the outer layer exhibit a more gradual helical structure, creating the perception of a longitudinal arrangement. The myenteric plexus contains nerve fibers and parasympathetic ganglia, located between the two layers of smooth muscle. The extensive network of nerves is present throughout the digestive system and provides the motor innervation to the smooth muscles that make up the outer layer of the entire gastrointestinal tract. The quantity of multipolar neurons present in the myenteric plexus is significant, surpassing 100 million neurons, and potentially surpassing the quantity of neurons found in the spinal cord. The gastrointestinal tract contains interstitial cells of Cajal, which are specialized cells found in the muscularis externa. These cells play a crucial role in maintaining normal gastrointestinal motility. The interstitial cells of Cajal are categorized into various subgroups of mesenchymal cells closely associated with components of the enteric nervous system and smooth muscle cells. A specific group of these cells is considered to be responsible for generating spontaneous slow peristaltic waves in the gastrointestinal muscles and serve as pacemaker cells. It is believed that other cells in this family are involved in relaxing smooth muscle, which is triggered by nitric oxide. The observed gastrointestinal movements, including gastric slow waves, segmentation waves of the small intestine, short and long-range peristaltic waves, and haustration of the colon, are believed to be controlled by the interaction between interstitial cells and the enteric nervous system. Furthermore, the muscularis externa exhibits forceful contractions known as migrating myoelectric contractions, which swiftly propel the contents of the stomach and small intestine into the colon. An analogous displacement of substances takes place in the colon.

7.2.7.26. Serosa

The muscularis externa is surrounded by a thin layer of loose connective tissue coated with a layer of mesothelial cells from the visceral peritoneum. The serosa of the intestinal wall is continuous with both sides of the mesentery at the point of attachment, enclosing connective tissue elements, blood vessels, and nerves. The duodenum is accompanied by an adventitia (Miller et al., 2021).

7.2.7.27. Ileocecal Junction

The lumen of the ileum and the large intestine are connected at the ileocecal junction. The lining of the digestive tract forms folds known as ileocecal valves located at the front and back. These valves comprise the mucosa and submucosa, surrounded by a thickening of the inner circular layer of the muscularis externa. The function of the ileocecal valves is to inhibit the premature passage of the contents of the ileum into the cecum and to prevent the retrograde flow of fecal matter from the colon into the ileum. Gastrin presence induces relaxation (dilation) of the ileocecal valve.

7.2.7.28. Large Intestine

The large intestine measures approximately 180 cm in length and is segmented into multiple regions. The cecum is connected to the ileum at the ileocecal junction and forms a closed sac at the beginning of the colon. The organism possesses an appendix, which is a diminutive and elongated diverticulum. The remaining portion of the colon is anatomically divided into ascending, transverse, descending, and sigmoid segments, which exhibit identical histological characteristics. The large intestine is connected to the rectum and anal canal, with the anal canal ending as the anus.

7.2.7.29. Mucosa

The mucosa of the large intestine shares some structural similarities with the small intestine, but it does not have villi and has a uniformly smooth inner surface. The lumen is coated with a straightforward columnar epithelium composed of enterocytes and goblet cells. The number of goblet cells increases towards the rectum, resulting in the distal region of the colon being primarily composed of goblet cells. The intestinal glands in the colon are longer and more densely arranged than those in the small intestine. They progressively increase in length towards the end, reaching their maximum depth of 0.7 mm in the rectum. The glands consist of a large number of goblet cells, endocrine cells, and proliferating and undifferentiated epithelial cells located in the lower half of the glands. Typically, Paneth cells are not present. The rate at which intestinal epithelial cells in the colon are replaced is approximately 6 days (Ostaszewska et al., 2018) (**Figure 7.8**).

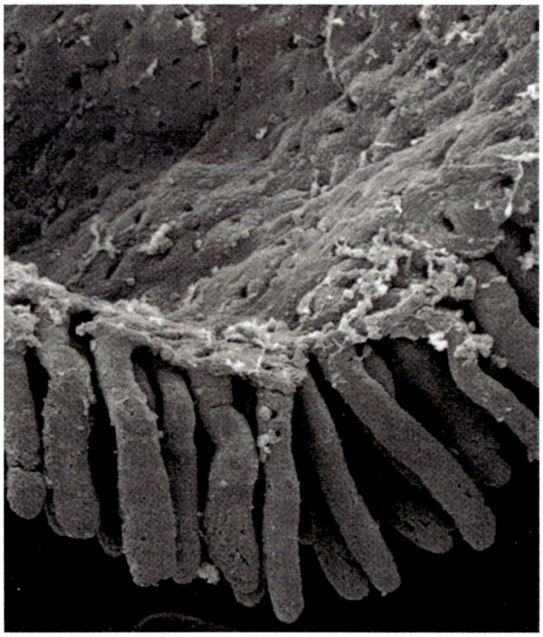

Figure 7.8. *This is a scanning electron micrograph showing a specific area of the colon's inner lining called the colonic mucosa. The image highlights the intestinal glands and their openings on the surface of the mucosa.*

Source: Photomicrograph courtesy of J. E. Magney, University of Minnesota.

The lamina propria and muscularis mucosae of the small intestine have an identical composition. There are lymphatic nodules spread out and may extend through the muscularis mucosae to be located in the submucosa. Consuming material enters the cecum in a partially liquid state and then solidifies in the colon. While the colon does not secrete digestive enzymes, some digestion occurs due to enzymes found in the developing fecal mass and the activity of bacterial flora typically found in the large intestine. Nevertheless, most of the process of breaking down and assimilating nutrients occurs prior to the ingesta reaching the colon. The primary functions of the large intestine are fluid absorption (sodium, chloride and water) and mucus secretion to protect the mucosa from abrasion by the developing feces. Out of the roughly 9 liters of fluid that enters the intestinal tract every day, only around 100 ml is excreted in the feces. The cellular mechanisms responsible for absorption and secretion in the colon's enterocytes are believed to be analogous to those observed in the enterocytes of the small intestine. The secretory functions of enterocytes in both regions of the gastrointestinal tract seem to be affected by the peptides guanylin and uroguanylin.

The latter, also found in significant amounts in the bloodstream, has been proposed to function as an intestinal natriuretic factor. It is widely recognized that the consumption of high quantities of salt leads to a significant and swift rise in salt excretion through urine. Intravenous administration of an equivalent quantity of salt results in minimal alterations in salt excretion through urine. Aldosterone and atrial natriuretic peptides do not seem to play a role in this phenomenon, indicating the presence of intestinal natriuretic factors like uroguanylin.

7.2.7.30. Submucosa

The submucosa of the colon bears resemblance to that of the small intestine and houses the larger blood vessels and the submucosal nerve plexus. Glands are not present. Similar to the rest of the digestive tube, blood vessels penetrate the muscularis externa and travel around the entire circumference of the intestinal wall. The major blood vessels provide branches that penetrate the muscular layer of the mucous membrane and create networks of small blood vessels in the connective tissue layer, surrounding the intestinal glands, and beneath the surface epithelium. The veins parallel the path of the arteries.

7.2.7.31. Muscularis Externa

The muscularis externa of the cecum and colon has a distinct outer coat different from the small intestine. This outer coat forms three longitudinal bands known as the taeniae coli. The muscle layer between the taeniae is comparatively thinner and may lack completeness. The inner circular layer is fully formed and resembles the structure found in the small intestine. The myenteric plexus components are located directly outside the circular layer, similar to their positioning in the small intestine. The wall of the colon forms haustra, which are outwardly bulging pockets, due to the tonus of the taeniae coli. The colon contains crescent-shaped folds known as plicae semilunares that extend into its lumen, located between the haustra.

7.2.7.32. Serosa

The serosa in the colon is not fully developed due to the retroperitoneal nature of the ascending and descending parts of the colon. The muscular wall of the colon is connected to nearby structures by an adventitia. If a serosa is present, it may contain appendices epiploicae, which are large lobules of fat that hang down (Ostaszewska et al., 2018).

7.2.7.33. Appendix

The appendix exhibits a similar structure to that of the colon, albeit in a smaller size. The lumen is diminutive and asymmetrical in shape, and taeniae coli are not present. The lamina propria is heavily infiltrated with lymphocytes, and the mucosa is frequently obscured by numerous lymphatic nodules that can occupy both the mucosa and submucosa.

7.2.7.34. Recto-Anal Junction

The rectum is a linear extension of the colon, measuring approximately 12 cm in length. The distal rectum contains three internal transverse rectal valves, also known as the valves of Houston. These permanent sickle-shaped structures are formed by the infoldings of the submucosa and the inner circular layer of the muscularis externa. The valves are responsible for separating flatus from the developing fecal mass. The mucosa of the initial segment of the rectum resembles that of the colon, except that the intestinal glands are slightly elongated and the lining epithelium is predominantly made up of goblet cells. The terminal portion of the rectum, measuring approximately 2 to 3 cm, constitutes the anal canal, terminating at the anus. Immediately proximal to the pectinate line, the intestinal glands become shorter and disappear. The simple columnar intestinal epithelium suddenly changes to noncornified stratified squamous epithelium at the pectinate line. After a short transition, the noncornified stratified squamous epithelium becomes continuous with the keratinized stratified squamous epithelium of the skin at the level of the external anal sphincter. The circumanal glands, which are simple tubular apocrine sweat glands, are located beneath the epithelium of this region. The mucosa of the anal canal forms rectal columns (of Morgagni), which are large longitudinal folds located proximal to the pectinate line. The distal extremities of the rectal columns are connected by transverse mucosal folds known as the anal valves. Each valve has a recess that creates a small anal sinus. The muscularis mucosae become discontinuous and subsequently disappears at the level of the anal valves. The anal canal's submucosa is composed of a multitude of veins that combine to create a substantial hemorrhoidal plexus. When the blood vessels become distended, or varicose they bulge into the mucosa above them and create internal hemorrhoids, also known as piles. The inner circular layer of the muscularis externa thickens and terminates as the internal anal sphincter. The taeniae coli converge in the distal rectum to form a continuous outer longitudinal layer surrounding the rectum. The outer layer of muscle, which is thin and runs lengthwise, breaks apart and merges with the nearby connective tissue and muscle of the pelvic diaphragm. The distal anal canal is surrounded by skeletal muscle fibers as it traverses the pelvic diaphragm. These fibers create the external anal sphincter, which can be consciously controlled (Pena et al., 2003).

7.2.8. Gastrointestinal Mucus

The gastric surface lining epithelium, Brunner's glands, and goblet cells secrete substances that combine to create a layer of mucus. This mucus forms a slippery and elastic gel, which lubricates the mucosal lining of the gastrointestinal tract. This layer is composed of a combination of glycoproteins, phospholipids, shed cells, different cellular and serum macromolecules, electrolytes, and water. The ability of gastrointestinal mucus to safeguard fragile underlying epithelial surfaces is primarily attributed to the gel-forming characteristics of its glycoprotein molecules known as mucins. The gastrointestinal mucus serves to safeguard the mucosal epithelial cells beneath it by upholding a beneficial pH gradient and preventing self-digestion from the lumen. The mucus secreting cells located throughout the gastrointestinal tract continuously produce and replenish a gel-like substance known as adhesive material. The unique characteristics of mucin glycoprotein molecules, such as their hydrophilic and viscoelastic properties, allow them to adhere to various substances in the gut, including undigested matter, sloughed cells, and inert particles. These molecules are then efficiently removed from the gut lumen through fecal flow, without causing any harm to the delicate mucosal surfaces. The mucus layer possesses both fluid-like properties, allowing it to flow under gentle shearing forces, and elastic properties, enabling it to bounce back from deformation stress and maintain its structural stability. The mucus layer has enough pores to facilitate the quick movement of nutrients and secretions between the underlying epithelial cells and the lumen. Mucins are believed to form an amorphous network by arranging themselves in loose, random coils due to their highly variable elongated branching oligosaccharide side chains. The interstices between clusters of these molecules are occupied by water, ions, serum proteins, lipids, enzymes, and other substances. The wide variety of carbohydrate units linked to these large mucin molecules offers a remarkable number of possible binding sites for disease-causing and mutually beneficial organisms in the lower part of the digestive system.

Certain mucin binding sites vie with microorganisms for the binding sites on the underlying epithelial cells, impeding the microorganisms' ability to reach the mucosal surface and aiding in their elimination. The resistance of the mucin glycoproteins in the mucus layer against luminal and bacterial enzymes that damage mucosal surfaces is believed to be a result of the structural arrangement of the mucin molecules. The glycoprotein molecules have a protective sleeve of oligosaccharide chains surrounding their protein core.

7.2.9. Liver

The liver, which weighs approximately 1.4 kg in an average adult, is the largest gland in the body. It functions as a dual gland, serving as both an endocrine and exocrine gland. It releases various substances directly into the bloodstream and secretes bile into the duct system. The liver plays a crucial role in conjugating lipid-soluble molecules such as steroids, bilirubin, and certain drugs with SO_3 or glucuronide. This process makes these molecules water-soluble, allowing their release into the bile and ultimately eliminated through the digestive system. The liver is positioned distinctively in relation to the venous blood flow coming from the gastrointestinal tract. The blood from the portal vein, responsible for draining the entire gastrointestinal tract and spleen, traverses through the liver before entering the systemic circulation. The smooth muscle in the wall of the portal vein is distinct from other parts of the blood vessels because it is characterized by phasic smooth muscle. Phasic smooth muscle can produce action potentials, which in turn cause rhythmic contractions that help propel blood towards the liver (Pena et al., 2003). The liver receives all substances absorbed by the gastrointestinal tract, except for certain lipids. Most lipids are transported by lymphatics to enter the bloodstream. The spleen, the main organ responsible for the removal and breakdown of old red blood cells, transports the byproducts of hemoglobin breakdown to the liver. Hepatic sinusoids receive tributaries from the portal vein, which drain into the hepatic veins. The configuration of a series of sinusoids between veins in the liver is referred to as the hepatic portal system. The liver receives blood from both the hepatic artery and the portal vein. This blood flows through the liver sinusoids and leaves through the hepatic vein.

7.2.9.1. Structural Organization

The liver is surrounded by a thin connective tissue capsule that is connected to the peritoneum. The capsule is composed of multiple elastic fibers and is enveloped by a mesothelium, except for a small exposed region where the liver comes into contact with the diaphragm. The liver consists of epithelial cells called hepatocytes, which are organized in branching and anastomosing plates that are separated by blood sinusoids. Both structures create a circular arrangement around a central vein, which is the smallest branch of the hepatic vein. The hepatic lobule is characterized by a radial arrangement of hepatic plates surrounding a central vein. This lobule has a somewhat hexagonal shape when viewed in cross-section, with the central vein located at the center and portal areas found at the corners. The liver is composed of approximately 1 million of these units. The portal area comprises a tributary of the portal vein, a tributary of the hepatic artery, a bile duct, and a lymphatic channel. All are surrounded by a shared investment of connective tissue. Hepatic artery and portal vein branches transport blood into the sinusoids, which are located between hepatocyte plates. The blood circulates sluggishly through the sinusoids towards the middle of the lobule and then leaves through the central vein. The hepatic artery branches transport oxygenated blood and contribute approximately 20% of the blood circulation within the hepatic sinusoids. On the other hand, the branches of the portal vein transport blood that is abundant in nutrients from the gastrointestinal tract and account for the remaining 80% of the blood flow in the sinusoids. Hepatocytes at the periphery of the lobule, near the portal vein and hepatic artery branches, receive blood with the highest levels of nutrients and oxygen. Both decrease as blood moves towards the central vein. The hepatic lobule can be divided into three distinct zones based on metabolic activity: a peripheral zone (zone 1) with continuous function, a central zone (zone 2) with intermittent activity, and a zone near the central vein (zone 3) with permanent rest. The boundaries of the hepatic lobule can be determined by observing the central vein and identifying the portal areas located at the corners of the lobule (Ray and Ringø, 2014).

Another component of the liver's blood supply is a smaller structure known as the liver acinus or functional unit. The liver acinus refers to the portion of hepatic tissue nourished by a terminal branch of the hepatic artery and portal vein and is drained by a terminal branch of the bile duct. The diamond-shaped area is depicted with central veins at two opposite corners. The blood vessels and bile ducts branch out between adjacent hepatic lobules to supply them. The extra lobule in the liver is involved in the exocrine secretion of bile. This structure is known as the portal lobule and contains a central portal canal. The structure comprises the hepatic tissue drained by the bile duct located in the portal area. A portal lobule is a triangular structure that encompasses portions of three neighboring hepatic lobules. There is a central vein situated at each corner of this unit. The bile secreted by hepatocytes moves in the opposite direction of blood towards the outer edge of the hepatic lobule (**Figure 7.9**).

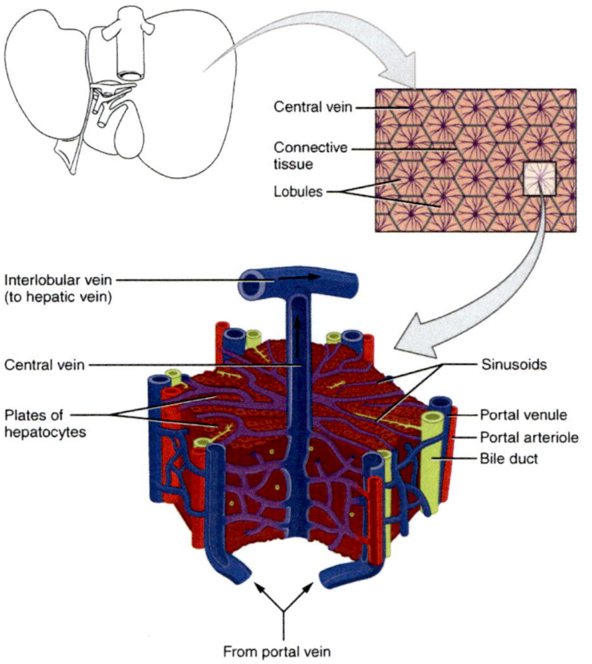

Figure 7.9. *A schematic diagram depicting the lobules of the liver.*

The liver parenchyma beneath the capsule is restricted by a subcapsular limiting plate, which consists of a solitary layer of small, dark hepatocytes. The periportal limiting plate, composed of hepatic cells, encloses the portal areas and is penetrated by branches of the hepatic artery, portal vein, lymphatic vessels, and bile ductules. The limiting plates of hepatocytes serve as a barrier that prevents blood from escaping from the classic hepatic lobules.

7.2.9.2. Hepatic Sinusoids

Hepatic sinusoids exhibit greater dimensions and a more irregular morphology compared to typical capillaries. The sinusoidal lining is composed of a single layer of flat epithelial cells, which is minimally supported by connective tissue (Ray and Ringø, 2014). The sinusoidal lining is composed of three types of cells: endothelial cells, stellate cells (also known as Kupffer cells or hepatic macrophages), and fat-storing cells (lipocytes). Endothelial cells are the primary cellular component of the sinusoidal lining and create an interrupted endothelium. The absence of a basal lamina results in a separation between cells through gaps measuring 0.2 to 0.5 μm in width. The endothelial cells also exhibit a multitude of intracellular fenestrations or pores. The sinusoidal lining is positioned adjacent to the liver cells, with a narrow perisinusoidal space (known as the space of Disse) separating them (**Figure 7.10**).

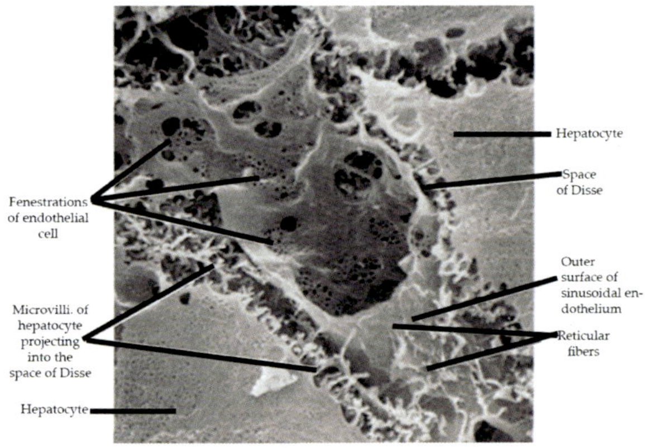

Figure 7.10. *A scanning electron micrograph illustrating a segment of a hepatic sinusoid.*

Source: Photomicrograph courtesy of G.H. Haggis, Ottawa, Canada.

Blood plasma circulates unimpeded through the endothelium and into the space, while the sinusoidal lining restricts the passage of erythrocytes. While there are some sporadic clusters of reticular fibers and delicate collagenous fibers in the perisinusoidal space, there is no underlying material, and the movement of blood plasma is unobstructed. Due to the direct connection between the plasma and the perisinusoidal space, the liver cells are consistently exposed to a fluid that contains a high concentration of nutrients absorbed by the intestines. Therefore, the perisinusoidal space plays a crucial role in the transfer of substances between the liver and plasma. The hepatocytes' plasmalemma that faces the perisinusoidal space is equipped with a large number of highly developed microvilli. These microvilli extend into the space, significantly expanding the surface area and enhancing absorption. The liver generates a significant quantity of lymph because not all of the formed tissue fluid is absorbed by the hepatocytes or returns to the sinusoidal lumen. The liver produces approximately 50% of the lymphatic fluid present in the thoracic duct. Lymph, similar to bile, circulates through the perisinusoidal space in the hepatic lobule, moving from the center toward the outer edges. The lymphatic vessels in the portal areas run parallel to the portal vein branches and eventually drain into the thoracic duct. The sinusoidal lining contains actively phagocytic cells, which are also known as hepatic macrophages or Kupffer cells. These cells are part of the sinusoidal lining and have irregular shapes. They expose most of their cytoplasm to the blood in the sinusoid and extend processes between the endothelial cells. In contrast to the adjacent endothelial cells, the cytoplasm of the hepatic phagocytes contains vacuoles, lysosomes, Golgi bodies, and small sections of granular endoplasmic reticulum. Phagocytized material may also be observed. These cells are a component of the mononuclear system of macrophages and originate from monocytes in the bone marrow (Rønnestad et al., 2013).

The third type of cell is situated on the side of the sinusoidal lining adjacent to the perisinusoidal space. This cell exhibits lipid accumulation and is most abundant in the peripheral and intermediate regions of the hepatic lobule. These cells are known as lipocytes, fat-storing, stellate, or interstitial cells, and their main role is to store vitamin A.

7.2.9.3. Hepatocytes

The liver's parenchyma comprises hepatocytes, which are large polyhedral cells organized in plate-like structures extending outward from the central vein. An individual hepatocyte's surfaces either come into contact with a neighboring liver cell or border a perisinusoidal space. The surface mentioned above contains a large number of highly developed microvilli. The hepatocytes' plates are upheld by a fragile stroma composed mainly of reticular fibers. Hepatocytes typically have large, round nuclei that are located in the central region of the cell.

Typically, there is one nucleus, although up to 25% of hepatocytes have two nuclei. The size of nuclei in hepatocytes varies significantly from cell to cell, which is due to the polyploid nature of these cells. Hepatocytes contain a substantial number of organelles in their cytoplasm, including abundant granular endoplasmic reticulum, a moderate amount of smooth endoplasmic reticulum, mitochondria, Golgi complexes, peroxisomes, and lysosomes. Common inclusions include glycogen and lipid. Glycogen frequently manifests as compact clusters (alpha particles) composed of smaller beta particles. The diameter of the alpha particles ranges from 20 to 30 nm. The cytoplasm exhibits variability in its appearance and undergoes alterations in response to the nutritional condition of the organ.

The bile canaliculi, which are small channels, run through the liver tissue between hepatocytes and terminate in the bile ducts located in the portal areas. Bile canaliculi are enlarged spaces between cells, with their walls formed by the neighboring hepatocytes' plasmalemma. The lumen is lined with short microvilli that extend from the cell membrane. The plasma membranes at the edges of the canaliculus are connected by occluding junctions, similar to the zonula occludens found in other epithelial tissues. They create a barrier to stop bile from leaking into the spaces between liver cells. The Golgi complexes of hepatocytes are frequently located next to the canaliculi. The bile canaliculi exhibit sporadic contractions (Rønnestad et al., 2013).

7.2.9.4. Hepatocyte Function

Hepatocytes are highly metabolically active cells that carry out a diverse range of functions. Hepatocytes play a role in the conversion of ammonium to urea, carry out gluconeogenesis (the conversion of lipids and amino acids into glucose), produce cholesterol, and also absorb immunoglobulin A (IgA) and secrete it as a form of IgA into the bile, which is then released into the small intestine. Hepatocytes have a significant role in carbohydrates, fats, and protein metabolism and storage.

Hepatocytes primarily store carbohydrates as glycogen. Hepatic glycogen serves the purpose of regulating blood glucose levels within the normal range of 70–100 mg/100 mL. Following the consumption of a meal high in carbohydrates, a rapid release of insulin leads to an elevation in the ratio of insulin to glucagon in the bloodstream. Increased insulin levels inhibit hepatic glucose production and enhance its uptake by insulin-dependent tissues. During high glucose concentrations, it is believed that glucokinase is translocated from the nucleus to the cytosol. This glucokinase then catalyzes the phosphorylation of glucose and facilitates the entry of glucose into hepatocytes. Insulin controls the activity of glucokinase in hepatocytes through both transcription and translocation. Glycogen, the storage form of glucose, is composed of glucose molecules connected by α 1, 4 glycosidic bonds. Glycogen synthase facilitates the formation of glycogen through a catalytic process. Glycogen degradation occurs during fasting and exercise, leading to a reduction in the ratio of insulin to glucagon and the release of epinephrine. The latter attaches to α- and β-adrenergic receptors on the hepatocytes. Hepatic glycogen phosphorylase breaks down liver glycogen into glucose-6-phosphate. This glucose-6-phosphate is then converted into free glucose by the enzyme glucose-6-phosphatase, which is found in the cisternae of the endoplasmic reticulum. The glucose-6-phosphate is transported into the lumen of the endoplasmic reticulum through a specialized glucose-6-phosphate transporter protein. Once inside, it is broken down into glucose and phosphate by the enzyme glucose-6-phosphatase. Glucose is conveyed from the endoplasmic reticulum to the plasmalemma of the hepatocyte through the use of glucose transport proteins. Hepatocytes are crucial in regulating blood lipid levels by absorbing fatty acids and converting them into triglycerides via esterification, which takes place in the smooth endoplasmic reticulum. The triglycerides are subsequently bound to proteins within the Golgi apparatus of hepatocytes to create a range of lipoproteins. Hepatocytes produce high-density lipoproteins (HDL) that aid in the transport of surplus cholesterol and triacylglycerides from the bloodstream to the liver for metabolic processing. Hepatocytes synthesize very-low-density lipoproteins (VLDL) containing high levels of triacylglycerides. These VLDLs are transported to skeletal muscle and fat cells, where the triacylglycerides are broken down into fatty acids by the enzyme lipoprotein lipase. Conversely, low-density lipoprotein (LDL) particles are abundant in cholesterol and transport cholesterol to cells in various body parts with LDL receptors (Suvarva et al., 2012). The liver deaminates amino acids to generate urea, which is subsequently excreted by the kidney. In addition to its primary functions, the liver also plays a role in protein metabolism, the production of fibrinogen, prothrombin, and albumin, as well as the storage of various vitamins, including vitamins A, D, B2, B3, B4, and B12. The enzymes present in hepatic peroxisomes possess the capability to metabolize alcohol. Conversely, enzymes linked to the smooth endoplasmic reticulum play a role in inactivating certain hormones, lipid-soluble drugs, and toxins, another crucial function of hepatocytes. Hepatocytes excrete detoxified materials into the bile, which are then transported through the biliary duct system to the intestinal tract for elimination. Bile is a multifaceted alkaline secretion produced by the liver. It consists of ions, water, bicarbonate, bile acids (taurocholic and glycocholic), bile pigment (bilirubin glucuronide), phospholipids, cholesterol, lecithin, and neutral fats. Bile acids/salts function as emulsifying agents and play a crucial role in digestion by breaking down fat into micelles in the intestinal lumen. Approximately 80% of bile acids are reabsorbed in the ileum and returned to the bile for secretion. The recycling of bile acids is known as the enterohepatic circulatory system. Bilirubin is produced in the spleen and liver because of the breakdown of the heme component of hemoglobin in damaged or old erythrocytes by macrophages at these locations. The bilirubin taken up by hepatocytes is then conjugated with glucuronic acid to form bilirubin glucuronide which is excreted into the bile. Upon entering the intestinal tract, bacterial activity transforms this molecule into urobilinogen. Of the urobilinogen formed, some are lost in the feces, some are absorbed and returned to the liver, and some are excreted by the kidneys.

7.2.9.5. Bile Ducts

Bile canaliculi merge with bile ducts in the portal canals through small, interconnected channels known as bile ductules. These structures are diminutive and possess delicate membranes, with tiny inner spaces enclosed by a low cuboidal layer of cells resting on a clearly defined basal lamina. The terminal ductules traverse the periportal limiting plate and drain into the interlobular bile ducts located in the portal areas. The diameter of the bile ducts expands as they move towards the outside, and the height of the lining epithelium increases. The interlobular ducts merge to create the extrahepatic ducts, where the layers of connective tissue surrounding them become thicker, and the lining epithelium becomes tall and columnar. The liver has two large extrahepatic ducts, known as the left and right hepatic ducts, which emerge from the liver lobes and join together to create the primary excretory duct of the liver, called the common hepatic duct. The common bile duct (ductus choledochus) is formed by the union of the cystic duct from the gallbladder, which drains into the duodenum.

The primary extrahepatic ducts are covered by a tall columnar epithelium that secretes mucus. The remaining part of the wall is composed of a substantial layer of connective tissue that is abundant in elastic fibers and frequently contains numerous lymphocytes and occasional migrating granulocytes. The common bile duct contains bundles of smooth muscle cells arranged in longitudinal and oblique orientations. These muscle cells form an incomplete layer that wraps around the inner space of the duct in a spiral pattern. Near the wall of the duodenum, the smooth muscle envelops the area completely and increases in thickness to create a small sphincter known as the sphincter choledochus. Beyond this area, the common bile duct and the major pancreatic duct combine as they traverse the intestinal wall and discharge through a shared structure called the hepatopancreatic ampulla. As the ducts penetrate the wall of the duodenum, they are encircled by a shared sphincter composed of smooth muscle. The liver produces bile constantly, which is then expeled from the organ through the extrahepatic duct system. Hepatocytes secrete approximately 500–900 ml of bile on a daily basis. Bile is compelled to enter the cystic duct and flow into the gallbladder due to resistance at the sphincters. The gallbladder then serves as a storage site for the bile. Bile formation predominantly takes place in two anatomical locations: bile canaliculi and bile ductules. Secretin stimulates the production of bile that contains a high concentration of bicarbonate in the ducts. Glucagon enhances the secretion of bile into the canalicular system.

7.2.9.5. Gallbladder

The gallbladder is a sacrosanct structure located on the lower surface of the liver, with dimensions of approximately 4 cm in width and 8 cm in length. The cystic duct, which has bundles of smooth muscle, connects to the common hepatic duct and is characterized by its mucous membrane with prominent spiraling folds. The spiral valve consists of these folds, which prevent the cystic duct from collapsing or expanding when there are abrupt changes in pressure. The gallbladder wall comprises a mucous membrane, a muscular layer, and a serosa or adventitia.

The gallbladder wall is composed of a single layer of columnar epithelial cells, and a layer of connective tissue called the lamina propria. The oval nuclei are positioned at the base of the cells, while the luminal surfaces exhibit a multitude of short microvilli. The uppermost points of neighboring cells are connected, close to the inner cavity, through characteristic zonula occludens junctions. The epithelium is supported by a thin basal lamina that acts as a barrier between it and the fragile connective tissue of the lamina propria. The lamina propria contains many small blood vessels. Glands are sometimes present in the lamina propria, particularly at the junction of the gallbladder and the cystic duct. These diminutive and uncomplicated tubuloacinar glands are believed to excrete mucus. The inner lining of the gallbladder, known as the mucosa, exhibits prominent and irregular folds called rugae. These rugae become flattened as the gallbladder fills with bile. The gallbladder lacks a submucosa. The muscularis layer of the gallbladder is composed of intertwined bundles of smooth muscle that form a spiral pattern around the inner cavity of the organ. Smooth muscle cells possess a multitude of receptors for cholecystokinin. The spaces between the smooth muscle bundles are occupied by collagenous, reticular, and elastic fibers. The gallbladder has a significant ability to expand due to its musculoelastic wall and rugae. The adventitia's surrounding fibroconnective tissue is relatively dense and seamlessly connects with the connective tissue of the liver capsule. The gallbladder's free surface, which is exposed to the abdominal cavity, is covered by a mesothelium, creating a serosa (Suvarva et al., 2012).

The gallbladder functions to store and concentrate bile, a substance that is continuously produced by the liver. The gallbladder in humans typically holds a volume of 30 to 50 milliliters of bile. Upon being stimulated by cholecystokinin, the gallbladder wall undergoes contraction while the sphincters of the common bile duct and ampulla relax, thereby facilitating the release of bile into the duodenum.

7.2.10. Pancreas

The pancreas is the second largest gland connected to the gastrointestinal tract. The human pancreas is a retroperitoneal organ measuring 20 to 25 cm long. It extends horizontally from the duodenum to the spleen, passing through the posterior abdominal wall. From a macroscopic perspective, the pancreas can be described as having a head located within the C-shaped curve of the duodenum, a slightly narrowed neck, and a body that makes up the majority of the organ. The pancreas does not have a distinct capsule, but it is surrounded by a thin layer of areolar connective tissue. This tissue extends thin partitions into dividing it into numerous small lobules. The septa contain blood vessels, nerves, lymphatics, and excretory ducts. The primary excretory duct extends throughout the entire length of the pancreas, gathering additional smaller branches along its path. The main pancreatic duct and its branches resemble the skeletal structure of a fish, providing internal support to the gland (Takei and Loretz, 2010).

The pancreas is composed of an exocrine section, which produces multiple digestive enzymes and bicarbonate, and an endocrine section, which releases substances that play a crucial role in carbohydrate metabolism. Unlike the liver, the pancreas carries out distinct exocrine and endocrine functions through separate groups of cells.

7.2.10.1. Exocrine Pancreas

The exocrine pancreas is a sizable, lobulated, complex tubuloacinar gland with tubular or flask-shaped secretory units. Each secretory unit is enveloped by an intricate network of reticular fibers, which also serve as the supporting stroma. An acinus is composed of a solitary layer of sizable pyramidal cells. These cells have slender apices that are adjacent to a central cavity, while their wide bases rest on a delicate basement membrane. The acinar cell contains a solitary, round nucleus positioned close to its base, and it may have one or more nucleoli. The cytoplasm surrounding the nucleus is densely packed with granular endoplasmic reticulum and mitochondria. The supranuclear region contains large Golgi complexes that play a role in the formation of zymogen granules. Fully developed zymogen granules are sizable, round, uniform structures enclosed by a membrane and frequently occupy the uppermost part of the cytoplasm. The pancreatic acinar cell is highly engaged in the production and secretion of proteins, specifically enzymes, as evident from its morphology. The pancreas produces digestive enzymes in the granular endoplasmic reticulum of the acinar cell. These enzymes then travel through the cisternae of this organelle to reach the Golgi complex in small transport vesicles. The Golgi complex membranes package precursor enzymes into zymogen granules. Subsequently, the granules are released into the uppermost part of the cell's cytoplasm, where they gather. During exocytosis, the granules move towards the outer surface of the cell membrane and release the enzymes into the acinar lumen. The granules' contents can also be released into small secretory canaliculi located between neighboring acinar cells connected to the acinar lumen. Pancreatic acinar cells release elastase, amylases, endopeptidases (lipases, trypsin, and chymotrypsin), which break central peptide bonds, and exopeptidases (carboxypeptidases A and B), which break terminal peptide bonds. These proteolytic enzymes work together to break down proteins in the intestine into smaller peptide fragments, which are then converted into amino acids before absorption.

Deoxyribonuclease and ribonuclease are also secreted by pancreatic acinar cells and specifically break down deoxyribonucleoprotein and ribonucleoprotein, respectively. Pancreatic amylase hydrolyzes starch and glycogen into disaccharides, while pancreatic lipase hydrolyzes fat micelles into fatty acids and glycerol.

7.2.10.2. Duct System

The pancreas contains a complex network of ducts. Initially, the ducts extend into the acini and are positioned between the acinar cells and the lumen. The ductal cells found in the pancreatic acini are referred to as centroacinar cells. These cells have a flattened shape, appear light in color, and have a limited number of organelles. The wall of the initial segment of the duct system, formed by centroacinar cells, remains unbroken as it extends from the secretory unit to the intercalated and intralobular ducts. The ducts mentioned are branches of the interlobular ducts located in the loose connective tissue between lobules. The transition between these ducts is gradual. The epithelial lining initially consists of a single layer of flat cells in the intercalated ducts, then becomes a layer of cube-shaped cells in the intralobular ducts, and finally transforms into a layer of column-shaped cells in the interlobular ducts. The ductal system contains scattered goblet cells and endocrine cells. The cells that cover the ducts exhibit faint staining, and their cytoplasm does not contain prominent organelles. Desmosomes are distributed sporadically along the sides of cells, and the uppermost parts of neighboring cells are connected by tight junctions. The uppermost surfaces are covered with microvilli. The intercalated and intralobular ducts are supported by sparse connective tissue primarily composed of reticular fibers. The interlobular and major secretory ducts are located within the interlobular septae and are, therefore, enveloped by a substantial amount of fibroconnective tissue. The interlobular ducts empty into both the primary and accessory pancreatic ducts. The main duct extends along the entire pancreas length, gradually becoming larger near the duodenum. At this point, it runs alongside the common bile duct and frequently has a shared opening at the greater duodenal papilla. The sphincter of the papilla regulates the openings of both ducts. A supplementary duct may be located near the primary duct and opens separately into the duodenal cavity. The exocrine pancreas is regulated by both the nervous system and hormones, resulting in the release of secretions. Cells in the intestinal mucosa release two polypeptide hormones, secretin, and cholecystokinin, which have an impact on exocrine pancreatic secretion. Secretin, produced by S cells in the lining of the duodenum and proximal jejunum, activates the pancreatic ducts to release a significant amount of fluid that contains a high concentration of bicarbonate. Within the intestinal lumen, an alkaline secretion is released to counteract the acidic chyme from the stomach. This secretion also inactivates the gastric enzyme pepsin, which functions best in an acidic environment with a pH of 2.0 (Takei and Loretz, 2010). Additionally, it creates the necessary neutraltoalkaline environment for the optimal functioning of pancreatic enzymes. Cholecystokinin, produced by I cells in the lining of the duodenum and jejunum, activates the secretory units of the pancreas to produce and release digestive enzymes. The proteolytic enzymes are released in the form of inactive precursors called zymogens. These zymogens are activated by enterokinase, an enzyme in the intestinal mucosa, which partially converts them into their active forms. Pancreatic amylase and lipase are known to be secreted in their fully functional states. Cholecystokinin additionally triggers the contraction of the gallbladder, which results in the release of bile. This bile helps to neutralize the contents of the intestine and contains bile acids that assist in breaking down neutral fats by acting as emulsifying agents.

7.2.10.3. Endocrine Pancreas

The pancreatic islets (of Langerhans) are irregular, elongated masses of pale-staining cells found within the pancreatic acini. These islets comprise the endocrine part of the pancreas. In humans, the number of these entities is approximately one million. The islets are distinguished from the adjacent exocrine pancreas by a fragile layer of reticular fibers, and like all endocrine glands, the islets are well-supplied with blood vessels. When examining regular tissue sections, the islets seem to consist of a uniform group of pale polygonal cells. However, using specific stains and electron micrographs makes it possible to distinguish several different types of cells within the islets (as shown in Table 7.3). Alpha and beta cells constitute most cells.

Alpha cells constitute approximately 20% of the islets and are typically situated at the outer edge of the islet. The granules found within them are large, dense, and have a spherical shape, enclosed by a membrane. Mitochondria exhibits an elongated and slender morphology, characterized by a distinctive internal organization. Several instances of granular endoplasmic reticulum are distributed throughout the cytoplasm, while Golgi bodies are typically located near the nucleus. The secretory granules have an average diameter of approximately 250 nm. Alpha cells synthesize the peptide hormone glucagon. Glucagon is secreted when blood sugar levels are low, and it affects the liver by converting stored glycogen into glucose. It also stimulates the liver to produce glucose from amino acids through gluconeogenesis. Additionally, glucagon prompts adipose tissue to release fatty acids, which are metabolized by the liver to produce keto acids. Glucagon secretion leads to an overall increase in blood levels of glucose, free fatty acids, and ketones. Therefore, glucagon is a significant hormone that mobilizes fuel (Wegner et al., 2009).

Beta cells constitute approximately 78% of the islet cells and are typically positioned near the central region of the islet. Their secretory granules exhibit a smaller size compared to the alpha cells. Beta cell granules are characterized by compact, minute crystals, which contribute to their unique visual appearance. The extent of the granular endoplasmic reticulum is reduced, while the Golgi complexes exhibit a more pronounced distinctiveness compared to alpha cells. Beta cells secrete insulin in response to high blood sugar levels, a condition known as hyperglycemia. Insulin then interacts with the plasmalemma of different cell types, particularly liver, muscle, and fat cells, to enhance glucose uptake into the cells, resulting in a decrease in blood glucose levels. Insulin additionally promotes fat production, hinders the breakdown of fats, and encourages the transportation of amino acids into cells and their formation into proteins. Insulin has an antagonistic effect to glucagon. Insulin functions as a hormone that stores fuel and reduces the levels of glucose, free fatty acids, and ketones in the blood.

A few additional types of endocrine cells exist in small quantities within the islets. Delta cells release the hormone somatostatin, which suppresses the secretion of hormones by neighboring alpha and beta endocrine cells in the pancreatic islet. Pancreatic polypeptide, released by PP cells, hinders the release of enzymes by the pancreatic acinar cells and the secretion of bicarbonate by the ductal system. Endocrine cells, such as alpha and beta cells, are also present in the ducts and acini of the exocrine pancreas. The number of distinct endocrine cells can vary depending on their specific locations within the head or body of the pancreas, which may be associated with the different origins of these two regions. The distribution of cells within the islets exhibits significant species variation. In humans, beta cells are typically situated in the central region of the islets, whereas alpha, delta, and PP cells are predominantly found at the outer edges of the islets.

Islet cells have a close relationship with the capillaries surrounding them, and the secretory granules are often found near the cell membrane next to the blood vessels. Islet cells release secretory granules through exocytosis into the adjacent blood vessels. The endothelium of the capillaries in the islets contains many fenestrations, which help the secretory products to enter the blood vessels. Unlike the fenestrated endothelium found in other capillaries, the endothelium of capillaries in the exocrine pancreas does not have pores. A considerable portion of the arterial blood flows into the pancreas through small interlobular and intralobular arteries, which initially provide blood to the islets. The arteries give rise to arterioles, which in turn give rise to capillaries at the periphery of the islets, specifically in the area where the alpha, delta, and PP-cells are located. Subsequently, the capillaries course towards the center of the islet, where they provide nourishment to the neighboring acinar cells of the exocrine pancreas. Therefore, the pancreatic islet cells can communicate with one another and impact the functioning of the exocrine pancreas.

Table 7.3. Endocrine Cell Types of the Pancreas

Cell Type	Hormonal Substance	Primary Function
A (alpha) cell	Glucagon	Increases blood sugar
B (beta) cell	Insulin	Decreases blood sugar
D cell	Somatostatin	Inhibitor of hormone secretion (paracrine function)*
PP cell	Pancreatic polypeptide	Opposes action of cholecystokinin
G cell Ψ	Gastrin	Increases HCL secretion in stomach

*Paracrine function. Secretion of somatostatin is directly into the intercellular space from which it diffuses to inhibit the secretion of adjacent endocrine cells. ΨG cells are present only in some species or restricted to fetal life in others.

7.2.11. Organogenesis

Once the three germ layers have developed, the embryo takes on the shape of a flattened disk, with the yolk sac protruding from its underside. The endoderm covers both the surface of the embryo and the interior of the yolk sac, serving as the lining for the entire digestive tract. Through subsequent growth, the embryo and gastrointestinal endoderm undergo a process of folding, resulting in the formation of a cylindrical shape. The folding process initiates at the extremities of the embryo, resulting in the formation of two endodermal tubes that lack an opening, and are connected to the inner cavity of the yolk sac at a specific region known as the intestinal portal. The proximal endodermal tube differentiates into the foregut, which develops into the oral cavity, pharynx, stomach, and proximal duodenum. The midgut is connected to the yolk sac and gives rise to the jejunum, ileum, cecum, appendix, ascending colon, and a portion of the transverse colon. The caudal tube transforms into the hindgut, which then undergoes differentiation to form the remaining portion of the large intestine (Wilson and Castro, 2010).

7.2.11.1. Oral Cavity

The lips initially develop as a thickened band called the labial lamina, which originates from the ectoderm and extends over the primitive jaw into the underlying mesenchyme. The labial lamina thickens, and as the central cells degenerate, splits to form the lips and gums. The cheeks arise by the fusion of the upper and lower lips at their lateral angles, thus reducing the original broad mouth opening. The skeletal muscle of the lip and cheeks originates from mesenchyme that migrates from the second branchial arch and positions itself between the mucosal and epidermal layers.

The tongue originates from the ventral extremities of the branchial arches. The tongue is composed of two parts: the ectoderm-covered oral part derived from the mandibular arches, and the endodermal pharyngeal part derived from the second branchial arch. The boundary between the outer layer of cells (ectoderm) and the inner layer of cells (endoderm) is located directly in front of the sulcus terminalis. Therefore, the fungiform and filiform papillae originate from the ectoderm, while the circumvallate papillae originate from the endoderm. Initially, the tongue is lined with cuboidal epithelium, which subsequently transitions into stratified squamous epithelium. Initially, all papillae develop as raised areas of the mucosa. Each circumvallate papilla is encircled by a thickened ring of epithelial tissue that extends into the surrounding mesenchyme and divides to create a trench surrounding each papilla. Epithelial cords extend from the base of the trench and generate von Ebner's glands. Taste buds form on the top of each circumvallate papilla, but they are later replaced by definitive buds on the sides of the papilla. Taste buds initially develop as localized thickenings of epithelium, where basal cells undergo elongation, migrate towards the surface, and differentiate into supporting and taste cells (Wilson and Castro, 2010).

The major and minor salivary glands are derived from ectodermal tissue. All begin from the epithelial surface as buds that grow and branch, treelike, forming a system of solid ducts. Terminal twigs, which eventually form intercalated ducts, round out at their ends to form secretory tubules and acini. Canalization of the duct follows. The sublingual gland differs slightly in that several buds form from the oral epithelium, and each remains a discrete gland. The parotid appears first, followed by the submandibular, sublingual, and, later still, minor salivary glands. Mesenchyme surrounding the epithelial primordia provides the capsule and septae of the salivary glands. Teeth have a dual origin: enamel arises from ectoderm; dentin, pulp, and cementum arise from mesoderm. Tooth development begins with the appearance of the dental lamina, a plate of epithelium on which knoblike swellings (enamel organs) appear at intervals. These give rise to enamel and act as molds for tooth development. The enamel organs grow into the mesenchyme to form inverted, cuplike structures invaginated at the bases by dental papillae. The latter are condensations of mesenchyme that give rise to the dentin and pulp of teeth. The enamel organ forms a double-walled sac, of which the outer and inner walls differentiate into outer and inner enamel layers, respectively. Loosely arranged cells lie between the two layers and form the enamel pulp. Cells of the inner layer become ameloblasts and produce enamel prisms, beginning at the interface with the dental papillae. Mesenchymal cells of the papillae next to the inner dental layer enlarge and differentiate into odontoblasts. These form a single layer of columnar cells whose apices face the ameloblasts. Odontoblasts produce predentin that soon calcifies to become definitive dentin. Mesenchyme central to the odontoblasts forms the dental pulp. Dentin is the first of the hard tissues to appear in the tooth. Thereafter, enamel and dentin are laid down, beginning at the apex and progressing toward the root. As the enamel and dentin layers thicken, the odontoblasts and ameloblasts gradually move away from each other. Ameloblasts migrate peripherally, remaining at the outer surface of the enamel, and eventually are lost from the tooth at eruption. Before they are lost, ameloblasts lay down an acellular layer called the enamel cuticle that covers the enamel, adhering tightly to it. This cuticle may persist for a considerable time after teeth erupt and the ameloblasts are lost. Odontoblasts progress centrally into the pulp cavity, where they persist. As they retreat, the odontoblasts trail fine cytoplasmic processes that extend through the dentin to the dentinoenamel junction. The entrapped processes form the dentinal fibers contained in fine dentinal tubules. Mesenchyme around the developing enamel organ differentiates into the loose connective tissue of the dentinal sac. Near the root, the inner cells of the sac become cementoblasts and cover the dentin with cementum. Cells at the exterior of the sac differentiate to produce the alveolar bone surrounding each tooth.

The connective tissue between the external and internal layers of the dental sac gives rise to the periodontal membrane. Before the tooth erupts, a small crater appears in the gingival epithelium and connective tissue, immediately above the crown. The crater, which expands to accommodate the tooth as it emerges, develops from focal pressure necrosis as the tooth grows upward, or by means of lytic activity of enzymes produced by the dental epithelium, or both (Won and Borski, 2013).

7.2.11.2. Alimentary Canal

The esophagus, stomach, small intestine, and colon are initially composed of an endodermal tube enveloped by a layer of splanchnic mesoderm. The endoderm is responsible for the development of the lining epithelium and all the glands associated with the digestive tube. On the other hand, the mesoderm differentiates into the supporting layers of the gastrointestinal tube. The esophagus originates as a concise conduit that links the pharynx and stomach. During the development of the neck region and thorax, the tube undergoes elongation. At first, the esophagus is covered by a layer of simple columnar epithelium, which gradually transforms into a thicker and stratified layer. Ciliated columnar cells and sporadic goblet cells are interspersed among the squamous cells. Ciliated cells may continue to exist until birth, after which the lining remains a moist stratified squamous epithelium.

The initial glands that emerge are the esophageal cardiac glands, succeeded by the esophageal glands proper, which undergo further development after birth. The ductal system of these glands is formed by outgrowths located at the base of the epithelium, while the secretory units develop from epithelial buds found on the terminal branches of the ducts. The stomach initially forms as an elongated expansion of the foregut, which is covered by a single layer of columnar epithelium that is either simple or pseudostratified and originates from the endoderm. Gastric pits form when the surface epithelium folds inward into the mesenchyme below. The formation of the pits initially occurs along the lesser curvature and subsequently progresses in other areas. Approximately three weeks later, they manifest in the pyloric and cardiac regions. Shortly after the formation of the pits, oxyntic glands emerge from epithelial buds located at the bottom of the pits. The development of pyloric and cardiac glands is similar but occurs later than the development of oxyntic glands. The development of the intestine typically follows a progression from the proximal (near the beginning) to the distal (near the end) regions, resulting in the formation of villi, glands, and various cell types. The gastrointestinal tract originates as a rudimentary endodermal tube that extends from the stomach to the cloaca. As the tube lengthens, a growth towards the tail indicates the early formation of the cecum, from which the appendix emerges due to very rapid growth at the closed end. The lumen of the duodenum is temporarily blocked due to a rapid increase in cell growth in the epithelial lining. Subsequently, vacuoles form within the epithelium, merge, and reinstate the openness of the lumen. Similar occurrences occur to a lesser extent in the rest of the small intestine and colon. The current lining epithelium comprises four to five layers of cells, with smooth surfaces facing both the lumen and the base, and is situated on a clearly defined basement membrane. The mesenchyme underlying has not undergone differentiation to form the lamina propria and submucosa. The rapid growth and multiplication of the epithelial cells, along with the inward folding of the connective tissue, results in the formation of folds or ridges in the inner lining of the mucous membrane. As these folds or ridges continue to multiply, the border of the inner lining becomes uneven. The initial formation of villi occurs because of the disintegration of the mucosal ridges. Due to the presence of different types of epithelium, namely stratified cuboidal and simple columnar, the thickness of these villi can vary. Following that, subsequent generations of villi are created as uncomplicated epithelium and connective tissue outgrowths, without the preceding formation of mucosal folds. The villi that form in the colon, cecum, and appendix undergo regression during the latter stages of fetal development. Intestinal glands form as uncomplicated tubular extensions of the epithelium located between villi. Duodenal glands originate from protrusions of the epithelium located on the intestinal floor, either between villi or from intestinal glands.

During the formation of villi, myoblasts undergo differentiation in the mesenchyme to establish the muscularis mucosae. Currently, epithelium is composed of a single layer of tall, cylindrical cells, and goblet and enteroendocrine cells form in a sequential manner from the head to the tail. Paneth cells exhibit a delayed appearance compared to other cell types. The muscularis externa of the small intestine originates prior to the muscularis mucosae, with the inner layer being the first to develop. The formation of this structure entails the process of differentiation and proliferation of smooth muscle cells originating from mesenchyme. This is then followed by hypertrophy, which is responsible for most of the ultimate thickness of the muscle coat. Plicae circulares develop later, after the formation of villi, and are characterized by their broad and elongated shape. After birth, the epithelial cells that line the villi in the distal ileum have a highly developed endocytic complex. The complex is composed of multiple vesicles and tubules that are created through invaginations of the cell membrane located between microvilli. These combine with vacuoles of different sizes that contain inclusions in the cytoplasm above the nucleus.

The complex is involved in the uptake of large molecules and antibodies during the initial weeks of breastfeeding. The muscularis externa of the entire gastrointestinal tract originates from the surrounding mesenchyme and undergoes differentiation to form the inner circular and outer longitudinal layers of smooth muscle cells. The initial development phase involves a period of high cell division activity and the transformation of mesenchymal cells into myoblasts. The inner circular layer is typically formed before the outer layer, which initially consists of a single layer of scattered, discontinuous myoblasts. The muscularis externa is a tissue that undergoes a slow renewal process, as evidenced by a consistently low rate of mitotic activity during development and into adulthood. Hypertrophy of the existing muscle layers is the second significant factor in the development of the muscularis externa. The innervation of the muscularis externa becomes functional during the early stages of muscle tissue development, which occurs around 6 weeks when smooth muscle cells are rapidly multiplying. Hypertrophy occurs following the establishment of the myenteric plexus. The neurons of the myenteric plexus (as well as the submucosal plexus) originate from the neural crest. Hirschsprung disease, also called colonic aganglionosis, is a congenital defect caused by the neural crest cells failing to migrate into the developing wall (muscularis externa) of the sigmoid colon and rectum to form the required plexus.

7.2.11.3. Liver and Pancreas

The formation of the liver primordium initiates as a thickening of the endodermal epithelium in the anterior intestinal portal, which will eventually become the duodenum, of the developing gastrointestinal tube. A ventral outgrowth, devoid of contents, emerges, covered by a layer of simple columnar epithelium that seamlessly connects with the lining of the duodenum. The hepatic diverticulum expands, extends into the vascular mesenchyme of the septum transversum, and splits into multiple parts. The cranial portion of the structure develops into the hepatic parenchyma and the intrahepatic bile ducts, while the caudal part gives rise to the common bile duct, cystic duct, gallbladder, and interhepatic bile ducts (Won and Borski, 2013). The adjacent mesenchyme gives rise to both the capsule and stroma. Initially, the hepatic cells are diminutive and asymmetrical in form, typically harboring a multitude of lipid droplets. The cords may arrange themselves in a non-uniform network, with islands of hematopoietic cells interspersed. However, there is a lack of distinct organization in well-defined plates and sinusoids. During the differentiation process, irregular clusters of cells emerge, projecting from the central veins towards the outer edges of each developing lobule, and sinusoids become visible. The lobulation observed in adult individuals is absent in developing embryos and is believed to be caused by the hemodynamics of blood circulation within the liver. The initial development of the liver is primarily driven by hyperplasia, although some hypertrophy is also observed. Hepatocytes experience lipid depletion, and hematopoietic activity diminishes and stops either before or shortly after birth. Bile canaliculi emerge at six weeks, preceding the initiation of bile secretion. Over the course of the next three to four weeks, the remaining part of the intrahepatic biliary system, specifically the bile ductules, develops from hepatocytes located near the limiting plate of the lobules. Subsequently, these bile ductules connect with the interlobular ducts found in the portal areas. The caudal hepatic diverticulum undergoes a transformation into a compact cluster of cells, which subsequently develops into the cystic duct and gallbladder. Epithelial cords and blood vessels extend into the connective tissue between lobules and transform into hepatic ducts that merge with bile ducts. The factors that determine how the two entities merge are currently unknown. The pancreas originates from endodermal outgrowths of the gastrointestinal tract wall, specifically in two locations on opposite sides of the duodenum. The ventral and dorsal pancreatic buds merge once the ventral bud has moved towards the dorsal side. The primary excretory ducts originate from the ventral bud, while the accessory duct forms from the dorsal bud. The initial structure of the pancreatic parenchyma is composed of a sequence of closed tubules made up of a single layer of columnar epithelial cells. These tubules then divide and enlarge within the neighboring mesenchyme tissue. Acini are formed at the terminal points of the tiniest ducts, while others are also generated as outgrowths from larger ducts. The formation of ducts and acini leads to the gradual development of lobes and lobules, which are defined by the surrounding connective tissue (Won and Borski, 2013). Certain acinar cells enlarge closer to the ducts, while some terminal ductal cells are assimilated into the acini as centroacinar cells. The proliferation of acinar cells primarily occurs through the division of differentiated cells and can continue into the later stages of postnatal development. Concurrently, islet cells undergo differentiation from progenitor cells derived from the endoderm within the ductal system. Islets primarily form at the terminations of ducts, although paratubular outgrowths can also occur. The secondary islets are formed as ducts and acini develop near the periphery of the lobules, causing the previously formed islets to become more centrally located in the lobule. Several islets maintain their association with the ductal epithelium from which they originated, but as the exocrine parenchyma grows, the connection between the islet and duct becomes less apparent. Several main islets are located outside the lobule, within the interlobular connective tissue. These cells are the initial endocrine cells that arise from the primary tubules before the formation of smaller ducts and acini. Individual endocrine cells or small clusters are still present throughout the ductal system or can be found between acinar cells, even in adulthood.

A Closer Look

The Liver

The liver is a vital organ situated in the upper right quadrant of the abdomen, weighing approximately 1.4 kilograms (3.1 pounds) in adults. It is the largest solid organ and serves a multitude of critical functions necessary for maintaining overall health. Anatomically, the liver is divided into two main lobes, each further subdivided into lobules, which are the functional units of the liver. These lobules are composed of hepatocytes, the liver's primary cell type, responsible for carrying out the majority of its functions. The liver is also richly vascularized, receiving blood from two primary **source**s: the hepatic artery, which supplies oxygen-rich blood, and the portal vein, which brings nutrient-rich blood from the gastrointestinal tract. This unique dual blood supply allows the liver to play a pivotal role in metabolism, detoxification, and digestion.

The liver's multifaceted functions can be categorized into metabolic, synthetic, and detoxifying roles. Metabolically, the liver is crucial in processing carbohydrates, proteins, and fats. It converts glucose to glycogen for storage, which can be mobilized back into glucose when energy is needed. In protein metabolism, the liver synthesizes various proteins, including albumin, which maintains blood volume and pressure, and clotting factors essential for hemostasis. Additionally, it is involved in lipid metabolism, converting excess carbohydrates and proteins into fatty acids and cholesterol. The liver also stores vital nutrients, such as vitamins A, D, E, K, and B12, as well as minerals like iron and copper, making it integral to overall nutritional balance.

Detoxification is another critical function of the liver. It filters harmful substances from the blood, including drugs, alcohol, and metabolic waste products. Hepatocytes contain enzymes that metabolize these substances into less toxic forms, which can then be excreted through bile or urine. The liver also plays a significant role in the metabolism of hormones, ensuring that they are maintained at appropriate levels in the body. This detoxifying capability helps to maintain homeostasis and protect the body from potential damage caused by accumulated toxins. Any dysfunction in these processes can lead to severe health consequences, highlighting the liver's importance in overall well-being.

Liver health is essential, but it can be compromised by various factors, including viral infections, excessive alcohol consumption, obesity, and metabolic disorders. Conditions such as hepatitis, cirrhosis, and fatty liver disease can significantly impair liver function. Early detection and management are crucial for preventing irreversible damage. Regular health check-ups, a balanced diet, moderate alcohol consumption, and vaccination against viral hepatitis are essential preventive measures. The liver's remarkable regenerative capacity allows it to recover from injury, but chronic damage can lead to scarring and liver failure. Thus, understanding the liver's functions and maintaining its health is vital for sustaining life and overall health.

Summary

The respiratory system's primary role is to facilitate gas exchange, providing oxygen to the bloodstream while removing carbon dioxide. It includes structures such as the nasal cavity, trachea, bronchi, and lungs, where the exchange occurs at the alveoli. This system not only supports cellular respiration but also plays a role in regulating blood pH and protecting against pathogens through mucous membranes and cilia.

The digestive system, on the other hand, is responsible for breaking down food, absorbing nutrients, and eliminating waste. It comprises a complex pathway, including the mouth, esophagus, stomach, intestines, liver, pancreas, and gallbladder. The digestive process begins with mechanical and chemical breakdown in the mouth and continues through various stages, where enzymes and acids further digest food. Nutrient absorption primarily occurs in the small intestine, while the large intestine reabsorbs water and compacts waste for excretion. Together, these systems ensure the body receives essential nutrients and oxygen, highlighting their interdependence for overall health and functioning.

References

1. Alves, A. P. C., Pereira, R. T., & Rosa, P. V. (2021). Morphology of the digestive system in carnivorous freshwater dourado *Salminus brasiliensis*. *Journal of Fish Biology, 99*(5), 1222–1235. https://doi.org/10.1111/jfb.14879.
2. Buddington, R. K., & Krogdahl, Å. (2004). Hormonal regulation of the fish gastrointestinal tract. *Comparative Biochemistry and Physiology Part A: Molecular & Integrative Physiology, 139*(3), 261–271. https://doi.org/10.1016/j.cbpb.2004.09.015.
3. Cao, X. J., & Wang, W. M. (2009). Histology and mucin histochemistry of the digestive tract of yellow catfish, *Pelteobagrus fulvidraco*. *Anatomia, Histologia, Embryologia, 38*(4), 254–261. https://doi.org/10.1111/j.1439-0264.2009.00930.x.
4. Carrassón, M., Grau, A., Dopazo, L. R., & Crespo, S. (2006). A histological, histochemical and ultrastructural study of the digestive tract of *Dextex dextex* (Pisces, Sparidae). *Histology and Histopathology, 21*(6), 579–593. https://doi.org/10.14670/HH-21.579.
5. Collie, N. L., & Ferraris, R. P. (1995). Nutrient fluxes and regulation in fish intestine. In P. W. Hochachka & T. Mommsen (Eds.), *Biochemistry and Molecular Biology of Fishes: Metabolic Biochemistry* (Vol. 4, pp. 221–239). Elsevier Science.
6. Gustafsson, J. K., & Johansson, M. E. V. (2022). The role of goblet cells and mucus in intestinal homeostasis. *Nature Reviews Gastroenterology & Hepatology, 19*(12), 785–803. https://doi.org/10.1038/s41575-022-00608-8.
7. Hernández, D. R., Pérez Gianeselli, M., & Domitrovic, H. A. (2009). Morphology, histology and histochemistry of the digestive system of South American catfish (*Rhamdia quelen*). *International Journal of Morphology, 27*(1), 105–111. https://doi.org/10.4067/S0717-95022009000100020.
8. Ji, H. S., Kim, J. K., & Kim, B. J. (2016). Molecular phylogeny of the families Pleuronectidae and Poecilopsettidae (Pisces, Pleuronectiformes) from Korea, with a proposal for a new classification. *Ocean Science Journal, 51*(3), 299–304. https://doi.org/10.1007/s12601-016-0027-6.

9. Kirschbaum, F., & Formicki, K. (2019). Digestive system. In *The Histology of Fishes* (pp. 88–115). CRC Press.

10. Lipscomb, T. N., Yanong, R. P., Ramee, S. W., & DiMaggio, M. A. (2020). Histological, histochemical and biochemical characterization of larval digestive system ontogeny in black tetra (*Gymnocorymbus ternetzi*) to inform aquaculture weaning protocols. *Aquaculture, 520*, 734957. https://doi.org/10.1016/j.aquaculture.2020.734957.

11. Miller, L. J., Harikumar, K. G., Wootten, D., & Sexton, P. M. (2021). Roles of cholecystokinin in the nutritional continuum: Physiology and potential therapeutics. *Frontiers in Endocrinology, 12*, 684656. https://doi.org/10.3389/fendo.2021.684656.

12. Ostaszewska, T., Krajnik, K., Adamek-Urbanska, D., Kasprzak, R., Rzepkowska, M., Luczynski, M., & Karczewska, A. T. (2018). Effect of feeding strategy on digestive tract morphology and physiology of lake whitefish (*Coregonus lavaretus*). *Aquaculture, 497*, 32–41. https://doi.org/10.1016/j.aquaculture.2018.08.021.

13. Pena, R., Dumas, S., Villalejo-Fuerte, M., & Ortiz-Galindo, J. L. (2003). Ontogenetic development of the digestive tract in reared spotted sand bass (*Paralabrax maculatofasciatus*) larvae. *Aquaculture, 219*(1–4), 633–644. https://doi.org/10.1016/S0044-8486(03)00016-0.

14. Ray, A. K., & Ringø, E. (2014). The gastrointestinal tract of fish. In *Aquaculture Nutrition: Gut Health, Probiotics and Prebiotics* (pp. 1–13). John Wiley and Sons.

15. Rønnestad, I., Yúfera, M., Ueberschär, B., Ribeiro, L., Sæle, Ø., & Boglione, C. (2013). Feeding behaviour and digestive physiology in larvae fish: Current knowledge, and gaps and bottlenecks in research. *Reviews in Aquaculture, 5*(S1), S59–S98. https://doi.org/10.1111/raq.12010.

16. Suvarva, S. K., Layton, C., & Bancroft, J. D. (2012). *Bancroft's Theory and Practice of Histological Techniques* (7th ed.). Churchill Livingstone.

17. Takei, Y., & Loretz, C. A. (2010). The gastrointestinal tract as an endocrine/neuroendocrine/paracrine organ: Organization, chemical messengers and physiological targets. *Fish Physiology, 30*, 261–317. https://doi.org/10.1016/S1546-5098(10)03005-8.

18. Wegner, A., Ostaszewska, T., & Rożek, W. (2009). The ontogenetic development of the digestive tract and accessory glands of sterlet (*Acipenser ruthenus* L.) larvae during endogenous feeding. *Reviews in Fish Biology and Fisheries, 19*(4), 431–444. https://doi.org/10.1007/s11160-009-9121-1.

19. Wilson, J. M., & Castro, L. F. C. (2010). Morphological diversity of the gastrointestinal tract in fishes. In M. Grosell, A. P. Farrell, & C. J. Brauner (Eds.), *Fish Physiology: The Multifunctional Gut of Fish* (pp. 1–55). Academic Press.

20. Won, E. T., & Borski, R. J. (2013). Endocrine regulation of compensatory growth in fish. *Frontiers in Endocrinology, 4*, 74. https://doi.org/10.3389/fendo.2013.00074.

Chapter 8

URINARY AND REPRODUCTIVE SYSTEM

Contents

Introduction

The urinary system, consisting of the kidneys, ureters, bladder, and urethra, primarily functions in waste excretion and fluid balance. The kidneys feature a complex histological structure with renal corpuscles (glomeruli and Bowman's capsules), proximal and distal convoluted tubules, loops of Henle, and collecting ducts. The glomeruli, located in the renal cortex, are composed of a network of capillaries surrounded by the Bowman's capsule, facilitating filtration. The tubules and loops are lined with epithelial cells specialized for reabsorption and secretion, ensuring efficient waste removal and fluid homeostasis.

In the reproductive system, histological examination varies significantly between males and females due to distinct organ structures. In males, the testes contain seminiferous tubules, where spermatogenesis occurs, supported by Sertoli cells and Leydig cells, which produce testosterone. The epididymis, vas deferens, and accessory glands, including the prostate, are lined with columnar epithelium and specialized cells for the maturation and transport of sperm (Andersen, 2017).

In females, the ovaries consist of follicles at various stages of development, surrounded by stroma and supported by theca and granulosa cells, which produce sex hormones. The uterine tubes, uterus, and vagina are lined with ciliated columnar and stratified squamous epithelium, facilitating the transport of ova and providing a site for implantation and fetal development. The cyclic changes in the endometrium, influenced by hormonal fluctuations, are critical for reproductive function. The histological complexity of the urinary and reproductive systems underscores their essential roles in maintaining homeostasis and reproductive health.

Orientation and Directional Terms

Term	Definition	Illustration
Urinary System	The organ system responsible for the production, storage, and elimination of urine, consisting of the kidneys, ureters, bladder, and urethra, and regulating fluid balance and waste removal.	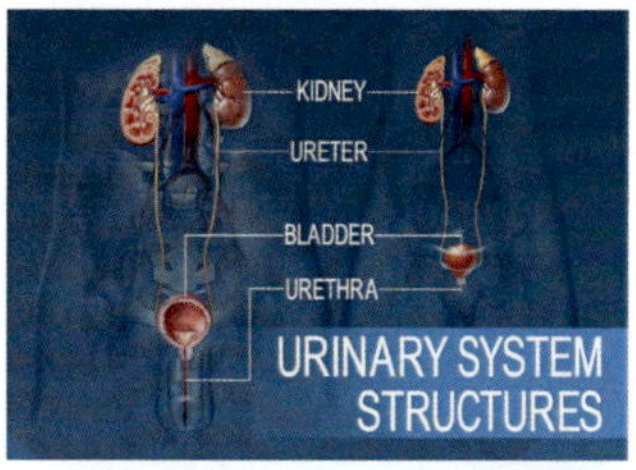
Testes	The male reproductive organs that produce sperm and hormones, primarily testosterone; they are located in the scrotum.	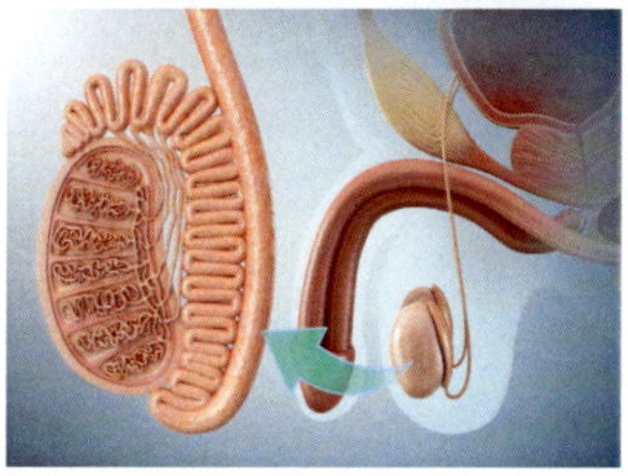
Ovaries	The female reproductive organs that produce eggs (ova) and hormones, including estrogen and progesterone; they are located in the pelvic cavity.	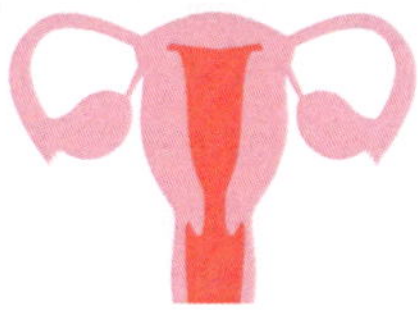
Oviducts	Also known as fallopian tubes, these are the tubes that transport eggs from the ovaries to the uterus; fertilization typically occurs within the oviducts.	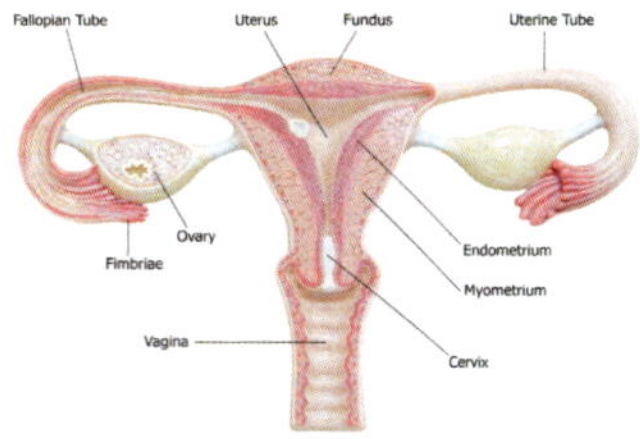
External Genitalia	The external structures of the reproductive system, including the penis and scrotum in males, and the vulva and clitoris in females; they play roles in reproduction and sexual function.	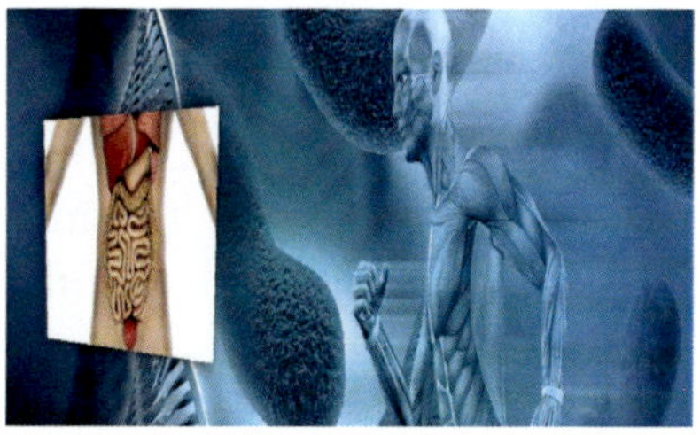

8.1. Urinary System

The total body water of an average person makes up about two-thirds of the total body weight. The total body water is subdivided into two major fluid compartments. An intracellular fluid compartment, the water contained within the cells of the body, accounts for about two-thirds of the total body water, while an extracellular fluid compartment makes up the remaining third. The extracellular fluid is further subdivided into the interstitial fluids and the plasma within the blood vascular system, which are linked by vessels of the lymphatic system.

Homeostasis of the extracellular fluid compartment is maintained in part by the urinary system. The urinary system consists of the kidneys, ureters, urinary bladder, and urethra. The ureters conduct urine from the kidneys to the bladder, where it is stored temporarily, and the bladder is drained by the urethra, through which the urine is ultimately voided from the body.

8.1.1. Kidneys

The kidneys are a pair of compound tubular glands that clear the blood plasma of metabolic wastes, regulate fluid osmolality and volume, regulate electrolyte balance, eliminate foreign chemicals, and help maintain the acid-base balance of the body. Excretion of metabolic products includes creatinine (from muscle creatine phosphate), uric acid (from nucleic acids), urea (from amino acids), metabolites of hormones and hemoglobin, as well as other substances. The kidneys also are instrumental in eliminating drugs, pesticides, and other environmental factors from the blood plasma. In addition to excretory functions, the kidneys have properties of endocrine organs and release two substances, renin and erythropoietin, directly into the bloodstream. Renin is important in regulating blood pressure and sodium ion concentration; erythropoietin influences hematopoietic activity. The kidneys also are important in activating circulating vitamin D to an active form, 1, 25- dihydroxyvitamin D3, necessary for normal absorption of calcium ion in the gastrointestinal tract (Andersen, 2017).

8.1.1.1. Macroscopic Features

Human kidneys are bean-shaped organs in a retroperitoneal position against the posterior abdominal wall, one on either side of the upper lumbar vertebrae. Each is contained within a thin but strong connective tissue capsule containing fat. The renal artery and nerves enter the kidney on the medial border at the hilum, a concavity that also serves as the point of exit for the renal vein, lymphatics, and ureter. The hilum is continuous with the renal sinus, a large central cavity surrounded by the parenchyma of the kidney and filled with loose areolar connective tissue that normally contains much fat. Nerves, lymphatics, and branches of the renal artery and vein run through the sinus. The renal pelvis is a funnel-shaped expansion of the ureter where it joins the kidney; it also passes through the sinus, dividing into two or three short tubular structures called the major calyces. These, in turn, divide into eight to twelve smaller units called minor calyces.

Each minor calyx forms a cylindrical attachment around a conical projection of renal tissue called a renal papilla. When a hemisection of the kidney is examined macroscopically, the organization of the parenchyma into two distinct regions can be seen readily. The darker, granular appearing outer region is the cortex, which forms a continuous layer beneath the capsule. The inner region, or medulla, is paler and smoother in texture and consists of 8 to 20 cone-shaped structures called medullary pyramids, which are separated from each other by inward extensions of cortical tissue. The cortex that separates adjacent medullary pyramids makes up a renal column. The bases of the pyramids are directed toward the overlying cortex, while their apices are oriented toward the renal sinus and form the renal papillae. From the bases of the pyramids, groups of tubules extend into the cortex, giving it a striated appearance. These striations represent a continuation of medullary tissue into the cortex and constitute the medullary rays. The arrangement of the cortex and medulla allows the subdivision of the kidney into smaller units, the lobes and lobules. A medullary pyramid, together with its closely associated cortical tissue, forms a renal lobe, while a medullary ray, together with its associated cortical tissue, forms a renal lobule. When the kidney consists of several lobes, it is referred to as a multilobular kidney; the kidneys of humans are this type.

8.1.1.2. Microscopic Features

Each renal lobule comprises numerous epithelial tubules called uriniferous tubules that collectively form the parenchyma of the kidney (**Figure 8.1**). Each uriniferous tubule can be divided into a nephron and a collecting duct. Each of these units has a different embryologic origin.

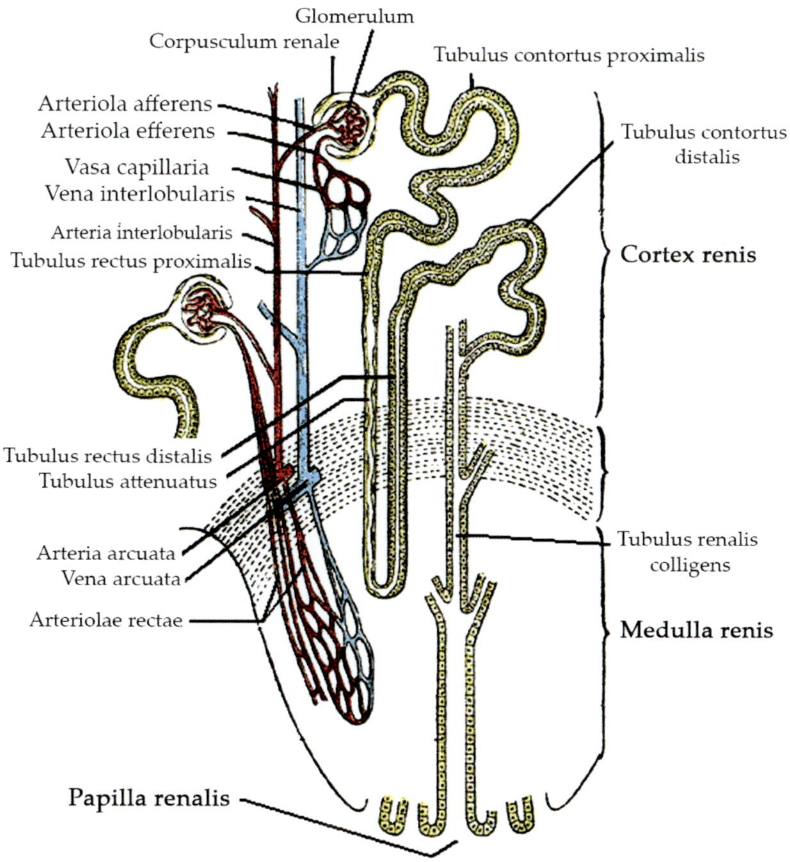

Figure 8.1. *Schematic drawing of a nephron.*

Source: *https://www.researchgate.net/profile/Daphne-Ijpelaar/publication/28650894/figure/fig1/AS:309913197793282@1450900472443/Schematic-drawing-of-a-nephron-Illustration-printed-with-permission-from-Elsevier-3.png.*

8.1.1.3. Nephron

There are 1 to 2 million nephrons in the human kidney, each representing a functional unit of the kidney. A nephron is a blindly ending epithelial tubule that can be subdivided into several components, each differing in structure, function, and position in the kidney. During urine formation, the various segments of a nephron take part in filtration, secretion, and resorption. A typical nephron consists of a renal corpuscle, a proximal tubule with convoluted and straight portions, a thin segment, and a distal tubule that also has straight and convoluted parts. Those segments of the nephron between the proximal and distal convoluted tubules (i.e., the straight descending part of the proximal tubule, the thin segment, and the straight ascending portion of the distal tubule) are collectively referred to as the loop of Henle (Andersen, 2017). The renal corpuscle and the proximal and distal convoluted tubules occur only in the cortex, whereas Henle's loop is generally confined to the medulla or to a medullary ray. The size of the nephrons and the length of their various segments vary according to the position of the parent renal corpuscle in the cortex. Renal corpuscles near the medulla are larger and the tubules are longer than are those of nephrons whose renal corpuscles are located in the periphery of the cortex. Nephrons from the subcapsular region have small renal corpuscles and their thin segments of the loop of Henle extend for a short distance into the medulla. Nephrons whose renal corpuscles occupy an intermediate position in the cortex show intermediate features.

8.1.1.4. Renal Corpuscle

A renal corpuscle is roughly spherical and measures 150 to 250 μm in diameter. It consists of a capillary tuft, the glomerulus, which projects into a blind expansion of the uriniferous tubule called the glomerular capsule (Bowman's capsule). The outer layer of the capsule surrounds the glomerulus as the parietal layer, which then reflects onto the glomerulus, where it is intimately applied to the glomerular capillaries to form a complete epithelial covering called the visceral layer of the glomerular capsule. The parietal layer is also known as the capsular epithelium, while the visceral layer is frequently referred to as the glomerular epithelium. The visceral and parietal layers of the capsule are separated by a narrow capsular space (Andersen, 2017) (Figures 8.2 and 8.3).

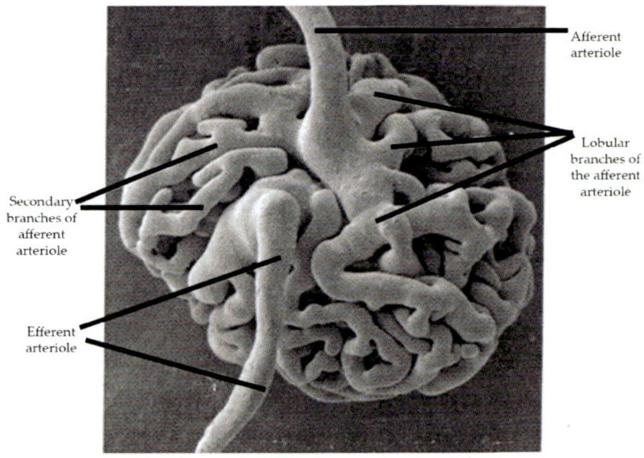

Figure 8.2. *A scanning electron micrograph of a cast made of a renal glomerulus.*

Source: Photomicrograph courtesy of T. Murakami, Okayama University.

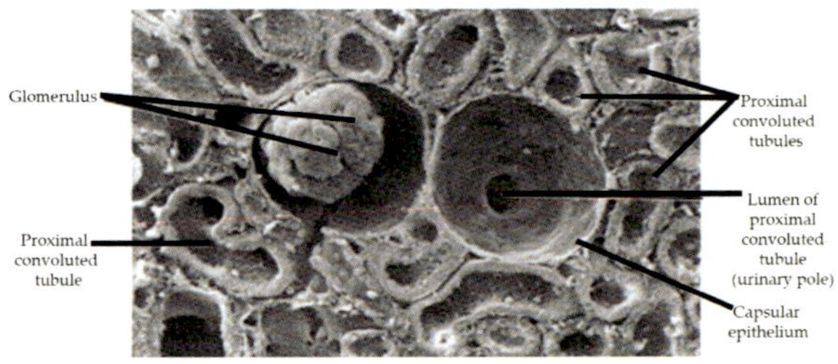

Figure 8.3. *A scanning electron micrograph of a fractured region of renal cortex illustrating the components of a renal corpuscle as well as several proximal convoluted tubules.*

Source: Photomicrograph courtesy of P. Andrews, Georgetown University.

The vascular pole is that area of the renal corpuscle at which the afferent and efferent arterioles enter and leave. As the afferent arteriole enters the renal corpuscle, it immediately divides into several primary branches, each forming a complex of capillaries (a capillary lobule) that then reunite to form the efferent arteriole. Each glomerulus is made up of several such capillary lobules. On the side opposite the vascular pole, the capsular space becomes continuous with the lumen of the proximal convoluted tubule; this region is known as the urinary pole. The parietal layer of the glomerular capsule consists of a single layer of tightly adherent squamous cells that contain few organelles. Near the urinary pole, there is an abrupt transition from this simple squamous form to the large pyramidal cells that line the proximal convoluted tubule. At the vascular pole, the simple squamous capsular epithelium changes to a specialized cell type called the podocyte that forms the glomerular epithelium. Podocytes are large, stellate cells whose bodies lie some distance from the underlying capillaries, separated from them by several cytoplasmic extensions called the primary processes. These processes wrap around the glomerular capillaries and give rise to numerous secondary foot processes (pedicles) that interdigitate with similar processes from adjacent podocytes to completely invest the capillary loops of the glomerulus (Baerwald et al., 2003). The plasmalemma of the foot processes exhibits a prominent glycocalyx rich in a sialoglycoprotein called podocalyxin. The narrow clefts between the interdigitating processes form the slit pores (filtration slits), which are about 25 nm wide. The gaps may be bridged by a thin slit membrane (diaphragm) (**Figure 8.4**).

The foot processes of the podocytes and the endothelial cells of the glomerular capillaries share a continuous common basal lamina that measures 0.1 to 0.5 μm thick. Ultra-structurally, the basal lamina consists of a central electron-dense lamina Densa, a lamina rara externa adjacent to the podocyte foot processes, and a lamina rara interna adjacent to the glomerular endothelium.

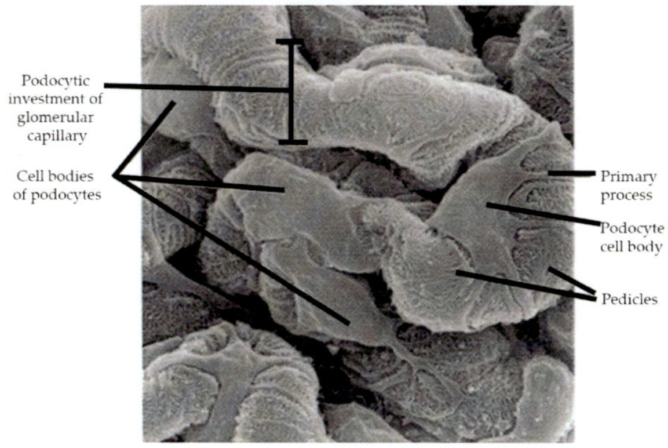

Figure 8.4. *A scanning electron micrograph of podocytes comprising the glomerular epithelium which form a complete investment around the glomerular capillaries.*

Source: Photomicrograph courtesy of P. Andrews, Georgetown University.

The lamina Densa consists of type IV collagen, laminin, and heparan sulfate proteoglycan. The lamina rara externa and interna consist primarily of fibronectin, which is thought to firmly attach epithelial and endothelial cells to the lamina Densa. Both cell populations are essential to establish the common basal lamina and, thereafter, continue to contribute to its production and maintenance.

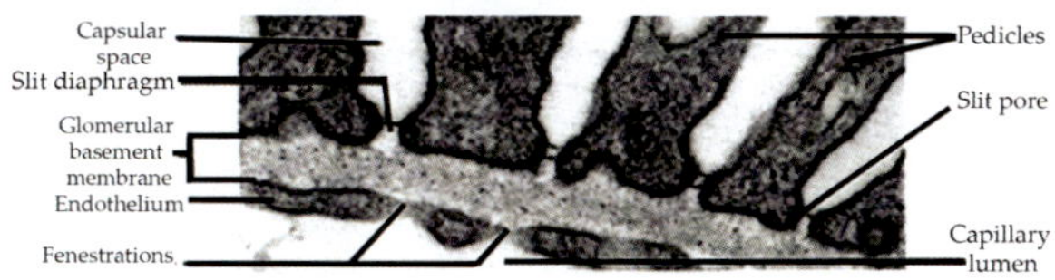

Figure 8.5. *A transmission electron micrograph illustrating the details of the renal filtration barrier.*

Source: *Photomicrograph courtesy of P. Andrews, Georgetown University.*

The glomerular capillaries are lined by a fenestrated glomerular endothelium. The attenuated squamous cells show numerous large pores (fenestrae) that measure 50 to 100 nm in diameter (Figures 8.5 and 8.6).

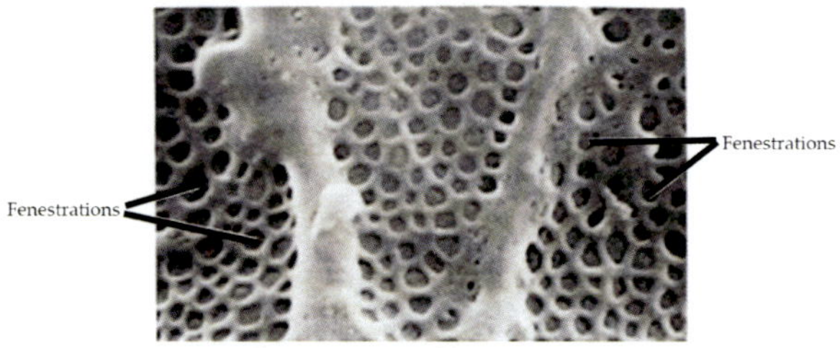

Figure 8.6. *A scanning electron micrograph of a portion of a fenestrated glomerular endothelial cell viewed from the capillary lumen.*

Source: Photomicrograph courtesy of P. Andrews, Georgetown University.

The renal corpuscle also shows stellate cells with long cytoplasmic processes that contain numerous filaments. These are mesangial cells, which occupy the area between the afferent and efferent arterioles at the vascular pole, where they lie in a matrix of amorphous material. These cells constitute the extraglomerular mesangium (Lacis cells) and are continuous with cells of similar appearance, the intraglomerular mesangial cells that lie between the glomerular endothelium and the basal lamina. The latter cells are thought to clear away large protein molecules that become lodged on the common basal lamina during filtration of blood plasma (Baerwald et al., 2003). Mesangial cells may participate in the removal of older portions of the basal lamina from the endothelial side as it is added to by the podocytes. Mesangial cells are contractile and respond to angiotensin II and other vasoconstrictors. They also have receptors for the atriopeptides. The contractile activity of the mesangial cells is thought to mediate blood flow through the glomerular capillaries. Mesangial cells are of clinical importance in some kidney diseases because they tend to proliferate. The renal corpuscle is the filter of the nephron. The fenestrated glomerular endothelium, the common basal lamina, and the foot processes of the glomerular epithelium form the filtration barrier of the renal corpuscle. This barrier permits passage of water, ions, and small molecules from the capillaries into the capsular space, but larger structures such as the formed elements of the blood and large, irregular molecules are retained. The capillary endothelial cells prevent the passage of formed elements; the common basal lamina restricts the passage of molecules with a molecular weight greater than 70,000. Substances of small molecular weight (40,000 or less) cross the basal lamina and pass through the filtration slits of the surrounding glomerular epithelium to enter the capsular space. Material that collects in the capsular space is not urine but a filtrate of blood plasma. Although materials with molecular weights larger than 45,000 or that have highly irregular shapes may pass through the endothelium and common basal lamina, they are unable to traverse the barrier provided by the foot processes of the podocytes. The filtration barrier limits the passage of materials not only on the basis of size and shape but also with respect to their charge. Anionic molecules are more restricted in their passage through the filtration barrier than are neutral molecules of similar size.

Heparan sulfate is a negatively charged (polyanionic) molecule of the glomerular basal lamina. The sialoprotein (podocalyxin) coats the podocyte foot processes and together with heparan sulfate gives the filtration barrier a net negative charge. The negatively charged glomerular basement membrane prevents or restricts the filtration of molecules such as albumin and other highly negatively charged molecules. Thus, the glomerular epithelium and the common basal lamina are important in limiting the materials that pass from the blood into the capsular space. The energy for the filtration process is supplied by the hydrostatic pressure of the blood in the glomerular capillaries. The pressure (about 70 mm Hg) provides sufficient force to overcome the colloidal osmotic pressure of substances in the blood (approximately 33 mm Hg) and the capsular pressure of the filtration membrane (about 20 mm Hg). The resulting filtration pressure (approximately 18 mm Hg) is great enough to force filtrable materials through all three layers of the filtration barrier and into the capsular space. The hydrostatic pressure exerted within the glomerular capillaries results from the unusual vascular arrangement of the glomerulus. Most vascular areas of the body are supplied by arterioles that form capillaries that then reunite into venules; but the glomerular capillaries are interposed between an afferent arteriole that conducts blood to the glomerulus and an efferent arteriole that conducts blood away from the glomerulus. This arrangement results in considerable pressure on the capillary walls and can be regulated by contraction of either arteriole. As more filtrate from the blood enters the capsular space, the rise in pressure forces the filtrate into the lumen of the proximal convoluted tubule. The capsular epithelium forms a tight seal around each renal corpuscle, preventing leakage of filtrate into the cortical tissue.

8.1.1.5. Proximal Tubule

The proximal tubule begins at the urinary pole of the renal corpuscle and is the largest segment of the human nephron. It is about 17 mm long and makes up most of the cortex. The proximal tubule is divided into a convoluted portion (pars convoluta) and a straight portion (pars recta). The convoluted portion is the longer of the two parts and is the one most frequently seen in sections of the cortex. After a tortuous course through the cortex in the region of its parent renal corpuscle, the proximal tubule takes a more direct route through the cortex to become the straight portion of the proximal tubule. It then enters the medulla or a medullary ray, where it turns toward a renal papilla as the first part of the loop of Henle (Baerwald et al., 2012).

The proximal convoluted tubule consists of a single layer of large, pyramidal cells with a well-developed microvillus (brush) border. The basolateral surfaces of these cells form an intricate system of interdigitating processes and ridges that often extend beneath neighboring cells to interdigitate with similar processes of adjacent cells. Tight junctions fuse the apices of the adjacent cells around the tubular lumen and clearly delineate apical and basolateral cell membrane domains. The resulting separation of transmembrane (transporter) proteins is vital to the function of proximal tubular cells. Thus, a complex labyrinth of cell membranes extends from the basal region of the epithelium to near the luminal surface between individual epithelial cells. Compartmentalization of the lateral and basal regions results in a greater surface area of cell membrane, which facilitates the transport of ions and other solutes. In typical tissue sections, profiles of proximal convoluted tubules are the most common structures seen in the cortex and usually show a stellate lumen bounded by a distinct brush border. Each cell of the proximal tubule has a large spherical nucleus, but in histologic sections, not all cells show a nucleus because of the large size of the cells. The cells contain a supranuclear Golgi complex and numerous rod-shaped mitochondria parallel to the long axis of the cell, closely associated with the lateral ridges and processes of the basolateral plasmalemma. The cytoplasm usually is darkly staining and granular. Structurally, the convoluted and straight parts of the proximal tubule are similar. Still, the cells of the straight portion are shorter, and the brush border and basolateral infoldings are less well-defined than in the convoluted part. Mitochondria are abundant but are smaller and more randomly scattered. One of the main functions of the proximal tubule is the absorption of the glomerular filtrate. The brush border, which consists of closely packed, elongated microvilli, increases the surface area available for absorption by about 30-fold. The microvilli are embedded in a coat of extracellular glycoprotein (glycocalyx). The apical surfaces of these cells absorb sugars and amino acids from the luminal contents in a manner similar to that of intestinal epithelial cells. Normally, all glucose in the glomerular filtrate is absorbed in the proximal convoluted tubule. If blood glucose levels exceed the absorptive capacity of the enzymes that control glucose absorption, the excess spills into the urine (glucosuria). Protein is absorbed in the proximal tubule by a system of invaginations called apical canaliculi that give rise to a series of small vesicles containing protein sequestered from the lumen. The tubular invaginations, the vesicles, and the vacuoles together make up the endocytic complex, which is actively involved in protein absorption. The vesicles coalesce to form large vacuoles that condense and fuse with lysosomes whose acid hydrolases reduce the protein to amino acids released back into the bloodstream. Over 65% of the sodium chloride and water of the glomerular filtrate is absorbed in the proximal tubule. Sodium ion is actively transported from the lumen, and chloride ion and water follow passively with no expenditure of energy by the cell to maintain the osmotic balance. Water passes through specialized protein channels called aquaporins. In the proximal tubule these are aquaporin-I channels which are not influenced by the presence of antidiuretic hormone (ADH). Aquaporin-I channels also are found in the descending thin limb of the loop of Henle. A key factor in proximal tubular cell reabsorption is a Na^+, K^+-ATPase enzyme pump located within the basolateral cell membranes that limit the complex intercellular space. The reabsorption of most substances, including water, is linked to the function of this Na^+, K^+-ATPase system. Glucose, amino acids, lactate, and phosphate are coupled to sodium entry across the apical plasmalemma of the cell by specific symporter (cotransport) and antiporter (countertransport) transmembrane proteins. Sodium is then moved out of the cell and into the intercellular space by the Na^+, K^+-ATPase mechanism, and glucose, amino acids, phosphate, and lactate follow by passive mechanisms. Glucose, amino acids, and lactate are usually completely removed from the tubular fluid in the first half of the proximal tubule by this mechanism. About 80% of the filtered bicarbonate is reabsorbed in the proximal tubule utilizing a Na^+/H^+- antiporter. Hydrogen ion is secreted into the lumen in exchange for bicarbonate ions. The remainder of the proximal tubule is involved primarily in the reabsorption of sodium chloride. Chloride ion concentration is high in this region because most bicarbonate, glucose, and organic anions have been preferentially reabsorbed proximally, resulting in an enriched chloride ion solution in the distal half of the proximal tubule. Here, sodium is reabsorbed with chloride by parallel Na^+-H^+ and Cl^--base- antiporter transmembrane proteins within the apical plasmalemma that also is dependent on the Na^+/K^+-ATPase enzyme system of the basolateral membranes. Sodium and chloride ions in this portion of the proximal convoluted tubule are also reabsorbed following a paracellular route between neighboring epithelial cells. Other inorganic ions (50% of potassium, 65% of ionized calcium, 15% of magnesium, 85% phosphate), urea, uric acid, and water-soluble vitamins (vitamin C and vitamin B complexes) also are absorbed by the proximal convoluted tubule. In addition to absorption, the proximal tubule secretes organic cations (creatine, dopamine, acetylcholine, and epinephrine) and anions (bile salts, fatty acids, urate, and para-aminohippurate) that are destined to be eliminated in the urine (Baerwald et al., 2012).

Hence, this region of the nephron serves as an exocrine gland. The proximal tubule is a major site of ammonia production in the nephron as component cells metabolize glutamine. Parathyroid hormone decreases phosphate resorption in the proximal convoluted tubule. Angiotensin II stimulates the sodium-hydrogen antiporter, which increases hydrogen ion secretion and, in addition, promotes sodium, chloride, and water reabsorption.

8.1.1.6. Thin Segment

The simple cuboidal epithelium of the straight descending part of the proximal tubule (the initial segment of the loop of Henle) changes abruptly in the thin segment to an attenuated simple squamous epithelium. The luminal diameter of the nephron also decreases markedly, from 65 μm in the descending proximal tubule to about 20 μm in the thin segment. The thin segment, largely confined to the medulla, forms the thin limb of the loop of Henle. The nuclei of the lining epithelial cells are centrally placed and cause this area of the cell to bulge into the lumen of the tubule. At the luminal surface, the brush border of the proximal tubule is replaced by short, scattered microvilli. Ultrastructurally, the cytoplasm shows fewer organelles; the lateral cell membranes have elaborate folds that interdigitate with those of adjacent cells. The cells are united at their apices by typical junctional complexes. The lateral interdigitations are less well-developed near the hairpin loops. The cells rest on a relatively smooth basal lamina of moderate thickness. The length of the thin segment varies with each nephron and depends on the position of the parent renal corpuscle in the cortex. Thin segments are short or even absent from nephrons whose renal corpuscle is located near the capsule and are longest when the renal corpuscle is situated near the medulla. In these nephrons, the thin segments may extend almost to the tip of a renal papilla (Baerwald et al., 2012).

8.1.1.7. Distal Tubule

The distal tubule is divided into a straight part (pars recta), a portion that contains the macula densa (pars maculata), and a convoluted portion (pars convoluta). The straight portion of the distal tubule begins as a gradual transition from the thin segment of the nephron. The epithelium becomes cuboidal, and while a few microvilli are present, the cells lack the brush border and apical canaliculi of the proximal tubule. Interdigitating processes are present along the basolateral surfaces of the cells, and these contain numerous mitochondria. The straight part of the distal tubule constitutes the thick ascending limb of the loop of Henle and completes the looping course of this structure as it ascends through the medulla. It then re-enters the cortex to return to the parent renal corpuscle. The thick ascending limb reabsorbs about 25% of the filtered load. Reabsorption of sodium, chloride, and potassium at this location is driven by a Na^+-K^+-2Cl- symporter located in the apical plasmalemma. Sodium chloride reabsorption by cells of the thick ascending limb relies on the Na^+/K^+-ATPase enzyme system confined to the basolateral cell membrane as well as a kidney-specific basolateral cell membrane chloride channel. Thus, the movement of sodium across the apical cell membrane and into the cell is controlled by the transmembrane protein (symporter) that couples the movement of sodium, chloride, and potassium ions. A specific ROMK channel (an inwardly- rectifying renal potassium channel) also located within the luminal plasmalemma of cells forming the thick ascending limb recycles potassium ion back into the tubular fluid. This is necessary to permit sustained Na^+-K^+-2Cl- cotransport activity in cells forming the thick ascending limb of the loop of Henle. A positive membrane potential (luminal voltage) is generated and maintained by the Na^+-K^+-2Cl- cotransporter and the ROMK channel. This established positive transepithelial voltage plays an important role in the paracellular movement of cations (Na^+, K^+, Ca^{++}, Mg^{++}) from the lumen of this region of the nephron. About 15% of the remaining bicarbonate is reabsorbed at this location, which is 25% of ionized calcium, 15% of sodium, 30% of potassium, and about 70% of magnesium from the remaining filtrate. As it reaches the renal corpuscle, the distal tubule establishes a close relationship with the afferent arteriole, and where it contacts the arteriole, the tubule contains a group of specialized cells that form the macula Densa (dense spot). This segment of the distal tube is called the pars maculata. The cells are taller and narrower than those in adjacent areas so that their nuclei are closer together, more prominent and lie just beneath the apical cell membrane. Cells of the macula Densa are polarized toward the basal surface, that is, the Golgi membranes, and occasional granules are found basal to the nucleus, facing the basal cell membrane. The macula Densa is related to a modified region of the afferent arteriole that contains the juxtaglomerular cells and is considered to represent an endocrine portion of the kidney. This feature and the polarization of the cell suggest that the macula Densa monitors the luminal fluid in the distal tubule. Cells of the macula Densa also are known to produce the enzyme nitric oxide synthase. The nitric oxide released by the macula Densa is thought to control the vascular tone of the afferent and/or efferent arterioles, thereby influencing kidney function. The macula Densa marks the division between the ascending and convoluted portion of the distal tubule. The convoluted portion runs a tortuous course in the cortex near the renal corpuscle of its origin. The distal convoluted tubule is shorter than the proximal convoluted tubule, so fewer sections of the distal tubule are seen in histologic preparations. The lumen of the distal tubule is generally wider than that of the proximal tubules; the cells are shorter and have lighter staining and nuclear profiles are usually seen in each cell, partly because many are binucleate. A brush border is lacking. Electron micrographs show deep, elaborate infoldings of the basolateral cell membrane associated with numerous elongated mitochondria that lie parallel to the long axis of the cell, producing the prominent basal striations of light microscopy. The cells of the distal tubules show a few luminal microvilli. The distal tubule is the site for further absorption of sodium chloride utilizing an apical thiazide-sensitive sodium-chloride transporter. This transporter is driven by low intracellular sodium and chloride concentrations created by Na^+/K^+ ATPase and a basolateral cell membrane chloride channel protein. Between 5 and 10% of the remaining filtered magnesium also is absorbed in the distal convoluted tubule utilizing a luminal magnesium channel and a basolateral cell membrane sodium-magnesium exchanger (Baker, 1965). Aldosterone acts on sodium channels to stimulate sodium reabsorption and on potassium channels in cells of the distal tubule to stimulate potassium secretion. About 90% of the bicarbonate in the glomerular filtrate has already been absorbed in the proximal tubule and loop of Henle. The distal tubule also is the site where ammonia is converted to ammonium ions. Thus, this segment of the nephron plays an important role in maintaining the acid-base balance of the body. Parathyroid hormone stimulates calcium ion reabsorption in cells forming the initial portion of the distal tubule. The last portion of the distal tubule can become permeable to water under the influence of antidiuretic hormone (ADH).

8.1.1.8. Loop of Henle

The loop of Henle is interposed between the proximal and distal convoluted tubules and consists of the straight portion of the proximal tubule, the thin segment, and the straight portion of the distal tubule. The loops descend in the medulla for variable distances, form hairpin loops, and then ascend through the medulla, parallel to the descending limb, to the cortex. The loop of Henle is essential for the production of hypertonic urine and is important in the conservation of body water. The loop consists of parallel limbs with tubular fluid flowing in opposite directions that act as a countercurrent multiplier system to aid in the concentration of urine. The descending thin segment is highly permeable to water but much less so to sodium and chloride ions and urea. In contrast, the ascending thin segment is impermeable to water but permeable to sodium chloride, which diffuses out of the tubule and contributes to the high osmolarity of the surrounding interstitium of the inner medulla passively. Some ions diffuse back into the lumen of the adjacent descending limb. Cells comprising the thick ascending limb (straight portion of the distal tubule) of the loop of Henle also are impermeable to water but actively transport sodium and chloride ions out of the tubule. Such activity results in a dilute tubular fluid and contributes to an increasing hyperosmotic interstitium. Urea follows a route similar to that of these ions and makes a significant contribution to the hyperosmolarity of the interstitium. Thus, sodium and chloride ions, as well as urea, are trapped in the interstitial substance of the medulla, resulting in an increase in the osmotic concentration around the tubules in the medulla. All three passively diffuse into the descending limb but either diffuse or are actively pumped out again by the ascending limb as the cycle repeats itself. Thus, the sodium chloride-urea trap establishes an osmotic gradient that increases strength toward the renal papillae. This gradient is important for the conservation of water and formation of hypertonic urine by the terminal portion of the distal tubule and the collecting ducts (Baker, 1965).

8.1.1.9. Collecting Ducts

The collecting ducts can be subdivided according to their location in the kidney. The initial segment is found in the cortex and includes short connecting portions that unite the distal tubules of cortical nephrons to collecting ducts and arched portions formed by the confluence of several connecting portions from juxtamedullary nephrons. The arched portions originate deep in the cortex, ascending through before arching to descend within a medullary ray. Medullary collecting ducts occur primarily in the medulla. As the ducts pass through the medulla, they converge to form larger, straight collecting ducts called papillary ducts, which end at the tip of a renal papilla. The numerous openings of the papillary ducts give a sieve-like appearance to the external surface of the papillae; this area has been called the area cribrosa. The external surfaces of the papillae are covered by transitional epithelium. The lining epithelium of the collecting ducts consists of principal and intercalated cells. Similar- appearing cells also are found in the last segment of the distal tubule. The principal (light) cells are generally cuboidal, with centrally placed, round nuclei and lightly staining cytoplasm with characteristic, distinct cell boundaries. Ultra structurally, the light cells show scattered, short microvilli on their apical surfaces, scattered mitochondria, and some infolding of the basal plasmalemma. They also possess a single, centrally located cilium (**Figure 8.7**).

Principal cells reabsorb sodium and water and secrete potassium ions. The activity of this cell type is dramatically influenced by antidiuretic hormone (ADH) in fluid/volume homeostasis. In the absence of ADH the apical plasmalemma is impermeable to water and urea. In contrast, the basolateral plasmalemma is freely permeable to both. An ADH receptor (an integral membrane glycoprotein), a stimulatory G-protein and a membrane-bound adenylate cyclase are present within the basolateral plasmalemma. In the presence of ADH, cytoplasmic vesicles containing aquaporin-2 channels for water and vesicles containing channels for urea are inserted into the luminal plasmalemma of these cells making the collecting tubule permeable to both water and urea. Thus, urea reabsorbed proximally in the proximal tubule or entering the descending limb of the thin segment can be recycled into the renal interstitium from the collecting tubule by this mechanism. The intercalated (dark) cells are scattered between the light cells, which have more mitochondria, stain more deeply, and show a large number of vesicles in the apical cytoplasm (Craig et al., 2007).

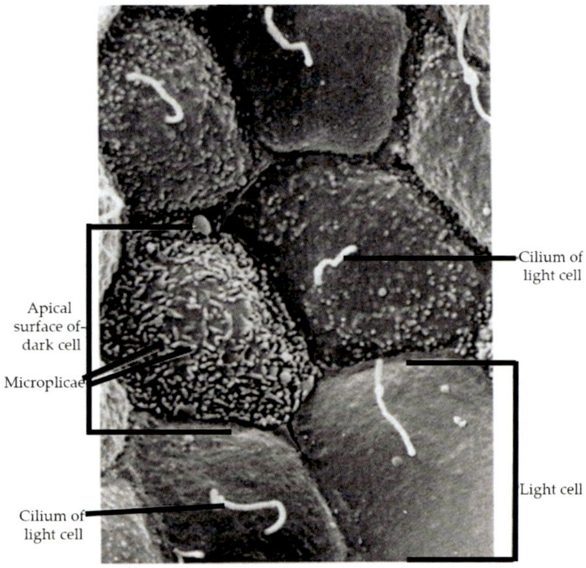

Figure 8.7. *A scanning electron micrograph of a portion of a human collecting tubule as viewed from the lumen demonstrating the surface features of light (principal) and dark (intercalated) cells.*

Source: Photomicrograph courtesy of P. Andrews, Georgetown University.

These cells lack central cilia; however, the apical plasmalemma exhibits microplicae. Some intercalated cells (α cells) secrete hydrogen ions in exchange for potassium ions using an H^+/K^+-ATPase located in the apical plasmalemma. For each hydrogen ion secreted into the tubular lumen, a bicarbonate ion is released from the basolateral cell membrane using a Cl^-/HCO_3^- antiporter. Thus, intercalated cells secrete H+ and reabsorb HCO_3^- and K^+ and, therefore, play an important role in regulating acid-base balance.

A small population of intercalated cells (β cells) have been observed that function opposite the α form and secrete potassium ions. As the collecting tubules pass through the medulla, the cells become tall columnar in the papillary ducts. The mechanism of ammonia excretion is complex and follows a circuitous route to be excreted indirectly. Glutamine is metabolized to ammonia (NH_3) and α-ketoglutarate by cells forming the proximal convoluted tubule. Intracellularly, NH_3 is converted to ammonium (NH_4^+), which is then transported into the tubular lumen via the Na^+-H^+ exchanger, with NH_4^+ substituting for H^+. As the luminal fluid reaches the thick ascending limb, much of the NH_4^+ is reabsorbed by the Na^+- K^+-$2Cl^-$ cotransporter in which case NH_4^+ is substituted for K^+. Within the surrounding medullary interstitium NH_4^+ and NH_3 contribute to the osmotic gradient maintained by high concentrations of sodium, chloride, and urea. The collecting duct, which passes back through the interstitium, contains α-intercalated cells that contain two hydrogen transporters (H^+-ATPase and H^+-K^+- ATPase) located in the luminal plasmalemma. As hydrogen ion is secreted into the tubular fluid, the lipid soluble NH_3 passes through cells of the collecting duct to enter the tubular fluid. Here, the NH_3 combines with secreted hydrogen ion to form the water-soluble NH_4^+ thereby effectively "trapping" the hydrogen ion for excretion in the urine. The amount of ammonia (hydrogen ion) secreted depends largely on the acid/base status of the extracellular fluids. The collecting ducts function to conserve water and produce hypertonic urine. As the ducts traverse the medulla to the tips of the pyramids, they pass through the increasingly hypertonic environment established by the loop of Henle. ADH controls the permeability of the collecting ducts to water. In the presence of ADH, water is drawn from the collecting ducts by osmosis because of the hypertonic environment maintained in the medullary interstitium. The loss of water from the tubular contents results in concentrated, hypertonic urine. If ADH is lacking due to injury or disease, the kidney is unable to concentrate urine, and copious amounts of dilute urine are produced, resulting in severe dehydration. This condition is known as diabetes insipidus (Craig et al., 2007).

The renal interstitium fills the spaces between the tubular elements of the kidney. The cortical interstitium is relatively scant except around blood vessels and consists of fine bundles of collagen, fibroblasts, and scattered phagocytes. The medullary interstitium is more plentiful, and its cells lie parallel to the long axis of the tubules. These interstitial cells possess long, branching processes that encircle adjacent tubules and blood vessels. Pleomorphic interstitial cells filled with small lipid droplets also occur in the medullary interstitium at regular intervals between the epithelial tubules and vessels. The cells are suspected to be endocrine cells and may secrete an antihypertension factor. The medullary interstitium contains an abundant intercellular ground substance and small groups of collagen fibers.

8.1.1.10. Juxtaglomerular Apparatus

The juxtaglomerular apparatus consists of the macula Densa of the distal tubule, the extraglomerular mesangium, and the juxtaglomerular cells in the wall of the afferent arteriole. The extraglomerular mesangium forms a loose mass of cells between the afferent and efferent arterioles. Component (Lacis) cells may contain granules, but their precise role in the function of the juxtaglomerular apparatus is unclear. The juxtaglomerular (JG) cells appear to be highly modified smooth muscle cells in the wall of the afferent arteriole as they enter the renal corpuscle. The cells contain a number of secretory granules, well-developed Golgi complexes, and abundant granular endoplasmic reticulum. The JG cells produce renin (a proteolytic enzyme), which, when released into blood, converts a plasma protein angiotensinogen (a α2-globulin from the liver) to angiotensin I. A converting enzyme in the blood (derived from endothelial cells lining capillaries of the lung) converts angiotensin I to the polypeptide angiotensin II, which acts on the zona glomerulosa of the adrenal cortex, and stimulates the release of aldosterone. Aldosterone secretion increases sodium ion absorption from the fluid within the terminal portion of the distal tubule and the cortical collecting ducts to the blood and increases movement of potassium ion from the blood to the tubular fluid. Angiotensin II also is a potent vasoconstrictor and elevates blood pressure. Within the kidney, it acts as a vasoconstrictor of the afferent and efferent arterioles and causes the contraction of mesangial cells. In addition, the juxtaglomerular apparatus has been implicated in the production of erythropoietin, an agent that stimulates erythropoiesis in the bone marrow. The location of the macula Densa, its basal polarization, and its orientation toward adjacent JG cells suggest that the three groups of cells may interact. The macular Densa may "sense" the ion (Na^+, K^+, Cl^-) concentration in the distal tubule and thereby influence the activity of JG cells. The tubuloglomerular feedback mechanism proposed suggests a concentration-dependent uptake of Na^+, K^+, and Cl- by a Na^+-K^+-$2Cl^-$ cotransporter located in the apical plasmalemma of macula Densa cells. This activity results in the generation of adenosine that activates an adenosine A1 receptor in the plasmalemma of extraglomerular mesangial cells. The activation of this receptor triggers an increase in cytoplasmic calcium, the resulting action potential of which is transmitted to the afferent arteriole by gap junctions resulting in vasoconstriction and inhibition of renin secretion (de Castro et al., 2016). Local angiotensin II, prostaglandins, and nitric oxide modulate this activity. The juxtaglomerular cells also act as baroreceptors and can function independently in the release of renin. Stimulation of renal sympathetic nerves results in the release of norepinephrine which also causes renin release.

8.1.1.11. Vascular Supply

The vascular pattern of the kidneys is complex and shows regional specializations related to the organization and function of the various parts of the nephron. About 20% of the cardiac output goes to the kidneys. The renal arteries arise from the abdominal aorta, and before reaching the renal sinus usually divide into branches that pass anterior and posterior to the renal pelvis to enter the renal sinus. Here, they give rise to segmental arteries, which also divide to form interlobar arteries that run between renal lobes. At the corticomedullary junction, these arteries divide into several arcuate arteries that arch across the base of each medullary pyramid and give off interlobular arteries that pass into the cortex between lobules. The interlobular arteries run peripherally in the cortex, giving rise to a system of intralobular arteries that enter renal lobules and provide afferent arterioles, which supply the glomeruli of renal corpuscles. As the efferent arteriole leaves the renal corpuscle of a cortical nephron, it immediately breaks into a peritubular capillary network that supplies the convoluted tubules. The main circulation of the renal cortex is unique in that the arterioles give rise to two distinct, sequential capillary beds: the glomerular and peritubular capillaries. Efferent arterioles from juxtamedullary nephrons, on the other hand, form several long, straight vessels, the vasa recta, that descend into the medullary pyramid and form hairpin loops. Like the loop of Henle, the loops of the vasa recta are staggered throughout the medulla. The walls of the vasa recta are thin, and the endothelium of the ascending (venous) limb is fenestrated. The vasa recta passes in close proximity to the loop of Henle, permitting passive interchange between the two elements. The vasa recta form a vascular countercurrent exchange system that removes excess water and ions. The medullary osmotic gradient is not disrupted due to the slower flow rate and the smaller volume (about 8% of the total renal blood flow) in the vasa recta and because the vasa recta also forms hairpin loops in which the blood flows down the descending side of the loop and then back up the ascending side of the loop. In addition to making the collecting tubules more permeable to water, the presence of ADH results in vasoconstriction of the vessels forming the vasa recta thereby reducing the flow rate even further and protecting the established interstitial osmotic gradient from being disrupted.

The venous drainage of the kidney is similar to and follows the same course as the arterial supply. However, there is no venous equivalent of the glomerulus or the afferent and efferent arterioles. The venous system of the medulla begins in the ascending limb of the vasa recta, which drains into interlobular or arcuate veins. In the peripheral cortex, capillaries unite to form small veins that assume a star-like pattern (stellate veins) as they drain into interlobular veins. The renal veins drain into the inferior vena cava. The left renal vein differs in that it is much longer and receives venous drainage from the left gonad.

8.1.2. Extrarenal Passages

The extrarenal passages consist of the minor and major calyces, renal pelvis, ureter, urinary bladder, and urethra. They convey urine to the outside of the body or store it temporarily in the case of the bladder. Except for the urethra, all have a similar basic structure with a mucosa, muscularis, and adventitia. The layers are thinnest in the minor calyces and increase in depth distally to reach their maximum development in the bladder.

8.1.2.1. Calyces, Renal Pelvis, Ureters, and Bladder

The thickness of the wall of the extrarenal passages gradually increases from the upper to lower parts; except for this, all parts of the extrarenal passages show a similar histologic structure. The lumen is lined by a mucosa consisting of transitional epithelium that rests on a lamina propria. There is no submucosa, and the lamina propria blends with the connective tissue of the well-developed muscular coat. Transitional epithelium covers the external surfaces of the renal papillae and reflects onto the internal surfaces of the surrounding minor calyces (de Castro et al., 2016). It also is continuous with the epithelium of the papillary ducts, thus providing a complete epithelial lining that prevents the escape of urine into the neighboring tissues. Transitional epithelium forms a barrier to the diffusion of salts and water into and out of the urine. In the major and minor calyces, the epithelium is two to three cells thick, increasing in the ureter to four or five layers and to six, eight, or more layers in the bladder.

The surface cells are large and rounded and in the relaxed bladder, have convex or dome-shaped borders that bulge into the lumen. The superficial cells sometimes contain large polyploid nuclei. The epithelium of the distended organ shows considerable changes in morphology. In the filled bladder, or as urine is propelled down the ureter, the epithelium is stretched and flattened and temporarily assumes the appearance of a thin stratified squamous epithelium. When the intraluminal pressure is relieved, the epithelium again assumes its nondistended appearance. In the relaxed bladder, the apical cytoplasm of the superficial cells contains fine filaments and fusiform vesicles limited by a membrane of the same thickness as the cell membrane. These vesicles are thought to represent reserve surface membranes for use during distension. Transitional epithelium lies on a very thin basement membrane that is usually not seen with a light microscope. The epithelium lies on a lamina propria that consists of a compact layer of fibroelastic connective tissue. Some diffuse lymphatic tissue also may be present. The muscularis of the urinary passageways consists of bundles of smooth muscle separated by abundant fibroconnective tissue and begins in the minor calyces as two thin layers of smooth muscle. The inner, longitudinal layer begins at the attachment of the minor calyces to the renal papillae; the outer circular layer of muscle spirals around the renal papilla forming a thin coat.

The walls of the minor calyces contract periodically around the renal papillae and aid in moving urine from the papillary ducts to the calyces and into the renal pelvis. The muscularis of the renal pelvis and upper two-thirds of the ureter consist of the same two layers and differ only in thickness. An additional outer, longitudinal layer of smooth muscle appears in the lower one-third of the ureter. The distal ends of the ureters, the intramural portions, pass obliquely through the bladder wall to empty into its lumen. The inner circular layer of smooth muscle disappears, and the contractions of the longitudinal layers help dilate the lumen of the distal ureter so that urine can enter the bladder. Peristaltic waves periodically pass along the ureter to convey urine to the bladder, emptying it in small spurts. As the bladder fills, the pressure of its contents keeps the intramural portions of the ureters closed due to their oblique course in the bladder wall.

The ureters open only when urine is forced through them. Reflux of urine into the ureters also is prevented by a valvelike flap of bladder mucosa that lies over the ureteral openings. The muscularis of the urinary bladder is moderately thick and consists of inner longitudinal, middle circular, and outer longitudinal layers of smooth muscle. The middle layer is the most prominent and spirals around each ureteral opening. Around the internal urethral orifice, the muscle increases in thickness to form the internal sphincter of the urethra. A coat of fibroelastic connective tissue, the adventitia, surrounds the muscularis and attaches the extrarenal passages to surrounding structures. In the renal pelvis, it blends with the kidney capsule. On the superior surface of the bladder, the fibroelastic coat is covered by the peritoneum. The adventitia contains numerous blood vessels, lymphatics, and nerves. Blood vessels pierce the muscularis, provide it with capillaries, and then form a plexus of small vessels in the lamina propria. A rich capillary layer lies immediately beneath the epithelium. Nerve fibers and small ganglia also occur in the adventitia and represent the sympathetic and parasympathetic divisions of the autonomic nervous system. Parasympathetic fibers are important for the control of micturition.

8.1.2.2. Male Urethra

In men, the urethra conveys urine from the bladder to the exterior and serves for the passage of seminal fluid during ejaculation. The male urethra is 18 to 20 cm long and has three segments. The first segment is 3 to 4 cm long and lies within the prostate, an accessory sex gland. This part forms the prostatic urethra (pars prostatica) and is lined by transitional epithelium similar to the bladder. The membranous urethra (pars membranacea) is very short (1.5 cm) and extends from the apex of the prostate to the root of the penis. The membranous urethra pierces the skeletal muscle of the urogenital diaphragm immediately before it enters the penis. The skeletal muscle surrounding this part of the urethra forms the external sphincter (sphincter urethrae) of the urethra and is under voluntary control during micturition. The third and longest segment, about 15 cm, is the penile urethra (pars cavernosa), which runs longitudinally through the corpus cavernosa urethrae to end at the tip of the glans penis. The membranous and penile parts of the urethra are lined by stratified or pseudostratified columnar epithelium. Stratified squamous epithelium often occurs in patches of the penile portion and also lines a distal enlargement, the fossa navicularis. The mucous membrane of the urethra shows small depressions or invaginations called the lacunae of Morgagni, which are continuous with the branched tubular glands of Littré. The epithelium lining these glands is the same as that found in the intraepithelial nests of clear, mucus-secreting cells within the urethral epithelium. The lamina propria beneath the urethral epithelium is a highly vascular, loose connective tissue rich in elastic fibers (Edson et al., 2009). The mucosa is bounded by inner longitudinal and outer circular layers of smooth muscle.

8.1.2.3. Female Urethra

The female urethra is shorter than the male (3 to 5 cm long) and is lined by stratified squamous epithelium, although patches of stratified or pseudostratified columnar may be found. Glands of Littré are present throughout its length. As in the male, the lamina propria is a vascular, fibroelastic connective tissue that contains numerous venous sinuses. The surrounding muscularis comprises an inner longitudinal layer of smooth muscle bundles and an outer circular layer. The female urethra is surrounded by the skeletal muscle of the urogenital diaphragm that forms the external urethral sphincter near its orifice.

8.1.3. Organogenesis

The urinary and reproductive systems arise in common from the mesoderm of the urogenital ridge. A nonfunctional pronephros, a mesonephros functional in the fetus, and a metanephros (the definitive kidney) arise successively from each caudal to the last with some overlapping. A functional pronephros occurs only in chordates such as Amphioxus and myxinoid fishes. Except for the lack of loops in Henle, pronephric and mesonephric nephrons resemble those of the metanephros. Although the nephron and collecting tubules form continuous structures in the definitive kidney, each has a separate origin, unlike other exocrine glands in which secretory and ductal units arise from the same primordium. Mesonephroi are drained by mesonephric ducts that regress in the female but in the male are incorporated into the reproductive tract. By a series of subdivisions, an outgrowth of the mesonephric duct, the uteric bud, gives rise to ureters, renal pelvis, major and minor calyces, papillary ducts, and collecting tubules. The ureteric bud extends into the metanephric blastema, a mass of mesoderm that gives rise to nephrons. The looser, more external layer of mesoderm forms the interstitial tissue and capsule of the kidney (Edson et al., 2009).

Proliferation of mesoderm in the subcapsular nephrogenic zone results in solid ovoid masses in which the mesenchymal cells that lie adjacent to collecting tubules form double-layered caps. The rest of the cell mass forms a primitive renal vesicle between a main collecting tubule and one of its branches. Cells of the renal vesicle and collecting tubule do not make contact. Each renal vesicle gives rise to a nephron unit. The single cell-layered vesicle lengthens and two indentations appear, transforming it into an S- shaped tubule. The space between the middle and distal limbs of the S fills with mesodermal cells and a capillary. Together, the vessel and the distal limb of the tubule evolve into a renal corpuscle. The capillaries lie immediately adjacent to the concave, external surface of the lower limb. As they expand into the tubule, they acquire an epithelial covering and form the glomerular capillaries. The parietal layer of the capsule, which originates from cells on the opposite side of the tubule, constricts around the point of entry of the capillary loops and establishes the vascular pole. Where the tubule surrounds the developing capillaries, the columnar cells and endothelial cells share a basal lamina. The provisional glomerular epithelial cells show numerous desmosomes and zonula adherens-like structures that maintain contact between the epithelial cells as the capillary loops expand. The attachments occur mainly along the central, lateral regions of the cell, rather than at their apices, thus maintaining cell-to-cell union as the glomerular epithelium changes from simple cuboidal to a layer of podocytes. The attachments are transitory and are lost as the podocytes differentiate. With development, podocytes become cuboidal and extend fingerlike processes from their basal surfaces toward adjacent cells. The cells begin to separate from one another, and their foot processes increase in size and mingle with others to cover the expanding capillaries. The opposite end of the S-shaped tubules unites with nearby collecting tubules, and the lumina becomes continuous. The tubules elongate, become U-shaped, and give rise to proximal and distal tubules and loops of Henle. The latter are the last segments to form and are not numerous until late in development. Initially, the development of the kidney is concerned with the formation of nephrons; this is followed by a period of growth and differentiation of established nephrons. In humans, nephronogenesis is complete by the thirty-fifth week. Renin-immunoreactive cells appear in the mesonephros by the sixth week of gestation and in the metanephros by the eighth week, suggesting that the renin-angiotensin system may be active even during early fetal life.

Early in development, the digestive and urogenital systems open into a common space, the cloaca. Later, a wedge of mesenchyme, the urorectal septum, divides the cloaca into a dorsal rectum and a ventral bladder, and a urogenital sinus. The endodermal lining of the newly formed bladder becomes stratified and the surrounding mesenchyme differentiates into the muscular wall of the bladder.

8.2. Male Reproductive System

The male reproductive system comprises the gonads (testes), their excretory ducts, the accessory sex glands, and the external genitalia. The testes produce male germ cells or gametes (sperm), conveyed to the exterior through an excretory duct system. The accessory sex glands contribute secretions that, along with the sperm, constitute semen.

8.2.1. Testes

The testes are compound tubular glands within a scrotal sac, suspended from the body by a spermatic cord. The testes are dual organs that act as exocrine glands producing a holocrine secretion, the sperm, and as endocrine organs that secrete the male sex hormone, testosterone. Each normal adult testis weighs between 12–15 gm and the right testis is commonly slightly larger and heavier than the left testis. Each testis is covered anteriorly and laterally by a simple squamous epithelium (mesothelium) called the visceral layer of tunica vaginalis. On the posterior aspect of the testis, this mesothelium reflects onto the scrotal sac and lines its interior as the parietal layer of the tunica vaginalis. The serous cavity between visceral and parietal layers allows the testes to move freely and reduces the chance of injury from increased pressure on the exterior of the scrotum. A thick, fibrous capsule, the tunica albuginea, lies beneath the visceral layer of tunica vaginalis, separated from it only by a basal lamina. Tunica albuginea is a dense fibroelastic connective tissue containing scattered smooth muscle cells. The muscle cells are concentrated in the posterior region, where the tunica albuginea thickens and projects into the testis to form the mediastinum testis. Connective tissue partitions, the septula testis, extend from the mediastinum into the interior of the testis and subdivide it into approximately 250 pyramid-shaped compartments called lobuli testis. The apices of the compartments are directed toward the mediastinum, and each lobule contains one to four convoluted seminiferous tubules that represent the exocrine portion of the testis. Their product is whole cells (spermatozoa). The inner region of the tunica albuginea, the tunica vasculosa, consists of loose connective tissue and contains numerous small blood vessels that supply the testis. The connective tissue extends into each lobule and fills the spaces between the seminiferous tubules, forming the interstitial tissue of the testis (Elvin et al., 2000). The interstitial tissue is rich in extracellular fluid and contains abundant small blood and lymphatic vessels that form a plexus around the seminiferous tubules. In addition to fibroblasts, the interstitial tissue contains macrophages, mast cells, mesenchymal cells, and large polyhedral cells 15 to 20 μm in diameter. These are the interstitial cells (of Leydig), which commonly occur in groups and make up the endocrine portion of the testis. They secrete the male steroid hormone testosterone. Interstitial cells usually contain single, large, spherical nuclei, but binucleate cells are not uncommon. Leydig cells are characterized by numerous LH receptors. In electron micrographs, the cytoplasm shows abundant smooth endoplasmic reticulum, well-developed Golgi complexes, and numerous mitochondria containing tubular rather than lamellar cristae. Morphologically, interstitial cells are characterized by large cytoplasmic crystals called the crystals of Reinke. These proteinaceous bodies are highly variable in shape and size but are readily seen with the light microscope. In electron micrographs they show a highly ordered structure. The crystals appear in the interstitial cells of most postpubertal individuals and vary considerably in number. Their significance is unknown. Most of the enzymes involved in testosterone synthesis are located in the smooth endoplasmic reticulum and mitochondria of interstitial cells. Only about 1 to 2% of circulating testosterone is in free form with the remainder being bound to a sex steroid-binding globulin or albumin produced by the liver. Testosterone and its metabolites are essential for the proliferation and differentiation of excretory ducts and male accessory sex glands and for maintaining these structures in a functional state. Metabolites of testosterone include two potent androgens. Dihydrotestosterone (DHT) is produced by the activity of the enzyme 5 α-reductase and 5 α-androstenediol due to the activity of the enzyme 3 α-reductase. Testosterone and its derivatives influence other tissues and are responsible for beard growth, low pitch of the voice, muscular build, and male distribution of body hair. Production of testosterone by the interstitial cells is controlled by a gonadotropic hormone called interstitial cell-stimulating hormone (ICSH) or LH, secreted by cells (gonadotrophs) located within the anterior pituitary.

8.2.2. Seminiferous Tubules

Each testicular lobule contains one to four highly convoluted seminiferous tubules that measure 150 to 250 μm in diameter and 30 to 70 mm long. Added together, the seminiferous tubules have a tubular length that exceeds 500 m. Each seminiferous tubule is organized into a non-branched closed loop, both ends of which open into the first portion of the excurrent duct system, the rete testis. A seminiferous tubule consists of a complex stratified germinal (seminiferous) epithelium surrounded by a layer of peritubular tissue. The peritubular tissue is separated from the germinal epithelium by a basal lamina and consists of collagenous fibers and flattened cells that, depending on the species, may contain numerous actin filaments. These are the myoid (peritubular) cells. In humans, the myoid cells are considered to be only moderately contractile. The production of testicular fluid by the germinal epithelium and its flow through the seminiferous tubules moves the spermatozoa into the excretory duct system. The germinal epithelium of the adult is unique among epithelia in that it consists of a fixed, stable population of supporting (Sertoli) cells and a proliferating population of differentiating spermatogenic cells. Developing germ cells slowly migrate upward along the lateral surfaces of the supporting cells to be released at the free surface into the lumen of the seminiferous tubule (Elvin et al., 2000).

8.2.2.1. Sertoli Cells

The Sertoli cell is a tall columnar cell that spans the germinal epithelium from the basal lamina to the luminal surface. The cell has an elaborate shape with numerous lateral processes with recesses or concavities surrounding differentiating spermatogenic cells. The apical portion of the cells also envelops developing germ cells and releases them into the lumen of the seminiferous tubule. The expanded portion of the cell contains an irregularly shaped nucleus distinguished by a large, prominent nucleolus that is readily seen with the light microscope. The basal cytoplasm contains abundant smooth endoplasmic reticulum, and a large, well-developed Golgi complex occupies the supranuclear region. The cytoplasm contains many lipid droplets, lysosomes, thin elongated mitochondria, scattered profiles of granular endoplasmic reticulum, and a sheath of fine filaments that envelops the nucleus and separates it from the organelles. Microtubules are present also, and their numbers depend on the state of activity of the cell. Human Sertoli cells feature membrane-bound inclusions called the crystalloids of Charcot- Böttcher; their function is unknown. Sertoli cells further characterized by FSH receptors. Tight junctions occur between adjacent Sertoli cells near their bases and subdivide the germinal epithelium into basal and adluminal compartments, each of which has a separate, distinct population of spermatogenic cells. The basal compartment extends from the basal lamina of the germinal epithelium to the tight junctions; the adluminal compartment lies between the tight junctions and the lumen of the tubule. The tight junctions between the Sertoli cells appear to form, at least in part, a blood-testis barrier (**Figure 8.8**).

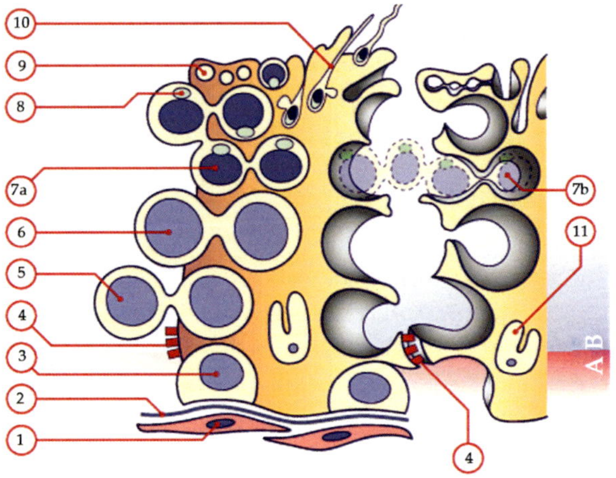

Figure 8.8. *A diagrammatic sketch of the germinal epithelium.*

Note: (1). Peritubular cells, (2). Basal membrane, (3). Spermatogonia, (4). Tight junction, (5). Spermatocyte I, (6). Spermatocyte II, (7a). Spermatids, (7b). Spermatids, (8). Acrosome, (9). Residual bodies, (10). Spermatozoas, (11). Cell nucleus of sustentacular cells (Sertoli) A Basal zone, B Adluminal zone.

Source: https://embryology.ch/en/media/multuse/u1l_sertoli.gif.

Germ cells in the basal compartment are contained within an environment that has access to substances in the blood plasma. In contrast, the germ cells in the adluminal compartment reside in a specialized milieu that is maintained and controlled by the Sertoli cells. A number of plasma proteins are present in the basal compartment that are not found in the luminal contents of the seminiferous tubule that is, however, rich in other amino acids and ions. Sertoli cells are thought to provide all the nutrients for the avascular germinal epithelium. In addition to secreting testicular fluid, Sertoli cells release androgen-binding protein, whose synthesis is stimulated by a pituitary gonadotropin, follicle-stimulating hormone (FSH). The androgen-binding protein binds testosterone, thus providing the adluminal compartment with the level of hormone needed for the normal differentiation and development of germ cells. The blood-testis barrier helps to confine the high concentration of testosterone to the adluminal compartment, thus allowing a different environment to be established in the basal compartment. Many of the developing germ cells in the adluminal compartment are haploid and might be regarded as foreign material by the body if released into surrounding tissues. The tight junctions between Sertoli cells are thought to prevent haploid germ cells from contacting general body tissues and thus prevent an autoimmune response to the individual's germ cells. Although tight junctions contribute to the blood-testis barrier, other factors may be involved. Sertoli cells phagocytize degenerating germ cells and take up the residual cytoplasm that normally is shed during the release of mature germ cells into the lumen of the seminiferous tubule. In addition to providing mechanical and nutritional support for developing sperm, Sertoli cells also control the epithelium to the lumen and are important in the release of germ cells into the lumen. The microtubules and actin filaments in the cytoplasmic processes of the Sertoli cells provide these processes with the mobility they need to carry out their functions (Frett et al., 2020). The numerous gap junctions that occur between adjacent Sertoli cells facilitate communication between cells along specific segments of a seminiferous tubule during migration and release of germ cells. Sertoli cells also secrete a glycoprotein known as inhibin. Inhibin suppresses the secretion of FSH by gonadotrophs in the anterior pituitary and, via this feedback loop, acts to control the rate of spermatogenesis. Likewise, the concentration of testosterone in the blood plasma is maintained at a specific concentration by circulating levels of this hormone that influence the secretion of pituitary gonadotrophs and gonadotrophin-releasing hormone (GnRH) containing neurons located in the arcuate nucleus of the hypothalamus via a negative feedback loop mechanism.

8.2.2.2. Spermatogenic Cells

The spermatogenic cells of the germinal epithelium consist of spermatogonia, primary and secondary spermatocytes, and spermatids. These are not separate cell types but represent stages in a continuous process of differentiation called spermatogenesis. The term includes the entire sequence of events in the transformation of diploid spermatogonia at the base of the germinal epithelium into haploid spermatozoa that are released into the lumen of the seminiferous tubule. Spermatogonia lie in the basal compartment of the germinal epithelium, immediately adjacent to the basal lamina. The cells are 10 to 20 μm in diameter and round or ellipsoidal, and the nucleus of each cell contains the diploid number of chromosomes. Two types of spermatogonia can be differentiated. Type A spermatogonia replicates by mitosis and provides a reservoir of stem cells for the formation of future germ cells. spermatogonia give rise to intermediate forms that eventually produce type B spermatogonia, which are committed to producing primary spermatocytes. The two types of spermatogonia can be differentiated by their nuclei. Type A spermatogonia have spherical or elliptical nuclei with a fine chromatin distribution and one or two nucleoli near the nuclear envelope. Many nuclei of this cell type also exhibit a clear nuclear vacuole. The lighter-stained, spherical nuclei of type B spermatogonia contain variably sized clumps of chromatin, most of which are arranged along the nuclear envelope. Only a single, centrally placed nucleolus is found. Primary spermatocytes at first resemble type B spermatogonia, but as they migrate from the basal lamina of the germinal epithelium, they become larger and more spherical, and the nucleus enters the initial stages of division. Primary spermatocytes usually are found in the central zone of the germinal epithelium. How these large cells pass from the basal to the adluminal compartment is unknown (Gershon and Dekel, 2020). The primary spermatocyte undergoes the first meiotic division to produce secondary spermatocytes. The homologous chromosomes have separated and the number is reduced by half, but the cells contain the diploid amount of DNA. Secondary spermatocytes lie nearer the lumen than the primary forms and are about half their size. Unlike the extended division of primary spermatocytes, secondary spermatocytes divide quickly in the second meiotic division to produce spermatids, which contain the haploid number of chromosomes and the haploid amount of DNA. Because they divide so quickly after being formed, secondary spermatocytes rarely appear in the germinal epithelium. Spermatids are about half the size of secondary spermatocytes. Numerous spermatids in different stages of maturation border the lumen of the seminiferous tubule. Early spermatids appear as small spherical cells with round, darkly stained nuclei. Late spermatids appear as tailed spermatozoa within the recesses of the Sertoli cell. The cell divisions that take place during formation of male germ cells are unique in that not only is the genetic material reduced by half; the division of the cytoplasm is incomplete. Thus, the cells resulting from a single spermatogonium remain in cytoplasmic continuity throughout the different stages of differentiation. The continuity is eventually broken as the spermatids are released from the Sertoli cells.

8.2.2.3. Spermiogenesis

The process by which spermatids differentiate into slender, motile sperm is called spermiogenesis. Newly formed spermatids are round cells with central, spherical nuclei, prominent Golgi complexes, numerous mitochondria, and a pair of centrioles. Each of these components undergoes significant changes during spermiogenesis. At the onset of spermiogenesis, many small granules appear in the Golgi membranes and eventually coalesce to form a single structure called the acrosome. The developing acrosome is bounded by a membrane, the acrosomal vesicle, which also is derived from the Golgi complex and is closely associated with the outer layer of the nuclear envelope. The acrosomal vesicle expands and then collapses over the anterior half of the nucleus to form the head cap. The acrosome, which contains hydrolytic enzymes, remains within the acrosomal membrane. As these events occur, the two centrioles migrate near the nucleus on the side opposite of the forming acrosome. Nine peripheral doublets plus a central pair of microtubules develop from the distal centriole and begin to form the axoneme of the tail. The proximal centriole becomes closely associated with a caudal region of the nucleus called the implantation fossa. As the axoneme continues to develop, nine longitudinal coarse fibers extend around it and blend with nine short, segmented columns that form the connecting piece, which unites the nucleus (head) with the tail of the spermatozoon. The annulus, a ringlike structure, forms near the centrioles and migrates down the developing flagellum. Randomly distributed mitochondria migrate to the flagellum and become aligned in a tight helix between the centrioles and the annulus (Gougeon, 1986). This spirally arranged mitochondrial sheath characterizes the middle piece of the tail of a mature spermatozoon. Simultaneously, marked changes occur in the nucleus: it condenses, elongates, and is slightly flattened. Together with the acrosome, it forms the sperm head. The bulk of the cytoplasm now is associated with the middle piece of the evolving spermatid, and as differentiation nears completion, the excess cytoplasm is shed as the residual body, leaving only a thin layer of cytoplasm to cover the spermatozoon. The residual cytoplasm is phagocytized by Sertoli cells as the spermatozoa are released into the lumen of the seminiferous tubule. Although morphologically, the spermatozoa appear mature, they are nonmotile and largely incapable of fertilization at this time. In most species, spermatids at specific stages of differentiation always are associated with spermatocytes and spermatogonia, which are also at specific stages of development. A series of such associations occur along the length of the same seminiferous tubule, and the distance between two identical germ cell associations is called a "wave" of the seminiferous epithelium. Human germinal epithelium exhibits a mosaic of such areas, and six different cell associations have been described. Such associations represent a fundamental pattern of cycling of the germinal epithelium during sperm production. The time taken for spermatogonia to become spermatozoa is relatively constant and species-specific: in humans, it is about 64 days. If germ cells fail to develop at their normal rate, they degenerate and are phagocytosed by adjacent Sertoli cells.

8.2.3. Excretory Ducts

The excretory ducts consist of a complex system of tubules that link each testis to the urethra, through which the exocrine secretion, semen, is conducted to the exterior during ejaculation. The duct system consists of the tubuli recti (straight tubules), rete testis, ductus efferentes, ductus epididymis, ductus deferens, ejaculatory ducts, and prostatic, membranous, and penile urethra.

8.2.4. Accessory Sex Glands

Male accessory sex glands include the seminal

vesicles, prostate, and bulbourethral glands. The secretion from each of these glands is added to the testicular fluid and forms a substantial part of the semen.

8.2.4.1. Seminal Vesicles

The seminal vesicles are elongated, saclike structures that lie posterior to the prostate gland. The duct of each vesicle joins with the distal end of the ductus deferens to form an ejaculatory duct. The mucosa of the seminal vesicles is thrown into numerous complex primary folds that give rise to secondary and tertiary folds. These project into the lumen and subdivide the seminal vesicle into many small, irregular compartments that give the lumen a honeycombed appearance. All the compartments communicate with a central lumen, although the impression is one of individual chambers in histologic sections. The mucosal folds are lined mainly by pseudostratified columnar epithelium consisting of rounded basal cells interposed between cuboidal or columnar cells. Regions of simple columnar epithelium may also be present. The mucosal cells contain numerous granules, some lipid droplets, and lipochrome pigment, which first appear at sexual maturity and increase with age. The ultrastructural features indicate a cell that is active in protein synthesis. The cytoplasm contains abundant granular endoplasmic reticulum, a prominent supranuclear Golgi complex, and conspicuous, dense secretory granules in the apical cytoplasm. The epithelium rests on a thin lamina propria of loose connective tissue with many elastic fibers. A muscular coat is present and consists of an inner layer of circularly arranged smooth muscle cells and an outer layer in which the smooth muscle cells have a longitudinal orientation. Both layers of muscle are thinner than those of the ductus deferens. External to the muscle coat is a layer of loose connective tissue (adventitia) rich in elastic fibers. Secretions from the seminal vesicles form a substantial part (65–70%) of the total ejaculate. It is a yellowish, viscid secretion that contains fructose, prostaglandins, and factors that increase sperm motility. It also contains components that suppress the immune response in the female reproductive tract and factors that clot and then liquefy semen in the vagina. Fructose is a **source** of energy for sperm. In contrast, prostaglandins are thought to stimulate smooth muscle contractions within the walls of the tubular structures of the female reproductive tract to aid in moving sperm to the site of fertilization. In sections, the secretions appear as deeply stained, coagulated masses, often with a netlike structure. The seminal vesicles depend on testosterone, and the removal of the hormone, as by castration, results in their involution and loss of secretory function (Gougeon, 1979).

8.2.4.2. Prostate

The prostate is the largest of the accessory sex glands in men and surrounds the urethra at its origin from the bladder. It is a composite gland, made up of 35 to 60 small, compound tubuloalveolar glands from which 20 or more ducts drain independently into the prostatic urethra. These small glands appear to form strata around the urethra and consist of the periurethral mucosal glands, submucosal glands, and the main or principal prostatic glands, which lie peripherally and make up the bulk of the prostate. The prostate is contained within a vascular, fibroelastic capsule with many smooth muscle cells in its inner layers. Broad septa extend into the prostate from the capsule and become continuous with dense fibroelastic tissue that separates the individual glandular elements. The secretory units of the glands are irregular and vary greatly in size and shape. The glandular epithelium varies between glands and even within a single alveolus. It is usually simple or pseudostratified columnar but may be low cuboidal or squamous in some of the larger saccular cavities. The epithelium is limited by an indistinct basal lamina and rests on a layer of connective tissue that contains dense networks of elastic fibers and numerous capillaries. The cells contain abundant granular endoplasmic reticulum and many apical secretory granules. The lumina of secretory units may contain spherical bodies, the prostatic concretions, that are thought to result from condensation of secretory material. The concretions appear to increase with age and may become calcified. The connective tissue surrounding the individual glandular units contains numerous smooth muscle cells (a fibromuscular stroma), which aids in the rapid discharge of prostatic fluid at ejaculation. The prostatic secretion is a thin, milky fluid of pH 6.5 that is rich in zinc, citric acid, phosphatase, factors that enhance sperm motility, and proteolytic enzymes, one of which, fibrinolysin, is important in the liquefaction of semen. Prostatic secretion accounts for about one-third of the total semen volume. Like the seminal vesicles, the development and functional maintenance of the prostate is dependent on testosterone and its metabolites. Blood levels of prostate-specific antigen (PSA) produced by the prostate is an important factor in screening for prostatic cancer.

8.2.4.3. Bulbourethral Glands

The bulbourethral glands (of Cowper) are a pair of pea-sized structures located in the urogenital diaphragm, close to the bulb of the penis. They are compound tubuloalveolar glands whose long ducts drain into the proximal part of the penile urethra. Each gland is limited by a connective tissue capsule from which septa, containing elastic fibers and smooth and skeletal muscle cells, extend into the glands, dividing them into lobules. The ducts and secretory portions are irregular in shape and size, and at their terminations, the secretory parts may form cyst like enlargements. The glandular epithelium varies from simple cuboidal to simple columnar depending on the functional state, but in distended alveoli, the epithelium may be flattened. Active cells show a lightly stained cytoplasm filled with mucin granules that confine the nucleus to the base of the cell. Excretory ducts are lined by simple columnar epithelium that becomes pseudostratified near the urethra. In smaller ducts, the epithelium appears to be secretory. The surrounding connective tissue contains an incomplete layer of circularly arranged smooth muscle. Bulbourethral glands produce a clear, syrupy fluid rich in amino sugars and containing sialoprotein. The glands secrete in response to erotic stimulation, and the secretion serves as a lubricant for the penile urethra.

8.2.4.4. Semen

The final product formed by the exocrine secretions of the testes and accessory sex glands is a whitish fluid called seminal fluid or semen. The average ejaculate of men is about 3 mL of semen which, in addition to about 300 million sperm, contains degenerating cells exfoliated by the ductal system, occasional wandering cells from connective tissues, pigment granules, and prostatic concretions. Hyaline bodies of unknown origin, lipid granules, fat, and protein are also present. In normal individuals, about 60% of the spermatozoa exhibit normal motility and about 60% show normal cytologic morphology (Guilhot et al., 2022).

8.2.5. External Genitalia

In men, the two structures that make up the external genitalia are the scrotum and penis.

8.2.5.1. Scrotum

The scrotum is a pendulous, cutaneous pouch situated at the base of the penis and below the symphysis pubis. It is divided into two compartments, each of which houses a testis, an epididymis, and the lower part of the spermatic cord. The scrotum consists only of skin and a closely associated tunica dartos. The scrotal skin is thin, pigmented, and commonly thrown into folds. It contains many sweat glands, sebaceous glands that produce an odorous secretion, and some coarse hair, the follicles of which are visible through the thin skin. The tunica dartos underlies the skin and forms the septum that divides the scrotum into its two compartments. It is firmly attached to the skin and consists largely of smooth muscle cells and collagenous connective tissue. The appearance of the scrotum varies with the state of contraction of the smooth muscle. Under the influence of cold, exercise, or sexual stimulation, the muscle contracts, and the scrotum become short and wrinkled. The spermatic cord consists of several thin layers of connective tissue acquired from the anterior abdominal wall as the testes descend from the abdominal cavity into the scrotal sac during development. It contains the ductus deferens, nerve fibers, lymphatic channels, testicular artery, and a pampiniform plexus of testicular veins. As the testicular artery nears the testis, it becomes highly convoluted and is surrounded by the venous plexus. The proximity of the surrounding, cooler venous blood causes the arterial blood to lose heat and provides a thermoregulatory (counter-current heat exchange) mechanism for precooling incoming arterial blood. In this way, the temperature of the testes is maintained a few degrees (2–3°C) below body temperature, a condition necessary for sperm production. The temperature can be elevated by drawing the testes closer to the abdominal wall by contraction of the layer of striated muscle (cremaster muscle) that invests the spermatic cord. In humans, failure of the testes to descend (cryptorchidism) results in sterility.

8.2.5.2. Penis

The penile urethra is a common channel for conducting urine and seminal fluid to the exterior. It is contained within a cylinder of erectile tissue, the corpus cavernosum urethrae (corpus spongiosum), that lies ventral to a pair of similar erectile bodies called the corpora cavernosa penis. Together the three structures make up the bulk of the penis, the copulatory organ of the male. The corpora cavernosa penis begin as separate bodies along the rami of the pubis on either side and join at the pubic angle to form the shaft of the penis. They are united by a common connective tissue septum called the pectiniform septum, and each corpus is surrounded by a thick, primarily collagenous sheath, the tunica albuginea. Trabeculae of collagenous and elastic fibers with numerous smooth muscle cells extend into the corpora from the tunica albuginea and divide the central regions of the corpora cavernosa into numerous cavernous spaces, those near the center being the larger. These spaces are endothelial-lined vascular spaces and are continuous with the arteries supplying them and draining veins. The cavernous tissue of each corpus cavernosum penis communicates with the other through numerous slitlike openings in the pectiniform septum. The ventrally placed corpus cavernosum urethrae (corpus spongiosum) ends in an enlargement, the glans penis, which forms a cap over the ends of the corpora cavernosa penis. Structurally, corpus spongiosum is similar to the corpora cavernosa penis, but the tunica albuginea is thinner and contains more elastic fibers and smooth muscle cells, and the trabeculae are thinner and contain more elastic tissue. The three corpora are bound together by subcutaneous connective tissue that contains numerous smooth muscle cells but lacks fat.

The shaft of the penis is covered by a thin, mobile skin that shows a slight increase in pigmentation. Unlike that of the root, the skin of the distal shaft lacks hair but does contain scattered sweat glands. The hairless skin of the glans penis is fused to the underlying connective tissue and is nonmobile. Unusual sebaceous glands not associated with hair follicles occur in this region (Holt et al., 2005).

The glans penis is covered by a fold of skin called the prepuce or foreskin, the inner surface of which is moist and resembles a mucous membrane. Numerous free nerve endings are present in the epithelium of the glans penis, prepuce, and subepithelial connective tissue of the urethra and skin. Meissner's corpuscles are associated with the epidermis of the genitals, and Vater-Pacini corpuscles are present in the deeper layers of the dermis.

8.2.5.3. Arterial Supply

The principal arterial supply to the penis is from two arteries that lie dorsal to the corpora cavernosa penis and deep arteries that run within the erectile tissue of these structures. Branches from the dorsal arteries penetrate the tunica albuginea and enter the cavernous tissue, where the arteries branch and either form capillary plexuses or course distally in the cavernous tissue. These helicine arteries are highly convoluted in the flaccid penis and take a spiral course through the trabeculae of the cavernous tissue. The intima of most of these arteries, even before they enter the cavernous tissue, have long, ridgelike thickenings that project into and partially occlude the lumina. These intimal ridges are most frequent where vessels branch. They consist of loose connective tissue that contains many smooth muscle cells. Blood from the large central lacunae drains peripherally toward the smaller vascular spaces and finally into a plexus of veins at the periphery. The veins run along the interior of the tunica albuginea, pierce the limiting tunica, and drain into the deep dorsal vein of the penis.

The arterial blood supply to the corpus spongiosum is similar to that of the corpora cavernosa penis, except for the venous drainage. Beginning at the lacunae, the veins of the corpus spongiosum have large openings and immediately penetrate the tunica albuginea to drain to the exterior. The structure and arrangement of the blood vessels in the cavernous tissues provide the mechanism for erection. During erotic stimulation, the smooth muscle of the arterial and trabecular walls relaxes, and blood pressure overcomes the elastic resistance of the arteries. The helicine arteries dilate and straighten, and the vascular spaces of the cavernous tissues quickly fill with blood. The lacunae, especially near the center of the cavernous bodies, become engorged with blood, thus compressing the small peripheral spaces and veins against the non-yielding tunica albuginea, retarding the egress of blood; the erectile tissues of corpora cavernosa penis become enlarged and rigid. During the erection, the intracavernous blood pressure may reach 1,100 and 1,200 mmHg in some individuals which is about 10 times normal blood pressure (Jain and Wotring, 2016). Corpus spongiosum does not become as rigid as the corpora cavernosa penis because there is less compression of the venous drainage, and the tunica albuginea is thinner and more yielding. The lesser rigidity of corpus spongiosum allows the urethra to remain patent, which is essential for the passage of semen during ejaculation. After cessation of sexual activity, the smooth muscle in the arteries and cavernous tissue regains its tone. The intimal ridges once again partially occlude the lumina of the arteries, thus reducing the volume of incoming blood. Excess blood in the vascular spaces of the erectile tissue is forced out by the contraction of smooth muscle cells in the trabeculae and by the recoil of surrounding elastic tissue. Gradually, the normal route of blood flow through the penis is restored, and the penis returns to the flaccid condition. Sexual reflexes of men can be triggered by a variety of stimuli and involve intricate coordination of both somatic and autonomic nerve pathways. During arousal, tactile (cutaneous) stimuli are transmitted to the sacral region (S2-S4) of the spinal cord by afferent somatic fibers within the dorsal penile nerve, a branch of the pudendal nerve. Impulses of efferent parasympathetic fibers via the pelvic splanchnic nerves result in vasodilatation of arteries supplying the erectile tissues, causing an erection. Efferent sympathetic fibers stimulate smooth muscle contraction within the following portions of the male reproductive system: epididymis, ductus deferens, prostate, and seminal vesicles. These contractions are coordinated with rhythmic contractions of skeletal muscle (primarily the bulbospongiosus) associated with the exterior of the penis that forcefully expel the ejaculate from the penile urethrae at emission. The muscle cells of these skeletal muscles are innervated by efferent somatic fibers of the pudendal nerve.

8.2.5.4. Spermatozoa

Spermatozoa that lie free in the lumina of seminiferous tubules consist of a head containing the nucleus and a tail, which eventually gives motility to the free cell. The chromatin of the nucleus is very condensed and reduced in volume, providing the functionally mature sperm with greater mobility. The condensed form of chromatin also protects the genome while the spermatozoon is en route to fertilize the ovum. The acrosomal cap covers the anterior two-thirds of the nucleus and contains enzymes important for penetration of the ovum at fertilization. The size and shape of the nucleus vary tremendously in different species. The sperm tail is about 55 μm long and consists of a neck, middle piece, principal piece, and end piece. The structural details of the different segments are best seen with the electron microscope. The neck is the region where the head and tail unite. It contains the connecting piece that joins the nine outer dense fibers of the tail to the implantation fossa of the nucleus. The region of the connecting piece that joins the implantation fossa is expanded slightly to form the capitulum. The middle piece extends from the neck to the annulus and consists of the axoneme, the nine coarse fibers, and the helical sheath of mitochondria. The principal piece is the longest part of the tail and consists of the axoneme and the nine coarse fibers (2 + 9 + 9 arrangement) enclosed by a sheath of circumferential fibers. The circumferential fibers join two longitudinal thickenings (columns) of this sheath on opposite sides. The end piece is the shortest tail segment and consists only of the axoneme surrounded by the plasmalemma (Jennings and Baker, 2000) (Figure 8.9).

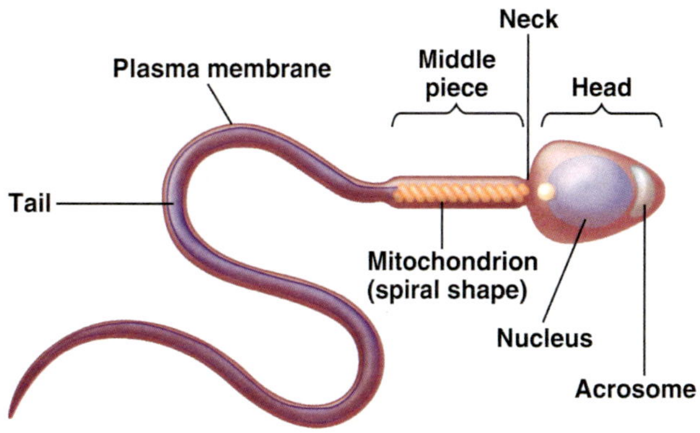

Figure 8.9. *A diagrammatic sketch illustrating the structure of a human spermatozoon.*

Source: https://www.biology.lifeeasy.org/?qa=blob&qa_blobid=3815661710730797871.

The last step in the physiologic maturation of spermatozoa takes place in the female reproductive tract and is called capacitation. This final activation occurs in the oviduct and is characterized by the removal of a glycoprotein coat and seminal proteins from the plasmalemma overlying the acrosome, by changes in the acrosomal cap, and by changes in the respiratory metabolism of the spermatozoa. Capacitation substantially increases the number of spermatozoa capable of fertilization, but the mechanism of this activation is not fully understood.

8.2.5.5. Tubuli Recti

Near the apex of each testicular lobule, the seminiferous tubules join to form short, straight tubules called the tubuli recti. The lining epithelium has no germ cells and consists only of Sertoli cells. This simple columnar epithelium lies on a thin basal lamina and is surrounded by loose connective tissue. The lumina of the tubuli recti is continuous with a network of anastomosing channels in the mediastinum, the rete testis.

8.2.5.6. Rete Testis

The rete testis is lined by simple cuboidal epithelium in which each cell component bears short microvilli and a single cilium on the apical surface. The epithelium lies on a delicate basal lamina. The channels of the rete testis are surrounded by a dense bed of vascular connective tissue (Koryak, 2014).

8.2.5.7. Ductuli Efferentes

In men, 10 to 15 ductuli efferentes emerge from the mediastinum on the posterosuperior surface of the testis and unite the channels of the rete testis with the ductus epididymis. The efferent ductules follow a convoluted course and, with their supporting tissue, make up the initial segment of the head of the epididymis. The luminal border of the efferent ductules shows a characteristic irregular contour due to the presence of alternating groups of tall and short columnar cells. Ciliated and nonciliated cells are present. Each contains the organelles normally associated with epithelia and supranuclear granules that are lysosomal in nature.

The nonciliated cells show numerous microvilli on their apical surfaces and are thought to absorb much of the testicular fluid in this part of the ductal system. Cilia on the other cell type beat toward the epididymis and help move the nonmotile sperm and testicular fluid in that direction. The epithelium lies on a basal lamina and is bounded by a layer of circularly arranged smooth muscle that thickens toward the duct of the epididymis. Cilia are not found beyond the ductuli efferentes, and the movement of sperm through the remainder of the duct system depends on the contractions of the muscular wall and fluid flow.

8.2.5.8. Ductus Epididymidis

The efferent ductules gradually unite to form a single ductus epididymidis that measures 5 to 7 m long. This highly coiled duct and its associated vascular connective tissue form the rest of the head, body, and tail of the epididymis. The epithelial lining is pseudostratified columnar and consists of principal and basal cells. Principal cells are the most numerous and are very tall (80 μm) in the proximal segment but gradually decrease in height distally to measure only 40 μm near the junction with the ductus deferens. Long, branched microvilli, inappropriately called stereocilia, extend from the apical surfaces of the principal cells. Like microvilli found elsewhere, they contain an axial bundle of actin microfilaments. The actin microfilaments extend from the stereocilia into the terminal web region of the principal cells. A very large Golgi complex takes up a supranuclear position in the cell, and an abundance of endoplasmic reticulum fills the basal region. Lysosomes, multivesicular bodies, and numerous coated vesicles also are present. One of the functions of the principal cell is absorption; together, the proximal portion of the ductus epididymidis and the ductuli efferentes absorb over 90% of the fluid produced by the seminiferous epithelium. Principal cells also phagocytose degenerate spermatozoa and residual bodies. Ubiquitin, a highly conserved protein molecule, is secreted by the principal cells of the epididymal epithelium. It forms covalently linked polyubiquitin chains on structures within the epididymal fluid, such as defective sperm and debris, during epididymal transit. These identified targets are recognized for endocytosis and removed from the epididymal fluid by the principal cells of the epididymal epithelium. The epithelium lining of the mid and distal regions of the ductus epididymis also secrete glycoproteins, sialic acid, and other factors that are believed to play a role in sperm maturation. Basal cells are small, round cells that lie on the basal lamina, interposed between the principal cells. They have a lightly staining cytoplasm with few organelles. Scattered intraepithelial lymphocytes often are present in the epithelium of the ductus epididymidis. The epididymal epithelium lies on a basal lamina and is surrounded by a thin lamina propria and a thin layer of circularly arranged smooth muscle cells. Near the ductus deferens, the muscle layer thickens and becomes three-layered (inner longitudinal, middle circular, outer longitudinal); it is continuous with the ductus deferens. The regional differences reflect differences in the mobility of the ductus epididymidis. Proximally, the duct shows spontaneous peristaltic contractions that slowly move spermatozoa through the epididymis; distally, the peristaltic contractions are reduced, and this region serves to store sperm. Spermatozoa become physiologically mature as they pass through the epididymis. Those entering the proximal part of the duct are mostly incapable of fertilization and swim in a weak, random fashion. Spermatozoa from the distal portion are capable of fertilizing ova and show strong, unidirectional motility. How the ductus epididymidis contributes to the maturation of spermatozoa is unknown. Transit time through the epididymis is about 3 weeks for humans.

8.2.5.9. Ductus Deferens

The ductus deferens unites the ductus epididymidis and the prostatic urethra. It is characterized by a wall consisting of a mucosa, a thick muscularis, and an adventitia. It is often referred to as the most muscular tube in the body. The mucosa is thrown into longitudinal folds that project into the lumen and is lined by a pseudostratified columnar epithelium resting on a thin basal lamina. The principal cells of the epithelium bear stereocilia on the luminal surface. The surrounding lamina propria is dense and contains numerous elastic fibers. The muscularis is the dominant feature of the ductus deferens and consists of three layers of smooth muscle cells arranged longitudinally in the inner and outer layers and circularly in the middle layer. The muscularis is surrounded by loose connective tissue (adventitia) that blends with neighboring structures and anchors the ductus deferens in place. Powerful contractions of the muscular wall propel sperm from the distal ductus epididymidis and rapidly transport them through the ductus deferens during ejaculation (Linossier et al., 2021). Near its termination, the ductus deferens dilates to form the ampulla. The lumen expands and the mucosa is folded, creating a labyrinth of pocket-like recesses. The lining epithelium is pseudostratified columnar. The muscular coat of the ampulla is thinner, and the layers are less distinct than those of other parts of the ductus deferens. Nearly all the smooth muscle in the muscularis of the ductus deferens is phasic smooth muscle characterized by distinct action potentials and rapid contraction. The autonomic nervous system innervates nearly every smooth muscle cell (multiunit innervation). This accounts for the rapid, forceful, pulse-like contractions of the ductus deferens during ejaculation.

8.2.5.10. Ejaculatory Duct

A short, narrow region of the ductus deferens extends beyond the ampulla and joins the duct of the seminal vesicle.

This combined duct forms the ejaculatory duct, which empties into the prostatic urethra. It is about 1 cm long and is lined by a pseudostratified or stratified columnar epithelium. The mucosa forms outpockets similar to, but not as well developed as, those in the ampulla. The remainder of the wall of the ejaculatory duct consists only of fibrous connective tissue.

8.2.5.11. Prostatic Urethra

The ejaculatory duct penetrates the prostate and

opens into the prostatic part of the urethra. The prostatic urethra is lined by a thin transitional epithelium and bears a dome-shaped elevation, the colliculus seminalis, on its posterior wall. A small blind diverticulum called the prostatic utricle lies on the summit of the colliculus and represents a remnant of the Müllerian duct in the male. The two ejaculatory ducts, one draining each testis, empty into the prostatic urethra on either side of the prostatic utricle. The numerous glands of the surrounding prostate also empty into this part of the urethra (Messinis, 2006).

8.2.6. Organogenesis

An indifferent gonad arises in the urogenital ridge, a thickened area of the mesoderm that contains the primordia for the kidneys and gonads. The proliferation of the peritoneal epithelium (mesothelium) on the ventromedial aspect of this ridge gives rise to a genital ridge, a longitudinal thickening several cells deep that runs parallel to the mesonephric ridge. The indifferent gonad consists of a superficial epithelium and an internal gonadal blastema made up of ill-defined cords of cells derived from the superficial epithelium. Male sexual development depends on the expression of a sex-determining region (SRY gene) of the Y-chromosome or a female phenotype will develop complete with ovary and oviduct. The SRY gene promotes the differentiation and development of the Sertoli and Leydig cells. In the XY genotypic male, the gonad rounds up, increases in size, and acquires a network of branching (testis) cords and a tunica albuginea, identifying it as a testis. With the appearance of the tunica albuginea, the germinal epithelium reverts to a typical peritoneal mesothelium and no longer plays a part in testicular development. Primordial germ cells migrate from the yolk sac during the fifth week of gestation and give rise to gonocytes, cells from the gonadal blastema form the testis cords. By the third month, fetal spermatogonia is present. The testis cords extend radially toward the mesorchium (gonadal mesentery) and a dense region that will become the rete testis. The two become continuous, and the testis cords elongate and differentiate into seminiferous tubules. Where they join the rete testis, the tubules remain straight and form the tubuli recti. The seminiferous tubules only contain only spermatogonia and Sertoli cells at this stage of development. During development, Sertoli cells elaborate Müllerian inhibitory factor (MIF), which inhibits further development of the paramesonephric (Müllerian) duct in the male fetus. The number of Sertoli cells remains constant from birth, but the spermatogonia increases markedly between about 10 years of age and puberty. The full sequence of spermatogenic cells from spermatogonia to spermatids does not appear until puberty. Thereafter, the single layer of columnar-shaped Sertoli cells prominent in the seminiferous tubules of the prepubertal testis is becomes hidden within the germinal epithelium due to the large number of spermatogenic cells. In old age, when the number of spermatogenic cells decreases, the Sertoli cell once again becomes a prominent feature of the seminiferous tubule.

The mesenchymal tissue in which the testis cords develop forms the septula testes, connective tissue of the mediastinum testis, and tunica albuginea. Cells within the mesenchymal stroma differentiate into interstitial cells (of Leydig). These are large and abundant from the 4th to the 6th months of development and produce large amounts of testosterone. They then regress after birth, only to increase again in number and size at puberty. Specific development of excurrent ducts does not occur in the male. As the mesonephric kidney degenerates and is resorbed, its ducts are incorporated into the male reproductive system and transformed into genital ducts. The cranial mesonephric tubules are modified and unite with tubules of the rete testis. These efferent ductules are continuous with mesonephric (Wolffian) ducts whose proximal region becomes highly convoluted to form the ductus epididymidis. Distally, the mesonephric duct remains straight, forming the ejaculatory duct and ductus deferens, which, near its distal end, dilates to form the ampulla. Just beyond the ampulla, the epithelium of the ductus deferens evaginates to provide the primordia for the seminal vesicles. Muscle coats are derived from the surrounding mesenchyme. The seminal vesicles attain the adult pattern by the seventh fetal month and slowly grow until puberty, after which the adult proportions are reached. Testosterone is essential in the normal development of the epididymis, ductus deferens, seminal vesicle and ejaculatory duct in the genotypic XY fetus. The prostate develops from multiple outgrowths of the urethral epithelium, above and below the entrance of the ejaculatory duct. Some 60 glands develop, organized into five groups that will become the lobes of the prostate. The mesenchyme into which the prostatic glands grow provides the fibromuscular stroma. The glands remain small until puberty, when, under the influence of testosterone, development is complete. The bulbourethral glands also arise as buds of ectodermal epithelium, but in the region of the urogenital sinus that forms the membranous urethra. The outgrowths evaginate through the investing mesenchyme to lie in the urogenital diaphragm. Mucous cells appear at about four months. The bulbourethral glands, which are also influenced by testosterone, grow throughout puberty. The urethral glands (of Littré) develop from outgrowths of the epithelium that lines the urethra. Early in the development of the external genitalia, the cloacal membrane becomes surrounded by mesenchyme and forms two folds that unite anteriorly to form the cloacal swelling. From the anterior part of the swelling, the genital (urethral) folds develop, while the posterior part forms the anal folds. The cloacal swelling increases in size, giving rise to a genital tubercle, at which time the genital swellings become visible just lateral to the genital fold. In males, the swellings are called scrotal swellings, which move caudally, fuse, and form the scrotum (Mishra and Luderer, 2019).

The genital tubercle elongates to form a phallus, pulling the genital fold forward as it does. The genital folds form the lateral walls of the urogenital groove, which extends along the caudal surface of the phallus. The genital folds close over, fuse, and form the penile urethra, the tip of which lacks an orifice. Ectodermal cells at the tip of the glans grow inwards as a solid cord that later canalizes to establish continuity with the remainder of the urethra. Corpora cavernosa penis and urethrae develop from paired and single columns of mesenchyme, respectively. The single column forms around the penile urethra within the shaft and also gives rise to the glans. The external genitalia develop slowly after birth, and then grow rapidly during puberty. Dihydrotestosterone is the primary mediator in growth of the prostate, penis, and scrotum. By the end of the second month of prenatal life, the differentiating testis lies on a common peritoneal fold called the urogenital fold which forms the gonadal ligaments. The cranial suspensory ligament develops between the testis and the dorsal abdominal wall near the 12th rib. The caudal ligament is known as the gubernaculum and links the developing testis to the scrotal swelling. In humans, the gubernaculum proper consists only of mesenchymal cells. Both are important in the descent of the testis. A period of transabdominal descent occurs due to rapid body growth and traction created by the gubernaculum. The testis descends beneath the peritoneum to reach the entrance of the presumptive inguinal canal by the third month of fetal life. Shortly before birth the testis completes its decent through the inguinal canal (trans-inguinal descent) and into the scrotum. A funnel-shaped outpocketing of the peritoneum called the processus vaginalis passes with the testis into the scrotal swelling along with other layers acquired from the abdominal wall. The processus vaginalis is obliterated with the exception of a small space that partially surrounds the testis. That region of the processus vaginalis that remains to line the scrotal cavity forms the parietal layer of the tunica vaginalis, that which is associated with the testis forms the visceral layer of the tunica vaginalis.

8.3. Female Reproductive System

The female reproductive system is composed of both internal and external structures. Internally, it includes the ovaries, oviducts (fallopian tubes), uterus, and vagina. Externally, it encompasses the external genitalia, which consists of the labia majora, labia minora, and clitoris. Additionally, the mammary glands, although not part of the reproductive organs, are important accessory structures.

During childhood, the reproductive organs of females remain immature, with growth mirroring that of the body overall. However, in the 2 to 3 years preceding the first menstrual period (menarche), these organs undergo significant changes, including an increase in size, breast enlargement, and the appearance of pubic and axillary hair.

After menarche, the female reproductive organs, including the ovaries, oviducts, uterus, vagina, and mammary glands, undergo cyclic changes in function and structure associated with the menstrual cycle and, later, pregnancy.

Menopause marks the end of the reproductive period, characterized by irregular menstrual cycles that eventually cease. In the postmenopausal period, the reproductive organs undergo atrophy (Mishra and Luderer, 2019).

8.3.1. Ovaries

The ovaries are paired oval bodies on each side of the uterus, suspended from the broad ligament by a mesentery, the mesovarium. The ovaries are homologous to the testes and are compound organs with exocrine and endocrine functions. The exocrine secretion consists of whole cells – the ova – thus the ovary can be classified as a holocrine or cytogenic gland. In cyclic fashion it secretes female sex hormones directly into the bloodstream and therefore is an endocrine gland.

8.3.1.1. Structure

Each ovary is covered by a mesothelium that is continuous with that of the mesovarium. As this membrane extends over the surface of the ovary, the squamous cells become cuboidal and form the surface epithelium of the ovary. Sections of the ovary show an outer cortex and an inner medulla, but the boundary between the two regions is indistinct. The stroma of the cortex consists of a compact feltwork of fine collagenous fibers and numerous fibroblasts. Elastic fibers are associated mainly with blood vessels and are rare in the cortex. Scattered throughout the cortical tissue are the ovarian follicles, whose size varies with their stage of development. Immediately beneath the surface epithelium, the connective tissue of the cortex is less cellular and more compact, forming a dense layer called the tunica albuginea. The stroma of the medulla consists of loose connective tissue that is less cellular than that of the cortex and contains many elastic fibers and smooth muscle cells. Numerous large, tortuous blood vessels, lymphatics, and nerves are also in the medulla.

8.3.2. Ovarian Follicles

The follicles are located in the cortex of the ovary, deep to tunica albuginea, and consist of an immature ovum surrounded by one or more layers of epithelial cells. At puberty, the human ovary contains 300,000 to 400,000 ova embedded in the cortical stroma, but only a few reach maturity and are ovulated. Approximately 300 to 400 ova are ovulated by a normal woman during her lifespan. During the menstrual cycle, several follicles (15–25) begin to grow and develop, but only one attains full maturity; the rest degenerate. The size of the follicle and the thickness of the epithelial envelope vary with the stage of development. During their growth, the follicles undergo a sequence of changes in which primordial, primary, secondary, and mature follicles can be distinguished.

8.3.2.1. Primordial Follicles

In the mature ovary, follicles are present in all stages of development. Most, especially in young women, are primordial or unilaminar follicles found in the peripheral cortex, just beneath the tunica albuginea. These follicles comprise an immature ovum surrounded by a single layer of flattened follicular cells resting on a basement membrane. At this stage, the ovum is a primary oocyte suspended in the diplotene stage of the meiotic prophase.

The primary oocyte is a large cell with a prominent vesicular nucleus and nucleolus. The Golgi apparatus is well developed, and spherical mitochondria tend to concentrate in the region of the centrosome. As the primordial follicle develops into a primary follicle, changes occur in the ovum, follicular cells, and adjacent connective tissue of the cortex.

8.3.2.2. Primary Follicles

During the growth of a primary follicle, the oocyte increases in size, and the Golgi complex, originally a single organelle next to the nucleus becomes a multiple structure scattered throughout the cytoplasm. Free ribosomes increase, mitochondria become dispersed, and granular endoplasmic reticulum, although not prominent, becomes more extensive. A few lipid droplets and lipochrome pigments appear in the cytoplasm, and yolk granules accumulate; these, however, are smaller and less numerous than in nonprimate species (Morgan et al., 2012). As the oocyte grows, a clear refractile membrane, the zona pellucida, develops between the oocyte and adjacent follicular cells. The zona pellucida consists of glycoproteins (ZP1, ZP2, ZP3) secreted primarily by the oocytes, although a lesser amount may be produced by surrounding granulosa cells. Microvilli extend from the oocyte into the zona pellucida. As the ovum grows, the flattened follicular cells of the primordial follicles become cuboidal or columnar and proliferate to form several layers. These cells are now referred to as granulosa cells, and the layer of stratified epithelium that they form is called stratum granulosum. Mitochondria, free ribosomes, and endoplasmic reticulum increase, and the Golgi element become prominent. Irregular, slender cytoplasmic processes extend from the granulosa cells and penetrate the zona pellucida to make contact with processes from the oocyte. The processes of the oocyte and granulosa cells are united by gap junctions. While these changes occur in the oocyte and follicular cells, the adjacent stroma becomes organized into a sheath or capsule, the theca folliculi, which surrounds the growing primary follicle. The theca folliculi is separated from the stratum granulosum by a distinct basement membrane. The cells differentiate into an inner secretory layer, the theca interna, and an outer fibrous layer, the theca externa, but the boundary between the layers is somewhat indistinct. The theca externa merges imperceptibly into the surrounding stroma. Many small blood vessels penetrate the theca externa to provide a rich vascular network to the theca interna. The stratum granulosum remains avascular until after ovulation. Follicle stimulating hormone (FSH) promotes the growth of a group of follicles, resulting in an increase in the production of estradiol and inhibin by the granulosa cells. As estradiol and inhibin levels rise, secretion of FSH is decreased. By the end of the first week of the cycle, falling FSH levels result in the selection of a dominant follicle, the one that is most sensitive to FSH. The dominant follicle continues to grow, produces large amounts of estradiol, and is destined to ovulate, while the others of the group are destined to become atretic. As estradiol levels increase, there is an increase in the amount of LH produced by gonadotrophs in the anterior pituitary that is not secreted.

8.3.2.3. Secondary Follicles

As the follicular cells proliferate, the growing follicle assumes an ovoid shape and gradually sinks deeper into the cortex. When the stratum granulosum has become 8 to 12 cell layers thick, fluid-filled spaces appear between the granulosa cells. The fluid, the liquor folliculi, increases in amount, and the spaces fuse to form a single cavity called the follicular antrum. Liquor folliculi contain several growth factors, steroids, gonadotrophic hormone, and other substances, many times their concentration in blood plasma. The follicle is now a secondary or antral follicle, and the oocyte has reached its full size and undergoes no further growth. The follicle, however, continues to increase in size, due in part to continued accumulation of liquor folliculi. The ovum is eccentrically placed in the follicle, surrounded by a mass of granulosa cells that projects into the fluid- filled antrum, forming the cumulus oophorus. The cells of the cumulus are continuous with those granulosa cells lining the antral cavity. Granulosa cells that immediately surround the oocyte form the corona radiata and are anchored to the zona pellucida by cytoplasmic processes (Morgan et al., 2012).

8.3.2.4. Mature Follicles and Ovulation

In women, a follicle requires 10 to 14 days to reach maturity. The dominant follicle continues to make more and more estradiol as the follicle continues to acquire an increase in the number of FSH and, later, LH receptors. In addition to estradiol, the growing follicle produces a small amount of progesterone. At maximum size, the follicle occupies the thickness of the cortex and bulges from the surface of the ovary. Fluid spaces appear between granulosa cells of the cumulus oophorus, and the connection between the ovum and stratum granulosum is weakened. The theca folliculi has attained its greatest development, and the theca interna assumes the cytologic characteristics of a steroid-secreting endocrine gland. Androstenedione and testosterone are important androgens secreted by the theca interna that serve as substrates for estrogen biosynthesis by the granulosa cells. The theca is thought to be influenced primarily by luteinizing hormone. An aromatase enzyme complex within the granulosa cells converts the substrates to estradiol, a form of estrogen. Estradiol then diffuses back across the limiting basement membrane of the stratum granulosum to enter the circulation via capillaries within the theca interna.

The oocyte completes the first meiotic division just before ovulation and gives off the first polar body. Thus, at ovulation a secondary oocyte is liberated. Rupture of the mature follicle and liberation of the ovum constitute ovulation, which normally occurs in the middle (day 14) of the menstrual cycle. Immediately before ovulation, further expansion of the follicle occurs due to increased secretion of liquor folliculi. Where the follicle bulges from the ovary, its wall becomes thinner, and a small, avascular, translucent area appears. This is the stigma or macula pellucida. The tunica albuginea thins out, and the surface epithelium of the ovary becomes discontinuous in this area. A collagenase produced by granulosa cells adjacent to the tunica albuginea appears responsible for the breakdown of collagen fibers at the site of the stigma. The stigma protrudes as a small blister and ruptures, and the ovum, with its surrounding zona pellucida and adherent corona radiata, is extruded along with follicular fluid. Ovarian contractility aids in ovulation. The released ovum measures about 120 μm in diameter.

8.3.2.5. Corpus Luteum

The maturing follicle that acquires LH receptors is one of the developing follicles that goes on to ovulate and is critical for subsequent corpus luteum formation after ovulation. Following ovulation, the follicle is transformed into a temporary endocrine structure, the corpus luteum, which elaborates estrogens, progesterone and inhibin. The walls of the follicle collapse, and the stratum granulosum is thrown inwards. Bleeding from capillaries in the theca interna may result in a blood clot in the center of the corpus luteum. At this time, it is sometimes referred to as a corpus hemorrhagicum. Granulosa cells increase greatly in size, take on a polyhedral shape, and transform into large, pale-staining granulosa lutein cells. Lipid accumulates in the cytoplasm of the cells, smooth endoplasmic reticulum becomes abundant, and mitochondria show tubular cristae. The theca interna cells also enlarge and become epithelioid in character to form theca lutein cells. The lutein cells derived from the theca interna are somewhat smaller than granulosa lutein cells. The process of formation of granulosa and theca lutein cells is called luteinization. With the depolymerization of the basement membrane between the theca interna and the granulosa cells, capillaries from the theca interna invade the lutein tissue to form a complex vascular network throughout the corpus luteum. Connective tissue from the theca interna also penetrates the mass of lutein cells and forms a delicate network around them. The fully formed corpus luteum secretes estrogens, inhibin, and progesterone; secretion of progesterone increases rapidly during luteinization, and high levels are maintained until the corpus luteum involutes. If the ovum is not fertilized, the corpus luteum persists for about 14 days and then undergoes involution. The cells decrease in size, accumulate much lipid, and degenerate. Hyaline material accumulates between the lutein cells and the corpus luteum and is gradually replaced by an irregular white scar of dense connective tissue, the corpus albicans (Navasiolava et al., 2011). Over the following months, the corpus albicans itself disappears. If fertilization occurs, the corpus luteum enlarges further and persists for about the first 6 months of pregnancy and then gradually declines. Following delivery, involution of the corpus luteum is accelerated, resulting in the formation of a corpus albicans. Estradiol, progesterone, and inhibin initially suppress FSH production by gonadotrophs in the anterior pituitary, but if pregnancy does not occur and the corpus luteum declines, FSH levels rise, and a new group of ovarian follicles is stimulated to develop and the cycle repeats.

8.3.2.6. Atresia of Follicles

During the early part of each menstrual cycle, several primordial follicles begin to grow, but usually only one attains full development and is ovulated. The remainder undergo a degenerative process called atresia, which may occur at any stage in the development of a follicle. In atresia of a primary follicle, the ovum shrinks, degenerates, and undergoes cytolysis; the follicular cells show similar degenerative changes. The follicle is resorbed, and the left space is rapidly filled by connective tissue from the stroma. Similar degenerative changes occur in larger follicles, but the zona pellucida may persist for a time after dissolution of the oocyte and follicular cells. Macrophages invade the atretic follicle and engulf the degenerating material, including fragments of the zona pellucida. Cells of the theca interna persist longer than those of the stratum granulosum but also show degenerative changes. The theca cells increase in size, lipid droplets appear in the cytoplasm, and the cells assume an epithelioid character, similar to that of lutein cells. The cells assume a cordlike arrangement, separating the cords by connective tissue fibers and capillaries. The basal lamina between granulosa cells and the theca interna frequently becomes thicker and forms a hyalinized, corrugated layer, the glassy membrane. This structure is characteristic of growing follicles that have undergone atresia and aids in distinguishing a large atretic follicle from a corpus luteum. Other differences include degenerative changes in the granulosa cells and the presence of fragments of zona pellucida at the center of a follicle without an associated oocyte. Ultimately, the degenerated remains of the follicle are removed, and a scar resembling a small corpus of albicans is left. This, too, eventually disappears into the stroma of the ovary. In some mammals, especially rodents, clusters of epithelioid cells are scattered in the stroma of the cortex. These interstitial cells contain small lipid droplets and bear a marked resemblance to luteal cells. These interstitial cells are thought to arise from the theca interna of follicles undergoing atresia. In humans, interstitial cells are most abundant during the first year of life, the period during which atretic follicles are most numerous. In women, they are present only in widely scattered, small groups. Their exact role in ovarian physiology is unknown; in humans they elaborate androgens. Other large epithelioid cells, the hilus cells, are found associated with vascular spaces and unmyelinated nerves in the hilus of the ovary. The cells appear similar to the interstitial cells of the testis and contain lipid, lipochrome pigments, and cholesterol esters. Hilus cells are most commonly found during pregnancy and at menopause, but their function is unknown (Navasiolava et al., 2011). Tumors arising from these cells have a masculinizing effect.

8.3.2.7. The Ovarian Cycle

During the ovarian cycle gonadotrophin-releasing hormone (GnRH) is synthesized by neurons in the arcuate nucleus of the hypothalamus and released in pulsatile fashion to stimulate follicle-stimulating hormone (FSH) and luteinizing hormone (LH) synthesis and release by gonadotrophs within the anterior pituitary. The receptor for GnRH on the gonadotrophs is a G-protein. The gonadotrophic hormones also are released in a pulsatile fashion corresponding to the GnRH pulses. Both the FSH and LH glycoprotein molecules bind to a G-protein linked cell-surface receptor which increases the production of cAMP in the appropriate cell. The maturation of ovarian follicles, their endocrine functions, and the phenomenon of ovulation are regulated by the follicle-stimulating and luteinizing hormones. Follicle-stimulating hormone is responsible for the growth of follicles and stimulates the aromatase enzyme complex within granulosa cells to produce estrogens and inhibin. Together with FSH, luteinizing hormone induces ripening of the mature follicle and ovulation. Alone, LH converts the ovulated follicle into a corpus luteum and induces it to secrete progesterone, estrogen, and inhibin. The cyclic nature of follicle formation and ovulation is the result of reciprocal interaction between the hypothalamic-pituitary axis and ovarian hormones. As the production of estrogens and inhibin by the granulosa cells increases, the release of FSH from the pituitary is inhibited, and the level of FSH falls below that needed for the maturation of new follicles. However, the rising level of estrogen does stimulates a surge in the release of LH from the pituitary, resulting in ovulation, formation of a corpus luteum, and secretion of progesterone, estrogen and inhibin by this structure. Increasing levels of progesterone from the corpus luteum now inhibit release of LH from the pituitary, and as the level of LH declines, the corpus luteum can no longer be maintained. With the decline of the corpus luteum, progesterone and estrogen levels diminish, the pituitary is no longer inhibited from secreting FSH, and a new cycle of follicle formation is initiated. The ovarian steroid hormones have only minor direct effects on the pituitary; their primary action is mediated through neurons in the hypothalamus. Both FSH and ovarian androgens stimulate granulosa cells to synthesize and release a glycoprotein called inhibin. Inhibin preferentially suppresses the synthesis and secretion of FSH by gonadotrophs in the anterior pituitary.

8.3.2.8. Age and the Ovary

The ovary looses its ability to produce viable ova with age. In women at 42 years of age the ability of the ovary to produce viable ova is reduced to about 50%. By 45 years of age ovarian failure in women is nearly 100%.

8.3.3. Oviducts

The oviducts (uterine tubes) are muscular tubes extending from the ovary to the uterus along the upper margin of the broad ligament. One end of the tube is closely related to the ovary and, at this end, is open to the peritoneal cavity. The other end communicates with the lumen of the uterus. The oviduct delivers the ovum, released at ovulation, to the uterine cavity and provides an environment for fertilization and initial segmentation of the fertilized ovum.

8.3.3.1. Structure

The oviduct is divided into several segments. The ovarian end, the infundibulum, is funnel-shaped, and its margin is drawn out in numerous tapering processes called fimbria. The infundibulum opens into the tortuous, thin-walled ampulla of the tube, which makes up slightly more than half the length of the oviduct. The ampulla is continuous with the isthmus, a narrower, cordlike portion that makes up about the medial one-third. The intramural (interstitial) part is the continuation of the tube, which passes through the uterine wall. As in other hollow viscera, the wall of the oviduct consists of several layers: an external serosa, an intermediate muscularis, and an internal mucosa.

8.3.3.2. Mucosa

The mucosa of the oviduct presents a series of longitudinal folds called plicae. In the ampulla the plicae have secondary and even tertiary folds to create a complex labyrinth of epithelial-lined spaces. In the isthmus, the plicae are shorter with little branching, while in the intramural part, the plicae form only low ridges. The plicae Throughout the tube consist of a single layer of columnar epithelial cells resting on an incomplete basement membrane and a lamina propria of richly cellular connective tissue containing a network of reticular fibers and fibroblasts. The epithelium decreases in height from ampulla to uterus and consists of ciliated and nonciliated cells. The ciliated cells are most numerous on the surface of the fimbria and progressively decrease in number through the ampulla, isthmus, and intramural portions. The nonciliated cells appear to be secretory and help establish an environment that is suitable for the survival and fertilization of the ovum and for the maintenance of the zygote. A third cell type, an undifferentiated cell with a darkly staining nucleus, may represent a precursor of the secretory cells or an exhausted secretory cell.

The epithelium shows cyclic changes associated with ovarian cycles. During the follicular phase, ciliated cells increase in height, reaching their maximum at about the time of ovulation, and there is evidence of increased activity in the secretory cells. In the luteal phase, ciliated cells decrease in height and lose their cilia, and there is augmented secretory activity by the secretory cells. Loss of cilia is greatest in the fimbria and least in the isthmus. The cilia are responsive to steroid hormones: estrogen appears responsible for the appearance and maintenance of cilia, while progesterone increases the rate at which they beat. Other ciliated cells located elsewhere in the body show no such hormone responsiveness.

8.3.3.3. Muscular Coat and Serosa

The mucous membrane rests directly on the muscle coat, with no submucosa. The muscle coat consists of two layers of smooth muscle cells, but the layers are not sharply defined. The inner layer is circular or closely spiraled; the outer layer of longitudinal muscle is thinner. The muscularis increases in thickness toward the uterus due to the increased depth of the inner layer. Externally, the oviduct is covered by a serosa that represents the peritoneal covering of the organ. Fertilization usually occurs in the ampulla of the oviduct (Otsuka et al., 2011).

8.3.4. Uterus

The human uterus is a single, hollow, pear-shaped organ with a thick muscular wall; it lies in the pelvic cavity between the bladder and rectum. The nonpregnant uterus varies in size depending on the individual but generally is about 7 cm long, 3 to 5 cm at its widest (upper) part, and 2.5 to 3.0 cm thick. It is slightly flattened dorsoventrally, and the luminal cavity corresponds to the overall shape of the organ. The uterus receives the fertilized ovum and nourishes the embryo and fetus throughout its development until birth.

8.3.4.1. Structure

Several regions of the uterus can be distinguished. The bulk of the organ consists of the body, which comprises the upper expanded portion. The dome-shaped part of the body between the junctions with the oviduct constitutes the fundus. Below, the uterus narrows and becomes more cylindrical in shape: this region forms the cervix, part of which protrudes into the vagina. The cervical canal passes through the cervix from the uterine cavity and communicates with the vaginal lumen at the external os. The uterine wall is made up of several layers that have specific names: the internal lining or mucosa is called the endometrium; the middle muscular layer forms the myometrium; and the external layer is referred to as the perimetrium. The perimetrium is the serosal or peritoneal layer that covers the body of the uterus, the supravaginal part of the cervix posteriorly, and the body of the uterus anteriorly (Otsuka et al., 2011).

8.3.4.2. Myometrium

The bulk of the uterine wall consists of the myometrium, which forms a thick coat about 15 to 20 mm in depth. The myometrium consists of bundles of smooth muscle cells separated by thin strands of connective tissue that contain fibroblasts, collagenous and reticular fibers, mast cells, and macrophages. The muscle forms several layers that are not sharply defined because of the intermingling of smooth muscle cells from one layer to another. Generally, however, internal, middle, and outer layers of smooth muscle can be distinguished. The internal layer is thin and consists of longitudinal and circularly arranged smooth muscle cells. The middle layer is the thickest and shows no regularity in the arrangement of the smooth muscle cells, which run longitudinally, obliquely, circularly, and transversely. This layer also contains many large blood vessels and has been called the stratum vasculare. The outer layer of smooth muscle consists mainly of longitudinally oriented cells, some extending into the broad ligament, oviducts, and ovarian ligaments. Elastic fibers are prominent in the outer layer but not in the inner layer of the myometrium except around blood vessels. In the nonpregnant uterus, the smooth muscle cells are 30 to 50 μm long, but during pregnancy, they hypertrophy to reach lengths of 500 to 600 μm or greater. New smooth muscle cells are produced in the pregnant uterus from undifferentiated cells and possibly from the division of mature cells also. The connective tissue of the myometrium also increases during pregnancy. Despite a total increase in muscle mass, the layers are thinned during pregnancy as the uterus becomes distended. After delivery, the muscle cells rapidly decrease in size, but the uterus does not regain its original, nonpregnant dimensions. The myometrium normally undergoes intermittent contractions that are not intense enough to be perceived. The intensity may increase during menstruation to result in cramps. The contractions are diminished during pregnancy, possibly in response to the hormone relaxin. At parturition, strong contractions of the uterine musculature occur, causing the fetus to be expelled. Uterine contractions increase in response to or after administration of oxytocin. This hormone is synthesized by neurons forming the supraoptic and paraventricular nuclei of the hypothalamus and released at the neurohypophysis. Uterine contractions also increase in response to prostaglandins. A rise in the level of prostaglandins occurs just prior to delivery.

8.3.4.3. Endometrium

The endometrium is a complex mucous membrane that, in women, undergoes cyclic changes in structure and function in response to the ovarian cycle. The cyclic activity begins at puberty and continues until menopause. In the body of the uterus, the endometrium consists of a thick lamina propria (endometrial stroma) and a covering epithelium. The stroma resembles mesenchymal tissue and consists of loosely arranged stellate cells with large, round or ovoid nuclei supported by a network of fine connective tissue where lymphocytes, granular leukocytes, and macrophages are scattered. There is no submucosa, and the stroma lies directly on the myometrium, which is firmly attached. The stroma is covered by a simple columnar epithelium containing ciliated and nonciliated secretory cells. The epithelium dips into the stroma to form numerous uterine glands that extend deeply into the stroma, occasionally penetrating into the myometrium. Most are simple tubular glands, but some may branch near the muscle. There are fewer ciliated cells in the glands than in the covering epithelium. A basement membrane underlies the glandular and surface epithelia. The endometrium can be divided into a stratum basale (basal layer) and a stratum functionale (functional layer), which differ in their structure, function, and blood supply. The stratum basale is the narrower, more cellular, and more fibrous layer and lies directly on the myometrium. Occasionally, small pockets of stratum basale may extend into the myometrium, between muscle cells. This layer undergoes a few changes during the menstrual cycle and is not shed at menstruation but serves as the **source** from which the functional layer is restored. The stratum functionale extends to the lumen of the uterus and is the part of the endometrium in which cyclic changes occur and is shed during menstruation. The stratum functionale is sometimes subdivided into the compacta, a narrow superficial zone, and the spongiosa, a broader zone that forms the bulk of the functionalis (Plehuna et al., 2022). The blood supply of the endometrium is unique and plays an important role in the events of menstruation. Branches of the uterine arteries penetrate the myometrium to its middle layer, where they furnish arcuate arteries that run circumferentially in the myometrium. One set of branches from these arteries supplies the superficial layers of the myometrium, while other branches, the radial arteries, pass inward to supply the endometrium. At the junction of myometrium and endometrium, the radial branches provide a dual circulation to the endometrium. Straight arteries supply the stratum basale, while the stratum functionale is provided by highly coiled spiral arteries. As the spiral arteries pass through the functional layer, they form terminal arterioles that unite with a complex network of capillaries and dilated vascular structures known as lacunae. The venous system forms an irregular network of venules and veins with irregular sinusoidal enlargements and then drains into a plexus at the junction of myometrium and endometrium. During menstrual cycles, the spiral arteries constrict periodically, subjecting the functional layer to intermittent periods of anoxia. The distal portions of the arterial supply in the functionalis undergo degeneration and regeneration with each menstrual cycle, whereas the straight arteries of the basal layer show no such changes (**Figure 8.10**).

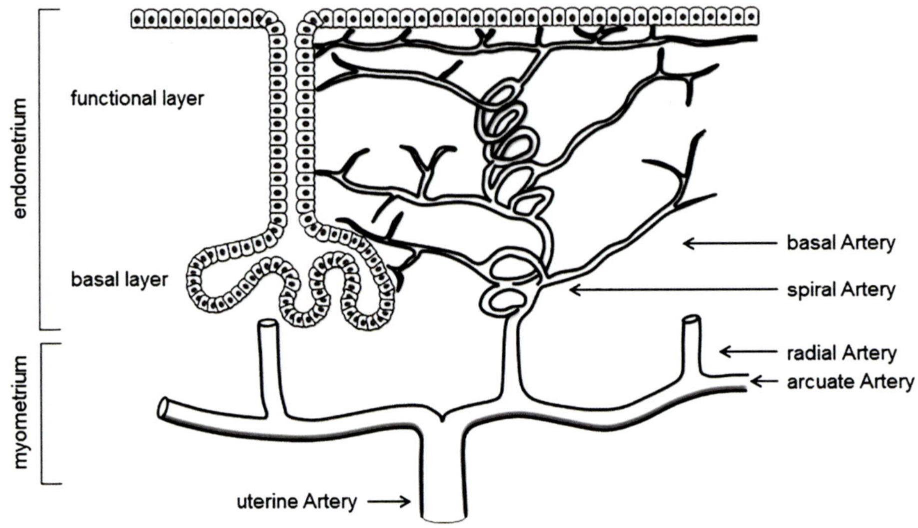

Figure 8.10. *A diagrammatic sketch illustrating the arrangement of blood vessels in the endometrium.*

Source: https://www.researchgate.net/publication/337466937/figure/fig3/AS:863617528365057@1582913872788/Schematic-diagram-of-the-endometrial-vascular-system-The-primate-endometrium-is.ppm.

8.3.4.4. Cyclic Changes in the Endometrium

During a normal menstrual cycle, the endometrium undergoes a continuous sequence of changes in which four phases can be described. The phases correlate with the functional activities of the ovaries and constitute the proliferative, secretory, ischemic (premenstrual), and menstrual phases (Plehuna et al., 2022). The proliferative phase begins at the end of the menstrual flow and extends to about the middle of the cycle. This stage is characterized by rapid regeneration and repair of the endometrium. Epithelial cells in the remnants of the uterine glands in the stratum basale proliferate and migrate over the raw surface of the mucosa; stromal cells also proliferate. In the early part of this period, the endometrium is of limited thickness, and its glands are sparse and fairly straight and have small lumina. The epithelium of the glands and surface is simple cuboidal to low columnar, and mitoses are present in the glandular lining. As the proliferative phase advances, the endometrial glands increase in number and length, become more tortuous and closely spaced, and the lumina widen. Toward the end of the proliferative phase (days 14–16), glycogen accumulates in the basal region of the glandular epithelium. The surface and glandular epithelia are tall columnar with fewer ciliated and more secretory cells. The secretory cells have large numbers of small mitochondria, but the endoplasmic reticulum and Golgi complex are poorly developed. Microvilli are present on the free borders of the cells. The nuclei are round or oval and contain finely granular chromatin with one or more nucleoli. The spiral arteries lengthen but are lightly coiled and do not extend into the superficial third of the endometrium. The proliferative phase corresponds to the maturation of the ovarian follicle up to the time of ovulation. Estrogen, secreted by the developing follicles, stimulates the growth of the endometrium; some growth may continue for a day or two after ovulation. During the secretory phase, the endometrium continues to increase in thickness due to hypertrophy of stromal and glandular cells, stromal edema, and increased vascularity.

The glands lengthen, become irregularly coiled and convoluted, and show wide, irregular lumina. The epithelial cells become larger, and their free surfaces show many long microvilli. Mitochondria are large, there is a rich endoplasmic reticulum, and the Golgi apparatus is prominent. Nuclei are enlarged and contain distinct nucleoli.

Glycogen and mucoid materials rapidly increase, first in the bases of the glandular cells, then in the apical portions of the cells, and then into the lumina of the glands. Elongation and coiling of the spiral arteries continue, and the vessels extend into the superficial part of the endometrium. The secretory phase is associated with the development of a corpus luteum and is maintained as long as the corpus luteum remains functional. Progesterone secreted by the corpus luteum is the steroid primarily responsible for the secretory changes in the endometrium. The ischemic (premenstrual) phase is characterized by intermittent constriction of the spiral arteries, resulting in vascular stasis and reduced blood flow to the functional layer. The outer zone of the endometrium is subjected to anoxia for hours at a time, resulting in the breakdown of the stratum functionale. The stroma becomes increasingly edematous and infiltrated by leukocytes. In the menstrual phase, the functional layer becomes necrotic and is shed. The spiral arteries also become necrotic, and blood is lost from the arteries and veins. Small pools of blood form and coalesce merge, and overlying patches of mucosa are detached, leaving a denuded stromal surface. Sloughing of the endometrium continues until the entire functional layer has been discarded. Blood oozes from veins torn during the shedding of the endometrial tissue. The menstrual discharge consists of arterial and venous blood, autolyzed and degenerated epithelial cells, and glandular secretions. The straight arteries of stratum Basale do not constrict during menstruation, thus preserving the basal layer to restore the endometrium during the following new proliferative stage. The onset of the menstrual cycle coincides with the beginning involution of a corpus luteum.

8.3.4.5. Cervix

The wall of the cervix differs considerably from that of the body of the uterus. Little smooth muscle is present, and the cervical wall consists mainly of dense connective tissue and elastic fibers. In the part that protrudes into the vaginal canal, smooth muscle is lacking. The cervical canal is lined by a mucosa, the endocervix, which forms complex, branching folds. The epithelial lining consists of tall, mucus-secreting columnar cells and a few ciliated columnar cells. Numerous large, branched cervical glands are present and lined by mucus-secreting columnar cells similar to those of the lining epithelium. The cervical canal usually is filled with mucus. Occasionally, the glands become occluded and filled with secretion, forming Nabothian cysts. The portion of the cervix that protrudes into the vaginal canal, the exocervix, is covered by a nonkeratinized stratified squamous epithelium whose cells contain much glycogen. The transition from the simple columnar epithelium of the cervical canal is abrupt and usually occurs near the external os. The cervical mucosa does not take part in the dramatic cyclic changes that occur in the endometrial lining of the body of the uterus and is not shed. However, the glandular elements show changes in secretory activity. At midcycle, there is a copious secretion of a thin alkaline fluid, probably the result of increased stimulation by estrogen. After ovulation and establishment of a corpus luteum, the amount of secretion decreases, and the mucus becomes thicker and more viscous (Rimon-Dahari et al.,

2016). The lumen of the cervix is usually less than 1 cm in diameter but will expand to 10 cm or more at the time of birth. The dilatation results from increased elasticity and a softening of the cervical stroma during labor. The changes that occur within the cervical stroma are complex and not completely understood. However, changes are known to occur with regard to the making up of glycosaminoglycans in the ground substance during labor. Hyaluronic acid levels increase, binding more water, whereas concentrations of dermatan sulfate decrease, reducing the number of cross-linkages between extracellular fibers within the stroma. The net result of these changes is a softening of the matrix with a separation of connective tissue fibers. In addition, the collagen and elastic fibers within the stroma are shortened and rearranged in such a way as to decreased tensile strength and resistance, allowing the dilatation to occur.

8.3.5. Vagina

The vagina is the lower-most portion of the female reproductive tract and is a muscular tube that joins the uterus to the exterior of the body.

It represents the copulatory organ of the female. Ordinarily the lumen is collapsed and the anterior and posterior walls make contact (Rimon-Dahari et al., 2016).

8.3.5.1. Structure

The vaginal wall consists of a mucosa, a muscularis, and an adventitia. The mucosa is thrown into folds (rugae) and consists of a thick surface layer of nonkeratinized stratified squamous epithelium overlying a lamina propria. The epithelial cells contain abundant glycogen, especially at midcycle. The glycogen of sloughed cells is broken down by commensal lactobacilli within the vaginal lumen and results in lactic acid being formed. The acid pH creates an environment favorable to the commensal bacterial flora and deters the growth of fungi (Candida albicans) and bacterial pathogens. The lamina propria consists of fairly dense connective tissue that becomes more loosely arranged near the muscle coat. Immediately beneath the epithelial lining, elastic fibers form a dense network. Diffuse and nodular lymphatic tissues are found occasionally, and many lymphocytes and granular leukocytes invade the epithelium. The vagina lacks glands, and the epithelium is kept moist by secretions from the cervix. The muscularis consists of bundles of smooth muscle cells arranged circularly in the inner layer and longitudinally in the outer layer. The longitudinally oriented smooth muscle cells become continuous with similarly oriented cells in the myometrium. The adventitia is a thin outer layer of connective tissue rich in elastic fibers. It merges imperceptibly into the surrounding loose connective tissue around other organs and acts to hold the vagina in place.

8.3.5.2. Cytology of the Cervical Canal

The nonkeratinized stratified squamous epithelium that lines the vagina and covers the exocervix is arranged in layers similar to those of the epidermis. The deepest is the basal layer (stratum germinativum), followed by an intermediate (spinous) layer and a superficial layer (stratum corneum) from which cells are shed. Desquamated cervical cells can be recovered from vaginal secretions, or cells can be obtained more directly by gentle abrasion of the exocervix. The cells can be studied in smear preparations, and examination of Papanicolaou's ("Pap") smears has become a standard procedure for early detection of cervical cancer. In normal women, four types of cells are usually recognized cytologically, loosely corresponding to the layers of the cervicovaginal epithelium. These include basal (lower basal) cells, parabasal (outer basal) cells, intermediate (precornified) squamous cells, and superficial (cornified) squamous cells. Germinal cells from the basal layer are exceedingly rare in smears from normal adults, and the basal and parabasal cells recognized cytologically are derived from different levels of the intermediate layer. They represent less mature cells, and their presence indicates that immature cells are at higher than normal levels in the epithelium. These cells are associated with a marked deficiency of estrogen and are common before puberty and during menopause. Basal cells arise from the lower levels of the transitional zone and are rounded or oval cells, about 4 to 5 times the size of a granular leukocyte. The central nucleus is deeply stained, but a pattern of fine chromatin granules and dense patches can be made. In some cells, a Barr body is distinctly visible. The moderate amount of basophilic cytoplasm stains deeply and evenly. Parabasal cells arise higher up in the transitional zone and are also round or oval cells, but they are larger than basal cells with a more abundant cytoplasm that is less basophilic and often shows a somewhat "blotchy" pattern. The central nucleus remains about the same size but may be denser than a basal cell. Intermediate squamous cells vary in size, but all appear as thin, polygonal plates with abundant transparent cytoplasm. The nucleus is smaller, vesicular, and centrally placed. The cytoplasm stains somewhat variably and may be lightly basophilic or show some degree of eosinophilia. Superficial squamous cells represent dead surface cells. They are large, with voluminous eosinophilic cytoplasm that is thin and transparent with sharply defined borders. Because of the thinness, the cytoplasm often is curled, wrinkled, and folded. The nucleus is very small – about one-half to one-third that of an intermediate squamous cell – and is densely stained and pyknotic. The superficial and intermediate squamous cells are the largest cells seen in a routine preparation and range from 40 to 50 μm in diameter. Occasionally, anucleate squamous cells may be found. They have a somewhat shriveled appearance, and the site of the nucleus is suggested by a pale central zone. They represent cells that are more completely keratinized. Cells that originate from the endocervix may also be present and often occur in small sheets or strips; their appearance depends on the orientation. From end on, the cells appear as groups or nests of small polyhedral or round cells with sharp cell boundaries and relatively large central nuclei. In the profile, the cells show their columnar shape with the nuclei close to one pole. Strips of these cells give a "picket fence" appearance.

8.3.6. External Genitalia

The external genitalia of the female consists of the labia, clitoris, and vestibular glands.

8.3.6.1. Labia

The labia majora consists of folds of skin covering an abundance of adipose tissue. In the adults, the outer surface is covered by coarse hair with many sweat and sebaceous glands. The inner surface is smooth and hairless and also contains sweat and sebaceous glands. The labia majora is the homolog of the scrotum in the male. The labia minora consist of a core of highly vascular, loose connective tissue covered by stratified squamous epithelium deeply indented by connective tissue papillae. The deeper layers of epithelium are pigmented. Both surfaces of the labia minora are devoid of hair, but large sebaceous glands are present (Robin et al., 2022).

8.3.6.2. Clitoris

The clitoris is an erectile body that corresponds to the dorsal penis. It consists of two corpora cavernosa enclosed in a layer of fibrous connective tissue and separated by an incomplete septum. The free end of the clitoris terminates in a small, rounded tubercle, the glans clitoridis, which consists of spongy erectile tissue. The clitoris is covered by a thin layer of nonkeratinized stratified squamous epithelium with high papillae associated with many specialized nerve endings. The clitoris has no corpus spongiosum and does not contain the urethra.

8.3.6.3. Vestibular Glands

The vestibule is the cleft between the labia minora, and in it are the vaginal and urethral openings. It is lined by stratified squamous epithelium and contains numerous small vestibular glands concentrated about the openings of the vagina and urethra. The glands contain mucous cells and resemble the urethral glands of the male. A pair of larger glands, the greater or major vestibular glands, are present in the lateral walls of the vestibule. They are compound tubuloalveolar glands that secrete a clear, mucoid lubricating fluid. The major glands correspond to the bulbourethral glands of the male (Rock and Fortney, 1984).

8.3.7. Pregnancy

Pregnancy begins with the implantation of a blastocyst into the prepared uterine endometrium, followed by the formation of a placenta that nourishes and maintains the developing embryo.

Prior to implantation, the ovum is fertilized, and the resulting zygote is cleaved in the ampulla of the oviduct.

8.3.7.1. Fertilization

Before an ovum can be fertilized, it must undergo maturational changes, the chief of which is the reduction of the chromosome complement to the haploid number. The oocyte passes through the early stages of the first meiotic division during fetal life, and it is only just before ovulation that the division is completed and the first polar body is given off. The resulting secondary oocyte immediately enters the second meiotic division, which, however, proceeds only to metaphase and is not completed until fertilization occurs. At the time of ovulation, the oviduct shows active movements that bring the infundibulum and fimbria close to the ovary (Ronca et al., 2014). Cilia on the surface of the fimbria sweep the ovum into the ampulla of the oviduct, where fertilization, if it is to occur, takes place. The human ovum remains fertile for between 24 and 48 hours, after which it degenerates if fertilization does not occur. Approximately 300 million sperm are released into the vaginal lumen during coitus, but it is estimated that only 300–500 spermatozoa reach the site of fertilization. These remain viable for about 72 hours. Muscular contractions within the walls of the uterus and oviduct propel the spermatozoa to the proximal region (ampulla) of the oviduct where fertilization occurs. The smooth muscle cells are thought to contract in response to prostaglandins and/or oxytocin released during sexual intercourse. Of the millions of sperm initially deposited in the female tract, only one penetrates the ovum. While random movement plays a major role in bringing sperm and ovum together, some studies suggest chemotactic factors may also be involved. The zona pellucida is important in fertilization as it provides sperm recognition sites for sperm binding and is the most efficient trigger of the sperm acrosome reaction. Both sperm binding and induction of the acrosome reaction are ligand-receptor interactions, the ligands located in the ZP3 glycoprotein of the zona pellucida. The acrosome reaction results in the release of acrosomal enzymes (acrosin and trypsin- like enzymes) needed to digest a hole in the zona pellucida. At the time of fertilization, when a spermatozoon pushes through the hole in the zona pellucida to enter the ovum, a period of hyperactivity of flagellar beat occurs, propelling the spermatozoon into the ovum. The entire spermatozoon is engulfed by the cytoplasm of the ovum. Thus, flagellar beat appears to be more important at the moment of fertilization rather than getting to the site of fertilization. Electron micrographs suggest that the plasma membranes of the sperm and ovum fuse, that of the spermatozoon being left at the surface of the ovum. Penetration is followed by the release of electron-dense cortical granules that underlie the plasmalemma of the ovum (cortical granule reaction) and by immediate changes in the permeability of the zona pellucida, which, thereafter, excludes entry by any additional competing sperm (polyspermy). The ovum now completes the second maturation division and extrudes the second polar body. The remaining chromosomes (23) reconstitute and form the female pronucleus. The nucleus (head) of the spermatozoon swells and forms the male pronucleus, and the sperm body and tail are resorbed. The two pronuclei move to the center of the cell, and two centrioles, supplied by the anterior centriole of the spermatozoon, appear. The chromatin of each pronucleus resolves into a set of chromosomes that align themselves on a spindle to undergo a normal mitotic division of the first cleavage. Each cell resulting from this division receives a full diploid set of chromosomes (Sandler and Winters, 1978).

8.3.7.2. Cleavage

The zygote undergoes a series of rapid divisions called cleavage that result in a large number of cells, the blastomeres. The cells are bounded by the zona pellucida, and a mulberry-like body, the morula, is formed. Cleavage is a fractionating process: no new cytoplasm is formed, and at each division, the cells become smaller until a normal, predetermined, cytoplasmic-nuclear ratio is reached. Thus, the total size of the morula is not increased. Cleavage occurs as the morula slowly moves along the oviduct by the waves of peristaltic contractions in the muscle coat. When the morula reaches the uterine cavity, it is at the 12- to 16-cell stage. At about this time, fluid penetrates the zona pellucida and diffuses between the cells of the morula. The fluid increases in amount, the intercellular spaces become confluent, and a single cavity, the blastocele, is formed. The morula has now become a blastocyst that forms a hollow sphere containing, at one pole, a mass of cells called the inner cell mass that will form the embryo proper. The capsule-like wall of the blastocyst consists of a single layer of cells, the trophoblast. After reaching a critical mass, the blastocyst breaks through the surrounding zona pellucida and remains free within the uterine cavity for about a day; then, it attaches to the endometrium, which is in the secretory phase. Encasement within the zona pellucida protects the forming blastocyst from the possible damaging effects of oviductal movements, possible adverse effects of oviductal and uterine secretions, and/or destruction by maternal tissues until it reaches a critical mass for survival. During cleavage, the zona pellucida progressively thins and coupled with the expansion of the blastocoele, the blastocyst hatches and crawls through and out of the surrounding zona pellucida. The hatched blastocyst makes contact with the maternal endometrial surface by apposing its trophectoderm to the uterine lining epithelial cells. The initial contact is mediated by cell surface oligosaccharides that play an important role in recognition, adhesion, and attachment to the uterine epithelium. Following these events, trophoblast cells penetrate between surface uterine epithelial cells and establish direct contact with underlying decidual cells (Tomilovskaya et al., 2019).

8.3.7.3. Implantation

At the time of implantation, the endometrium is in the secretory phase and, having been under the influence of progesterone from the corpus luteum for several days, has reached its greatest thickness and development. Implantation is initiated by a close approximation of the trophoblast to the microvilli and surface projections of the uterine epithelial cells. At the points of contact, the cytoplasm of the trophoblast contains clusters of coated vesicles and numerous lysosomes. The microvilli shorten and disappear, and the trophoblast extends finger-like processes between the uterine epithelial cells, and the two layers become closely locked by numerous tight junctions that develop between them. The uterine epithelial cells degenerate and are engulfed by the trophoblast, the cellular debris appearing in phagosomes within the trophoblast cytoplasm. Where it is fixed to the endothelium, the trophoblast proliferates to form a cellular mass between the blastocyst and maternal tissues. No cell boundaries can be made out in this cell mass, called the syncytial trophoblast. The syncytium continues to erode the endometrium at the point of contact, creating a ragged cavity into which the blastocyst sinks, gradually becoming more deeply embedded until it lies entirely within the endometrial stroma. The surface defect in the endometrium is closed temporarily by a fibrin plug. Later, the proliferation of surrounding cells restores the surface continuity of the endometrial lining. As the blastocyst sinks into the endometrium, the syncytial trophoblast rapidly increases in thickness at the original attachment site and progressively extends to cover the remainder of the blastocyst. When completely embedded, the entire wall of the blastocyst consists of a thick outer syncytial trophoblast and an inner cytotrophoblast, composed of a single layer of cells with well-defined boundaries. The cytotrophoblast shows active mitosis and contributes cells to the syncytial trophoblast, where they fuse with and become part of that layer. The syncytial trophoblast continues to erode the uterine tissues, opening up the walls of maternal blood vessels. Spaces appear in the syncytial trophoblast and these lacunae expand, become confluent, and form a labyrinth of spaces. Many spaces contain blood from eroded maternal blood vessels; this blood supplies nourishment for the embryo and represents the first step in the development of uteroplacental circulation.

8.3.7.4. Placenta

As the lacunae enlarge, intervening strands of trophoblast form the primary villi that cover the entire periphery of the blastocyst. Each villus consists of a core of cytotrophoblast covered by a layer of syncytial trophoblast. Trophoblastic cells at the tips of the villi apply themselves to the endometrium and form a lining for the cavity in which the blastocyst lies. When the embryonic germ layers have been established, the mesoderm emerges from the embryo as the chorion and forms a lining for the trophoblast surrounding the blastocyst. Mesoderm extends into the primary villi to form a core of connective tissue and convert the primary villi to secondary villi. The deeply embedded portion of the chorion constitutes the chorionic plate from which numerous villi project to form the chorion frondosum. Villi on that part of the chorion facing the uterine cavity grow more slowly and are less numerous; ultimately, these villi disappear; leaving a smooth surface that forms the chorion laeve. Blood vessels develop in the mesenchymal cores of the secondary villi and soon make connection with the fetal circulation. With vascularization, the secondary villi become the definitive or tertiary placental villi (Tou et al., 2002). At parturition, all but the deepest layers of the endometrium are shed; thus, the superficial part of the endometrium is called the decidua. A feature of the stroma is the alteration of its cells to form enlarged, decidual cells that contain much glycogen. According to the relationship with the implantation site, three areas of the decidua are recognized. The decidua capsularis is the part that lies over the surface of the blastocyst, while the decidua basalis underlies the implantation site and forms the maternal component of the placenta. The endometrium lining the remainder of the pregnant uterus is the decidua parietalis. As the embryo grows, the decidua capsularis becomes increasingly attenuated. Eventually, the decidua capsularis makes contact with decidua parietalis on the opposite surface of the uterus, and the uterine cavity is obliterated. The mature placenta consists of maternal and fetal components. The maternal part is decidua basalis; the fetal portion consists of the chorionic plate and the villi arising from it. Maternal blood circulates through the intervillous spaces and bathes the villi, of which there are two types. Some pass from the chorionic plate to decidua basalis as anchoring villi from which secondary and tertiary branches float in the intervillous spaces as the floating villi. Both types of villi consist of a core of loose connective tissue in which lie fetal capillaries. Covering each villus is an inner layer of cytotrophoblast cells with large nuclei and lightly basophilic cytoplasm containing considerable glycogen. External to the cytotrophoblast is a layer of syncytial trophoblast of variable thickness. The cells of the cytotrophoblast decrease in number in the latter half of pregnancy, and only a very few are present at term. The syncytial trophoblast also thins out to form a narrow layer (**Figure 8.11**).

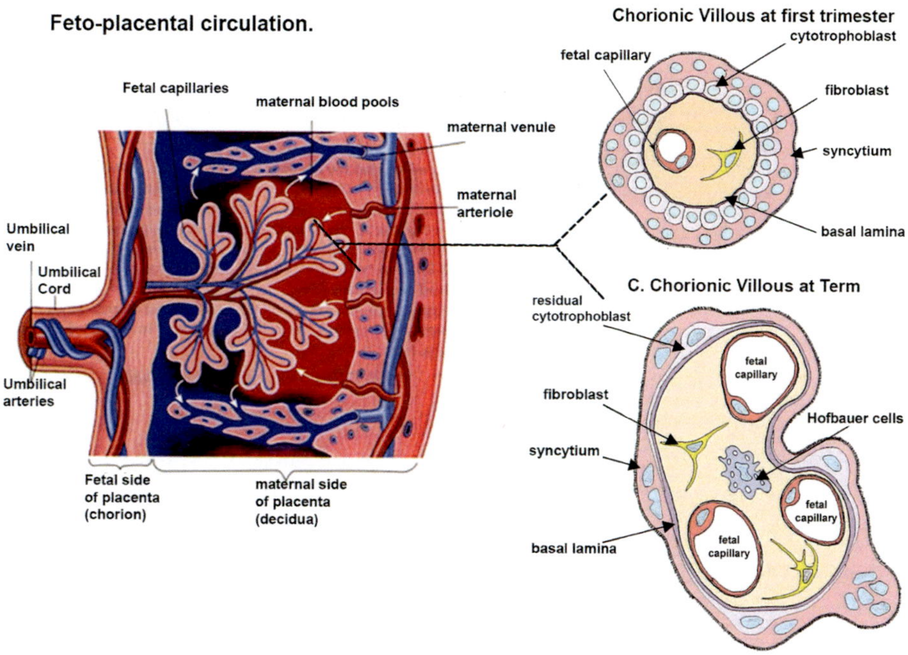

Figure 8.11. *Schematic representation of a human placenta.*

Note: (A) A representative drawing of the fetal placental circulation. Note the dotted line, which shows the position from which drawings of a section through the chorionic villous at ~10 weeks (B) and term (C) are taken. (B) Chorionic villous with the presence of syncytiotrophoblast, a layer of cytotrophoblast cells, connective tissue of the villus containing fibroblasts and the fetal capillaries. (C) At term, in some areas, the placental membrane is so thin, such that the syncytiotrophoblast comes into direct contact with the fetal capillary endothelium, and is thus called the vasculo-syncytial membrane.

Source: Adapted and modified from http://imueos.wordpress.com/2010/05/25/placenta-function/.

The placenta transfers oxygen and nutrients from the maternal to the fetal circulation and waste products from the fetal to the maternal circulation. Although maternal and fetal circulations are closely apposed, they remain separated by the syncytial trophoblast (and early in pregnancy by the cytotrophoblast also), a basement membrane, the connective tissue of the villi, and the wall of the fetal blood vessels. Transport of material between fetal and maternal blood appears to be regulated by the syncytial trophoblast. Without cell boundaries and intercellular spaces, any materials passing into or out of the fetal blood must pass through the cell membranes and cytoplasm of the syncytium. Electrolytes, steroids, fatty acids, oxygen, and carbon dioxide traverse the syncytial trophoblast by passive diffusion. Other substances, such as glucose, cross this barrier by carrier molecules. In addition, the syncytial trophoblast plasmalemma contains receptors for macromolecules such as transferrin, insulin, and immunoglobulins that are taken in by receptor-mediated endocytosis and cross the epithelial barrier in transport vesicles. The cytotrophoblast continues to serve as the source of cells for the syncytial trophoblast. The placenta also is a multipotential endocrine organ essential for maintaining pregnancy. The trophoblast secretes a glycoprotein, human chorionic gonadotrophin that can be detected by the end of the first week after fertilization. It increases in amount to the fifth week of pregnancy and maintains and stimulates the corpus luteum to secrete estrogens and progesterone during early pregnancy (Tou et al., 2004). The placenta also secretes estrogens and progesterone that aid in maintaining the uterine environment for continued fetal development. At about 9 weeks' gestation, the placenta takes over progesterone production. A variety of other factors, similar to releasing hormones of the hypothalamus and pituitary-like hormones, are synthesized and released by the placenta into the maternal blood. One of these, human chorionic somatomammotropin or hCS (also referred to as human placental lactogen) is important in breast development and lactation and in making glucose available from the maternal circulation for both the placenta and fetus. Human chorionic somatomammotropin imparts a condition of insulin resistance to the mother so that glucose, rather than being rapidly removed from the circulation by maternal tissues, is available for the developing fetus.

8.3.8. Breasts (Mammary Glands)

Mammary glands are present in both sexes, but in men, they remain rudimentary throughout life. In women, the size, shape, and structure vary with age and functional status. Prior to puberty, the female breasts are undeveloped but enlarge rapidly at puberty due mainly to the accumulation of adipose tissue. They reach their greatest development during late pregnancy and lactation. In women, the breasts are variably hemispherical and conical in shape, each surmounted by a cylindrical projection, the nipple. Surrounding the nipple is a slightly raised, circular area of hairless pigmented skin, the areola. The mammary glands are compound tubuloalveolar glands of cutaneous origin, representing modified apocrine sweat glands.

8.3.8.1. Structure of the Resting Gland

Each breast consists of 15 to 20 individual pyramid-shaped lobes that radiate from a nipple. The lobes are divided by septa of dense connective tissue. Each lobe represents an individual mammary gland and contains glandular tissue drained by its own ductal components, embedded in connective tissue. The proportions of glandular and non-glandular tissue vary with functional status. In the resting gland, the principal glandular elements are the ducts, which are grouped to form lobules. The smallest branches of the ductal system are lined by simple cuboidal epithelium, but the lining increases in height as the ducts unite and pass toward the nipple. Just beneath the areola, the ducts expand to form the lactiferous sinuses lined by a two-layered stratified cuboidal epithelium. As the duct ascends through the nipple, it becomes lined by stratified squamous epithelium. Secretory units consist of clusters of alveoli surrounding a small duct. The alveolar wall consists of simple cuboidal epithelium resting on a basement membrane. Between the epithelial cells and the basement membrane are highly branched myoepithelial cells whose long, slender processes embrace the alveolus in a basket-like network. Alveoli are not prominent in the resting gland, it is uncertain whether they are present at all. When present, they usually occur as small, budlike extensions of the terminal ducts. The intralobular connective tissue around the ductules and alveoli is loosely arranged and cellular, whereas that surrounding the larger ducts and lobes (interlobular connective tissue) is variably dense and contains much adipose tissue (Vitt et al., 2000).

8.3.8.2. Nipple and Areola

The nipple is covered by keratinizing stratified squamous epithelium continuous with that of the skin overlying the breast. The dermis projects deeply into the epithelium, forming unusually tall dermal papillae. The skin of the nipple is pigmented and contains many sebaceous glands but is devoid of hair and sweat glands. The nipple is traversed by many lactiferous ducts, each draining a lobe and emptying onto the tip of the nipple. The outer parts of the ducts also are lined by keratinizing stratified squamous epithelium. The dense collagenous connective tissue of the nipple contains bundles of elastic fibers, and smooth muscle. The smooth muscle cells are arranged circularly and radially and, on contraction, produce an erection of the nipple. The areola is the pigmented area of skin that encircles the base of the nipple. During pregnancy, the areola enlarges and darkens in color. It contains sweat, sebaceous, and areolar glands. The latter appears to be intermediate in structure between apocrine sweat glands and true mammary glands.

8.3.8.3. Pregnancy and Lactation

During pregnancy, mammary glands undergo extensive development in preparation for their role in lactation. During the first half of pregnancy, the terminal portions of the ductal system grow rapidly, branch, and develop terminal buds that expand to become alveoli. Glandular tissue proliferates while fat and stromal connective tissue decrease. The connective tissue becomes infiltrated with lymphocytes, plasma cells, and granular leukocytes. During late pregnancy, the proliferation of glandular tissue subsides, but the alveoli expand and begin to form secretory materials (Watenpaugh, 2016). The first secretion, colostrum, is thin and watery. It is poor in lipids but contains a considerable amount of immunoglobulin that provides passive immunity to the newborn. True milk secretion begins a few days after parturition, but not all the breast tissue is functioning simultaneously. In some areas, the alveoli are distended with milk, the epithelial lining is flattened, and the lumen is distended; in other areas, the alveoli are resting and are lined by tall columnar epithelial cells. Secreting cells have abundant granular endoplasmic reticulum, moderate numbers of relatively large mitochondria, and supranuclear Golgi complexes. Milk proteins are elaborated by the granular endoplasmic reticulum and associated with the Golgi body form membrane-bound vesicles. These are carried to the apex of the cell, where the contents are released by exocytosis. Lipid arises as cytoplasmic droplets that coalesce to form large spherical globules. The droplets and globules reach the apex of the cell and protrude into the lumen. Ultimately, they pinch off, surrounded by a thin film of cytoplasm and the detached portion of the plasmalemma. This method of release is a form of apocrine secretion, but only minute amounts of cytoplasm are lost. Immunoglobulins in milk are synthesized by plasma cells in the connective tissue surrounding the alveoli of the mammary glands. The secreted immunoglobulin is taken up by receptor-mediated endocytosis along the basolateral plasmalemma of mammary gland epithelial cells and transported in small vesicles to the cell apex, where it is discharged into the lumen by exocytosis. The passage of milk from alveoli into and through the initial ductal segments is due to the contraction of myoepithelial cells. The average milk production by a woman breast-feeding a single infant is about 1,200 ml/day. Milk consists of about 88% water, 6.5% carbohydrate, 3.3% lipid, and 1.5% protein. Lactose is the primary carbohydrate, and casein, is the primary protein. In addition, immunoglobulins (IgE and IgA), electrolytes ($Na+$, $K+$, Cl^-), minerals (Ca^{++}, Fe^{++}, Mg^{++}), and other substances occur in milk. Women in the fourth and fifth months of lactation may secrete as much as 0.5 g of immunoglobulin per day in their milk. Such immunoglobulins are important in the resistance of enteric infections and provide the infant with considerable passive immunity. With weaning, lactation soon ceases, and the glandular tissue returns to its resting state. However, regression is never complete, and not all the alveoli completely disappear.

8.3.8.4. Hormonal Control

Before puberty, the growth of the mammary gland parallels general body growth, but as the ovaries become functional, the mammary tissue comes under the influence of estrogen and progesterone. While some structural changes can be observed, the cyclic response of the breast is minor. During pregnancy, the glands are continuously stimulated by estrogen and progesterone from the corpus luteum and placenta. Generally, growth of the ductal system depends on estrogen, but for alveolar development, both progesterone and estrogen are required. To attain full development in pregnancy, other hormones -somatotropin, prolactin, adrenal corticoids, and human chorionic somatomammotropin – appear necessary. At the end of pregnancy, following birth, circulating estrogen and progesterone levels fall abruptly. In the absence of their inhibition, there is an increased output of prolactin by cells of the adenohypophysis. Prolactin is a powerful lactogenic stimulus, and full lactation is established in a few days after birth. Maintenance of lactation requires continuous secretion of prolactin, which results from a neurohormonal reflex established by suckling. Periodic suckling also causes the release of oxytocin from the neurohypophysis, which stimulates the contraction of myoepithelial cells, resulting in the release of milk from alveoli and into the ducts (milk letdown).

8.3.9. Organogenesis

Early development of the female reproductive tract is related closely to that of the urinary system and the male reproductive tract. All arise in the mesoderm of the urogenital ridges within epithelial thickenings on each side of the midline. Initially, the ovaries and testes are indistinguishable and form a primitive, indifferent gonad that does not acquire male or female morphology until the seventh week of development. The first indication of gonads appears at four weeks, when a pair of longitudinal ridges, the gonadal ridges, appear. These are divided into lateral and medial parts and only the medial portion gives rise to the ovary. No germ cells are present in the gonadal ridges until the sixth week of development. The epithelium of the gonadal ridge proliferates, and in places, clumps of cells become thickened to form a number of cellular gonadal cords that penetrate the underlying mesenchyme. The cords at the periphery form a primary ovarian cortex, while centrally; proliferation of mesenchyme establishes a primary medulla. The gonadal cords break up into irregular clusters separated by strands of mesenchyme, an extension of which cuts off the cell clusters from the surface epithelium and eventually forms the tunica albuginea. A second proliferation of the surface epithelium gives rise to new cellular cords that invade the primary cortex, dissociate into isolated clusters, and form the definitive cortex. The cell clusters surround one or more primitive germ cells (primary oocytes) that enter the prophase of the first meiotic division. The primary medulla is replaced by a fibroelastic stroma to establish a permanent medulla (Zhang et al., 2016). Primordial germ cells, which give rise to the definitive oogonia, are segregated early in development. They appear first in the yolk sac, then migrate to the dorsal mesentery and genital ridges. It is uncertain whether the primordial cells arise from a group of special blastomeres during cleavage or as clones of a single blastomere. Their early association with endoderm has suggested this as the tissue of origin. The forming ovary contains 6–7 million oogonia at 20 weeks gestation. The number of oogonia drops to between 1–2 million by the time of birth. By 6 weeks' gestation, male and female embryos have paired mesonephric and paramesonephric ducts. In the female embryo, paramesonephric ducts become predominant, giving rise to oviducts, the uterus, and possibly, vagina. Unlike males, mesonephric ducts do not contribute to the female reproductive system. Mesonephric ducts regress, except for a few remnants. Paramesonephric ducts begin to form at about 35- or 36-days gestation. Each duct begins as an invagination on the lateral side of the mesonephric ridge. The ingrowing mesothelium forms a short groove that sinks beneath the surface and seals off to form a tube. The anterior end develops first and opens into the coelomic cavity as a funnel-shaped structure that gives rise to the fimbriated and ampullary parts of the oviduct. Caudally, the paramesonephric ducts from each side lengthen and descend, then turn medially to meet each other and form a single structure, the utero-vaginal canal. At first, the two lumina are separate, but the intervening walls degenerate, forming a single cavity. The descending part forms the body and cervix of the uterus. Mesenchyme surrounding the utero-vaginal canal supplies the endometrial stroma and myometrium. The vagina develops from an epithelial proliferation known as the sinovaginal bulb on the posterior wall of the urogenital sinus. It is not certain whether this epithelium is true sinus epithelium or epithelium of the mesonephric duct that descended into this region. The proliferating epithelium extends cranially as a solid bar that forms the vaginal plate. Beginning at the caudal end, cells in the center of the plate degenerate, and a vaginal lumen is formed. Canalization is complete by the fifth month. The fetal vaginal epithelium is under the influence of maternal hormones and, in late fetal life, becomes markedly hypertrophied. It regresses after birth and assumes its inactive childhood form. The external genitalia also pass through an indifferent stage before they develop their definitive sexual characteristics. The caudal end of the primitive hindgut is closed by a cloacal membrane around which the urogenital folds develop. The folds unite at their cranial ends to form the genital tubercle, which, in the female, elongates only slightly to give rise to the clitoris. A pair of genital swellings develop along each side of the genital folds; in the female develop along each side of the genital folds; in females, these remain separate and form the labia majora. Similarly, the urogenital folds do not fuse in the female, give giving rise to the labia minora (Zhang et al., 2016).

A Closer Look

Organogenesis

Organogenesis is a critical phase of embryonic development in which the three germ layers—ectoderm, mesoderm, and endoderm—differentiate into specific organs and tissues. This intricate process begins after gastrulation, when the basic body plan is established. During organogenesis, cellular differentiation, proliferation, and morphogenetic movements work in concert to form functional structures. Each organ system arises from specific germ layers, with unique signaling pathways and genetic programs guiding development. Understanding organogenesis not only sheds light on normal developmental processes but also provides insights into congenital disorders and regenerative medicine.

The process of organogenesis is characterized by a series of tightly regulated events that ensure proper organ formation. For instance, in vertebrates, organogenesis starts with the development of the heart and circulatory system, which is crucial for delivering nutrients and oxygen to other developing organs. The heart arises from mesodermal precursors and undergoes a complex series of morphogenetic changes, including folding, fusion, and chamber formation. Following cardiac development, other organs such as the lungs, kidneys, and liver begin to form through similar processes. Each organ's formation is orchestrated by intricate signaling networks, including pathways involving fibroblast growth factors (FGFs), bone morphogenetic proteins (BMPs), and hedgehog proteins, which provide essential cues for cell fate determination and spatial organization.

Cellular interactions play a pivotal role in organogenesis. The process often involves not only the intrinsic genetic programming of cells but also extrinsic signals from neighboring tissues. For example, during the development of the kidney, mesenchymal cells interact with ureteric bud cells, leading to reciprocal signaling that promotes kidney morphogenesis. These interactions can result in a variety of cellular responses, including proliferation, differentiation, and apoptosis, which are essential for shaping the developing organ. The formation of organ systems is also influenced by mechanical forces and the physical environment, which can affect cellular behavior and tissue architecture. Understanding these dynamics is vital for deciphering the complexity of organ development and its regulation.

Despite the remarkable efficiency of organogenesis, disruptions can lead to congenital anomalies and organ dysfunction. Research into the genetic and environmental factors that influence organ development has revealed that variations in signaling pathways or mutations in key developmental genes can result in significant developmental disorders. For instance, mutations in the genes responsible for heart development can lead to congenital heart defects, one of the most common birth anomalies. Moreover, advances in stem cell research and tissue engineering have opened new avenues for regenerative medicine, allowing scientists to harness the principles of organogenesis to create functional tissues and organs for transplantation. This intersection of developmental biology and clinical application underscores the importance of understanding the mechanisms of organogenesis and their implications for health and disease.

Therefore, organogenesis is a fundamental biological process that establishes the complex architecture of multicellular organisms. It involves a highly coordinated interplay of genetic, cellular, and environmental factors that guide the formation of organs from embryonic tissues. As researchers continue to unravel the intricacies of organogenesis, the knowledge gained holds the potential to revolutionize approaches in regenerative medicine, offering hope for the treatment of various congenital and acquired diseases. The ongoing exploration of organogenesis not only enhances our understanding of human development but also paves the way for innovative therapeutic strategies that can address organ dysfunction and promote tissue regeneration.

Summary

The urinary system plays a critical role in maintaining fluid and electrolyte balance, regulating blood pressure, and removing waste products from the bloodstream. The kidneys filter blood to produce urine, which is then transported and stored until excretion. This system is essential for homeostasis, helping to maintain the body's internal environment despite external changes.

The chapter also explores the reproductive system, which includes distinct structures in males and females. In males, the system involves the testes, vas deferens, prostate, and penis, primarily focusing on sperm production and delivery.

In females, the system includes the ovaries, fallopian tubes, uterus, and vagina, highlighting the processes of ovulation, fertilization, and gestation.

The reproductive systems are governed by complex hormonal regulation, influencing sexual development and reproductive cycles. Together, the urinary and reproductive systems underscore the body's intricate processes for waste management and reproduction, essential for survival and species continuation.

References

1. Andersen, C. Y. (2017). Inhibin-B secretion and FSH isoform distribution may play an integral part of follicular selection in the natural menstrual cycle. *Molecular Human Reproduction, 23*(1), 16–24. https://doi.org/10.1093/molehr/gaw073.
2. Baerwald, A. R., Adams, G. P., & Pierson, R. A. (2003). A new model for ovarian follicular development during the human menstrual cycle. *Fertility and Sterility, 80*(1), 116–122. https://doi.org/10.1016/S0015-0282(03)00547-X.
3. Baerwald, A. R., Adams, G. P., & Pierson, R. A. (2012). Ovarian antral folliculogenesis during the human menstrual cycle: A review. *Human Reproduction Update, 18*(1), 73–91. https://doi.org/10.1093/humupd/dmr039.
4. Baker, T. G. (1963). A quantitative and cytological study of germ cells in human ovaries. *Proceedings of the Royal Society of London. Series B, Biological Sciences, 158*(972), 417–433. https://doi.org/10.1098/rspb.1963.0055.
5. Craig, J., Orisaka, M., Wang, H., Orisaka, S., Thompson, W., Zhu, C., Kotsuji, F., & Tsang, B. K. (2007). Gonadotropin and intra-ovarian signals regulating follicle development and atresia: The delicate balance between life and death. *Frontiers in Bioscience, 12*, 3628–3639. https://doi.org/10.2741/2334.
6. de Castro, F. C., Cruz, M. H. C., & Leal, C. L. V. (2016). Role of growth differentiation factor 9 and bone morphogenetic protein 15 in ovarian function and their importance in mammalian female fertility—A review. *Asian-Australasian Journal of Animal Sciences, 29*(8), 1065–1074. https://doi.org/10.5713/ajas.15.0435.
7. Edson, M. A., Nagaraja, A. K., & Matzuk, M. M. (2009). The mammalian ovary from genesis to revelation. *Endocrine Reviews, 30*(6), 624–712. https://doi.org/10.1210/er.2009-0012.
8. Elvin, J. A., Yan, C., & Matzuk, M. M. (2000). Growth differentiation factor-9 stimulates progesterone synthesis in granulosa cells via a prostaglandin E2/EP2 receptor pathway.

Proceedings of the National Academy of Sciences, 97(18), 10288–10293. https://doi.org/10.1073/pnas.170289597.

9. Frett, T., Green, D. A., Mulder, E., Noppe, A., Arz, M., Pustowalow, W., Petrat, G., Tegtbur, U., & Jordan, J. (2020). Tolerability of daily intermittent or continuous short-arm centrifugation during 60-day 6° head down bed rest (AGBRESA study). *PLOS ONE, 15*(10), e0239228. https://doi.org/10.1371/journal.pone.0239228.

10. Gershon, E., & Dekel, N. (2020). Newly identified regulators of ovarian folliculogenesis and ovulation. *International Journal of Molecular Sciences, 21*(13), 4565. https://doi.org/10.3390/ijms21134565.

11. Gougeon, A. (1979). Qualitative changes in medium and large antral follicles in the human ovary during the menstrual cycle. *Annales de Biologie Animale, Biochimie, Biophysique, 19*(6), 1461–1468. https://doi.org/10.1051/rnd:19791006.

12. Gougeon, A. (1986). Dynamics of follicular growth in the human: A model from preliminary results. *Human Reproduction, 1*(2), 81–87. https://doi.org/10.1093/oxfordjournals.humrep.a136367.

13. Guilhot, C., Fovet, T., Delobel, P., Dargegen, M., Jasmin, B. J., Brioche, T., & Chopard, A., & Py, G. (2022). Severe muscle deconditioning triggers early extracellular matrix remodeling and resident stem cell differentiation into adipocytes in healthy men. *International Journal of Molecular Sciences, 23*(10), 5489. https://doi.org/10.3390/ijms23105489.

14. Holt, J. A., Macias, B. R., Schneider, S. M., Watenpaugh, D. E., Lee, S. M. C., Chang, D. G., & Hargens, A. R. (2016). WISE 2005: Aerobic and resistive countermeasures prevent paraspinal muscle deconditioning during 60-day bed rest in women. *Journal of Applied Physiology, 120*(10), 1215–1222. https://doi.org/10.1152/japplphysiol.00484.2015.

15. Jain, V., & Wotring, V. E. (2016). Medically induced amenorrhea in female astronauts. *NPJ Microgravity, 2*, 16008. https://doi.org/10.1038/npjmgrav.2016.8.

16. Jennings, R. T., & Baker, E. S. (2000). Gynecological and reproductive issues for women in space: A review. *Obstetrical & Gynecological Survey, 55*(2), 109–116. https://doi.org/10.1097/00006254-200002000-00023.

17. Koryak, Y. A. (2014). Influence of simulated microgravity on mechanical properties in the human triceps surae muscle *in vivo*. I: Effect of 120 days of bed-rest without physical training on human muscle musculo-tendinous stiffness and contractile properties in young women. *European Journal of Applied Physiology, 114*(5), 1025–1036. https://doi.org/10.1007/s00421-014-2833-4.

18. Linossier, M. T., Peurière, L., Fernandez, P., Normand, M., Beck, A., Bareille, M. P., Bonneau, C., Gauquelin-Koch, G., & Vico, L. (2022). DI-5-Cuffs: Bone remodeling and associated metabolism markers in humans after five days of dry immersion to simulate microgravity. *Frontiers in Physiology, 13*, 801448. https://doi.org/10.3389/fphys.2022.801448.

19. Messinis, I. E. (2006). From menarche to regular menstruation: Endocrinological background. *Annals of the New York Academy of Sciences, 1092*(1), 49–56. https://doi.org/10.1196/annals.1365.005.

20. Mishra, B., & Luderer, U. (2019). Reproductive hazards of space travel in women and men. *Nature Reviews Endocrinology, 15*(12), 713–730. https://doi.org/10.1038/s41574-019-0257-1.

21. Morgan, J. L. L., Zwart, S. R., Heer, M., Ploutz-Snyder, R., Ericson, K., & Smith, S. M. (2012). Bone metabolism and nutritional status during 30-day head-down-tilt bed rest. *Journal of Applied Physiology, 113*(10), 1519–1529. https://doi.org/10.1152/japplphysiol.00674.2012.

22. Navasiolava, N. M., Custaud, M. A., Tomilovskaya, E. S., Larina, I. M., Mano, T., Gauquelin-Koch, G., Gharib, C., & Kozlovskaya, I. B. (2011). Long-term dry immersion: Review and prospects. *European Journal of Applied Physiology, 111*(9), 1235–1260. https://doi.org/10.1007/s00421-010-1750-x.

23. Otsuka, F., McTavish, K. J., & Shimasaki, S. (2011). Integral role of GDF-9 and BMP-15 in ovarian function. *Molecular Reproduction and Development, 78*(1), 9–21. https://doi.org/10.1002/mrd.21265.

24. Plehuna, A., Green, D. A., Amirova, L. E., Tomilovskaya, E. S., Rukavishnikov, I. V., & Kozlovskaya, I. B. (2022). Dry immersion induced acute low back pain and its relationship with trunk myofascial viscoelastic changes. *Frontiers in Physiology, 13*, 1039924. https://doi.org/10.3389/fphys.2022.1039924.

25. Rimon-Dahari, N., Yerushalmi-Heinemann, L., Alyagor, L., & Dekel, N. (2016). Ovarian folliculogenesis. In *Results and Problems in Cell Differentiation* (Vol. 58, pp. 167–190). Springer. https://doi.org/10.1007/978-3-319-31973-5_7.

26. Robin, A., Navasiolava, N., Gauquelin-Koch, G., Gharib, C., Custaud, M. A., & Treffel, L. (2022). Spinal changes after 5-day dry immersion as shown by magnetic resonance imaging (DI-5-CUFFS). *American Journal of Physiology-Regulatory, Integrative and Comparative Physiology, 323*(2), R310–R318. https://doi.org/10.1152/ajpregu.00112.2022.

27. Rock, J. A., & Fortney, S. M. (1984). Medical and surgical considerations for women in spaceflight. *Obstetrical & Gynecological Survey, 39*(8), 525–535. https://doi.org/10.1097/00006254-198408000-00003.

28. Ronca, A. E., Baker, E. S., Bavendam, T. G., Beck, K. D., Miller, V. M., Tash, J. S., & Jenkins, M. (2014). Effects of sex and gender on adaptations to space: Reproductive health. *Journal of Women's Health, 23*(11), 967–974. https://doi.org/10.1089/jwh.2014.4912.

29. Sandler, H., & Winters, D. (1978). Physiological responses of women to simulated weightlessness: A review of the significant findings of the first female bed rest study (NASA SP-340). NASA Scientific and Technical Information Office.

30. Tomilovskaya, E., Shigueva, T., Sayenko, D., Rukavishnikov, I., & Kozlovskaya, I. (2019). Dry immersion as a ground-based model of microgravity physiological effects. *Frontiers in Physiology, 10*, 284. https://doi.org/10.3389/fphys.2019.00284.

31. Tou, J. C. L., Grindeland, R. E., & Wade, C. E. (2004). Effects of diet and exposure to hindlimb suspension on estrous cycling in Sprague-Dawley rats. *American Journal of Physiology-Endocrinology and Metabolism, 286*(3), E425–E433. https://doi.org/10.1152/ajpendo.00381.2003.

32. Tou, J., Ronca, A., Grindeland, R., & Wade, C. (2002). Models to study gravitational biology of mammalian reproduction. *Biology of Reproduction, 67*(6), 1681–1687. https://doi.org/10.1095/biolreprod67.6.1681.

33. Vitt, U., Hayashi, M., Klein, C., & Hsueh, A. (2000). Growth differentiation factor-9 stimulates proliferation but suppresses the follicle-stimulating hormone-induced differentiation of

cultured granulosa cells from small antral and preovulatory rat follicles. *Biology of Reproduction, 62*(2), 370–377. https://doi.org/10.1095/biolreprod62.2.370.

34. Watenpaugh, D. E. (2016). Analogs of microgravity: Head-down tilt and water immersion. *Journal of Applied Physiology, 120*(4), 904–914. https://doi.org/10.1152/japplphysiol.00986.2015.

35. Zhang, S., Zheng, D., Wu, Y., Lin, W., Chen, Z., Meng, L., Liu, J., & Zhou, Y. (2016). Simulated microgravity using a rotary culture system compromises the *in vitro* development of mouse preantral follicles. *PLOS ONE, 11*(3), e0151062. https://doi.org/10.1371/journal.pone.0151062.

INDEX

FSC
www.fsc.org
MIX
Papier | Fördert
gute Waldnutzung
FSC® C083411

Kolibri 360 GmbH
Ferdinand-Jühlke-Straße 7
99095 Erfurt, Deutschland
produktsicherheit@kolibri360.de